Neuromodulation in Psychiatry

Neuromodulation in Psychiatry

EDITED BY

Clement Hamani

Paul Holtzheimer

Andres M. Lozano

Helen Mayberg

WILEY Blackwell

Registered Office
John Wiley & Sons, Ltd, The Atrium, Southern Gate, Chichester, West Sussex, PO19 8SQ, UK

Editorial Offices
9600 Garsington Road, Oxford, OX4 2DQ, UK
The Atrium, Southern Gate, Chichester, West Sussex, PO19 8SQ, UK
111 River Street, Hoboken, NJ 07030-5774, USA

For details of our global editorial offices, for customer services and for information about how to apply for permission to reuse the copyright material in this book please see our website at www.wiley.com/wiley-blackwell

Library of Congress Cataloging-in-Publication Data

Neuromodulation in psychiatry / edited by Clement Hamani, Paul Holtzheimer, Andres Lozano & Helen Mayberg.
p. ; cm.
Includes bibliographical references and index.
ISBN 978-1-118-80104-8 (hardback)
I. Hamani, Clement, editor. II. Holtzheimer, Paul E., editor. III. Lozano, A. M. (Andres M.), 1959– , editor. IV. Mayberg, Helen S. (Helen Susan), 1956– , editor.
[DNLM: 1. Mental Disorders–therapy. 2. Electric Stimulation Therapy. 3. Mental Disorders–surgery. 4. Radiosurgery. 5. Transcranial Magnetic Stimulation. WM 400]
RC485
616.89′122–dc23

2015034735

A catalogue record for this book is available from the British Library.

Wiley also publishes its books in a variety of electronic formats. Some content that appears in print may not be available in electronic books.

Cover image: ©agsandrew/gettyimages

Set in 10/12.5pt Meridien by SPi Global, Pondicherry, India

1 2016

Contents

Contributors

Joshua P. Aronson, MD
Department of Neurosurgery, Massachusetts General Hospital, Boston, USA

Naazia H. Azhar, MD
Washington University School of Medicine in St. Louis, Department of Psychiatry, St. Louis, Missouri, USA

Malek Bajbouj, MD
Professor, Psychiatry and Affective Neuroscience, Affective Neuroscience, Charité and Freie Universitaet Berlin, Berlin, Germany

Gordon Baltuch, MD, PhD
University of Pennsylvania Health System, Philadelphia, USA

Mera S. Barr, PhD
Temerty Centre for Therapeutic Brain Intervention, Biobehavioural Addictions and Concurrent Disorders Research Laboratory (BACDRL); Campbell Family Research Institute, Centre for Addiction and Mental Health, Department of Psychiatry, University of Toronto, Toronto, Canada

Marcelo Batistuzzo, Psy.D., PhD
University of São Paulo Medical School, São Paulo, Brazil

Daniel M. Blumberger, MD, FRCPC
Temerty Centre for Therapeutic Brain Intervention, Toronto, Canada

André Russowsky Brunoni, MD, PhD
Service of Interdisciplinary Neuromodulation and Interdisciplinary Center for Applied Neuromodulation, Department and Institute of Psychiatry, University of São Paulo, São Paulo, Brazil

Charles R. Conway, MD
Washington University School of Medicine in St. Louis, Department of Psychiatry, St. Louis, Missouri, USA

Anna Cyriac, HBS
University Health Network, Toronto, Canada

Zafiris J. Daskalakis, MD, PhD, FRCPC
Temerty Centre for Therapeutic Brain Intervention, Toronto, Canada

Karen D. Davis, PhD
Professor, Department of Surgery and Institute of Medical Science, University of Toronto; Senior Scientist and Head; Division of Brain, Imaging and Behaviour – Systems Neuroscience, Toronto Western Research Institute, University Health Network, Tornato, Canada

Antônio A.F. De Salles, MD, PhD
Professor of Neurosurgery and Radiation Oncology, Department of Neurosurgery, Head of Stereotactic Surgery Section, University of California Los Angeles, Los Angeles, USA

Damiaan Denys, MD, PhD
Department of Psychiatry, Academic Medical Center, University of Amsterdam; The Netherlands Institute for Neuroscience, an Institute of the Royal Netherlands Academy of Arts and Sciences, Amsterdam, The Netherlands

Darin D. Dougherty, MD
Department of Psychiatry, Massachusetts General Hospital, Boston, USA

Jonathan Downar, MD, PhD
Assistant Professor, Department of Psychiatry and Institute of Medical Science, Faculty of Medicine, University of Toronto; Scientist, Toronto Western Research Institute, University Health Network; Director, MRI-Guided rTMS Clinic, Toronto Western Hospital, University Health Network, Toronto, Canada

Emad N. Eskandar, MD
Director of Stereotactic and Functional Neurosurgery; Professor of Neurosurgery, Harvard Medical School, Department of Neurosurgery, Massachusetts General Hospital, Boston, USA

Martijn Figee, MD, PhD
Department of Psychiatry, Academic Medical Center, University of Amsterdam, Amsterdam, The Netherlands

Joseph J. Fins, MD, MACP
The E. William Davis, Jr., M.D. Professor of Medical Ethics, Chief, Division of Medical Ethics, Professor of Medicine, Professor of Health Care Policy and Research, Professor of Medicine in Psychiatry, Weill Medical College of Cornell University, New York, USA

Kelly D. Foote, MD
Department of Neurosurgery, University of Florida, Gainesville, USA

Felipe Fregni, MD, PhD, MPH
Laboratory of Neuromodulation, Spaulding Rehabilitation Hospital, Harvard Medical School, Boston, USA

Andre Felix Gentil, MD, PhD
University of São Paulo Medical School, São Paulo, Brazil

Peter Giacobbe, MD, MSc, FRCPC
Department of Psychiatry, University of Toronto, University Health Network, Toronto, Canada

Michael Giffin, MSc
Department of Psychiatry, Academic Medical Center, University of Amsterdam, Amsterdam, The Netherlands

Alessandra A. Gorgulho, MD
HCOR NEUROSCIENCE, Department of Neurosurgery and Department of Radiation Oncology, São Paulo, Brazil; David Geffen School of Medicine, University of California Los Angeles, Los Angeles, USA

Britt M. Gott, MS
Washington University School of Medicine in St. Louis, Department of Psychiatry, St. Louis, Missouri, USA

Robert E. Gross, MD, PhD
Professor, Departments of Neurosurgery, Neurology and Biomedical Engineering, Emory University School of Medicine, Atlanta, USA

Suzanne N. Haber, PhD
Department of Pharmacology and Physiology, University of Rochester, Rochester, USA

Clement Hamani, MD, PhD
Division of Neurosurgery, Toronto Western Hospital, University of Toronto, Toronto, Canada

Professor Marwan Hariz, MD, PhD
Unit of Functional Neurosurgery, UCL Institute of Neurology, London, UK; Department of Clinical Neuroscience, Umeå University, Umeå, Sweden

Sarah R. Heilbronner, PhD
Department of Pharmacology and Physiology, University of Rochester, Rochester, USA

Sarah Hescham, BSc
Departments of Neurosurgery and Neuroscience, Maastricht University Medical Center, Maastricht, The Netherlands; Department of Stereotactic and Functional Neurosurgery, University of Cologne, Cologne, Germany

Marcelo Queiroz Hoexter, MD, PhD
University of São Paulo Medical School, São Paulo, Brazil

Paul Holtzheimer, MD
Departments of Psychiatry and Surgery, Geisel School of Medicine at Dartmouth, Hanover, USA

Kristopher G. Hooten, MD
Department of Neurosurgery, University of Florida, Gainesville, USA

David Huie, A.B.
Department of Neurosurgery, Massachusetts General Hospital, Boston, USA

Willard S. Kasoff, MD, MPH
Assistant Professor, Division of Neurosurgery, University of Arizona College of Medicine, Tucson, USA

Sidney H. Kennedy, MD, FRCPC
Department of Psychiatry, University of Toronto, St Michael's Hospital, University Health Network, Arthur Sommer-Rotenberg Chair in Suicide Studies, St Michael's Hospital, Toronto, Canada

Jean-Pascal Lefaucheur, MD, PhD
Department of Physiology, EA 4391, Henri Mondor Hospital, Assistance Publique – Hôpitaux de Paris, Faculty of Medicine, Paris Est Créteil University, Créteil, France

Scott Lempka, PhD
Center for Neurological Restoration, Cleveland Clinic Neurological Institute, Research Service, Louis Stokes Cleveland VA Medical Center, Cleveland, USA

Sarah Hollingsworth Lisanby, MD
Department of Psychiatry and Behavioral Sciences, Duke University School of Medicine; Department of Psychology and Neuroscience, Duke University School of Arts and Sciences, Durham, USA

Colleen Loo, MD
School of Psychiatry, University of New South Wales, Psychiatry, St George Hospital, Black Dog Institute, Wesley Hospital, Sydney, Australia

Antonio Carlos Lopes, MD, PhD
University of São Paulo Medical School, São Paulo, Brazil

Andres M. Lozano, MD, PhD
Division of Neurosurgery, Toronto Western Hospital, University of Toronto, Toronto, Canada

Andre Machado, MD, PhD
Center for Neurological Restoration, Cleveland Clinic Neurological Institute, Cleveland, USA

Donel Martin, PhD
School of Psychiatry, University of New South Wales, Advanced Neuropsychological Treatment Services, Sydney, Australia

Caio Matias, MD
Center for Neurological Restoration, Cleveland Clinic Neurological Institute, Cleveland, USA

Helen Mayberg, MD
Departments of Psychiatry and Behavioral Science and Neurology, Emory University School of Medicine, Atlanta, USA

W. Vaughn McCall, MD, MS
Professor and Chair, Department of Psychiatry and Health Behavior, Medical College of Georgia, Georgia Regents University, Augusta, USA

Shane J. McInerney, MB, MSc, MRC Psych
Department of Psychiatry, University of Toronto, St Michael's Hospital, University Health Network, Toronto, Canada

Maartje Melse, MD
Departments of Neurosurgery and Neuroscience, Maastricht University Medical Center, Maastricht, The Netherlands; Department of Stereotactic and Functional Neurosurgery, University of Cologne, Cologne, Germany

Euripedes Constantino Miguel, MD, PhD
University of São Paulo Medical School, São Paulo, Brazil

Andrada D. Neacsiu, PhD
Department of Psychiatry & Behavioral Sciences, Duke University School of Medicine, Durham, USA

Seth F. Oliveria, MD, PhD
Department of Neurosurgery, University of Florida Gainesville, USA

Gaby S. Pell, PhD
Department of Life Sciences, Ben Gurion University, Beer Sheva, Israel

Jared Pisapia, MD, MTR
University of Pennsylvania Health System, Philadelphia, USA

Barbara R. Pohl, MA
Research Assistant, Weill Cornell Medical College, New York, USA

Alexandra M. Rodman, AM
Department of Psychology, Harvard University, Cambridge, USA

Peter B. Rosenquist, MD
Professor and Vice Chair, Department of Psychiatry and Health Behavior, Medical College of Georgia, Georgia Regents University, Augusta, USA

Yiftach Roth, PhD
Department of Life Sciences, Ben Gurion University, Beer Sheva, Israel

Ziad Safadi, PhD
Department of Pharmacology and Physiology, University of Rochester, Rochester, USA

Sandarsh Surya, MBBS
Chief Resident, Department of Psychiatry and Health Behavior, Medical College of Georgia, Georgia Regents University, Augusta, USA

Yasin Temel, MD, PhD
Departments of Neurosurgery and Neuroscience, Maastricht University Medical Center, Maastricht, The Netherlands; Department of Stereotactic and Functional Neurosurgery, University of Cologne, Cologne, Germany

Veerle Visser-Vandewalle, MD, PhD
Department of Stereotactic and Functional Neurosurgery, University of Cologne, Cologne, Germany

Abraham Zangen, PhD
Department of Life Sciences, Ben Gurion University, Beer Sheva, Israel

CHAPTER 1

History of invasive brain stimulation in psychiatry: Lessons for the current practice of neuromodulation

Marwan Hariz
UCL Institute of Neurology, London, UK
Umeå University, Umeå, Sweden

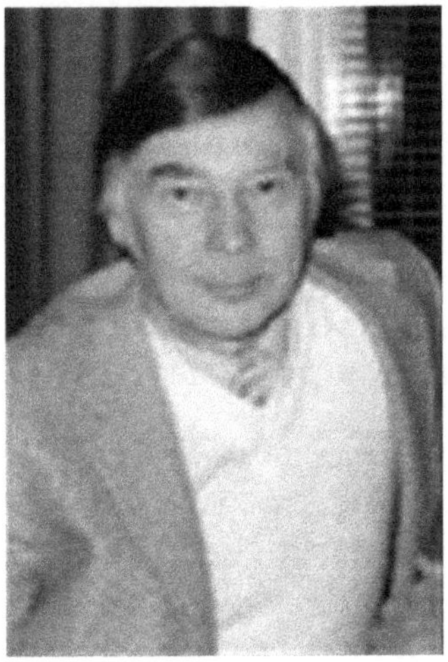

The basic problem of psychosurgery is psychiatric. Therefore, the initiative in considering surgical treatment must be taken by the psychiatrist. As soon as he is sure that conservative treatment by every available method cannot cure the patient, he should consult the neurosurgeon. Psychosurgery will remain experimental for years. Therefore, its use should be concentrated and restricted to psychosurgical research units having strong and intimate affiliation with scientists from many disciplines.

Lauri V. Laitinen, 'Ethical Aspects of Psychiatric Surgery', 1977 [1]

The International Neuromodulation Society defines neuromodulation as the alteration of nerve activity through the delivery of electrical or electromagnetic stimulation, chemical agents or light (optogenetics) to targeted sites of the central or peripheral nervous system. The aim of neuromodulation is to modulate (aka normalize) pathological nerve function. Some examples of various means to provide 'neuromodulation' to treat various illnesses and symptoms are functional electrical stimulation, spinal cord stimulation, peripheral nerve stimulation, intrathecal drug delivery systems, occipital nerve stimulation, motor cortex stimulation, repetitive transcranial magnetic stimulation, sacral nerve stimulation, transcranial direct current stimulation, vagus nerve stimulation and deep brain stimulation (DBS).

Thus, it appears that electricity has been and still is the main agent used to provide 'neuromodulation', starting in antiquity with the electrical fish and gaining a momentum with the so-called 'electrotherapy' in the 18th and 19th centuries when electrotherapy was used for the 'treatment' of a variety of illnesses, including epilepsy, paralysis, chorea, deafness, blindness, rheumatism, glandular enlargement and also for artificial respiration and resuscitation [2].

Neuromodulation in Psychiatry, First Edition. Edited by Clement Hamani, Paul Holtzheimer, Andres M. Lozano and Helen Mayberg.

According to the web site of the International Neuromodulation Society (http://www.neuromodulation.com/brief-history-of-neuromodulation consulted on 14 January 2014), 'The modern era of neuromodulation began in the early 1960s, first with deep brain stimulation which was soon followed (in 1967) by spinal cord stimulation, both for otherwise intractable pain'. In the opinion of this author, this is a rather selective way of writing history! In fact, the modern era of neuromodulation began at least a decade before 'the early 1960s' and it was not 'for otherwise intractable pain'. It is true that the *main* application of deep brain stimulation in the late 1960s and 1970s was for the treatment of chronic pain, and it is true that Medtronic trademarked the term 'DBS' with respect to chronic subcortical stimulation for pain in the mid-1970s [3]. However, scholar sources show that the history of deep brain stimulation before it was called 'DBS', that is, the history of *electrical stimulation of subcortical structures delivered through chronically implanted electrodes*, started in the early 1950s soon after the introduction of the method of human stereotactic surgery. It is also evident that subcortical brain stimulation was not initially intended to treat pain but rather was applied in psychiatry and to modify behaviour. In order to be able to fully grasp the 'lessons learned for current practice', as is suggested by the title of this chapter, one has to understand how DBS unfolded historically and why do we today need, in the first place, to 'learn lessons' from the 'history of neuromodulation in psychiatry'.

In the contemporary discourse about the history of DBS, there is a commonly held belief that DBS was initiated for surgical treatment of movement disorders in 1987 [4], and entered the realm of psychiatry first in 1999 [5, 6]. Indeed, it was the paper by Veerle Vandewalle *et al.* on DBS for Tourette syndrome published in *The Lancet* in February 1999 [5], and the publication of Nuttin *et al.* on DBS for obsessive–compulsive disorder (OCD), also in *The Lancet* in October 1999 [6], that heralded the most recent era of DBS in psychiatry. As the field of psychiatric neuromodulation has literally exploded in the last decade, at least judging by the number of publications in the field, with new psychiatric applications of DBS on an ever-increasing number of brain targets [7], perhaps a sober look at past experience in this field may provide some clues about what is to be expected and what can go wrong in this specific area of psychiatric neuromodulation, aka *psychiatric surgery*.

The main aim of this chapter is thus to review the historical applications and trials of DBS in the realm of psychiatry and behaviour, and to summarize what lessons, if any, can be learned from these previous practices.

The birth, rise and fall of the 20th-century psychiatric DBS

Human stereotactic neurosurgery was initially and purposely devised with the intent to avoid the devastating side effects of the crude frontal lobotomy by allowing to perform anatomically focused tiny lesions in psychiatric patients. Thus, in the same way, as human stereotactic *ablative* surgery was applied at its inception in 1947 in the psychiatric domain [8], human subcortical brain stimulation was also first proposed in the realm of psychiatry: in 1952, neurophysiologist and neurobehaviourist José Delgado and his colleagues [9] described a technique of electrode implantation for chronic recording and stimulation to evaluate 'its possible therapeutic value in psychotic patients'. The following year, the Mayo Clinic organized a symposium on 'intracerebral electrography'. The proceedings of that meeting were published and included a paper on 'Neurosurgical and neurologic applications of depth electrography', where one could read: 'An observation that may have some practical significance was that several of our psychotic patients seem to improve and become more accessible in the course of stimulation studies lasting several days' [10]. The authors thought that a likely explanation for this effect 'was that the local stimulation was having a therapeutic effect comparable to that of electroshock' and concluded that '... this aspect of localized stimulation studies requires further investigation since it may lead to a most specific, less damaging, and more therapeutically effective electrostimulation technic than can be achieved by the relatively crude extracranial stimulation methods in use at present' [10]. One of the authors in this paper was Carl Wilhelm Sem-Jacobsen, a Norwegian neurophysiologist and neuropsychiatrist who was a fellow at the Mayo Clinic and who continued to work with chronic subcortical stimulation for psychiatric illness when he returned to Norway (see further next).

Also in the early 1950s, a team at Tulane University in New Orleans, led by psychiatrist Robert Heath, had started chronic depth electrode stimulation, including stimulation of the 'septal area' in schizophrenic and other psychotic patients [11].

Furthermore, already in 1961, Daniel Sheer, Professor of psychology at the University of Houston, edited a book entitled *Electrical Stimulation of the Brain – An Interdisciplinary Survey of Neurobehavioral Integrative Systems* [12]. As the title indicates the main focus of electrical stimulation was on neurobehaviour and the authors of the chapters of that book discussed the use of subcortical recording and stimulation in epilepsy, obesity, aggressive behaviour and other neurological and behavioural conditions. Hence, from its very beginning, the technique of chronic stimulation of deep brain structures was intended and applied for behavioural and psychiatric studies and occasionally in the treatment of mental disorders.

What went wrong?

Studying the literature on old psychiatric DBS from the mid-1950s to the 1970s, it appears that DBS was used more for exploration and modification of behaviour, and less for the treatment of true psychiatric illness: those scarce publications detailing the few attempts to treat psychiatric illnesses with DBS were authored mainly by neurosurgeons, whereas the non-neurosurgeons were more prolific publishers on DBS mainly as a means to study and alter personality. To give few examples: in 1972, Mexican neurosurgeon Escobedo *et al.* [13] implanted quadripolar electrodes bilaterally in the head of the caudate nucleus in two patients with epilepsy, mental retardation and destructive aggressive behaviour, and described vegetative, motor and behavioural responses to stimulation. In 1979, West-German neurosurgeon Gert Dieckmann [14] performed unilateral stimulation of the non-dominant thalamus using a quadripolar Medtronic 'deep brain stimulation electrode' to treat a woman with phobia. The electrode contacts extended over 12 mm and were aimed at the parafascicular and rostral intralaminar areas. Stimulation was delivered intermittently at a low frequency (5 Hz) and resulted in disappearance of the phobias, while attempts at stimulation with 50 Hz 'was experienced as being very disagreeable'. A possible reason for the scarcity of neurosurgical papers on psychiatric DBS as a treatment of psychiatric illness during the 1960s and 1970s was that during that period, which saw the demise of the previously popular lobotomy, focused stereotactic ablative procedures (anterior capsulotomy and cingulotomy) were gaining momentum and were the preferred surgical method to treat psychiatric illness, since the DBS hardware and technology of that period were quite cumbersome and not user-friendly.

On the other hand, there is a wealth of publications on DBS from the 1950s through the 1970s, authored by very few psychiatrists and neurophysiologists, in which DBS was not mainly a tool to treat psychiatric disease, but rather to study the brain and to alter human behaviour, as stated earlier. The scholar literature reveals three main workers, a neurophysiologist, a psychiatrist and a neurophysiologist-psychiatrist, who, independently of each other, devoted much of their career to study the effect of DBS in humans and sometimes to promote its use for aims beyond psychiatric disease.

José Delgado, a Spanish neurophysiologist and neurobehaviourist who moved from Spain to Yale University in 1950 and worked there with Fulton, is probably best known for a motion picture showing a bull whose charge in the arena could be stopped through remote brain stimulation. Delgado worked extensively with chronic subcortical stimulation in rats, goats and monkeys and then in humans. In a lecture delivered in 1965 titled *Evolution of Physical Control of the Brain*, he reported: 'Monkeys may learn to press a lever in order to stimulate by radio the brain of another aggressive animal and in this way to avoid his attack'. Heterostimulation in monkey colonies demonstrates the possibility of 'instrumental control of social behaviour' [15]. He concluded, 'Autonomic and somatic functions, individual and social behaviour, emotional and mental reactions may be evoked, maintained, modified, or inhibited, both in animals and in man, by electrical stimulation of specific cerebral structures. Physical control of many brain functions is a demonstrated fact…' [15]. Delgado's enthusiasm for this new technology and its possible effects on behaviour led him to publish in 1969 a book titled *Physical Control of the Mind: Towards a Psychocivilized Society* [16]. This book's title provoked a storm of critic and Delgado was compelled to negate the impression that mind control could be achieved by electrodes wired into people's brain. He emphasized that the technique of 'Electrical Stimulation of the Brain (ESB)', as he called it, was meant as a research tool to study and understand the human mind. Delgado then developed a technique of subcortical stimulation using chronically implanted electrodes connected to a subcutaneous receiver implanted in the scalp that he labelled 'Stimoceiver', which could be remotely controlled by radio waves. This technique of 'radio communication with the brain' was developed by Delgado explicitly for use in psychiatric patients [16–18], although there are no testimonies in the scholar literature to its results in 'real' patients. Anecdotically, Harvard physician turned writer Michael Crichton described in his semi-fictive and famous book *The Terminal Man* first published in 1972 [19] a patient whose personality and behaviour were changed by stimulation through several electrodes implanted in various parts of his brain initially for control of epilepsy, but who also suffered from psychosis. Some of the stimulation effects experienced by the hero of this novel bear strange resemblance to the DBS experiments conducted on real people by another psychiatrist, Robert Heath, at Tulane University in New Orleans.

Robert Heath was a psychiatrist at Tulane University, New Orleans. He implanted a multitude of electrodes in several subcortical nuclei and pathways to study the effect of stimulation on behaviour and probably pioneered the concept of electrical 'self-stimulation'[20]. Heath started a program of DBS to treat schizophrenia as well as pain and epilepsy in the early 1950s [21]. There were no benefits in schizophrenic patients, but Heath made the interesting observation that some patients described the experience of self-stimulation as 'pleasant', 'jovial' or 'euphoric'. In these patients, the electrodes were located in the septal area [21, 22]. This pleasurable response obtained from the 'septal area' came to dominate Heath's further research on DBS applications. He reported relief from physical pain by stimulation of 'this pleasure-yielding area of the brain' and extended studies of this brain area during sexual arousal and orgasm [21–23].

In 1972, Moan and Heath [24] described the use of septal stimulation to induce heterosexual behaviour in a homosexual man. The individual was shown a pornographic video, then a female prostitute was introduced to him in the laboratory and following stimulation to his septal area, the individual and the woman had a sexual intercourse culminating in the subject's orgasm and description of the experience as 'pleasurable'. The authors wrote that during these sessions the individual 'stimulated himself to a point that he was experiencing an almost overwhelming euphoria and elation, and had to be disconnected, despite his vigorous protests' [24]. Two electrodes, each with six contacts, had been implanted in this individual and the paper contains two figures from the Atlas of Schaltenbrand and Bailey depicting their location: one electrode lay in the 'septal area' (close to the nucleus accumbens) and the other in the region of the centromedian nucleus of the thalamus. Heath pursued similar and other experiments through the 1970s and received sponsorship from the US military who were interested in his experiments. Incidentally, and interestingly, in an article published in *Nature* on 12 November 2013, titled 'Implant aims to track brain signals in real time. Device that zaps neurons and monitors electrochemical changes could reveal secrets of deep-brain stimulation therapy', Helen Shen wrote: 'The results come at a time of great excitement in the DBS field. More recently, the US government's Defense Advanced Research Projects Agency (DARPA) announced a 5-year, US$70-million initiative to support development of the next generation of therapeutic brain-stimulating technologies' (http://www.nature.com/news/implant-aims-to-track-brain-signals-in-real-time-1.14153) (accessed 14 January, 2014).

One of Heath's last publications in the 1970s was 'Modulation of emotion with a brain pacemaker. Treatment for intractable psychiatric illness' [25] featuring an illustration showing the commonly used DBS system at the time consisting of a pulse sender with an antenna placed above the skin of the pectoral area where the receiver was implanted (the Xtrel Medtronic system). 'Modulation of emotion' by DBS, an issue widely criticized in the 1970s [22], re-emerged 30 years later from the pen of another psychiatrist Luc Mallet from Paris who published a paper titled: 'La stimulation cérébrale profonde: un outil pour la modulation thérapeutique du comportement et des emotions' (Deep brain stimulation: a tool for therapeutic modulation of behavior and emotions) [26].

The third main proponent of DBS in psychiatry during the 1950–1970s was the Norwegian physiologist-psychiatrist mentioned earlier, Carl Wilhelm Sem-Jacobsen who was a fellow at the Mayo Clinic in the early 1950s [10]. In 1963, he published an article about depth-electrographic observations in psychotic patients [27] in which he stated: 'electrical stimulation in some regions of the ventro-medial part of the frontal lobe resulted in a temporary improvement to complete freedom from symptoms'. The specific aim of his studies was 'to use chronic implanted electrodes in the target area in an attempt to improve the leucotomy operation' [28]. In 1972, he reported that 213 patients had been treated with his 'depth-electrographic stereotactic neurosurgical technique'; of these, 123 patients were suffering from mental disorders [28]. Sem-Jacobsen's technique using chronically implanted electrodes aimed merely to study brain activity and perform intermittent chronic stimulation of various brain targets before subsequent lesioning.

DBS in psychiatry and behaviour never gained momentum, and, similarly to lobotomy, became increasingly discredited and abandoned. In the 20 years between the paper of Dieckmann published in 1979 on DBS in a patient with phobia [14], and the first paper of the 'new' DBS era about DBS in OCD in 1999 [6], one cannot find a single paper on DBS in psychiatry. In fact, it was the misuse of this technique for dubious indications in the 1960–1970s, especially at the hands of the Heath and the Tulane team [21], that contributed to its demise.

In that respect, it is interesting to note that, already in 1977, Finnish neurosurgeon Laitinen commented on the questionable ethics of one of Heath's papers [23]. Laitinen wrote: 'There is no doubt that in this study all standards of ethics had been ignored. The ethical responsibility of the editors who accept reports of this kind for publication should also be discussed' [1]. Laitinen was not against the use of DBS as a therapeutic tool in psychosurgery; in that same paper he wrote, 'After implantation of chronic electrodes, long-term depth recordings and repeated electrical stimulations enable the psychosurgeon to accumulate knowledge about the pathophysiology of the brain and to improve the treatment of the patient in question. It may even be possible to treat the patient with repeated electrical stimulation without macroscopic destruction of brain tissue' [1], and Laitinen proposed a 'model of controlled trial', whereby eligible patients are randomized to receive either the best available conservative therapy or stereotactic surgery and stated, 'Psychosurgery will remain an experimental therapy for years. Therefore its use should be concentrated and restricted to psychosurgical research units having strong and intimate affiliation with scientists from many disciplines' [1]. Neurosurgeon Laitinen's public suggestion to set up a randomized trial of stereotactic psychosurgery versus 'best available conservative therapy' fell on deaf ears at that time, probably because psychosurgery altogether was already doomed and psychiatrists were no longer interested. In any case, this is a historical testimony that it was in fact a pioneer neurosurgeon who was first to suggest a scientific approach to psychosurgery, which contradicts the often repeated contemporary claims that neurosurgeons of the past were those responsible of the 'errors of the past' or were those who were 'acting alone' [29].

In 2000, Heath's experiments were analysed in depth by psychologist Baumeister in a paper titled 'The Tulane Electrical Brain Stimulation Program a historical case study in medical ethics', published in the *Journal of the History of the Neurosciences* [21]. Baumeister reviewed three decades of DBS work performed at Tulane University and concluded by this verdict: '... the Tulane electrical brain stimulation experiments had neither a scientific nor a clinical justification... The conclusion is that these experiments were dubious and precarious by yesterday's standards']21].

The contemporary discourse on psychiatric neuromodulation

Contemporary DBS started in 1987 in the surgical treatment of movement disorders [4]. Since the turn of the century, and ongoing, the field of psychiatric neuromodulation by DBS is witnessing a frenetic activity, whereby DBS is being tried in no less than nine brain targets for Gilles de la Tourette, eight brain targets for OCD and seven brain targets for depression [7, 30], and the search for the ideal target(s) for these conditions is still ongoing, and none of the psychiatric indications in none of the brain targets for DBS is as yet considered as 'established' (Figure 1.1). The number of published papers about psychiatric DBS probably exceeds even the number of operated patients. In parallel, a plethora of publications by ethicists, psychologists, neurologists, psychiatrists, sociologists, philosophers and others have suddenly started to appear dealing with ethics, reviews, guidelines and so forth for conduct of DBS in mental illness. Many of these articles have kept repeating the obvious mantra that the novel era of DBS in psychiatry should not repeat 'the errors of the past', should 'avoid the abuses of that earlier era' [29] and should

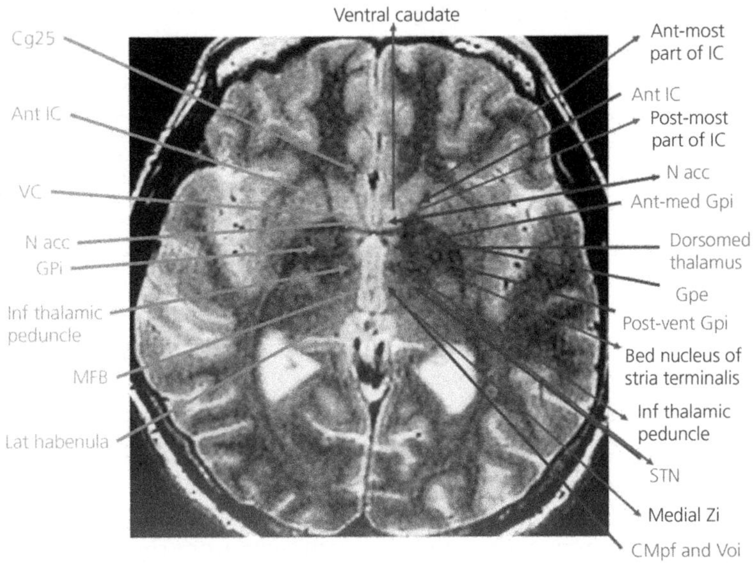

Figure 1.1 Published brain targets submitted to DBS for depression (green) OCD (red), and Tourette (blue). Some targets are overlapping between these three conditions. Note: Not all targets are visible on this axial slice at the level of anterior–posterior commissural plane. Ant-med, anteromedial; Ant-most, anteriormost; Cg25, Cingulum area 25; CMPf, centre median parafascicular nucleus of thalamus; Dorsomed, dorsomedial; GPe, globus pallidus externus; GPi, globus pallidus internus; IC, internal capsule; Inf, inferior; Lat, lateral; MFB, medial forebrain bundle; N acc, Nucleus accumbens; Post-most, posteriormost; Post-vent, posteroventral; STN, subthalamic nucleus; VC, ventral caudate; Voi, nucleus ventralis oralis internus of thalamus; Zi, zona incerta. (*See insert for color representation of the figure.*)

be multidisciplinary. One publication from 2006 stated outright that 'It is ethically untenable for this work to proceed by neurosurgeons in isolation without psychiatrists determining the diagnosis and suitability of patients for treatment'[29]. This latest statement, implying that neurosurgeons have been or are conducting surgery for psychiatric illness 'in isolation' from psychiatrists, merits a few comments.

1 'Abuses of that earlier era' [29] alludes mainly to the unrestricted lobotomies practised by Walter Freeman, who was a neurologist not a neurosurgeon; in fact, 'his' neurosurgeon, James Watts, abandoned him because of Freeman's all too liberal indications for lobotomy [31, 32].
2 In the modern era, it was indeed a neurosurgeon, Alim-Louis Benabid, the father of contemporary DBS, who was the first to take the initiative to seek ethical review on the use of DBS in psychiatry by asking 'the French commission to consider the ethics of using neurostimulation on OCD patients'[33].
3 A search of PubMed using the search words 'ethics' and 'deep brain stimulation' reveals that the first article ever dealing with the ethics of DBS was published in 1980 and authored by three neurosurgeons [34]. That article, titled 'Indications and ethical considerations of deep brain stimulation', was published 7 years before the start of the modern DBS era; at that time, DBS was mostly used to treat chronic pain.
4 After that paper from 1980, the next publication dealing with ethics of DBS did not appear until the year 2000 [35] discussing DBS in impaired consciousness. Then, it was in 2003 that the first paper discussing ethics

of DBS in psychiatry was published [36]. Hence, it was first when modern DBS moved from neurology and movement disorders towards psychiatry and behaviour, that ethics of modern DBS became a matter of concern, which implies that between 1987 and 1999, when modern DBS was used only for Parkinson's, tremor and dystonia, there did not seem to be any ethical considerations worth discussing and publishing.

5 The September 2009 issue of the *Archives of General Psychiatry* featured an article titled 'Scientific and ethical issues related to deep brain stimulation for disorders of mood, behavior and thoughts' [37]. This article summarized a 2-day conference that was convened to examine scientific and ethical issues in the application of DBS in psychiatry in order to 'establish consensus among participants about the design of future clinical trials of DBS for disorders of mood, behaviour and thought' and to 'develop standards for the protection of human subjects participating in such studies'. None of the 30 participants at the meeting, 19 of whom are authors of the article, was a neurosurgeon.

Twenty-first century DBS: a tool for enhancement and social control?

Today DBS is perceived as reversible, and because stereotactic ablative surgery for psychiatric illness suffered and still suffers from the legacy of the lobotomy era, DBS is considered as a more 'legitimate' and acceptable tool for surgical treatment of psychiatric illnesses. This neuromodulation technique has opened further avenues for its applications in other behavioural disorders such as substance addiction and eating disorders, and in cognition.

Recently, notwithstanding the fact that no psychiatric neuromodulation procedure is as yet 'established' despite 15 years of intense activity in the field, DBS is witnessing a qualitatively different and potentially alarming jump, whereby DBS is being discussed for purposes beyond disease: for cognitive enhancement of healthy people and as a means to 'treat' antisocial behaviour: a survey of North American neurosurgeons published in 2011 revealed that more than 50% of those who answered the survey saw no ethical issue in using DBS to provide surgical memory enhancement to healthy people who request it [38]. Furthermore, in February 2012, *Brain* published an uncommented article titled 'Functional and clinical neuroanatomy of morality' [39], in which the authors wrote that 'understanding the dysfunctional brain structures underlying abnormal moral behaviour can lead to specific treatments nowadays using deep brain stimulation or other new non-invasive neuromodulation techniques'. Then, the authors assert 'evidence that subcortical structures intervene in morality' and suggest that 'deep brain stimulation might be used in...pathological antisocial behavior or violence...' and for 'shaping individual morality'. This proposal of a possible use of DBS for such indications, even if the authors acknowledge that this 'raises intriguing ethical issues that should prompt the development of treatment guidelines' is not without provoking a strong sense of déjà vu.

Lessons learned for current practice

When asked in 1972 about what can be learned from the experience of the French Revolution, Mr. Zhou En Lai, China's prime minister between 1949 and 1976, replied: 'It is too early to tell'. Similarly, and in light of the above, it is perhaps still too early today to grasp the 'Lessons learned for Current Practice' from the history of neuromodulation in psychiatry. Besides, what is exactly the 'current practice' of 'neuromodulation in psychiatry' to start with?

According to WHO, psychiatric illness is by far much more prevalent in the world, and carries a much higher burden, than Parkinson's disease (PD) and other movement disorders. Also, it is a fact that the number of clinically active psychiatrists worldwide very highly exceeds the number of clinically active functional neurosurgeons. So how come that in the last 14 years since the introduction of DBS in psychiatry, so very few patients have received this neuromodulative therapy? Is the very rare use of DBS in psychiatry due to the lessons drawn from the practices of the past? Be it as it may, eventual 'lessons learned' from past history play in fact a minor role in the paucity of patients operated. Psychiatrists active in the field of psychiatric DBS, judging by names on publications, can be counted on the fingers of both hands. They are a microscopic minority compared with the number of neurologists active in the field of neurological DBS. There are, in absolute and relative terms, almost infinitely more functional neurosurgeons interested in psychiatric DBS than there are interested psychiatrists. In fact, most psychiatrists, including biological psychiatrists, seem to have very poor idea as to what DBS entails, to the extent that the Chair of the 'Task Force on Brain Stimulation' of the World Federation of Societies of Biological Psychiatry had to literally specify in a guidelines publication in *The World Journal of Biological Psychiatry* in 2010 that 'the term deep brain stimulation refers to methods where electrodes are implanted deep in the brain under the dura' [40].

The criteria for patient selection for DBS in PD and other movement disorders have been for a long time, and still are in most centres, the severity, chronicity and refractoriness of the symptoms. These same selection criteria do indeed apply for the many more available patients who suffer from depression or OCD. Yet, very few patients are referred/recruited for surgery. Unlike in PD patients, where the L-DOPA test usually predicts the outcome of DBS, there are no predictive tests for the outcome of DBS in OCD and depression. Unlike tremor patients, for example, in whom it is established in which brain target(s) DBS should be located to be efficient, we are still far from sure which brain areas are best to target with DBS for depression and OCD. As of today, there is a total of 10–12 different brain targets, the indications for which are overlapping between OCD, depression and Tourette syndrome, such that the same brain target may be used for any of these three illnesses. So, unlike DBS for PD, especially DBS in the STN, it is evident that DBS in psychiatry has not had a breakthrough yet, in any brain target and for any indication. Hence, we do not have today a 'current practice' of DBS in psychiatry. What we have are case reports, very small series and ongoing trials. One of these completed trials on DBS in ventral striatum–ventral capsule versus sham stimulation in 30 patients with major depression showed that DBS was not better than sham stimulation at 4 months blinded follow up, and in the open-phase stimulation at 8–12 months only 21% of patients were 'responders' [41]. In another double-blind trial of STN DBS for OCD, published in 2008, the results were mitigated by the frequency of side effects and the follow up after surgery was 3 months [42], and so far no publication has been made available about the fate of this cohort of patients at longer follow up. These publications using 'evidence-based' methodology are not something that will convince psychiatrists to start referring patients with severe OCD or depression for DBS on a mass scale. Even in trials, one of the problems is the low recruitment of eligible patients, the difficulty to program stimulation parameters in psychiatric patients, the compliance of patients with the trials if it involves sham stimulation, the necessary length of follow up, the lack of disease-specific evaluation tools pertaining to the quality of life and social (re)integration of patients, and many other issues, so in summary one cannot claim that there is any current 'practice' of DBS in psychiatry.

In fact, the main lessons of past historical experience of psychiatric neuromodulation are that there are now about 15 different publications providing ethical guidelines for the conduct of psychiatric DBS, starting with the first published in 2003 [43] and the last just published online [44]. These publications from partly overlapping authors and centres share the same fundamental main ethical requirements for the conduct of DBS in psychiatry. The main guidelines from these publications are summarized as follows, and they are discussed and commented in light of previous historical as well as contemporary practices:

a DBS in any brain target tried so far, and for any psychiatric or behavioural disorder, still remains at an investigational stage.

Interestingly, when FDA approved DBS for OCD as a humanitarian device exemption (HDE) in 2011, that decision was questioned and criticized as a 'misuse' of the HDE by the very pioneers of DBS for OCD, surgeons, psychiatrists and ethicists [45].

b Researchers are encouraged to design randomized controlled trials, based on scientific rationale for DBS in various psychiatric diseases and various brain targets.

Here it is of interest to reiterate what was stated earlier in this chapter that, already in 1977, Laitinen had proposed a similar approach for stereotactic ablative psychosurgery but apparently nobody was interested at that time [1].

c An experienced multidisciplinary team is mandatory for the safe and ethical conduct of any psychiatric neurosurgery.

As shown previously, published guidelines about 'Scientific and ethical issues related to DBS for disorders of mood, behaviour and thought' by 19 authors and co-authors [37] included all disciplines (neurology, psychiatry, ethics, etc.) except neurosurgeons. So much for modern multidisciplinarity!

Besides, the multidisciplinarity that is so important today in all functional neurosurgeries did also exist in the previous era of lesional stereotactic surgery. The father of cingulotomy, neurosurgeon Thomas Ballantine from Massachusetts General Hospital in Boston, was praised by neuroethicist Joe Fins in a paper in 2003, in which Fins wrote about the role of Ballantine in promoting a multidisciplinary approach to stereotactic psychosurgery, whereby 'decisions to operate were to be made in conjunction with a psychiatrist, who would also make psychiatric follow-up available, and patients and family were to be informed of potential risks and benefits' [36].

d Severity, chronicity and refractoriness of patients submitted to DBS must be documented.

e There should be proper consent procedures that respect patient's capacity and autonomy.

f Evaluation should rely on validated and multifaceted scales and tools preoperatively as well as at long term after surgery.

g There should be a comprehensive reporting of all effects and side effects for *all* patients submitted to DBS.

With respect to this last guideline, it appears that even in contemporary practice, multidisciplinarity in psychiatric DBS and ethical awareness may still not be enough to ensure a truly ethical and honest conduct of DBS in psychiatry. There has been at least one example where a DBS trial failed to live up to this fundamental rule, that is, that all patients included in that trial should be accounted for [46]: Two of the very first patients operated upon with DBS for OCD, one of whom was included in the first trial ever performed in DBS for OCD, were never reported, neither in the pioneer paper describing the first four patients, published in *Lancet* in October 1999 [6], nor in subsequent publications, despite the very rigorous ethical standards advocated in the ethical guidelines published by that same group in 2002 [43]. The first mention ever about the existence of these two missing patients is to be found in a paper by Greenberg *et al.* in 2010 [47] in which one laconic sentence reads: 'Two patients operated in Stockholm had no clear benefit'.

Be it as it may with respect to 'lessons' learned or not learned, and as has been discussed earlier, the real issues facing psychiatric neuromodulation with DBS are that very few psychiatrists are interested in DBS. One reason may be that no DBS procedure for any psychiatric illness in any of the multitude of brain targets tried so far has shown a breakthrough during the 15 years of trials of DBS in psychiatry. For a comparison, it did not take 15 years, or 10 or even 5 years before STN DBS or pallidal DBS was endorsed by virtually the whole world community of movement disorders neurologists as a surgical treatment for PD. In the opinion of this author, successful treatment of chronic complicated severe psychiatric illness such as depression or OCD, by modulating pathological brain circuitries with DBS, leading to an improvement that will allow chronic, refractory and severely ill patients to reintegrate society and lead a normal life, is unfortunately still very far away. The technique of DBS involves implantation of hardware in generally young patients, with the need to deliver high energy stimulation, with the need for frequent visits to hospital, with the need of frequent changes of battery over life time, with a cumulative risks of hardware infection and with possible rebound of symptoms in patients who do well when the battery is depleted or when it has to be explanted, aside from many other issues well described recently by the Okun team in Florida [48]. Hence, this technique may perhaps not be ideal in patients with OCD or depression, unless any of the ongoing trials of DBS in OCD or depression shows a real unequivocal and long-term breakthrough in terms of safety and efficacy.

One wonders whether one main 'lesson' of historical psychiatric surgery praxis is that stereotactic lesional surgery (capsulotomy and cingulotomy) has been unnecessarily and unjustly too much denigrated so that almost nobody uses it or even discusses it today, despite its more or less documented long-term efficacy [49–51]. Also the corollary 'lesson' is that DBS is presented today not only as promising (it has been labelled constantly as 'promising' during the last 15 years), but also as safe, reversible, adjustable, adaptable and non-destructive, so much so that it is not even being considered as a surgical treatment: a title published in *The Harvard Mental Health Letter* reads, 'Treating obsessive–compulsive disorder. Options include medication, psychotherapy, surgery, and deep brain stimulation'. [52]. So at Harvard, DBS for OCD is different from 'surgery'!

With this in mind, the commentary of Rhode Island neurologist Joseph H. Friedman from 2004 is worth to meditate about: 'Now that DBS means that psychosurgery is reversible, we no longer have to worry about permanent harm. On the other hand, now that psychosurgery could be readily available, potentially for a large number of conditions, we have a lot more to worry about' [53].

Conclusions

In the last 15 years, neuromodulation, using mainly the technique of DBS, is being increasingly trialled as a potential treatment for various psychiatric and behavioural disorders. The contemporary ethical discourse on psychiatric neuromodulation insists on avoiding the 'abuses' and 'errors' of the past without stating explicitly what is meant by abuses and errors of the past. The modern literature insists on the need for multidisciplinarity and strict ethical conduct in psychiatric surgery, as if ethics and multidisciplinarity were unknown in the past. A study of the historical scholar literature shows that the use of DBS in psychiatry is almost as old as human stereotactic surgery itself, and that principles of ethics and multidisciplinarity did indeed exist, but they were simply ignored by some workers in this field.

Therefore, it is important that those involved in the field of neuromodulation for psychiatric illness properly acknowledge history and keep in mind the following: (i) While it is certainly 'untenable that neurosurgeons act alone' [29], the scholar literature shows that 'acting alone' was not at all restricted to neurosurgeons. (ii) Multidisciplinarity in psychosurgery is not new. It has been the rule, not the exception, in the stereotactic lesional era of psychosurgery. (iii) Multidisciplinarity, per se, is not a guarantee against the excesses or the malpractice of psychosurgery, and proper moral or ethical values are not necessarily better or worse within one particular medical profession, as compared with another. (iv) 'Lessons learned for current practice' will not be learned fully before acknowledging that 'neuromodulation in psychiatry' can also become 'neuromanipulation' and that DBS is not the only and holy surgical approach available for the treatment of severe refractory psychiatric illnesses such as OCD and depression.

Acknowledgements

Marwan Hariz and the Unit of Functional Neurosurgery at the UCL Institute of Neurology are supported by the Parkinson Appeal UK and by the Monument Trust.

The author dedicates this chapter to the memory of a pioneer neurosurgeon 'of the past', Lauri Laitinen, who insisted on, and advocated, the ethical, multidisciplinary, scientific and evidence-based conduct of stereotactic psychosurgery.

Disclosures

Marwan Hariz has occasionally received travel expenses and honoraria from Medtronic and St Jude Medical for speaking at meetings.

References

1 Laitinen LV. Ethical aspects of psychiatric surgery. In Sweet WH, Obrador S, Martín-Rodríguez JG (eds.) Neurosurgical Treatment in Psychiatry, Pain, and Epilepsy. University Park Press: Baltimore, MD, 1977: 483–488.
2 Fodstad H, Hariz M. Electricity in the treatment of nervous system disease. Acta Neurochir Suppl 2007; 97: 11–19.
3 Coffey RJ. Deep brain stimulation devices: a brief technical history and review. Artif Organs 2009; 33: 208–220.
4 Benabid AL, Pollak P, Louveau A, Henry S, de Rougemont J. Combined (thalamotomy and stimulation) stereotactic surgery of the VIM thalamic nucleus for bilateral Parkinson disease. Appl Neurophysiol 1987; 50: 344–346.
5 Vandewalle V, van der Linden C, Groenewegen HJ, Caemaert J. Stereotactic treatment of Gilles de la Tourette syndrome by high frequency stimulation of thalamus. Lancet 1999; 353: 724.
6 Nuttin B, Cosyns P, Demeulemeester H, Gybels J, Meyerson B. Electrical stimulation in anterior limbs of internal capsules in patients with obsessive-compulsive disorder. Lancet 1999; 354: 1526.
7 Hariz M. Twenty-five years of deep brain stimulation: celebrations and apprehensions. Mov Disord 2012; 27: 930–933.
8 Spiegel EA, Wycis HT, Marks M, Lee AJ. Stereotaxic apparatus for operations on the human brain. Science 1947; 106: 349–350.
9 Delgado JM, Hamlin H, Chapman WP. Technique of intracranial electrode implacement for recording and stimulation and its possible therapeutic value in psychotic patients. Confin Neurol 1952; 12: 315–319.
10 Bickford RG, Petersen MC, Dodge HW Jr, Sem-Jacobsen CW. Observations on depth stimulation of the human brain through implanted electrographic leads. Proc Staff Meet Mayo Clin 1953; 28: 181–187.
11 Heath RG. Depth recording and stimulation studies in patients. In: Winter A (ed.) The Surgical Control of Behavior. Charles C Thomas: Springfield, IL, 1971: 21–37.
12 Sheer DE. Electrical Stimulation of the Brain. An Interdisciplinary Survey of Neurobehavioral Integrative Systems. University of Texas Press: Austin, TX, 1961.

13 Escobedo F, Fernández-Guardiola A, Solís G. Chronic stimulation of the cingulum in humans with behaviour disorders. In: Laitinen LV, Livingstone KE (eds.) Surgical Approaches in Psychiatry. Medical and Technical Publishing Co: Lancaster, 1973: 65–68.
14 Dieckmann G. Chronic mediothalamic stimulation for control of phobias. In: Hitchcock ER, Ballantine HT Jr, Meyerson BA (eds.) Modern Concepts in Psychiatric Surgery. Elsevier: Amsterdam, 1979: 85–93.
15 Delgado JMR. Evolution of physical control of the brain. In: *James Arthur Lecture on the Evolution of the Human Brain*, No. 34. American Museum of Natural History: New York, pp. 1–54, 1965.
16 Delgado JMR. Physical Control of the Mind: Towards a Psychocivilized Society. Harper and Row: New York, 1969.
17 Delgado JMR. Therapeutic programmed stimulation in man. In Sweet WH, Obrador S, Martín-Rodríguez JG (eds.) Neurosurgical Treatment in Psychiatry, Pain, and Epilepsy. University Park Press: Baltimore, MD, 1977: 615–637.
18 Delgado JMR, Obrador S, Martín-Rodríguez JG. Two-way radio communication with the brain in psychosurgical patients. In: Laitinen LV, Livingstone KE (eds.) Surgical Approaches in Psychiatry. Medical and Technical Publishing Co: Lancaster, 1973: 215–223.
19 Crichton M. The Terminal Mak.k.n. Knopf Publishing Group, New Work, 1972.
20 Heath RG. Electrical self-stimulation of the brain in man. Am J Psychiatry 1963; 120: 571–577.
21 Baumeister AA. The Tulane Electrical Brain Stimulation Program a historical case study in medical ethics. J Hist Neurosci 2000; 9: 262–278.
22 Valenstein ES. Brain Control. A Critical Examination of Brain Stimulation and Psychosurgery. John Wiley & Sons, Inc.: New York, 1973.
23 Heath RG. Pleasure and brain activity in man. Deep and surface electroencephalograms during orgasm. J Nerv Ment Dis 1972; 154: 3–18.
24 Moan CE, Heath RG. Septal stimulation for the initiation of heterosexual behaviour in a homosexual male. J Behav Ther Exp Psychiatry 1972; 3: 23–30.
25 Heath RG. Modulation of emotion with a brain pacemaker. Treatment for intractable psychiatric illness. J Nerv Ment Dis 1977; 165: 300–317.
26 Mallet L. La stimulation cérébrale profonde: un outil pour la modulation thérapeutique du comportement et des emotions. Encéphale 2006; 32: S44–S47.
27 Sem-Jacobsen CW. Depth-electrographic observations in psychotic patients. Acta Psychiatr Scand Suppl 1959; 34: 412–416.
28 Sem-Jacobsen CW, Styri OB. Depth-electrographic stereotaxic psychosurgery. In: Hitchcock E, Laitinen L, Vaernet K (eds.) Psychosurgery. Charles C Thomas: Springfield, IL, 1972: 76–82.
29 Fins JJ, Rezai AR, Greenberg BD. Psychosurgery: Avoiding an ethical redux while advancing a therapeutic future. Neurosurgery 2006; 59: 713–716.
30 Krack P, Hariz MI, Baunez C, Guridi J, Obeso JA. Deep brain stimulation: from neurology to psychiatry? Trends Neurosci 2010; 33: 474–484.
31 El-Hai J. The Lobotomist. John Wiley & Sons, Inc.: Hoboken, NJ, 2005.
32 Hariz MI, Blomstedt P, Zrinzo L. Deep brain stimulation: 1947–1987. Neurosurg Focus 2010; 29: E1.
33 Goodman S. France wires up to treat obsessive disorder. Nature 2002; 417: 677.
34 Siegfried J, Lazorthes Y, Sedan R. Indications and ethical considerations of deep brain stimulation. Acta Neurochir Suppl (Wien) 1980; 30: 269–274.
35 Fins JJ. A proposed ethical framework for interventional cognitive neuroscience: a consideration of deep brain stimulation in impaired consciousness. Neurol Res 2000; 22: 273–278.
36 Fins JJ. From psychosurgery to neuromodulation and palliation: history's lessons for the ethical conduct and regulation of neuropsychiatric research. Neurosurg Clin N Am 2003; 14: 303–319.
37 Rabins P, Appleby BS, Brandt J, DeLong MR, Dunn LB, Gabriëls L, Greenberg BD, Haber SN, Holtzheimer PE III, Mari Z, Mayberg HS, McCann E, Mink SP, Rasmussen S, Schlaepfer TE, Vawter DE, Vitek JL, Walkup J, Mathews DJ. Scientific and ethical issues related to deep brain stimulation for disorders of mood, behaviour, and thought. Arch Gen Psychiatry 2009; 66: 931–937.
38 Lipsman N, Mendelsohn D, Taira T, Bernstein M. The contemporary practice of psychiatric surgery: results from a survey of North

American functional neurosurgeons. Stereotact Funct Neurosurg 2011; 89: 103–110.
39 Fumagalli M, Priori A. Functional and clinical neuroanatomy of morality. Brain 2012; 135: 2006–2021.
40 Schlaepfer TE, George MS, Mayberg H; WFSBP task force on brain stimulation. WFSBP guidelines on brain stimulation treatments in psychiatry. World J Biol Psychiatry 2010; 11: 2–18.
41 Dougherty D, Carpenter L, Bhati M, Howland R, O'Reardon J, Denko T, Jacobs KJ, Pandya MM, Price LH, Tyrka AR, Evans K, Rezai AR, Baltuch G, Machado AG, Eskandar EN, Kondziolka D, Cusin C, Malone DA. A randomized sham-controlled trial of DBS of the VC/VS for treatment-resistant depression. *Society of Biological Psychiatry 67th Annual Scientific Convention*, 2012. http://goo.gl/PGTpo (accessed 18 January 2014).
42 Mallet L, Polosan M, Jaafari N, Baup N, Welter ML, Fontaine D, du Montcel ST, Yelnik J, Chéreau I, Arbus C, Raoul S, Aouizerate B, Damier P, Chabardès S, Czernecki V, Ardouin C, Krebs MO, Bardinet E, Chaynes P, Burbaud P, Cornu P, Derost P, Bougerol T, Bataille B, Mattei V, Dormont D, Devaux B, Vérin M, Houeto JL, Pollak P, Benabid AL, Agid Y, Krack P, Millet B, Pelissolo A; STOC Study Group. Subthalamic nucleus stimulation in severe obsessive-compulsive disorder. N Engl J Med 2008; 359: 2121–2134.
43 OCD-DBS Collaborative Group Deep brain stimulation for psychiatric disorders. Neurosurgery 2002; 51: 519.
44 Nuttin B, Wu H, Mayberg H, Hariz M, Gabriëls L, Galert T, Merkel R, Kubu C, Vilela-Filho O, Matthews K, Taira T, Lozano AM, Schechtmann G, Doshi P, Broggi G, Régis J, Alkhani A, Sun B, Eljamel S, Schulder M, Kaplitt M, Eskandar E, Rezai A, Krauss JK, Hilven P, Schuurman R, Ruiz P, Chang JW, Cosyns P, Lipsman N, Voges J, Cosgrove R, Li Y, Schlaepfer T. Consensus on guidelines for stereotactic neurosurgery for psychiatric disorders. J Neurol Neurosurg Psychiatry, 2014; 85: 1003–1008.
45 Fins JJ, Mayberg HS, Nuttin B, Kubu CS, Galert T, Sturm V, Stoppenbrink K, Merkel R, Schlaepfer TE. Misuse of the FDA's humanitarian device exemption in deep brain stimulation for obsessive-compulsive disorder. Health Aff (Millwood) 2011; 30: 302–311.
46 Hariz MI. Psychosurgery, deep brain stimulation, and the re-writing of history. Neurosurgery 2008; 63: E820.
47 Greenberg BD, Gabriels LA, Malone DA Jr, Rezai AR, Friehs GM, Okun MS, Shapira NA, Foote KD, Cosyns PR, Kubu CS, Malloy PF, Salloway SP, Giftakis JE, Rise MT, Machado AG, Baker KB, Stypulkowski PH, Goodman WK, Rasmussen SA, Nuttin BJ. Deep brain stimulation of the ventral internal capsule/ventral striatum for obsessive-compulsive disorder: worldwide experience. Mol Psychiatry 2010; 15: 64–79.
48 Vora AK, Ward H, Foote KD, Goodman WK, Okun MS. Rebound symptoms following battery depletion in the NIH OCD DBS cohort: clinical and reimbursement issues. Brain Stimul 2012; 5: 599–604.
49 Bingley T, Leksell L, Meyerson BA, Rylander G. Long-term results of stereotactic anterior capsulotomy in chronic obsessive-compulsive neurosis. In: Sweet WH, Obrador S, Martín-Rodríguez JG (eds.) Neurosurgical Treatment in Psychiatry, Pain, and Epilepsy. University Park Press: Baltimore, MD, 1977: 287–299.
50 Christmas D, Eljamel MS, Butler S, Hazari H, MacVicar R, Steele JD, Livingstone A, Matthews K. Long term outcome of thermal anterior capsulotomy for chronic, treatment refractory depression. J Neurol Neurosurg Psychiatry 2011; 82: 594–600.
51 Sheth SA, Neal J, Tangherlini F, Mian MK, Gentil A, Cosgrove GR, Eskandar EN, Dougherty DD. Limbic system surgery for treatment-refractory obsessive-compulsive disorder: a prospective long-term follow-up of 64 patients. J Neurosurg 2013; 118: 491–497.
52 Anonymous. Treating obsessive-compulsive disorder. Options include medication, psychotherapy, surgery, and deep brain stimulation. Harv Ment Health Lett 2009; 25: 4–5.
53 Friedman JH. DBS. Med Health R I 2004; 87: 62.

CHAPTER 2
Ethics of neuromodulation in psychiatry

Joseph J. Fins[1] and Barbara R. Pohl[2]
[1] *The E. William Davis, Jr., Weill Medical College of Cornell University, New York, USA*
[2] *Division of Medical Ethics, Weill Cornell Medical College, New York, USA*

Introduction

Neuropsychiatric conditions pose profound moral dilemmas within the health care system. Many individuals suffering from severe psychiatric illnesses do not receive treatments that respond to their clinical needs and many others suffer from the pervasive stigma attached to mental illness [1]. Given the marginalization of patients with psychiatric illness, neurosurgeons, neurologists, psychologists and psychiatrists have an ethical obligation to assist this population by pursuing novel therapeutic interventions. Neuromodulation, especially through deep brain stimulation (DBS), offers just this opportunity for patients with refractory conditions that do not respond to conventional pharmacological therapies or psychotherapy [2]. The most promising areas of research for DBS as a novel therapeutic are for patients with severe depression and obsessive–compulsive disorder (OCD), suggesting that it could become a standard therapy for these two conditions [3].

The ethical principles governing the use of neuromodulation in psychiatry will seek to protect this underserved and vulnerable population from harm and support research that enhances its welfare. These commitments draw upon the basic tenets of research and clinical ethics, as electrical stimulation of the brain for psychiatric disorders straddles both the therapeutic and investigational divide, as well as the emerging domain of *neuroethics* with its inherent concerns, which hind upon mind and personhood, about interventions in the brain.

We will begin this consideration with a brief historical recapitulation of the ethical issues that attended antecedent periods of research and practice involving psychosurgery and then move into the modern era of neuromodulation for neuropsychiatric disorders.

A brief history

While neuromodulation continues to grow as an established science holding great therapeutic promise for individuals with psychiatric conditions, it follows a history of treatment for psychiatric illnesses riddled with controversy. Some of these ethical issues arose in the mid-20th century with the development of ablative surgery and electrical stimulation in the brain. Briefly examining the legacy of psychosurgery provides a cautionary note for our consideration of neuromodulation in modern psychiatric practice and research [4].

Electricity has played a role in treating and understanding neuropsychiatric illnesses since the 19th century. Early experiments in animals used electricity as a means of understanding epilepsy, and neurosurgeons Harvey Cushing and Wilder Penfield continued such explorations during the first half of the century

Neuromodulation in Psychiatry, First Edition. Edited by Clement Hamani, Paul Holtzheimer, Andres M. Lozano and Helen Mayberg.

[5]. By 1947, neurosurgery had advanced with the significant development of how to localize the brain in three dimensions with the advent of stereotactic neurosurgery. This facilitated the placement of electrodes on targets deep in the brain without open craniotomies but by their passage through burr holes [6].

While these developments in the electrical stimulation of the brain are an important part of the history leading to DBS and neuromodulation, they were neither the only one nor the most controversial. Instead, it was the ablative lineage of psychosurgery that destroyed tissue in the service of health that most shaped public perceptions of any form of intervention in the brain. Initially welcomed as a treatment of refractory psychoses and for the shell shock of returning veterans from World War II, psychosurgery would eventually be perceived with disdain and outrage with which it was zealously promoted by its adherents [4, 7].

But make no mistake about it, psychosurgery constituted a major therapeutic breakthrough. Before the Portuguese Egas Moniz pioneered the lobotomy as an effective therapy for severe mental illness in 1935, physicians could only manage patients with psychoses by committing them to mental institutions that deprived patients of their freedom, their community and dignity. When Moniz subsequently won the Nobel Prize for his contribution to medicine and physiology in 1949, the award partially signified the public perception that this therapeutic option had great clinical utility. Contemporaries commenting on novel and experimental therapeutics, such as Cornell's psychiatry chair Oskar Diethelm, argued that physicians should acknowledge the uncertainty surrounding such intervention and to safeguard patients from harm [8].

This admonition, however, did not translate to the work of those who followed Moniz and who pursued dangerous, irreversible procedures with little scientific proof of its efficacy [4]. Indeed, Walter Freeman's disturbing crusade performing frontal lobotomies using an ice pick, without training as a neurosurgeon, as well as the advent of major tranquilizers in the early 1950s, led to the rapid decline of ablative procedures by mid-decade [9].

The work of Jose M.R. Delgado, beginning in the 1950s, continued at the basic and applied level in studies geared to understand neurophysiology. Delgado advanced work in the electrical stimulation of the brain, designing a brain implant, what he called a 'stimoceiver' that he controlled with a remote control. He famously implanted the electrode into the caudate nucleus of a Spanish fighting bull and demonstrated an ability to stem the animal's aggressive charges [10]. His work became controversial because it aroused fears of mind control by third parties who would use the stimoceiver. Delgado courted further controversy because he advocated these technologies to 'psychocivilize society', an objective that was perceived as necessary by some during the tumultuous 1960s [11]. Although many feared how these technologies could threaten civil liberties, Delgado imagined that their use would quell aggression and promote liberty and autonomy within a more civil community [4, 11].

The worry that interventions such as Delgado's and other forms of psychosurgery would be used for behavioural control pervaded the public's distrust for such measures. Some experts argued for the use of psychosurgery to control violence within American cities, basing this recommendation on the correlation between brain disorders such as epilepsy and violent behaviours and, despite reports suggesting evidence to the contrary, many assumed that American prisons commonly used psychosurgery to control its inmates, although this was not the case [12]. Artistic works such as Michael Crichton's *The Terminal Man* fuelled the worry that law enforcement might use electrical stimulation to treat violent individuals [4, 13]. In response to the public's growing objection to psychosurgery, as well as the emergence of a bioethics movement during this same period, the

National Commission for the Protection of Human Subjects of Biomedical and Behavioral Research issued a report on psychosurgery [14]. This report was one of many others, including one from the Hastings Center that explored the ethical dimensions of psychosurgery at that time [4, 12].

In 1977, the National Commission published its report on psychosurgery – defined to include both electric stimulation and ablative surgery. The report acknowledged the therapeutic efficacy of certain surgical procedures such as cingulotomy and concluded that, with rigid regulatory structures in place, clinicians could study and utilize psychosurgery for therapeutic purposes, not as a form of social control [4]. In advocating for strict regulation of psychotherapy, the National Commission suggested that institutional review boards (IRBs) comprised of experts in neurology, neurosurgery, psychiatry and psychology assess the safety, efficacy and utility of any psychotherapeutic procedure performed on an individual [4, 14].

This recommendation entailed concerns for acquiring adequate informed and voluntary consent from those participating in such research. The report excluded a variety of individuals – children, mentally ill, prisoners and people the courts deemed incompetent or who clinicians deemed incapacitated – from participating in psychosurgery. While this provision respected the vulnerability of many populations whose researchers might otherwise exploit (a safeguard steeped in the then recent exposure of scandals such as the Tuskegee syphilis study) [15], it also denied patients with psychiatric conditions that may influence their decision-making capacity the opportunity of participating in research of interest to them [4].

History with a difference

Although the National Commission's report on psychosurgery may have foreshadowed many normative commitments relevant to neuromodulation in psychiatry, it was forgotten until one of us (JJF) brought it back into the current literature on neuromodulation [4]. This omission is striking given that many modern clinicians, researchers and neuroethicists also possess a balanced enthusiasm for psychiatric neurosurgery [9]. So why was the report lost to history? It would seem that until the modern era of neuromodulation, it was easier to see the excesses of these interventions in isolation without due appreciation of their therapeutic potential. There was no need to have a balanced view of the harms if the putative benefits were unappreciated. But once the potential for these therapies is realized, differences between past and present, ablative and neuromodulatory approaches become salient [4, 16].

First, neuromodulation, unlike surgery, is reversible. Whether electroconvulsive therapy, transcranial magnetic stimulation or deep-brain stimulation, an individual can switch the source of stimulation on or off and even can remove the electrodes without great risk [4, 17, 18]. Second, while some classical psychosurgery procedures (such as lobotomy) lacked experimental evidence demonstrating their therapeutic success, a number of research studies have begun to demonstrate its safety and efficacy in the treatment of psychiatric or neurological illnesses or injuries [19–21]. Third, unlike past psychosurgeries performed without stringent selection criteria, modern DSM nosology and proper longitudinal regard for side effects, current studies must now meet rigorous specifications and interdisciplinary teams must perform long-term follow ups [22]. Finally, a vast neuroethical cannon has accompanied its development and encouraged a culture that responds to both the 'promise and perils' of technological interventions in the brain [7, 23]. With these differences in mind, it is possible to revive the National Commission's tempered endorsement of psychosurgery and reflect upon some of the more fundamental ethical concerns.

Any form of intervention in the brain raises philosophical concerns about free will, autonomy and personal identity, in turn, bearing on the more practical need for the best ways of obtaining voluntary, informed consent [5, 9, 24]. Given the complexities of the brain itself, technologies that probe this organ often complicate existing boundaries between research and therapy and make proportionality assessments all the more difficult. These ethical issues point to a need for a regulatory climate that allows clinician-investigators to use these devices to advance the basic scientific understanding of the brain itself while also developing meaningful therapies for patients with psychiatric illnesses. Moreover, these ethical concerns raise the possibility for adopting the focus of palliative care: using neuromodulation to alleviate suffering associated with psychiatric illness. This chapter will discuss each of these elements in turn.

Autonomy and the self

Part of what made psychosurgery so contentious, as we have seen, was that it entailed the act of operating on the brain. As a *Lancet* editorial written in 1972 explained, to enter the brain 'surgically carries a peculiar penumbra of sacrilege' [25]. The act of intervening in the brain through neuromodulation continues to worry many individuals today because it raises a unique series of ethical questions dealing with subjective experience and autonomy [5]. The brain is, indeed, an exceptional organ that is integral to lived experience and to the formation of an individual's sense of self. Any intervention that involves the brain's structure or function implicates brain states and personhood. Electrical stimulation of the brain has the possibility to alter, albeit reversibly, an individual's actions, thoughts and thus personality leading to great concerns over the use of technologies such as DBS. But neuromodulation neither appears to fundamentally undermine any of the 'capacities constitutive for personhood', including self-consciousness, free will, episodic memory, dispositions, preferences and so on [3], nor differs in its effects of mind from those of drugs, illness and even education.

A naturalistic understanding of the self can allay concerns about the device's potential to alter personal identity in troubling ways. Such a view does not understand the person, or self, as a non-physical entity, but instead as a 'biological–cognitive representational system' with the capacity to construct a subjective experience [22]. This account eschews dualism, and conceptualizes personality as the manifestation of complex interactions between more basic sensorimotor and higher level emotional processes. Neuromodulation, in this view, can induce changes in personality on multiple levels and to varying degrees. When used as a therapy for psychiatric illness, for example, the goal of neuromodulation is precisely to alter basic sensorimotor and higher level emotional processes that have been altered by illness and to induce constructive changes in mood and behaviour in the service of normative improvement. [22].

One aspect of introducing positive alterations to personality is its ability to restore autonomy. Philosophers have long recognized that autonomy entails both the ability to act and agency over the 'conscious and unconscious mental states that move one to act' [26]. A neurological injury or psychiatric illness may cause an individual to experience a loss of autonomy, lacking control over his or her thoughts or actions [27]. Neuromodulation through its intercession may paradoxically promote autonomy by 'restoring the neural functions mediating the relevant mental and physical capacities', allowing an individual to regain control over his or her own actions; in the case of a psychiatric condition such as OCD, electrical stimulation may reduce the frequency of repetitive behaviours and enable an individual to act as he or she chooses [26].

Not only does neuromodulation have the potential to enhance an individual's Maslowian self-actualization, it may also lead to changes in personal relationships. Since the milieu in which an individual lives shapes his or her identity – impacting his or her choices, preferences and desires – any intervention that impacts autonomy will have a bearing on others within his or her lived experience. If we transcend the atomistic model of the autonomous self and accept a more molecular configuration of reciprocal relationality, we will soon appreciate that changes to an individual's self-conception may have constructive or destructive consequences in his or her interpersonal relationships. Certain studies of DBS with Parkinson's disease have demonstrated changes in a subject's mood and behaviour rendering these consequences worthy of consideration [27].

Society may also seek to invest in those technologies that assist in individuals realizing their potential and maximizing their participation in communal life [27]. Much like a civil rights framework can advocate for marginalized patients with severe brain injury who 'remain sequestered' from advances in neuroscience that may promote their rehabilitation and recovery, the same pushes for integration can ground a societal investment in neuromodulation research intended to restore the autonomy of patients with severe psychiatric conditions [28, 29].

Informed consent

In order to respect the autonomy of a patient or research subject, a clinician or researcher must acquire their informed consent [3]. Such a requirement is consistent with the Belmont Report's respect for persons principle, although this connection is perhaps over asserted [29, 30]. A successful informed consent process will contain an explicit discussion of the risks and benefits of an intervention, along with an acknowledgement of any uncertainties and a clear statement of the expected result [27]. In the case of neuromodulation for psychiatric illness, it is especially important that this process be a longitudinal one, and revisited at different points in time [9].

The nature of this conversation will also differ based on whether it occurs in a research or clinical context, as the norms governing either diverge. An investigator intends for an experimental intervention to enhance scientific knowledge for the community's benefit while a clinician must offer a therapeutic intervention that he or she reasonably expects will benefit the individual patient [31]. When obtaining consent for participating in a clinical trial, an investigator should ensure that patients do not conflate the investigation with receiving a therapy that is the standard of care, avoiding what is known as the *therapeutic misconception* [32].

While the marginalization of patients with psychiatric illnesses and their past abuses in clinical research warrant protections restricting their participation, the prevailing view that they are 'less able to give informed consent' than other individuals with chronic illnesses does not hold [9]. This stigma comes from the view that some psychiatric patients may express preferences shaped by their condition itself, leading perhaps to desperate pursuits of interventions such as DBS [22]. For this reason, assessing the decision-making capacity of individuals is necessary. Many patients diagnosed with severe depression retain decision-making capacity to participate in clinical trials [33]. Given that patients with psychiatric disorders are still a stigmatized and vulnerable population, some recommend that IRBs approve the capacity assessment tool used in the consenting process [34–37].

There are currently many restrictions on individuals who do not have the capacity to consent to research. In 1998, the National Bioethics Advisory Commission issued a report, which was never enacted into law, entitled *Research Involving Mental Disorders That May Affect Decisionmaking Capacity*, proposing stringent guidelines for allowing surrogates to consent for patients who lack decision-making capacity as a result of a psychiatric illness [38]. Some have argued that these protections further stigmatized those with psychiatric conditions as opposed to other chronic, life-threatening diseases [39]. Moreover, by denying incapacitated individuals with neuropsychiatric ailments access to clinical trials, these restrictions hinder the research efforts that would ultimately help them [18, 39, 40]. The New York State Task Force on Life and the Law has begun to respond to such inequities, devising a report that offers guidance for institutions involved in conducted research with decisionally incapacitated patients [41].

Proportionality: weighing individual benefits and harms

As observed in the many constraints placed on the informed consent process for people with psychiatric illness, the legacy of psychosurgery has encouraged the development of an ethical framework that seeks to prevent this population from exploitation and suffering. This protective stance has encouraged cautious investment in research that is expected to benefit patients with severe illnesses that are recalcitrant to other therapies. Adhering to the principle of beneficence, or promoting 'the good', entails a commitment to research that maximizes the benefits and minimizes the harms to a population with psychiatric illness [42, 43].

When assessing the benefits and harms of a technology such as DBS, one must first recognize that it is an intrusive procedure requiring facilities and physicians with great resources and skill, with clinical effects that may manifest over many years [9]. According to the principle of beneficence, an appropriate use of DBS for a psychiatric patient will afford her an 'actual benefit' defined not only in biological terms but also in personal terms; an individual may benefit from DBS if it enhances her autonomy and allows her to pursue 'personally valuable goals' [22]. Calculating possible therapeutic benefits is difficult for psychiatric conditions, as their aetiology likely hinges upon various biological, personal and social factors, and a variety of different classifications based on different group of symptoms exists [22].

Implanting an electrode in any location in the brain comes with risk, although some carry a greater level than others, and many side effects can accompany the stimulation [34]. Some of these side effects include changes in self-perception [44–46]. An awareness of an impairment or of an undesired change may threaten a patient's sense of self, a state Eric Cassell describes as suffering [47]. When determining whether an intervention such as DBS poses an unacceptable harm to a patient, such a possibility must be compared with the relative harm of not pursuing the intervention if it is a vetted therapy [22].

Weighing these risks and benefits is ethically more fraught in the psychiatric arena than in addressing DBS for improving motor function of patients with Parkinson's disease, as such a discussion requires choosing between decreased motor functionality with the potential risk of changes in 'states of mind' [48]. In the case of investigations of the use of DBS for psychiatric disorders, the relevant quality-of-life assessments may not be as clear in advance. It is important that such studies utilize 'core assessment protocols' to compare and contrast the risks and benefits associated with various approaches in order to assist in future research [3]. These assessments may be useful when devising standard inclusion criteria for clinical trials examining the therapeutic effects of neuromodulation for different psychiatric conditions; currently, the main suggested criteria are that a patient be old enough to provide independent informed consent, be diagnosed with a severe psychiatric disorder for at least 5 years, and has not responded to other pharmacological, behavioural or ECT therapies [9]. A rigorous selection process will ensure that the benefits appropriately outweigh the risks for a particular individual, and thus can exclude patients for whom it is not reasonable to expect a benefit [49].

Distinguishing research from therapy

While DBS holds therapeutic potential for many psychiatric illnesses, it remains in the investigational phase for conditions such as major depressive disorder and has been approved under Humanitarian Device Exemption for OCD. For an intervention such as DBS to become a standard therapy, it requires a majority of physicians to agree that an intervention adequately mitigates symptoms with a degree of risk that does not exceed the expected benefits [2, 34]. In order for DBS to adopt a therapeutic classification, safety and efficacy trials (double-blind, randomized control trials being the gold standard) must generate a sufficient body of evidence. Many of the ethical principles applying to neuromodulation in psychiatry are specific to the research context. As in any form of clinical research, an IRB must oversee the investigations of DBS for different psychiatric disorders. These regulatory bodies will promote valid informed consent processes, accurate proportionality calculations and encourage rigorous selection of participants [2]. In some cases, a Data Safety Monitoring Board should be established to evaluate adverse events and therapeutic outcomes if the study is blinded.

Since neuromodulation remains largely investigational, a great deal of uncertainty surrounds the safety and efficacy of its use for various psychiatric conditions. Clinician-researchers ought to abide by a 'precautionary principle' when contemplating an innovative insertion of an electrode for a particular condition without wholly 'stifling' their creative instinct [50, 51]. Since a basal level of risk accompanies any novel surgical intervention, neurosurgeons and other experts must balance their precautions with the potential therapeutic benefits. Before bringing a patient to the operating room, any surgeon calculates whether the benefits will be greater than the risks given his proximity to the patient's outcome [51].

The history of psychosurgery should temper the blind pursuit of innovation, as it reminds clinician researchers to maintain their humility and exercise caution when performing such risk–benefit calculations [16]. Cultivating an interdisciplinary approach to neuromodulation offers one way of avoiding such errors; it allows neurosurgeons to take responsibility for the limits of their competence and to encourage psychiatrists and psychologists to participate in meaningful clinical examinations of such interventions [52].

Determining when a technology passes from the investigational context to the clinical context, however, is still a difficult business. Inserting a device into the brain is a highly individualized process, meaning that it is harder to orchestrate rigorous clinical trials that can demonstrate safety and efficacy; researchers instead must generalize from a variety of individualized findings [53]. The small sample size makes it difficult for 'establishing a threshold for vetted treatment' [54]. For this reason, DBS often straddles the line between investigative and therapeutic – necessitating federal regulations that are sensitive to its mosaicism [24].

Neuromodulation research and the marketplace

The aforementioned arguments outline the principles needed to protect vulnerable psychiatric patients and/or research subjects and the related principles encouraging researchers and clinicians to exercise caution and humility while pursuing neuromodulation within psychiatry. Although these recommendations intend to constrain activity to ensure ethical conduct, they do not intend to promote an entirely nihilistic view about neuromodulation or hinder the research that will advance its progress in psychiatry. A second set of normative commitments establishes how clinical investigators and the regulatory environment ought to promote the fruits of responsible research on ways neuromodulation can treat psychiatric illnesses.

The ethical commitment to protect patients from harm within the therapeutic context may deprive patients who lack capacity access to neuromodulation. This exclusion stems from existing FDA regulations categorizing DBS or other like devices solely as therapies, shortchanging their role in broadening our scientific understanding of the brain's neural circuitry [24]. Before researchers have the opportunity to employ a device in trials that would expand the knowledge base, they are approved as therapies and prematurely commodified, limiting the opportunity for additional discovery of the circuitry underlying neuropsychiatric conditions [24, 55].

Manufacturers can avoid such gridlock through the humanitarian device exemption that allows them to bring these devices to market without first conducting a clinical trial in certain cases. This exemption is meant to meet the need of patient populations with rare conditions that might not interest industry to fund expensive, rigorous clinical trials, but the profitability of developing devices may have subverted this original goal [56]. For example, the FDA through the HDE mechanism may have problematically approved DBS for severe OCD; this approval failed to recognize that the 'equivalent use' of an electrode depends on where it is placed in the brain and did not recognize the need to monitor for adverse events and collect data on the safety of the intervention [57].

In order to avoid encouraging practices that undermine the welfare of patients with neuropsychiatric conditions who might benefit from neuromodulation, regulatory frameworks ought to regard such devices as both investigational and therapeutic and fronts for additional recovery [21, 58]. It is problematic to rush the application of devices to the marketplace as it fails to cultivate such valuable scientific work [54].

To conceptualize devices as both investigative and therapeutic is consistent with both principles of beneficence and justice. Investigators (and referring clinicians) may possess a fiduciary obligation to encourage participation in rigorous double-blind trials with the potential to enhance our understanding of the pathophysiology of psychiatric conditions and eventually yield novel therapies. As suggested earlier, patients with severe psychiatric conditions remain in need of alternatives to drugs. Encouraging the advancement of knowledge surrounding the application of neuromodulation for psychiatric conditions may address inequities in care. Patients with psychiatric illnesses deserve sufficient investment in promising research in order to maximally integrate them into the community as consistent with the emerging field of disability rights [59].

One way of adhering to this justice principle is to ensure that existing regulations do not deny the population a meaningful opportunity to participate in research by prematurely classifying devices as therapeutic. The existing intellectual property laws represent one opportunity for reformation. While the Bayh–Dole Act of 1980 – allowing academic research institutions and investigators to profit from their discoveries – may have been responsible for the flourishing biotechnology industry, it has contributed to the narrow therapeutic focus of DBS research; more theoretical work has less value in the marketplace [60]. Moreover, this commodification of devices developed for therapeutic purposes can engender conflicts of interest for researchers who may reap financial benefits from the basic science that they continue to explore [55, 61]. For this reason, delaying IP transfer until after a phase I trial has demonstrated that a device is efficacious may help in the development of new interventions without attendant conflicts of interest once ideas are commodified [60].

In order to conform to the principle of justice, however, the medical establishment must have adequate infrastructure to support participants in clinical trials or patients receiving any form of neuromodulation. Such support must take the form of adequate physician–patient conversations about the indications, risks and benefits of placing electrodes and adequate infrastructure to maintain the device once inserted for therapeutic or investigational purposes. A patient who receives a device must have access to a skilled team of clinicians to continue monitoring his progress. For patients involved in clinical trials, the long-term maintenance of their device remains precarious given the regulatory environment described earlier. Establishing such an infrastructure is consistent with the principle of non-abandonment [62].

A palliative care ethos

Rather than merely considering the ethics of neuromodulation within psychiatry using principles specific to either research or therapy, it is appropriate to also apply the principles of palliative care. A palliative care ethic promotes the mitigation of a patient's and families' pain and suffering associated with an illness through shared decision-making and supportive measures [63]. This framework applies to neuromodulation in the case of psychiatric illness, as we can conceptualize these interventions as masking symptoms associated with psychiatric disorders. Technologies such as DBS are prosthetic, restoring the functionality of impaired neural circuitry and thereby promoting an individual's autonomy and agency [26].

As part of alleviating suffering, a palliative ethic promotes the patient's participation in directing his or her care. After patients with neuropsychiatric disorders have an electrode implanted, they can assist in monitoring the amount of stimulation, as is done in patient-controlled analgesia within the realm of palliative care. Granting patients this power to manipulate their own device is another way of enhancing their autonomy and self-determination. Given the historical association of Delgado's stimoceiver with behavioural control, following principles that promote a patient's control over their stimulators can allay such concerns [4].

When understood through the lens of palliative care, the insertion of a device such as DBS is only one component of the comprehensive care needed to restore a patient to agency and alleviate suffering. Interdisciplinary teams of neurologists, neurosurgeons, psychiatrists and psychologists can monitor the care of the patient over the long term – assessing changes in the quality of life, mood and behaviour – and even assist the patient (or subject) in taking control over his or her care. In this manner, the technologies associated with neuromodulation would emphasize this population's positive entitlement to comprehensive care that meets its longitudinal needs. Indeed, cultivating the use of interdisciplinary teams to promote the welfare of neuropsychiatric patients is consistent with the famed neurosurgeon Wilder Penfield's own 'organizational ethic' and his observation that, in scientific discovery and clinical care, *No Man is Alone* [7].

Conclusion

An ethical framework governing the use of neuromodulation in psychiatry ought to be sensitive to the past dilemmas that arose in the era of psychosurgery, the potential vulnerability of patients with and stigmas attached to psychiatric illness, and the obligation for experts to provide this population with access to available therapies and research. Since technologies associated with neuromodulation remain in the fairly nascent stages of development, the relevant ethical considerations derive from both the investigative and clinical context. For patients with psychiatric illnesses, the use of invasive therapies with the potential to alter their preferences, thoughts and behaviour raises concerns about the self and personhood, issues often discussed in the field of neuroethics. Adopting the prevailing sentiments of a palliative care ethos may cogently unite principles to protect this population from harm while encouraging their participation in meaningful research that will likely offer great benefits.

References

1 Becker AE, Kleinman A. Mental Health and the Global Agenda. N Engl J Med. 2013;369(1): 66–73.

2 Nuttin B, Hemmings W, Mayberg HS, Hariz M, Gabriels L, Galter T, *et al.* Consensus on Guidelines for Stereotactic Neurosurgery for Psychiatric Disorders. J Neurol Neurosurg Psychiatry. 2014: 85(9):1003–8.

3 Merkel R, Boer G, Fegert J, Galert T, Hartmann D, Nuttin B, and Rosahl S. Intervening in the Brain: Changing Psyche and Society. Berlin Heidelberg: Springer; 2007.

4 Fins JJ. From Psychosurgery to Neuromodulation and Pallation: History's Lessons for the Ethical Conduct and Regulation of Neuropsychiatric Research. Neurosurg Clin N Am. 2003;14: 303–19.

5 Fins JJ. Neuromodulation, Free Will and Determinism: Lessons from the Psychosurgery Debate. Clin Neurosci Res. 2004;4:113–8.

6 Gildenberg PL, Krauss JK. History of Stereotactic Neurosurgery. In: Lozano AM, Gildenberg PL, Tasker RR, editors. Textbook of Stereotactic and Functional Neurosurgery. New York: Springer; 2009.

7 Fins JJ. A Leg to Stand On: Sir William Osler and Wilder Penfield's 'Neuroethics'. Am J Bioethics. 2008;8(1):37–46.

8 Diethelm O. An Historical Review of Somatic Therapy in Psychiatry. Am J Psychiatry. 1939;95(4):1165–79.

9 Mathews D, Rabins P, Greenberg B. Deep Brain Stimulation for Treatment-Resistant Neuropsychiatric Disorders In: Illes J, Sahakian BJ, editors. The Oxford Handbook of Neuroethics. New York: Oxford University Press; 2011.

10 Osmundsen JA. 'Matador' With a Radio Stops Wired Bull: Modified Behavior in Animal Subjects of Brain Study. The New York Times. May 17, 1965; 1.

11 Delgado JM, Anshen RN, editors. Physical Control of the Mind: Toward a Psychocivilized Society. New York: Harper and Row; 1969.

12 Blatte H. State Prisons and the Use of Behavior Control. Hastings Cent Rep. 1974; 4(4):661–74.

13 Crichton M. The Terminal Man. New York: Ballatine Books; 1998.

14 The National Commission for the Protection of Human Subjects of Biomedical and Behavioral Research. Use of Psychosurgery in Practice and Research. Report and Recommendations of National Commission for the Protection of Human Subjects of Biomedical and Behavioral Research, Washington, DC. Federal Register, 1977.

15 Jones JH. Bad Blood: The Tuskegee Syphilis Experiment. New York: The Free Press; 1993.

16 Heller CA, Amar AP, Liu CY, Apuzzo MLJ. Surgery of the Mind and Mood: A Mosaic of Issues in Time and Evolution. Neurosurgery. 2006;59:720–39.

17 Fins JJ. Deep Brain Stimulation. In: Post S, editor. Encyclopedia of Bioethics 3rd Edition. New York: MacMillan Reference; 2004. pp. 629–34.

18 Fins JJ. A Proposed Ethical Framework for Interventional Cognitive Neuroscience: A Consideration of Deep Brain Stimulation in Impaired Consciousness. Neurol Res. 2000; 22(3):273–8.

19 Nuttin B, Cosyns P, Demeneulemeester H, Gybels J, Meyerson B. Electrical Stimulation in Anterior Limbs of Internal Capsules in Patients with Obsessive-Compulsive Disorder. Lancet. 1999;354:1526.

20 Mayberg HS, Lozano AM, Voon V, McNeely HE, Seminowics D, Hamani C, *et al.* Deep Brain Stimulation for Treatment-resistant Depression. Neuron. 2005;45:651–60.
21 Schiff N, Giacino J, Kalmar K, Victor J, Baker K, Gerber M, *et al.* Behavioral Improvements with Thalamic Stimulation After Severe Traumatic Brain Injury. Nature. 2007;448:600–3.
22 Synofzik M, Schlaepfer TE. Stimulating Personality: Ethical Criteria for Deep Brain Stimulation in Psychiatric Patients and for Enhancement Purposes. Biotechnol J. 2008;3: 1511–20.
23 Fins JJ. Neuroethics and the Lure of Technology. In: Illes J, Sahakian BJ, editors. Oxford Handbook of Neuroethics. New York: Oxford University Press; 2011.
24 Fins JJ. Deep Brain Stimulation as a Probative Biology: Scientific Inquiry and the Mosaic Device. AJOB Neurosci. 2012;3(1):4–8.
25 Editorial. Psychosurgery. Lancet. 1972;7767(2): 69–70.
26 Glannon W. Neuromodulation, Agency and Autonomy. Brain Topogr. 2014;27:46–54.
27 Montgomery J, Baldwin T, Burls A, Furness P, Gallagher A, Gill R, *et al.* Novel Neurotechnologies: Intervening in the Brain. London: Nuffield Council on Bioethics, 2013.
28 Fins JJ. Minds Apart: Severe Brain Injury. In: Freeman M, editor. Law and Neuroscience: Current Legal Issues, vol. 13(ch 18), pp. 367–84. New York: Oxford University Press; 2010.
29 Fins JJ. Constructing an Ethical Stereotaxy for Severe Brain Injury: Balancing Risks, Benefits and Access. Nat Rev Neurosci. 2003;4:323–7.
30 The National Commission for the Protection of Human Subjects of Biomedical and Behavioral Research. Principles and Guidelines for the Protection of Human Subjects of Research. Washington, DC: US Department of Health, Education, and Welfare, 1979.
31 Faden R, Beauchamp TL. A History and Theory of Informed Consent. New York: Oxford University Press; 1986.
32 Applebaum PS, Roth LH, Lidz C. The Therapeutic Misconception: Informed Consent in Psychiatric Research. Int J Law Psychiatry. 1982;5:319–29.
33 Appelbaum PS, Grisso T, Frank E, O'Donnell S, Kupfer DJ. Competence of Depressed Patients for Consent to Research. Am J Psychiatry. 1999; 156:1380–4.
34 Rabins P, Appleby BS, Brandt J, DeLong M, Dunn L, Gabriels L, *et al.* Scientific and Ethical Issues Related to Deep Brain Stimulation for Disorders of Mood, Behavior, and Thought. Arch Gen Psychiatry. 2009;66(9):931–7.
35 Dunn LB, Holtzheimer PE, Hoop JG, Mayberg HS, Roberts LW, Appelbaum PS. Ethical Issues in Deep Brain Stimulation Research for Treatment-Resistant Depression: Focus on Risk and Consent. AjOB Neurosci. 2011;2(1): 29–36.
36 Christopher PP, Leykin Y, Appelbaum PS, Holtzheimer PE, Mayberg HS, Dunn LB. Enrolling in Deep Brain Stimulation Research For Depression: Influences on Potential Subjects' Decision Making. Depress Anxiety. 2012;29:139–46.
37 Bell E, Racine E, Chiasson P, Dufourcq-Brana M, Dunn LB, Fins JJ, *et al.* Beyond Consent in Research: Revisiting Vulnerability in Deep Brain Stimulation for Psychiatric Disorders. Camb Q Healthc Ethics. 2014;23:361–8.
38 Research Involving Persons with Mental Disorders that may Affect Decisionmaking Capacity. National Bioethics Commission, Washington, D.C.: U.S. Government Printing Office; 1998.
39 Fins JJ, Miller FG. Protecting Vulnerable Research Subjects Without Unduly Constraining Neuropsychiatric Research. Arch Gen Psychiatry. 1999;56:701.
40 Fins JJ, Miller FG. Enrolling Decisionally Incapacitated Subjects in Neuropsychiatric Research. CNS Spectr. 2000;5(10):32–42.
41 Koch VG, Han SA. 'Of Vital Importance': The New York State Task Force on Life and the Law's Report and Recommendations for Research with Human Subjects Who Lack Consent Capacity. NYSBA Health Law J. 2014;19(1):27–37.
42 Fins JJ, Schlaepfer TE, Nuttin B, Kubu CS, Galert T, Sturm V, *et al.* Ethical Guidance for the Management of Conflicts of Interest for Researchers, Engineers and Clinicians Engaged in the Development of Therapeutic Deep Brain Stimulation. J Neural Eng. 2011;8:1–7.
43 Beauchamp TL, Childress JF. Principles of Biomedical Ethics. Sixth Edition. New York: Oxford University Press; 2008.
44 Mathews DJ. Deep Brain Stimulation, Personal Identity and Policy. Int Rev Psychiatry. 2011; 23(5):486–92.

45 Florin E, Muller D, Pfeifer J, Barbe MT, Fink GR, Timmermann L. Subthalamic Stimulation Modulates Self-Estimation of Patients with Parkinson's Disease and Induces Risk-Seeking Behavior. Brain. 2013;136(Pt 11):3271–81.
46 Gilbert F. The Burden of Normality: From 'Chronically Ill' to 'Symptom Free'. New Ethical Challenges for Deep Brain Stimulation Postoperative Treatment. J Med Ethics. 2012;38(7): 408–12.
47 Cassell E. The Nature of Suffering and the Goals of Medicine. New York: Oxford University Press; 1991.
48 Glannon W. Stimulating Brains, Altering Minds. J Clin Ethics. 2009;35:289–92.
49 Clausen J. Ethical Brain Stimulation – Neuroethics of Deep Brain Stimulation in Research and Clinical Practice. Eur J Neurosci. 2010;32:1152–62.
50 Holm S, Harris J. Precautionary Principle Stifles Discovery. Nature. 1999;400:398.
51 Fins JJ. Surgical Innovation and Ethical Dilemmas: Precautions and Proximity. Cleve Clin J Med. 2008;75(6):S7–12.
52 Fins JJ. Psychosurgery: Avoiding an Ethical Redux While Advancing a Therapeutic Failure. Neurosurgery. 2006;59(4):713–6.
53 Fins JJ, Shapiro ZE. Deep Brain Stimulation, Brain Maps and Personalized Medicine: Lessons from the Human Genome Project. Brain Topogr. 2014;27:55–62.
54 Fins JJ, Dorfman GS, Pancrazio JJ. Challenges to Deep Brain Stimulation: A Pragmatic Response to Ethical, Fiscal, and Regulatory Concerns. Ann NY Acad Sci. 2012;1265:80–90.
55 Fins JJ, Schiff ND. Conflicts of Interest in Deep Brain Stimulation Research and the Ethics of Transparency. J Clin Ethics. 2010;21(2): 125–32.
56 Bernad DM. Humanitarian Use Device and Humanitarian Device Exemption Regulatory Programs. Expert Rev Med Devices. 2009; 6(2):137–45.
57 Fins JJ, Mayberg HS, Nuttin B, Kubu CS, Galert TG, Sturm V, *et al.* Misuse of the FDA's Humanitarian Device Exemption in Deep Brain Stimulation for Obsessive-Compulsive Disorder. Health Affairs. 2011;30(2):302–11.
58 Schiff N. Recovery of Consciousness After Brain Injury: A Mesocircuit Hypothesis. Trends Neurosci. 2010;33(1):1–9.
59 Fins JJ. Rights Come to Mind: Ethics and the Struggle for Consciousness. New York: Cambridge University Press, 2015.
60 Fins JJ. Deep Brain Stimulation, Free Markets and the Scientific Commons: Is it Time to Revisit the Bayh-Dole Act of 1980? Neuromodulation. 2009;10(13):153–9.
61 Fins JJ, Schachter M. Investigators, Industry, and the Heuristic Device. Ethics, Patent Law, and Clinical Innovation. Acc Res. 2001;8(3): 219–33.
62 Fins JJ. Deep Brain Stimulation, Deontology and Duty: The Moral Obligation of Non-Abandonment at the Neural Interface. J Neural Eng. 2009;6:1–4.
63 Fins JJ. A Palliative Ethic of Care: Clinical Wisdom at Life's End. Sudbury, MA: Jones and Bartlett Publishers; 2006.

CHAPTER 3

Neurocircuits commonly involved in psychiatric disorders and their stimulation and lesion therapies

Sarah R. Heilbronner, Ziad Safadi and Suzanne N. Haber
University of Rochester, Rochester, USA

Introduction

While the pathophysiology of psychiatric disorders remains incompletely understood, converging lines of evidence point to abnormalities in the prefrontal cortico-basal ganglia circuit. This is particularly evident in imaging studies that show abnormalities in the orbital frontal cortex (OFC), ventral medial prefrontal cortex (vmPFC), dorsal anterior cingulate cortex (dACC), dorsolateral prefrontal cortex (DLPFC), striatum in obsessive–compulsive disorder (OCD), and addiction to drugs of abuse, depression and schizophrenia. Not surprisingly, neuromodulatory interventions for psychiatric disorders target these networks. Understanding the circuits that link disease-related structures together requires translating results from detailed primate anatomical studies to human neuroimaging. In this chapter, we will review the circuits central to dysfunction in and stimulation and lesion treatment of OCD, addiction, depression and schizophrenia. These circuits are composed primarily of specific areas within the PFC, striatum and associated white matter (WM). In this chapter, we will first address the functional anatomy of the regions most implicated in these disorders: OFC, vmPFC, dACC, DLPFC and striatum. Second, we will review the organization of specific WM pathways that carry PFC fibres and are known to be abnormal in psychiatric disorders: the anterior limb of the internal capsule (ALIC), cingulum bundle (CB), uncinate fasciculus (UF) and corpus callosum (CC). Finally, we will discuss the circuits most likely affected by neuromodulatory stimulation and lesion therapies for OCD, addiction, depression and schizophrenia. These therapies include deep brain stimulation (DBS), with a focus on two targets, the ALIC and subcallosal WM; lesion therapies, including capsulotomy and cingulotomy; and transcranial magnetic stimulation (TMS) and transcranial direct current stimulation (tDCS) in the DLPFC.

Circuits of OCD, depression, schizophrenia and addiction

The prefrontal cortex

The vmPFC, OFC and rostral dACC mediate different aspects of affective processes. In contrast, the DLPFC and caudal dACC are associated with cognitive and executive functions, and

Neuromodulation in Psychiatry, First Edition. Edited by Clement Hamani, Paul Holtzheimer, Andres M. Lozano and Helen Mayberg.

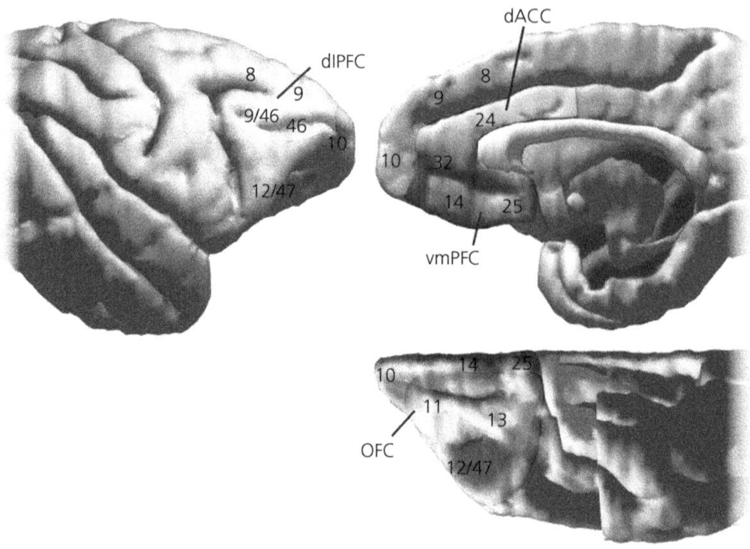

Figure 3.1 Schematic illustrating key PFC regions associated with OCD, addiction, depression and schizophrenia, displayed on the macaque brain. dACC = yellow; DLPFC = green; OFC = orange; vmPFC = red. Source: From Haber and Behrens [1]. Reproduced with permission of Elsevier. (*See insert for colour representation of the figure.*)

the DLPFC in particular is thought to provide cognitive control over motivational and emotional behaviours. Different prefrontal cortical areas and corresponding striatal regions (see later) are involved in various aspects of OCD, addiction, depression and schizophrenia. Here, we briefly review the connectivity, function and disease-related changes associated with the OFC, vmPFC, dACC and DLPFC (see Figure 3.1 for illustration of these regions).

Orbital frontal cortex

The OFC (areas 11, 12, 13 and 12/47, orbital proisocortex and orbital periallocortex) is highly intra-connected. In addition, patches throughout the OFC are connected to various cingulate cortex, PFC, amygdala and temporal lobe regions. From a functional perspective, there is a general caudal and rostral connectional distinction. The caudal OFC receives input from all of the sensory modalities as well as particularly strong amygdala input and is considered important for integrating emotionally relevant input from multisensory regions [2–7]. In contrast, the rostral OFC not only receives highly processed sensory information but is also connected to cognitive areas of the frontal lobe, including the frontal pole and DLPFC [8].

In monkey physiology, human lesion and neuroimaging studies, the OFC is closely related to reward processing [9–13]. This cortical region is particularly involved in linking sensory stimuli with outcomes [14, 15]. Consistent with its connections, both sensory and abstract rewards can recruit the OFC, with sensory rewards activating more posterior OFC regions, and abstract rewards activating more anterior OFC regions [16]. Patients with OCD, addiction, schizophrenia and depression show abnormalities in OFC and in OFC-linked behavioural traits. OCD patients have pronounced hypermetabolism of the OFC [17]. This hyperactivity is enhanced by symptom provocation [18]. During reversal learning, however, OCD patients have reduced the activation of OFC, perhaps reflecting a failure to update stimulus–outcome associations [19]. Indeed, OCD patients demonstrate an over-reliance on habits in a controlled laboratory setting [20]. The OFC is hyperactive in response to drug-related cues in addiction (reminiscent of its responses to symptom provocation in OCD) and is associated with drug craving and expectation [21, 22]. The OFC is also abnormal in schizophrenia, both in size and shape [23, 24]. Consistent with this region's normal role in reward learning, OFC volume abnormalities are associated with negative symptoms (such as anhedonia) in schizophrenia [25]. The OFC is also one of several affective regions dysregulated in depression [26, 27], although its functional role in this disorder is not clear.

Ventral medial prefrontal cortex

The medial orbital areas and the subgenual cingulate cortex are collectively referred to as the vmPFC (areas 32, 25 and 14). vmPFC contains strong links to visceral and emotional processing stations, in particular, the hypothalamus, amygdala and the shell of the nucleus accumbens (NAccS) [28–30]. Inputs from the hypothalamus, hippocampus and amygdala terminate most densely in caudal parts of the vmPFC. In turn, the caudal vmPFC projects densely to the hypothalamus, amygdala and NAccS [30]. Thus, these strong reciprocal connections, input from the hippocampus and a projection to the NAccS are special features of vmPFC. Taken together, the vmPFC is in a pivotal position to track internal states for the purpose of emotional processing.

Disruptions in vmPFC are associated with dysregulated emotional states in psychiatric disorders, especially depression, addiction, schizophrenia and, to a lesser extent, OCD. The vmPFC plays a role in monitoring correct responses based on previous experience and the internal milieu [31–33]. vmPFC activation is related to transient sadness and depression [34–36]. Furthermore, depression remission is typically accompanied by vmPFC deactivation [37]. A hyperactive vmPFC may be involved in the generation of negative affect in depression, or in rumination and negative self-reflection more broadly [38]. vmPFC activity also increases in response to drug-related cues and craving in addiction [39, 40], and decreases with successful regulation of craving [41]. In contrast to the vmPFC hyperactivation observed in depressed patients and addiction, schizophrenia is associated with vmPFC hypoactivation [42]. As in depression, vmPFC pathologies are thought to reflect abnormal self-reflective processing. Whether this area plays a critical role in the pathophysiology of OCD remains unclear.

Dorsal anterior cingulate cortex

Vogt and colleagues [43] have systematically divided dACC (area 24 in monkeys and 24 and dorsal 32 in humans) into three distinct components: rostral, anterior mid-cingulate and posterior mid-cingulate. Receptor architecture [44] and neuroimaging results [45] suggest that each of these has a distinct function: the rostral dACC is thought to be involved in emotion processing; the central dACC is associated with cognitive functions and the posterior dACC is associated with motor functions. The rostral dACC is connected primarily to the vmPFC, OFC, medial area 9, the rostral temporal cortex and the amygdala [46, 47]. These connections support its association with emotion processing. However, it is also linked to DLPFC, and thus is in a pivotal position to connect emotion processes and cognitive control. Central dACC is widely connected with DLPFC and parietal cortex [48, 49]. Thus, this region is tightly linked to cognitive control regions. Finally, caudal dACC has the strongest connections with motor control regions and limited ones with OFC and PFC areas 10 and 9. These are not abrupt divisions based on anatomical connectivity; rather, there is a continuum of connections [47]. Thus, the dACC is in a pivotal position within the frontal cortex to link emotion, cognition and motor control areas of frontal cortex.

The dACC is a unique part of frontal cortex, containing diverse frontal lobe functions, including motivation, cognition and motor control. However, the overall role of the dACC appears to be involved in monitoring these functions in conflicting or volatile situations [50–53]. It is also prominently dysregulated in OCD, addiction, depression and schizophrenia. OCD patients show enhancements in dACC activity, both during symptom provocation and in response to errors or conflict [54–56]. Such hyperactivity may reflect overactive monitoring processes, or conflict between task-related and compulsion-related demands. In addiction, dACC activity increases as cravings subside [41]. Addicts make more errors during inhibitory control tasks, likely because of dACC hypoactivation [57]. dACC also shows abnormal activity in depressed patients (although the pattern is less consistent than what is observed in OCD and addiction) and is typically associated with abnormal emotion regulation [58, 59]. Similarly, neuroimaging studies of the dACC in schizophrenia are somewhat contradictory [60, 61], but it is clear that the dACC does not properly monitor and adjust to conflict in the schizophrenic patient [62].

Dorsolateral prefrontal cortex

The DLPFC (areas 9 and 46) connects with dACC, posterior cingulate, superior temporal cortex, premotor regions and OFC, as well as the lateral and medial parietal cortex [63, 64]. Through these connections, the DLPFC has access to highly processed visual and auditory information, and can influence motor output. This suggests that the DLPFC is involved in online monitoring of sensory and motor information for working memory [63]. Indeed, physiology, lesion and neuroimaging findings implicate the DLPFC in working memory and cognitive control [65–70], and these capacities are most critical when multiple options must be held in mind for evaluation, comparison and selection. Thus, the vmPFC, OFC, dACC and DLPFC may work together in a complementary fashion to compare valued options and choose among them. They then channel that choice into a course of action that promotes acquiring the most valuable option and learning from the subsequent outcome [15, 71, 72].

The DLPFC is central to a variety of psychiatric disorders. DLPFC activity negatively correlates with activity in affective regions such as vmPFC. Thus, DLPFC potentially acts as a regulator of negative affect. Depression may involve an abnormal reduction in regulatory control over such emotions. For example, while vmPFC displays heightened activity to negative stimuli in depressed patients, DLPFC has reduced activity [27, 73]. DLPFC and vmPFC also have a negative relationship in addiction. DLPFC activity increases as cravings subside (while vmPFC activity decreases), particularly as subjects exert control over their actions by considering long-term consequences [41]. Although its functions in schizophrenia are more specific to working memory, it is clear that DLPFC abnormalities are also critical to schizophrenia pathophysiology. Specifically, its activation during working memory is impaired in schizophrenia patients [74]. DLPFC's role in OCD is less clear, but may involve a dysfunctional attentional disengagement process [75, 76].

Striatum

The basal ganglia work in concert with the frontal cortex to orchestrate and execute motivated, planned behaviours requiring limbic, cognitive and motor control systems. The cortico-basal ganglia circuit has been described in detail elsewhere (e.g. [77–81]. Briefly, the striatum is the main input structure of the basal ganglia. Corticostriatal topography forms a general ventromedial to dorsolateral gradient of projections from limbic, cognitive and motor control areas, respectively [28, 82]. However, despite this general topography, there is extensive convergence of fibres from functionally diverse cortical areas. For example, within the limbic circuits, dense projections from the dACC and OFC regions do not occupy completely separate territories, but converge. This convergence exists most extensively at rostral levels, rostral to the anterior commissure. In this area, dense projections from dACC and OFC also converge with inputs from the DLPFC. These areas of convergence provide an anatomical substrate for integration between different processing circuits and may represent 'central nodes' for plasticity and adaptation. Abnormalities in these prefrontal–striatal nodes may lead to psychiatric conditions; if so, the rostral striatum should be disrupted in these disorders.

Indeed, overall, striatal abnormalities are central to OCD. OCD patients have enhanced metabolic rates in the striatum [17]; this increases even further during symptom provocation [83, 84]. This effect reduces with successful therapeutic intervention [85]. Interestingly, the striatal effects for OCD are largely observed in the rostral striatum where prefrontal inputs converge (see previous text). Resting state studies have revealed that OCD patients have increased functional connectivity between the ventral PFC (vPFC) and the striatum [86–88], providing further evidence that prefrontal cortico-striatal networks are central to this disorder. The striatum also plays a critical, but complex, role in the neural basis of addiction. Dopamine release in the striatum is associated with subjective hedonic aspects of drug intake [89], but concentrations of striatal dopamine are reduced in drug abusers [90]. As drug use becomes compulsive, striatal activation shifts from a ventral to dorsal position, particularly within the rostral striatum [91, 92]. Similarly, it is in the rostral striatum that dopamine hyperactivity has long been associated with schizophrenia onset and severity [93–96]. This finding was central to the modified dopamine hypothesis of schizophrenia, which generally posited enhanced striatal dopamine activity and reduced prefrontal dopamine activity [97]. Striatal hyperdopaminergia was thought to be tightly linked with the positive symptoms of schizophrenia, such as delusions and hallucinations, while hypodopaminergia and hypoactivity in the PFC were associated with negative symptoms. Although these mechanisms appear increasingly complex, striatal hyperdopaminergia in schizophrenia may be caused specifically by aberrations in presynaptic dopamine release [98]. Finally, although the striatum does not appear to be broadly abnormal in depression, it does show reduced abnormal reward-related activation in patients [99, 100]. Together, these findings implicate the rostral striatum in particular in psychiatric disorders, indicating that the areas of prefrontal convergence found in this region may be key to the aetiology of OCD, addiction, schizophrenia and depression.

WM pathways

Connectivity between the OFC, vmPFC, dACC and DLPFC forms a complex neural network. Delineating this connectivity is the basis for understanding how these different brain regions work together to evaluate environmental stimuli, transform that information into actions and adapt future actions based on learned associations. It is also essential for elucidating the pathophysiology of psychiatric diseases associated with these cortical regions, including OCD, addiction, depression and schizophrenia. With the advent of diffusion-weighted magnetic resonance imaging (dMRI), it is possible to non-invasively image human WM pathways, in both patient and healthy populations, and to generally relate WM abnormalities in disease states with specific connections. Moreover, several neuromodulatory therapies for OCD and depression (and, to a lesser extent, schizophrenia and addiction) – specifically stimulation, and lesions – target primarily WM tracts. The clinical outcomes following these treatments will depend on which fibres are captured at each target. However, animal studies provide the foundation for understanding and interpreting neuroimaging results by helping to identify the origins and end points of axons within WM, and demonstrating possible false positives (dMRI connections not seen in anatomical tracing experiments) and false negatives (connections observed in anatomical tracing experiments, but not using dMRI).

In the sections that follow, we first discuss four WM bundles central to OCD, addiction, depression and schizophrenia: ALIC, CB, CC and UF. We review their position, shape and location, as well as the organization of PFC pathways through them, based on animal tracing experiments. Next, we compare this organization to that seen with dMRI in monkeys and humans and to observed WM changes in psychiatric disorders. Finally, we analyse which pathways are likely to be affected by lesion and stimulation interventions for OCD, addiction, depression and schizophrenia.

Anterior limb of the internal capsule

Overview of the ALIC

The ALIC is the major WM bundle that connects the PFC to the thalamus and brainstem (Figure 3.2a). Rostrally, the ALIC forms at the rostral appearance of the putamen. It is surrounded medially by the caudate nucleus, and laterally by the putamen and the rostral pallidum. While the classical ventral border has been the nucleus accumbens and anterior commissure [103], recent evidence has demonstrated that the small WM bundles that travel through the ventral striatum are also part of the ALIC [101].

PFC-ALIC projections: Anatomy

Axons from the vmPFC and OFC (collectively referred to as the vPFC) travel through the ventral portion of the ALIC, including within the small fascicles embedded in the striatum and anterior commissure. vPFC fibres show medial–lateral topography as they travel to and within the ALIC [101]. To reach the ALIC, fibres from vmPFC and the medial OFC (mOFC) travel dorsally from the orbital surface. These fibres enter the ALIC ventrally. In contrast, central OFC (cOFC) and lateral OFC (lOFC) fibres travel dorsally, then curve medially through the WM to enter the ALIC at its dorsolateral edge. Thus, medial vPFC fibres enter the ALIC ventrally, while lateral vPFC fibres enter the ALIC dorsally.

Within the ALIC, fibres from the medial vPFC travel ventrally to those from the lateral vPFC (Figure 3.2b). Thus, vmPFC fibres are the most ventral within the ALIC; mOFC fibres are located ventral to cOFC fibres and cOFC fibres are ventral to lOFC fibres. Importantly, vPFC bundles from a given region are also organized within the ALIC according to their destinations. Corticothalamic vPFC fibres travel dorsally within the ALIC to fibres terminating in the subthalamic nucleus, midbrain and medulla. Just caudal to the anterior commissure, the corticothalamic bundles split off from the capsule, while brainstem fibres continue descending ventrally and caudally (Figure 3.2b).

Like lateral vPFC axons, dACC and DLPFC fibres enter the ALIC dorsally, then travel to the thalamus, subthalamic nucleus and brainstem [104, 105]. Preliminary evidence indicates that, as in vPFC pathways, dACC and DLPFC bundles are also organized according to their origins and destinations, in that corticothalamic bundles travel dorsally to brainstem bundles [106].

PFC-ALIC projections: dMRI and disease

With the exception of fibres from vmPFC, the organizational principles of vPFC fibres in the ALIC can be replicated in monkeys and humans using dMRI [102]. The relative positions in the ALIC from the medial to lateral OFC are preserved across species. In macaque anatomical tract-tracing, vmPFC pathways travelled ventrally within the ALIC to cOFC pathways, and cOFC pathways travelled ventrally to lOFC pathways (mOFC seeds were not included in the dMRI study). dMRI replicates cOFC fibres travelling ventrally within the ALIC to lOFC fibres. In addition, dMRI in both monkeys and humans replicates the splitting of vPFC ALIC fibres into a dorsal bundle targeting the thalamus and a ventral one targeting the brainstem. However, the routes taken by vmPFC fibres to and within the ALIC do not replicate with dMRI. In monkey tracing experiments, vmPFC fibres

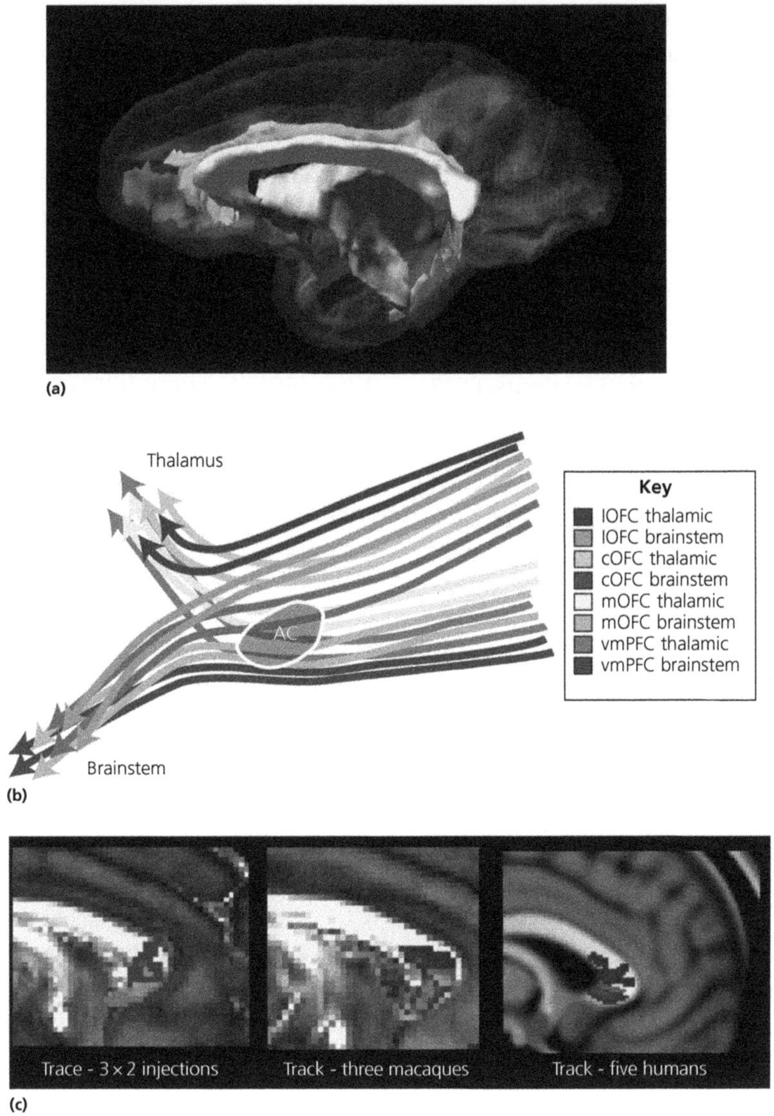

Figure 3.2 WM pathways central to psychiatric disorders. (**a**) 3D renderings of the CC (white), UF (red), ALIC (purple) and CB (yellow) in the monkey brain. (**b**) In the ALIC, vmPFC fibres travel ventral to mOFC fibres, which are ventral to cOFC fibres, which are ventral to lOFC fibres. Each set of axons splits into two bundles in the ALIC: the dorsal bundle travels to the thalamus, while the ventral bundle continues to the brainstem. Adapted from Ref. 101. (**c**) The ventral–dorsal gradient in vPFC fibres in the CC, as seen in monkey tracing (left), monkey dMRI (middle) and human dMRI (right) studies. Source: From Jbabdi et al. [102]. Reproduced with permission of Society for Neuroscience. (*See insert for colour representation of the figure.*)

can be found crossing ventrally through the anterior commissure or travelling in the small fascicles embedded in the striatum. dMRI streamlines fail to follow those fibres in their ventral position. This false negative is likely attributable to resolution lower than the small fascicles. Although ALIC axons from many PFC regions travel in small fascicles, this is the main route by which ALIC axons travel to and through the ALIC. Instead of taking a ventral route, vmPFC dMRI streamlines are found crossing dorsally to the anterior commissure, similar to cOFC fibres. These streamlines represent a false positive.

Anatomical and dMRI-derived maps of the pathways in the ALIC can help determine the connections underlying WM abnormalities in psychiatric diseases. Reduced fractional anisotropy (FA) values have been demonstrated in the ventral ALIC of depressed patients [107, 108]. These abnormalities may reflect changes in the vPFC fibre pathways described earlier, especially vmPFC and mOFC [101, 102], since these occupy the ventral portion of the ALIC in both humans and monkeys. By contrast, OCD and schizophrenia patients have shown a reduction in FA values in the central and dorsal portions of the ALIC, respectively [109–111]. These may reflect abnormalities in dACC and DLPFC fibre pathways travelling to the thalamus and/or brainstem [106].

Cingulum bundle

Overview of the CB

The CB is one of the brain's major limbic pathways, linking the frontal, parietal and temporal lobes. The CB is positioned laterally to the dorsal cingulate gyrus and ventrally to the cingulate sulcus. At its posterior end, it curves ventrally and rostrally into the temporal lobe. Early studies suggested that the CB was made up of 'relays' of axons that exit within a short distance of their origins [112]. However, while many fibres from adjacent cortex are continually leaving the CB, others project long distances within it [113]. These fibres travel both anteriorly and posteriorly [114]. Rostrally, the CB extends both towards the frontal pole and ventrally towards subcallosal cingulate. Not surprisingly (given its position), the CB is particularly strongly linked with cingulate cortex [113, 115, 116]. The medial position of the CB within the brain coupled with its connections with the medial temporal lobes (MTL) and cingulate cortex places the CB as one of the primary bundles of the limbic circuit [113].

PFC-CB projections: Anatomy

The CB contains both fibres from adjacent cingulate cortex continually entering and leaving the CB and long association axons projecting extensive distances within the bundle [113, 114]. Striatal, thalamic/brainstem and commissural bundles course laterally from cingulate cortical regions across the CB to reach their targets. These fibres join with other WM bundles, including Muratoff's bundle, internal capsule and the CC. Other fibres project long distances within the CB. Importantly, these include axons from both cingulate and non-cingulate regions. OFC, vmPFC, dACC and DLPFC axons, along with those from other cortical and subcortical areas, join the CB and travel rostrally and caudally to cingulate, MTL, PFC and precuneus [104, 105, 117]. Thus, many cortical and subcortical fibres that travel through the CB neither originate nor terminate in cingulate cortex [105, 117–119]. As such, this bundle is not simply a pathway for cingulate fibres, but represents a much broader connecting system.

PFC-CB projections: dMRI and disease

Like the ALIC, PFC fibres coursing through the CB can be non-invasively identified in both monkeys and humans using dMRI [102, 120–122], making this bundle an ideal object of study for psychiatric disorders. Although it is clear that the CB is abnormal in OCD, depression, addiction and schizophrenia, the precise connections involved are unknown. Patients with OCD show reduced mean diffusivity [109], as well as abnormal asymmetry (left > right) in FA, in the dorsal portion of the CB [123]. Another study found reduced FA within the rostral portion of the dorsal CB [124]. Women at risk for depression show reduced FA in the subgenual portion of the CB [125], and adolescents with major depressive disorder have reduced FA in the anterior

CB [126]. Schizophrenia has been associated with reduced FA in the anterior CB [127, 128]. The anterior CB may also be abnormal in addiction [129].

Abnormalities in various illnesses that are limited to distinct portions of the CB are likely to involve different sets of fibres. We recently demonstrated that the CB can be segmented into four distinct portions on the basis of frontal and subcortical fibres travelling through each segment of the bundle [117]. The segments are subgenual, rostral dorsal, caudal dorsal and temporal. For example, the rostral dorsal segment is distinguished from the caudal dorsal segment in part by the presence of amygdala fibres in the former. Based on this segmentation, abnormalities in the rostral dorsal CB (but not the caudal dorsal CB) may reflect abnormalities in amygdala connections with dACC [117]. Thus, our segmentation into four regions can be leveraged to identify the connections that underlie WM abnormalities.

Uncinate fasciculus

Overview of the UF

The UF is a plate-like bundle underlying the orbital cortex that, caudally, curves into the temporal lobe. Traditionally, the UF has been thought of as a bidirectional long association bundle connecting the medial and orbital cortex to the rostral temporal cortex [130–132]. However, in addition to the fibres connecting the PFC and temporal lobe, the UF also contains fibres connecting distinct vPFC regions to one another, and vPFC fibres travelling to other bundles, such as the CC and the CB [101, 103, 133].

PFC-UF projections: Anatomy

vPFC fibres use the UF in three ways: (i) to reach other vPFC regions, (ii) to reach other WM bundles and (iii) to travel to the temporal lobe. All of these fibres are intermixed within the UF. vmPFC and mOFC fibres in particular travel substantial distances through the UF to reach other WM bundles, including the CB, the CC and the superior longitudinal fasciculus. cOFC and lOFC bundles cut directly through the UF, without travelling long distances within it, to reach these bundles [101].

PFC-UF projections: dMRI and disease

The organization within the UF is difficult to observe using dMRI due to the extensive fibre crossings [102, 134]. Nonetheless, as a whole, dMRI does show abnormalities in psychiatric disorders. For example, FA values are reduced in the UF in patients with depression [126, 135, 136], schizophrenia [137] and addiction [129, 138, 139], but increased in patients with OCD [140].

Corpus callosum

Overview of the CC

The CC is the major connection between the cortical hemispheres [112, 114]. The CC is divided into three regions: in the rostral portion, the genu (forceps minor); the body; and in the caudal portion, the splenium (forceps major). The body of the CC sits between the genu (anterior) and splenium (posterior). The CC is organized rostral-caudally, with the most rostral portions connecting frontal regions, and caudal portions connecting parietal, temporal and occipital projections [141, 142]. Cortical projections in the CC travel to both contralateral cortex and striatum [143, 144].

PFC-CC projections: Anatomy

Fibres from various subdivisions of the PFC, including vmPFC, OFC, dACC and DLPFC, travel through the rostral half of the CC, including both the rostral body and the genu [145, 146]. Some dACC fibres travel slightly caudally and overlap with axons coming from the premotor and motor areas. Although there are not strict boundaries, fibres from limbic vPFC and dACC regions travel rostrally and ventrally within the genu to more dorsal and lateral regions, such as DLPFC [147]. Moreover, we found that axons originating in vPFC fibres from more medial cortical regions travel ventrally to those from more lateral cortical regions: vmPFC and mOFC fibres lie ventral to cOFC and lOFC fibres [101].

PFC-CC projections: dMRI and disease

Generally, the rostral–caudal topography of the CC is maintained across species and methods [102, 148, 149]. Thus, similar to anatomical tract-tracing studies in monkeys have shown, dMRI studies in both monkeys and humans demonstrate frontal fibres crossing in the rostral CC, followed caudally by parietal, temporal and occipital fibres [148, 150]. In addition, like anatomical tract-tracing, dMRI in monkeys and humans shows a dorsal–ventral gradient within vPFC fibres: lOFC fibres are positioned dorsal to cOFC fibres; cOFC fibres are positioned dorsal to vmPFC fibres (Figure 3.2c).

Because of established left–right asymmetries in emotion processing (e.g. [151]), several investigators hypothesized that the CC might be abnormal in depression. However, these studies consistently show normal CC measures in depressed patients [136, 152–154]. OCD and addiction patients, however, show reduced FA in rostral regions of the CC [155–159], and schizophrenia patients may have reduced FA in the splenium [160, 161].

Stimulation and lesion therapeutic approaches for psychiatric illnesses

DBS, TMS and tDCS are three relatively new stimulation methods being investigated for the treatment of severe (DBS) and less severe (TMS and tDCS) psychiatric disorders. Despite the potential effectiveness of these therapies, their mechanisms of action are not well understood. Nonetheless, they are thought to act primarily on WM [162–164]. Two older and invasive approaches for psychiatric treatment are cingulotomy and capsulotomy. While both include grey matter, their primary goal is to disconnect frontal regions by severing specific WM bundles [165, 166]. Since both stimulation and lesion approaches target specific WM, determining the precise connections that are involved at each site is critical for understanding and interpreting clinical outcomes and for adjusting the target locations, if necessary. Thus, it may well be that differences in the effectiveness of these approaches across patients is related to the specific connections that are involved at each site [166, 167].

Deep brain stimulation

Several DBS targets are currently under investigation, including the ALIC, the subgenual WM, the nucleus accumbens, the lateral habenula and the subthalamic nucleus [168–171]. The later three, while targeting specific structures, most likely involve the WM embedded within (the nucleus accumbens target) or surrounding it (subthalamic nucleus and lateral habenula target). For example, the nucleus accumbens target is positioned near or partially within the ALIC. Moreover, as described earlier, descending vPFC fibres are embedded within this area of the striatum. Thus, this target is likely to be quite similar to the ALIC target in that it will involve descending and ascending thalamic and brainstem fibres passing through parts of the ALIC. The two DBS targets most widely studied are the ALIC and the subcallosal WM positions. The ALIC target is located at the caudal nucleus accumbens, just rostral to or at the border of the anterior commissure. The subcallosal target is located in WM adjacent to areas 25 and 32 in the vmPFC.

ALIC stimulation

The ALIC site is used to treat both depression and OCD. This target does not involve direct corticocortical connections. Instead, it includes primarily corticothalamic and cortico-brainstem fibres (Figure 3.3b). Nevertheless, the affected ALIC pathways originate in PFC regions that have been shown to be abnormal in OCD and depression—vmPFC, OFC, dACC and DLPFC. Consistent with this view, Rauch and colleagues

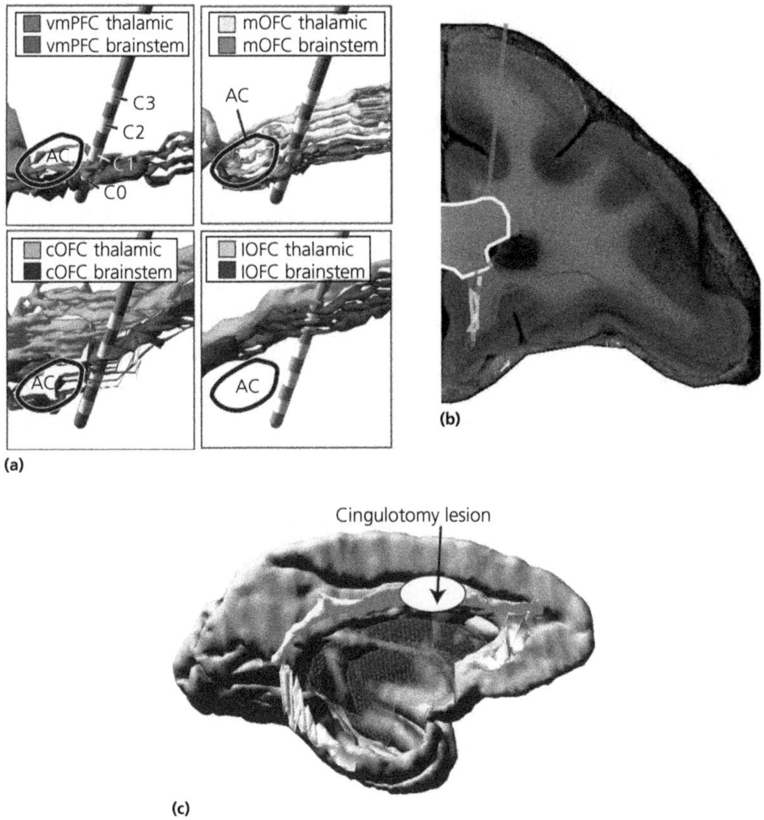

Figure 3.3 WM pathways central to neuromodulatory interventions for psychiatric disorders. (**a**) Each contact on the ALIC electrode intersects a unique set of vmPFC, mOFC, cOFC and lOFC fibres. Adapted from Ref. 101. (**b**) The subcallosal DBS electrode intersects the UF (red), CB (yellow) and CC (white). Adapted from Ref. 117. (**c**) The cingulotomy lesion intersects the dACC and the WM of the anterior portion of the dorsal CB. Source: From Heilbronner and Haber [117]. Reproduced with permission of Society for Neuroscience. (*See insert for colour representation of the figure.*)

[172] imaged OCD patients and found that acute ALIC DBS was associated with increased activity (relative to the DBS-off condition) in mOFC, vmPFC, striatum and the globus pallidus. Moreover, high-frequency stimulation in a rat homolog of the ALIC DBS target causes changes in OFC, medial PFC and striatum [173].

Each contact in the ALIC site involves a different combination of PFC thalamic and/or brainstem bundles [101] (Figure 3.3a). The organizational principles we have described can help elucidate which fibres are present at each contact point. For example, contact 0 (the most ventral contact) essentially centres stimulation on vmPFC and mOFC brainstem bundles, while contact 1 centres on thalamic fibres from vmPFC, along with cOFC brainstem axons. Contact 2 captures cOFC thalamic fibres and some dACC fibres. Contact 3 (the most dorsal contact) captures brainstem and thalamic fibres originating in more caudal dACC, cOFC, rostral DLPFC and frontal pole, along with brainstem fibres from lOFC. Thus, each contact centres on a different subset of fibres, each of which include both thalamic and brainstem axons [101, 174].

Subcallosal stimulation

Stimulation at the subgenual site (used to treat depression, but not OCD) captures all cortical and subcortical projections from and to the area surrounding each contact location (Figure 3.3b). As outlined earlier, vmPFC has unique connections to visceral and emotion processing centres, including the hypothalamus, amygdala and nucleus accumbens. However, this subcallosal stimulation site also affects fibres of passage via the UF, CB and CC. In other words, this location contains fibres originating and terminating outside of the vmPFC. These include axons travelling in the UF, connecting the vmPFC and OFC to each other as well as to the medial forebrain bundle, CB, superior longitudinal fasciculus and CC [101]. Furthermore, some subcortical fibres (such as amygdala axons) are present at the subcallosal DBS site. These fibres travel within the subcallosal portion of the CB and then project dorsally to the dorsal portion of the CB [117]. From there, they travel to dACC and dorsomedial frontal cortex. These CB pathways to dACC and dorsomedial frontal cortex may be critical to the efficacy of DBS. In a recent dMRI case study, the therapeutically effective electrode contact point was found to intercept subgenual CB tracts that extended to the dorsal CB, whereas the non-therapeutic contact point did not [175]. This suggests that the subcallosal DBS electrode may need to intercept both vmPFC axons and fibres of passage travelling to dACC and dorsomedial frontal cortex. In linking together affective, self-reflective and cognitive control systems, the dACC, vPFC and amygdala may be critical to depression pathology [176]. DBS efficacy may depend on targeting this dorsal system via subcallosal fibres.

Lesions: Capsulotomy and cingulotomy

Capsulotomy procedures preceded and formed the basis for the ALIC DBS target. A recent study [177] examined neural changes in patients who had undergone either ALIC DBS or capsulotomy. Both groups showed similar post-treatment changes in the vmPFC, OFC, striatum and thalamus. The metabolic differences were more pronounced in the capsulotomy group, perhaps indicating that this lesion method impacts a larger WM area than DBS.

The cingulotomy site, by contrast, is located in a very different portion of the cingulate WM than the subcallosal DBS site (Figure 3.3c). Cingulotomies target the dACC and the dorsal portion of the CB. While the lesion will certainly have a substantial impact on adjacent dACC subareas, it is also in a position to affect fibres of passage in the WM of the CB. Thus, a cingulotomy may impact both cingulate and non-cingulate fibres travelling to both cingulate and non-cingulate targets. These include axons connecting amygdala, thalamus, prefrontal cortices and neurotransmitter systems with cingulate, dmFC and precuneus. Intriguingly, more rostral cingulotomy lesions may be more effective at treating depression [178]. Amygdala axons are present in the rostral, but not caudal, CB, suggesting that the effectiveness of the lesion may depend on capturing amygdala fibres [117].

TMS and tDCS in the DLPFC

Both TMS and tDCS are relatively new neuropsychiatric tools for OCD [179], depression [180, 181], addiction [182–184] and schizophrenia [185] therapy. Both techniques can be safely applied in awake, alert adults, and both have been shown to quickly alter neuronal function both directly at the coil position and in connected brain regions [186–189], with their strongest impacts on the cortical surface. As described earlier, depression has been consistently associated with hypoactivation of the DLPFC and, due to its location on the dorsal and lateral surface, is a viable candidate for TMS and tDCS. In contrast, deep cortical regions, including the vmPFC, OFC, dACC and striatum, cannot be directly or selectively stimulated with traditional TMS or tDCS. However, they can be indirectly modulated via their connections with the DLPFC.

Following TMS to the DLPFC, significant differences in functional connectivity have been seen in a variety of cortical and subcortical regions, including the vmPFC. For example, TMS on the left DLPFC induced a significant reduction in dopamine D2 receptor binding potential in the ipsilateral subgenual and pregenual ACC and medial OFC [190]. The more effective stimulation site in the left DLPFC is significantly more anticorrelated with the vmPFC compared with a less effective site [191], suggesting that the relationship between DLPFC and vmPFC is critical to the efficacy of TMS. However, anatomical studies have shown that direct DLPFC connections with vmPFC are inconsistent and sparse, and tend to be concentrated in area 32 [3, 63]. Although these two areas are functionally connected, they may not be strongly structurally connected. Thus, a third brain region that connects to both the vmPFC and the DLPFC, such as the dACC, may mediate functional connectivity between these two regions.

Conclusions

Linking anatomical studies in animals with human neuroimaging is a powerful way to gain insight into brain regions associated with psychiatric illnesses. As imaging techniques are refined, we will be able to use results from those studies to explore in depth the underpinnings of co-activation or temporal activation of structures that appear unrelated. dMRI allows us to visualize connectivity in humans, and thus promises to further bridge the gap between primate structure and human function and dysfunction [102, 192–194]. When combined with careful anatomical studies, dMRI and fMRI allow us to identify the specific connections that are abnormal in psychiatric disorders, such as OCD, depression, addiction and schizophrenia. These results can then be used to determine the white and grey matter structures that are affected by neuromodulatory interventions, as well as to identify new targets. As our maps of the functional neuroanatomy of the vmPFC, OFC, dACC, DLPFC and striatum, as well as their associated WM pathways, evolve, logical new targets for lesion, DBS, TMS or tDCS may become clear.

References

1 Haber SN, Behrens TE. The neural network underlying incentive-based learning: implications for interpreting circuit disruptions in psychiatric disorders. Neuron. 2014;83(5):1019–39.

2 Barbas H. Organization of cortical afferent input to orbitofrontal areas in the rhesus monkey. Neuroscience. 1993;56:841–64.

3 Barbas H, Pandya DN. Architecture and intrinsic connections of the prefrontal cortex in the rhesus monkey. J Comp Neurol. 1989;286:353–75.

4 Carmichael ST, Price JL. Sensory and premotor connections of the orbital and medial prefrontal cortex of macaque monkeys. J Comp Neurol. 1995;363:642–64.

5 Barbas H. Architecture and cortical connections of the prefrontal cortex in the rhesus monkey. In: Chauvel P, Delgado-Escueta AV, editors. Advances in Neurology. New York: Raven Press, Ltd; 1992. p. 91–115.

6 Morecraft RJ, Geula C, Mesulam M-M. Cytoarchitecture and neural afferents of orbitofronal cortex in the brain of the monkey. J Comp Neurol. 1992;323:341–58.

7 Ghashghaei HT, Hilgetag CC, Barbas H. Sequence of information processing for emotions based on the anatomic dialogue between prefrontal cortex and amygdala. NeuroImage. 2007 Feb 1;34(3): 905–23.

8 Carmichael ST, Price JL. Limbic connections of the orbital and medial prefrontal cortex in macaque monkeys. J Comp Neurol. 1995 Dec 25;363(4):615–41.

9 Padoa-Schioppa C, Assad JA. Neurons in the orbitofrontal cortex encode economic value. Nature. 2006 May 11;441(7090):223–6.

10 Roesch MR, Olson CR. Neuronal activity related to reward value and motivation in primate frontal cortex. Science. 2004 Apr 9;304(5668):307–10.

11 Rolls ET. The orbitofrontal cortex and reward. Cereb Cortex. 2000;10(3):284–94.
12 Bechara A, Damasio AR, Damasio H, Anderson SW. Insensitivity to future consequences following damage to human prefrontal cortex. Cognition. 1994;50:7–15.
13 O'Doherty J, Kringelbach ML, Rolls ET, Hornak J, Andrews C. Abstract reward and punishment representations in the human orbitofrontal cortex. Nat Neurosci. 2001 Jan;4(1): 95–102.
14 Schoenbaum G, Roesch M. Orbitofrontal cortex, associative learning, and expectancies. Neuron. 2005 Sep 1;47(5):633–6.
15 Rushworth MF, Noonan MP, Boorman ED, Walton ME, Behrens TE. Frontal cortex and reward-guided learning and decision-making. Neuron. 2011 Jun 23;70(6):1054–69.
16 Kringelbach ML, Rolls ET. The functional neuroanatomy of the human orbitofrontal cortex: evidence from neuroimaging and neuropsychology. Prog Neurobiol. 2004 Apr;72(5):341–72.
17 Baxter LR, Jr., Schwartz JM, Mazziotta JC, Phelps ME, Pahl JJ, Guze BH, et al. Cerebral glucose metabolic rates in nondepressed patients with obsessive-compulsive disorder. Am J Psychiatry. 1988 Dec;145(12):1560–3.
18 Adler CM, McDonough-Ryan P, Sax KW, Holland SK, Arndt S, Strakowski SM. fMRI of neuronal activation with symptom provocation in unmedicated patients with obsessive compulsive disorder. J Psychiatr Res. 2000 Jul–Oct;34(4–5):317–24.
19 Chamberlain SR, Menzies L, Hampshire A, Suckling J, Fineberg NA, del Campo N, et al. Orbitofrontal dysfunction in patients with obsessive-compulsive disorder and their unaffected relatives. Science. 2008 Jul 18;321(5887): 421–2.
20 Gillan CM, Papmeyer M, Morein-Zamir S, Sahakian BJ, Fineberg NA, Robbins TW, et al. Disruption in the balance between goal-directed behavior and habit learning in obsessive-compulsive disorder. Am J Psychiatry. 2011 Jul;168(7):718–26.
21 Sell LA, Morris JS, Bearn J, Frackowiak RS, Friston KJ, Dolan RJ. Neural responses associated with cue evoked emotional states and heroin in opiate addicts. Drug Alcohol Depend. 2000 Aug 1;60(2):207–16.
22 Kufahl P, Li Z, Risinger R, Rainey C, Piacentine L, Wu G, et al. Expectation modulates human brain responses to acute cocaine: a functional magnetic resonance imaging study. Biol Psychiatry. 2008 Jan 15;63(2):222–30.
23 Nakamura M, Nestor PG, McCarley RW, Levitt JJ, Hsu L, Kawashima T, et al. Altered orbitofrontal sulcogyral pattern in schizophrenia. Brain. 2007 Mar;130(Pt 3):693–707.
24 Nakamura M, Nestor PG, Levitt JJ, Cohen AS, Kawashima T, Shenton ME, et al. Orbitofrontal volume deficit in schizophrenia and thought disorder. Brain. 2008 Jan;131(Pt 1):180–95.
25 Lacerda AL, Hardan AY, Yorbik O, Vemulapalli M, Prasad KM, Keshavan MS. Morphology of the orbitofrontal cortex in first-episode schizophrenia: relationship with negative symptomatology. Prog Neuropsychopharmacol Biol Psychiatry. 2007 Mar 30;31(2):510–6.
26 Arnone D, McIntosh AM, Ebmeier KP, Munafo MR, Anderson IM. Magnetic resonance imaging studies in unipolar depression: systematic review and meta-regression analyses. Eur Neuropsychopharmacol. 2012 Jan;22(1):1–16.
27 Groenewold NA, Opmeer EM, de Jonge P, Aleman A, Costafreda SG. Emotional valence modulates brain functional abnormalities in depression: evidence from a meta-analysis of fMRI studies. Neurosci Biobehav Rev. 2013 Feb;37(2):152–63.
28 Haber SN, Kim KS, Mailly P, Calzavara R. Reward-related cortical inputs define a large striatal region in primates that interface with associative cortical connections, providing a substrate for incentive-based learning. J Neurosci. 2006 Aug 9;26(32):8368–76.
29 Rempel-Clower NL, Barbas H. Topographic organization of connections between the hypothalamus and prefrontal cortex in the rhesus monkey. J Comp Neurol. 1998 Aug 31;398(3): 393–419.
30 Ongur D, An X, Price JL. Prefrontal cortical projections to the hypothalamus in macaque monkeys. J Comp Neurol. 1998 Nov 30;401(4): 480–505.
31 Bouret S, Richmond BJ. Ventromedial and orbital prefrontal neurons differentially encode internally and externally driven motivational values in monkeys. J Neurosci. 2010 Jun 23;30(25):8591–601.
32 Hare TA, Camerer CF, Rangel A. Self-control in decision-making involves modulation of the

vmPFC valuation system. Science. 2009 May 1;324(5927):646–8.
33 Craig AD. How do you feel? Interoception: the sense of the physiological condition of the body. Nat Rev Neurosci. 2002 Aug;3(8): 655–66.
34 Mayberg HS, Liotti M, Brannan SK, McGinnis S, Mahurin RK, Jerabek PA, et al. Reciprocal limbic-cortical function and negative mood: converging PET findings in depression and normal sadness. Am J Psychiatr. 1999;156(5):675–82.
35 Milad MR, Quinn BT, Pitman RK, Orr SP, Fischl B, Rauch SL. Thickness of ventromedial prefrontal cortex in humans is correlated with extinction memory. Proc Natl Acad Sci U S A. 2005 Jul 26;102(30):10706–11.
36 Milad MR, Wright CI, Orr SP, Pitman RK, Quirk GJ, Rauch SL. Recall of fear extinction in humans activates the ventromedial prefrontal cortex and hippocampus in concert. Biol Psychiatry. 2007 Sep 1;62(5):446–54.
37 Goldapple K, Segal Z, Garson C, Lau M, Bieling P, Kennedy S, et al. Modulation of cortical-limbic pathways in major depression: treatment-specific effects of cognitive behavior therapy. Arch Gen Psychiatry. 2004 Jan;61(1):34–41.
38 Koenigs M, Grafman J. The functional neuroanatomy of depression: distinct roles for ventromedial and dorsolateral prefrontal cortex. Behav Brain Res. 2009 Aug 12;201(2):239–43.
39 Goudriaan AE, De Ruiter MB, Van Den Brink W, Oosterlaan J, Veltman DJ. Brain activation patterns associated with cue reactivity and craving in abstinent problem gamblers, heavy smokers and healthy controls: an fMRI study. Addict Biol. 2010 Sep 14;15(4):491–503.
40 Seo D, Lacadie CM, Tuit K, Hong KI, Constable RT, Sinha R. Disrupted ventromedial prefrontal function, alcohol craving, and subsequent relapse risk. JAMA Psychiatry. 2013 Jul;70(7): 727–39.
41 Kober H, Mende-Siedlecki P, Kross EF, Weber J, Mischel W, Hart CL, et al. Prefrontal-striatal pathway underlies cognitive regulation of craving. Proc Natl Acad Sci U S A. 2010 Aug 17;107(33): 14811–6.
42 Kuhn S, Gallinat J. Resting-state brain activity in schizophrenia and major depression: a quantitative meta-analysis. Schizophr Bull. 2013 Mar;39(2):358–65.
43 Vogt BA. Pain and emotion interactions in subregions of the cingulate gyrus. Nat Rev Neurosci. 2005 Jul;6(7):533–44.
44 Palomero-Gallagher N, Vogt BA, Schleicher A, Mayberg HS, Zilles K. Receptor architecture of human cingulate cortex: evaluation of the four-region neurobiological model. Hum Brain Mapp. 2009 Aug;30(8):2336–55.
45 Bush G, Luu P, Posner MI. Cognitive and emotional influences in anterior cingulate cortex. Trends Cogn Sci. 2000 Jun;4(6):215–22.
46 Ongur D, Price JL. The organization of networks within the orbital and medial prefrontal cortex of rats, monkeys and humans. Cereb Cortex. 2000;10(3):206–19.
47 Morecraft RJ, Stilwell-Morecraft KS, Cipolloni PB, Ge J, McNeal DW, Pandya DN. Cytoarchitecture and cortical connections of the anterior cingulate and adjacent somatomotor fields in the rhesus monkey. Brain Res Bull. [Research Support, N.I.H., Extramural]. 2012 Mar 10;87(4–5): 457–97.
48 Vogt BA, Pandya DN. Cingulate cortex of the Rhesus monkey: II. Cortical afferents. J Comp Neurol. 1987;262:271–89.
49 Cavada C, Goldman-Rakic PS. Posterior parietal cortex in rhesus monkey: II. Evidence for segregated corticocortical networks linking sensory and limbic areas with the frontal lobe. J Comp Neurol. 1989;287(4):422–45.
50 Walton ME, Bannerman DM, Alterescu K, Rushworth MF. Functional specialization within medial frontal cortex of the anterior cingulate for evaluating effort-related decisions. J Neurosci. 2003 Jul 23;23(16): 6475–9.
51 Paus T. Primate anterior cingulate cortex: where motor control, drive and cognition interface. Nat Rev Neurosci. 2001 Jun;2(6):417–24.
52 Vogt BA, Vogt L, Farber NB, Bush G. Architecture and neurocytology of monkey cingulate gyrus. J Comp Neurol. 2005 May 9;485(3):218–39.
53 Behrens TE, Woolrich MW, Walton ME, Rushworth MF. Learning the value of information in an uncertain world. Nat Neurosci. 2007 Sep;10(9):1214–21.
54 Ursu S, Stenger VA, Shear MK, Jones MR, Carter CS. Overactive action monitoring in obsessive-compulsive disorder: evidence from

functional magnetic resonance imaging. Psychol Sci. [Research Support, U.S. Gov't, P.H.S.]. 2003 Jul;14(4):347–53.

55 Fitzgerald KD, Welsh RC, Gehring WJ, Abelson JL, Himle JA, Liberzon I, et al. Error-related hyperactivity of the anterior cingulate cortex in obsessive-compulsive disorder. Biol Psychiatry. 2005 Feb 1;57(3):287–94.

56 Nakao T, Nakagawa A, Yoshiura T, Nakatani E, Nabeyama M, Yoshizato C, et al. Brain activation of patients with obsessive-compulsive disorder during neuropsychological and symptom provocation tasks before and after symptom improvement: a functional magnetic resonance imaging study. Biol Psychiatry. 2005 Apr 15;57(8):901–10.

57 Kaufman JN, Ross TJ, Stein EA, Garavan H. Cingulate hypoactivity in cocaine users during a GO-NOGO task as revealed by event-related functional magnetic resonance imaging. J Neurosci. 2003 Aug 27;23(21):7839–43.

58 Rive MM, van Rooijen G, Veltman DJ, Phillips ML, Schene AH, Ruhe HG. Neural correlates of dysfunctional emotion regulation in major depressive disorder. A Syst Rev Neuroimaging Stud Neurosci Biobehav Rev. 2013 Dec;37(10 Pt 2):2529–53.

59 Beauregard M, Paquette V, Levesque J. Dysfunction in the neural circuitry of emotional self-regulation in major depressive disorder. Neuroreport. [Research Support, Non-U.S. Gov't]. 2006 May 29;17(8):843–6.

60 Braus DF, Weber-Fahr W, Tost H, Ruf M, Henn FA. Sensory information processing in neuroleptic-naive first-episode schizophrenic patients: a functional magnetic resonance imaging study. Arch Gen Psychiatry. 2002 Aug;59(8): 696–701.

61 Ngan ET, Lane CJ, Ruth TJ, Liddle PF. Immediate and delayed effects of risperidone on cerebral metabolism in neuroleptic naive schizophrenic patients: correlations with symptom change. J Neurol Neurosurg Psychiatry. 2002 Jan;72(1): 106–10.

62 Kerns JG, Cohen JD, MacDonald AW, III, Johnson MK, Stenger VA, Aizenstein H, et al. Decreased conflict- and error-related activity in the anterior cingulate cortex in subjects with schizophrenia. Am J Psychiatry. 2005 Oct;162 (10):1833–9.

63 Petrides M, Pandya DN. Dorsolateral prefrontal cortex: comparative cytoarchitectonic analysis in the human and the macaque brain and corticocortical connection patterns. Eur J Neurosci. 1999;11(3):1011–36.

64 Selemon LD, Goldman-Rakic PS. Common cortical and subcortical targets of the dorsolateral prefronal and posterior parietal cortices in the rhesus monkey: evidence for a distributed neural network subserving spatially guided behavior. J Neurosci. 1988;8(11):4049–68.

65 Fletcher PC, Henson RN. Frontal lobes and human memory: insights from functional neuroimaging. Brain. 2001 May;124(Pt 5):849–81.

66 Smith EE, Jonides J. Working memory: a view from neuroimaging. Cogn Psychol. 1997;33(1): 5–42.

67 Passingham D, Sakai K. The prefrontal cortex and working memory: physiology and brain imaging. Curr Opin Neurobiol. 2004 Apr;14(2): 163–8.

68 Blumenfeld RS, Ranganath C. Dorsolateral prefrontal cortex promotes long-term memory formation through its role in working memory organization. J Neurosci. 2006 Jan 18;26(3): 916–25.

69 Fuster JM. Prefrontal neurons in networks of executive memory. Brain Res Bull. 2000;52(5): 331–6.

70 Goldman-Rakic PS. The prefrontal landscape: implications of functional architecture for understanding human mentation and the central executive. Philos Trans R Soc Lond Ser B Biol Sci. 1996;351(1346):1445–53.

71 MacDonald AWr, Cohen JD, Stenger VA, Carter CS. Dissociating the role of the dorsolateral prefrontal and anterior cingulate cortex in cognitive control. Science. 2000;288:1835–9.

72 Ridderinkhof KR, Ullsperger M, Crone EA, Nieuwenhuis S. The role of the medial frontal cortex in cognitive control. Science. 2004 Oct 15;306(5695):443–7.

73 Hamilton JP, Etkin A, Furman DJ, Lemus MG, Johnson RF, Gotlib IH. Functional neuroimaging of major depressive disorder: a meta-analysis and new integration of base line activation and neural response data. Am J Psychiatry. 2012 Jul 1;169(7):693–703.

74 Barch DM, Carter CS, Braver TS, Sabb FW, MacDonald A, III, Noll DC, et al. Selective

deficits in prefrontal cortex function in medication-naive patients with schizophrenia. Arch Gen Psychiatry. 2001 Mar;58(3):280–8.
75 Remijnse PL, Nielen MM, van Balkom AJ, Cath DC, van Oppen P, Uylings HB, et al. Reduced orbitofrontal-striatal activity on a reversal learning task in obsessive-compulsive disorder. Arch Gen Psychiatry. 2006 Nov;63(11): 1225–36.
76 Gu BM, Park JY, Kang DH, Lee SJ, Yoo SY, Jo HJ, et al. Neural correlates of cognitive inflexibility during task-switching in obsessive-compulsive disorder. Brain. 2008 Jan;131(Pt 1):155–64.
77 Haber SN. The primate basal ganglia: parallel and integrative networks. J Chem Neuroanat. 2003 Dec;26(4):317–30.
78 Haber SN. Integrative networks across basal Ganglia circuits. In: Steiner H, Tseng K-Y, editors. Handbook of basal ganglia structure and function. London: Academic; 2010. p. 409–27.
79 Alexander GE, Crutcher MD. Functional architecture of basal ganglia circuits: neural substrates of parallel processing. Trends Neurosci. 1990;13:266–71.
80 Parent A, Hazrati L-N. Anatomical aspects of information processing in primate basal ganglia. Trends Neurosci. 1993;16:111–5.
81 Selemon LD, Goldman-Rakic PS. Longitudinal topography and interdigitation of corticostriatal projections in the rhesus monkey. J Neurosci. 1985;5:776–94.
82 Calzavara R, Mailly P, Haber SN. Relationship between the corticostriatal terminals from areas 9 and 46, and those from area 8A, dorsal and rostral premotor cortex and area 24c: an anatomical substrate for cognition to action. Eur J Neurosci. 2007 Oct;26(7):2005–24.
83 Rauch SL, Jenike MA, Alpert NM, Baer L, Breiter HC, Savage CR, et al. Regional cerebral blood flow measured during symptom provocation in obsessive-compulsive disorder using oxygen 15-labeled carbon dioxide and positron emission tomography. Arch Gen Psychiatry. 1994 Jan;51(1):62–70.
84 Simon D, Kaufmann C, Musch K, Kischkel E, Kathmann N. Fronto-striato-limbic hyperactivation in obsessive-compulsive disorder during individually tailored symptom provocation. Psychophysiology. [Research Support, Non-U.S. Gov't]. 2010 Jul 1;47(4):728–38.
85 Baxter LR, Jr., Schwartz JM, Bergman KS, Szuba MP, Guze BH, Mazziotta JC, et al. Caudate glucose metabolic rate changes with both drug and behavior therapy for obsessive-compulsive disorder. Arch Gen Psychiatry. 1992 Oct;49(9):681–9.
86 Harrison BJ, Soriano-Mas C, Pujol J, Ortiz H, Lopez-Sola M, Hernandez-Ribas R, et al. Altered corticostriatal functional connectivity in obsessive-compulsive disorder. Arch Gen Psychiatry. 2009 Nov;66(11):1189–200.
87 Sakai Y, Narumoto J, Nishida S, Nakamae T, Yamada K, Nishimura T, et al. Corticostriatal functional connectivity in non-medicated patients with obsessive-compulsive disorder. Eur Psychiatry. 2011 Oct;26(7):463–9.
88 Fitzgerald KD, Welsh RC, Stern ER, Angstadt M, Hanna GL, Abelson JL, et al. Developmental alterations of frontal-striatal-thalamic connectivity in obsessive-compulsive disorder. J Am Acad Child Adolesc Psychiatry. 2011 Sep;50(9): 938 e3–48 e3.
89 Volkow ND, Wang GJ, Telang F, Fowler JS, Logan J, Childress AR, et al. Cocaine cues and dopamine in dorsal striatum: mechanism of craving in cocaine addiction. J Neurosci. 2006 Jun 14;26(24):6583–8.
90 Volkow ND, Wang GJ, Fowler JS, Logan J, Gatley SJ, Hitzemann R, et al. Decreased striatal dopaminergic responsiveness in detoxified cocaine-dependent subjects. Nature. 1997 Apr 24;386(6627):830–3.
91 Everitt BJ, Robbins TW. Neural systems of reinforcement for drug addiction: from actions to habits to compulsion. Nat Neurosci. 2005 Nov;8(11):1481–9.
92 Porrino LJ, Lyons D, Smith HR, Daunais JB, Nader MA. Cocaine self-administration produces a progressive involvement of limbic, association, and sensorimotor striatal domains. J Neurosci. 2004 Apr 7;24(14):3554–62.
93 Laruelle M, Abi-Dargham A, Gil R, Kegeles L, Innis R. Increased dopamine transmission in schizophrenia: relationship to illness phases. Biol Psychiatry. 1999;46(1):56–72.
94 Howes OD, Montgomery AJ, Asselin MC, Murray RM, Valli I, Tabraham P, et al. Elevated striatal dopamine function linked to prodromal signs of schizophrenia. Arch Gen Psychiatry. 2009 Jan;66(1):13–20.

95 Abi-Dargham A, Gil R, Krystal J, Baldwin RM, Seibyl JP, Bowers M, et al. Increased striatal dopamine transmission in schizophrenia: confirmation in a second cohort. Am J Psychiatry. 1998 Jun;155(6):761–7.
96 McGowan S, Lawrence AD, Sales T, Quested D, Grasby P. Presynaptic dopaminergic dysfunction in schizophrenia: a positron emission tomographic [18F]fluorodopa study. Arch Gen Psychiatry. 2004 Feb;61(2):134–42.
97 Davis KL, Kahn RS, Ko G, Davidson M. Dopamine in schizophrenia: a review and reconceptualization. Am J Psychiatry 1991;148(11):1474–86.
98 Howes OD, Kapur S. The dopamine hypothesis of schizophrenia: version III – the final common pathway. Schizophr Bull. 2009 May;35(3):549–62.
99 Pizzagalli DA, Holmes AJ, Dillon DG, Goetz EL, Birk JL, Bogdan R, et al. Reduced caudate and nucleus accumbens response to rewards in unmedicated individuals with major depressive disorder. Am J Psychiatry. 2009 Jun;166(6):702–10.
100 Epstein J, Pan H, Kocsis JH, Yang Y, Butler T, Chusid J, et al. Lack of ventral striatal response to positive stimuli in depressed versus normal subjects. Am J Psychiatry. 2006 Oct;163(10):1784–90.
101 Lehman JF, Greenberg BD, McIntyre CC, Rasmussen SA, Haber SN. Rules ventral prefrontal cortical axons use to reach their targets: implications for diffusion tensor imaging tractography and deep brain stimulation for psychiatric illness. J Neurosci. 2011 Jul 13;31(28):10392–402.
102 Jbabdi S, Lehman JF, Haber SN, Behrens TE. Human and monkey ventral prefrontal fibers use the same organizational principles to reach their targets: tracing versus tractography. J Neurosci. 2013 Feb 13;33(7):3190–201.
103 Dejerine J. Anatomie des centres nerveux. Paris: Rueff; 1895.
104 Mufson EJ, Pandya DN. Some observations on the course and composition of the cingulum bundle in the rhesus monkey. J Comp Neurol. 1984 May 1;225(1):31–43.
105 Morris R, Pandya DN, Petrides M. Fiber system linking the mid-dorsolateral frontal cortex with the retrosplenial/presubicular region in the rhesus monkey. J Comp Neurol. 1999 May 3;407(2):183–92.
106 Safadi Z, Haber S. Rules prefrontal pathways use in the anterior limb of the internal capsule: implications for neuroimaging and deep brain stimulation. Poster presented at the annual meeting of the American College of Neuropsychopharmacology, Hollywood, FL. 2013.
107 Jia Z, Huang X, Wu Q, Zhang T, Lui S, Zhang J, et al. High-field magnetic resonance imaging of suicidality in patients with major depressive disorder. Am J Psychiatry. 2010 Nov;167(11):1381–90.
108 Zhu X, Wang X, Xiao J, Zhong M, Liao J, Yao S. Altered white matter integrity in first-episode, treatment-naive young adults with major depressive disorder: a tract-based spatial statistics study. Brain Res. 2010 Oct 31.
109 Lochner C, Fouche JP, du Plessis S, Spottiswoode B, Seedat S, Fineberg N, et al. Evidence for fractional anisotropy and mean diffusivity white matter abnormalities in the internal capsule and cingulum in patients with obsessive-compulsive disorder. J Psychiatry Neurosci. [Research Support, U.S. Gov't, Non-P.H.S.]. 2012 May;37(3):193–9.
110 Zou LQ, Xie JX, Yuan HS, Pei XL, Dong WT, Liu PC. Diffusion tensor imaging study of the anterior limb of internal capsules in neuroleptic-naive schizophrenia. Acad Radiol. 2008 Mar;15(3):285–9.
111 Rosenberger G, Nestor PG, Oh JS, Levitt JJ, Kindleman G, Bouix S, et al. Anterior limb of the internal capsule in schizophrenia: a diffusion tensor tractography study. Brain Imaging Behav. 2012 Sep;6(3):417–25.
112 Beevor C. On the course of the fibers of the cingulum and the posterior parts of the corpus callosum and fornix in the marmoset monkey. Philos Trans R Soc Lond B. 1891;182:135–99.
113 Yakovlev PI, Locke S. Limbic nuclei of the thalamus and connections of limbic cortex. III. Corticocortical connections of the anterior cingulate gyrus, the cingulum, and the ubcallosal bundle in monkey. Arch Neurol. 1961;5:364–400.
114 Mettler R. Corticofugal fiber connections of the cortex of Macaca mulatta. The frontal region. J Comp Neurol. 1935;61:509–42.

115 Cajal S. Histologie du système nerveux de l'homme et des vertébrés. Translated into French by L. Azoulay. Paris: Maloine. Translated into English by N. Swanson N and L.W. Swanson as Histology of the nervous system of man and vertebrates. New York: Oxford University Press; 1995.
116 Adey WR, Meyer M. An experimental study of hippocampal afferent pathways from prefrontal and cingulate areas in the monkey. J Anat. 1952 Jan;86(1):58–74.
117 Heilbronner SR, Haber, SN. Frontal cortical and subcortical projections provide a basis for segmenting the cingulum bundle: implications for neuroimaging and psychiatric disorders. J Neurosci. 2014; 34:10041–54.
118 Goldman-Rakic PS, Selemon LD, Schwartz ML. Dual pathways connecting the dorsolateral prefronal cortex with the hippcampal formation and parahippocampal cortex in the rhesus monkey. Neuroscience. 1984;12(3): 719–43.
119 Mufson EJ, Mesulam MM. Thalamic connections of the insula in the rhesus monkey and comments on the paralimbic connectivity of the medial pulvinar nucleus. J Comp Neurol. 1984;227:109–20.
120 Croxson PL, Johansen-Berg H, Behrens TE, Robson MD, Pinsk MA, Gross CG, et al. Quantitative investigation of connections of the prefrontal cortex in the human and macaque using probabilistic diffusion tractography. J Neurosci. 2005 Sep 28;25(39):8854–66.
121 Makris N, Worth AJ, Sorensen AG, Papadimitriou GM, Wu O, Reese TG, et al. Morphometry of in vivo human white matter association pathways with diffusion-weighted magnetic resonance imaging. Ann Neurol. 1997 Dec;42(6):951–62.
122 Gong G, Jiang T, Zhu C, Zang Y, Wang F, Xie S, et al. Asymmetry analysis of cingulum based on scale-invariant parameterization by diffusion tensor imaging. Hum Brain Mapp. 2005 Feb;24(2):92–8.
123 Cannistraro PA, Makris N, Howard JD, Wedig MM, Hodge SM, Wilhelm S, et al. A diffusion tensor imaging study of white matter in obsessive-compulsive disorder. Depress Anxiety. 2007;24(6):440–6.
124 Szeszko PR, Ardekani BA, Ashtari M, Malhotra AK, Robinson DG, Bilder RM, et al. White matter abnormalities in obsessive-compulsive disorder: a diffusion tensor imaging study. Arch Gen Psychiatry. 2005 Jul;62(7):782–90.
125 Keedwell PA, Chapman R, Christiansen K, Richardson H, Evans J, Jones DK. Cingulum white matter in young women at risk of depression: the effect of family history and anhedonia. Biol Psychiatry. [Research Support, Non-U.S. Gov't]. 2012 Aug 15;72(4): 296–302.
126 Cullen KR, Klimes-Dougan B, Muetzel R, Mueller BA, Camchong J, Houri A, et al. Altered white matter microstructure in adolescents with major depression: a preliminary study. J Am Acad Child Adolesc Psychiatry. 2010 Feb;49(2):173 e1–83 e1.
127 Wang F, Sun Z, Cui L, Du X, Wang X, Zhang H, et al. Anterior cingulum abnormalities in male patients with schizophrenia determined through diffusion tensor imaging. Am J Psychiatry. 2004 Mar;161(3):573–5.
128 Sun Z, Wang F, Cui L, Breeze J, Du X, Wang X, et al. Abnormal anterior cingulum in patients with schizophrenia: a diffusion tensor imaging study. Neuroreport. 2003 Oct 6;14(14): 1833–6.
129 Romero MJ, Asensio S, Palau C, Sanchez A, Romero FJ. Cocaine addiction: diffusion tensor imaging study of the inferior frontal and anterior cingulate white matter. Psychiatry Res. 2010 Jan 30;181(1):57–63.
130 Petrides M, Pandya DN. Efferent association pathways from the rostral prefrontal cortex in the macaque monkey. J Neurosci. 2007 Oct 24;27(43):11573–86.
131 Petrides M, Pandya DN. Association fiber pathways to the frontal cortex from the superior temporal region in the rhesus monkey. J Comp Neurol. 1988;273(1):52–66.
132 Ungerleider LG, Gaffan D, Pelak VS. Projections from inferior temporal cortex to prefrontal cortex via the uncinate fascicle in rhesus monkeys. Exp Brain Res. 1989;76(3):473–84.
133 Nauta W. Some efferent connections of the prefrontal cortex in the monkey. In: Waren J, Akert K, editors. The Frontal Granular Cortex and Behavior. New York: McGraw-Hill; 1964. p. 397–409.
134 Schmahmann JD, Pandya DN, Wang R, Dai G, D'Arceuil HE, de Crespigny AJ, et al. Association fibre pathways of the brain:

parallel observations from diffusion spectrum imaging and autoradiography. Brain. 2007 Mar;130(Pt 3):630–53.
135 Taylor WD, MacFall JR, Gerig G, Krishnan RR. Structural integrity of the uncinate fasciculus in geriatric depression: relationship with age of onset. Neuropsychiatr Dis Treat. 2007;3(5): 669–74.
136 Zhang A, Leow A, Ajilore O, Lamar M, Yang S, Joseph J, et al. Quantitative tract-specific measures of uncinate and cingulum in major depression using diffusion tensor imaging. Neuropsychopharmacology. [Research Support, N.I.H., Extramura]. 2012 Mar;37(4):959–67.
137 Hubl D, Koenig T, Strik W, Federspiel A, Kreis R, Boesch C, et al. Pathways that make voices: white matter changes in auditory hallucinations. Arch Gen Psychiatry. 2004 Jul;61(7): 658–68.
138 Lim KO, Wozniak JR, Mueller BA, Franc DT, Specker SM, Rodriguez CP, et al. Brain macrostructural and microstructural abnormalities in cocaine dependence. Drug Alcohol Depend. 2008 Jan 1;92(1–3):164–72.
139 Upadhyay J, Maleki N, Potter J, Elman I, Rudrauf D, Knudsen J, et al. Alterations in brain structure and functional connectivity in prescription opioid-dependent patients. Brain. 2010 Jul;133(Pt 7):2098–114.
140 Zarei M, Mataix-Cols D, Heyman I, Hough M, Doherty J, Burge L, et al. Changes in gray matter volume and white matter microstructure in adolescents with obsessive-compulsive disorder. Biol Psychiatry. 2011 Dec 1;70(11): 1083–90.
141 Sunderland S. The projection of the cerebral cortex on the pons and cerebellum in the macaque monkey. J Anat. 1940 Jan;74(Pt 2): 201–26 1.
142 Pandya D, Seltzer B. The topography of commissural fibers. In: Lepore F, Jasper H, Ptito M, editors. Two hemispheres-one brain: functions of the corpus callosum. New York: Wiley; 1986. p. 47–73.
143 Cavada C, Goldman-Rakic PS. Topographic segregation of corticostriatal projections from posterior parietal subdivisions in the macaque monkey. Neuroscience. 1991;42(3): 683–96.
144 Locke S, Angevine JB, Yakovlev PI. Limbic nuclei of the thalamus and connections of the limbic cortex. VI. Thalamocortical projection of lateral dorsal nucleus in cat and monkey. Arch Neurol. 1964;11:1–12.
145 Pandya DN, Dye P, Butters N. Efferent cortico-cortical projections of the prefrontal cortex in the rhesus monkey. Brain Res. 1971;31: 35–46.
146 Barbas H, Pandya DN. Topography of commissural fibers of the prefronal cortex in the rhesus monkey. Exp Brain Res. 1984;55:187–91.
147 Bayer SA. Neurogenetic and morphogenetic heterogeneity in the bed nucleus of the stria terminalis. J Comp Neurol. 1987;265(1):47–64.
148 Hofer S, Merboldt KD, Tammer R, Frahm J. Rhesus monkey and human share a similar topography of the corpus callosum as revealed by diffusion tensor MRI in vivo. Cereb Cortex. 2008 May;18(5):1079–84.
149 Aboitiz F, Scheibel AB, Fisher RS, Zaidel E. Fiber composition of the human corpus callosum. Brain Res. 1992 Dec 11;598(1–2):143–53.
150 Hofer S, Frahm J. Topography of the human corpus callosum revisited – comprehensive fiber tractography using diffusion tensor magnetic resonance imaging. NeuroImage. 2006 Sep;32(3): 989–94.
151 Davidson RJ. Anterior cerebral asymmetry and the nature of emotion. Brain Cogn. 1992 Sep;20(1):125–51.
152 Lacerda AL, Brambilla P, Sassi RB, Nicoletti MA, Mallinger AG, Frank E, et al. Anatomical MRI study of corpus callosum in unipolar depression. J Psychiatr Res. 2005 Jul;39(4):347–54.
153 Lammers CH, Doraiswamy PM, Husain MM, Figiel GS, Lurie SN, Boyko OB, et al. MRI of corpus callosum and septum pellucidum in depression. Biol Psychiatry. 1991 Feb 1;29(3): 300–1.
154 Brambilla P, Nicoletti M, Sassi RB, Mallinger AG, Frank E, Keshavan MS, et al. Corpus callosum signal intensity in patients with bipolar and unipolar disorder. J Neurol Neurosurg Psychiatry. 2004 Feb;75(2):221–5.
155 Oh JS, Jang JH, Jung WH, Kang DH, Choi JS, Choi CH, et al. Reduced fronto-callosal fiber integrity in unmedicated OCD patients: a diffusion tractography study. Hum Brain Mapp. 2011 Sep 16;33(10):2441–52.
156 Saito Y, Nobuhara K, Okugawa G, Takase K, Sugimoto T, Horiuchi M, et al. Corpus callosum

in patients with obsessive-compulsive disorder: diffusion-tensor imaging study. Radiology. 2008 Feb;246(2):536–42.
157 Bora E, Yucel M, Fornito A, Pantelis C, Harrison BJ, Cocchi L, et al. White matter microstructure in opiate addiction. Addict Biol. 2012 Jan;17(1):141–8.
158 Moeller FG, Hasan KM, Steinberg JL, Kramer LA, Dougherty DM, Santos RM, et al. Reduced anterior corpus callosum white matter integrity is related to increased impulsivity and reduced discriminability in cocaine-dependent subjects: diffusion tensor imaging. Neuropsychopharmacology. 2005 Mar;30(3):610–7.
159 Salo R, Nordahl TE, Buonocore MH, Natsuaki Y, Waters C, Moore CD, et al. Cognitive control and white matter callosal microstructure in methamphetamine-dependent subjects: a diffusion tensor imaging study. Biol Psychiatry. 2009 Jan 15;65(2):122–8.
160 Ardekani BA, Tabesh A, Sevy S, Robinson DG, Bilder RM, Szeszko PR. Diffusion tensor imaging reliably differentiates patients with schizophrenia from healthy volunteers. Hum Brain Mapp. 2011 Jan;32(1):1–9.
161 Foong J, Symms MR, Barker GJ, Maier M, Miller DH, Ron MA. Investigating regional white matter in schizophrenia using diffusion tensor imaging. Neuroreport. 2002 Mar 4;13(3): 333–6.
162 McIntyre CC, Hahn PJ. Network perspectives on the mechanisms of deep brain stimulation. Neurobiol Dis. 2010 Jun;38(3):329–37.
163 Terao Y, Ugawa Y. Basic mechanisms of TMS. J Clin Neurophysiol. 2002 Aug;19(4):322–43.
164 Di Lazzaro V, Ranieri F, Profice P, Pilato F, Mazzone P, Capone F, et al. Transcranial direct current stimulation effects on the excitability of corticospinal axons of the human cerebral cortex. Brain Stimul. 2013 Jul;6(4):641–3.
165 Greenberg BD, Price LH, Rauch SL, Jenike MA, Malone D, Friehs G, et al. Neurosurgery for intractable obsessive-compulsive disorder and depression: critical issues. Neurosurg Clin N Am. 2003 Apr;14(2):199–212.
166 Greenberg BD, Rauch SL, Haber SN. Invasive circuitry-based neurotherapeutics: stereotactic ablation and deep brain stimulation for OCD. Neuropsychopharmacology. [Review]. 2010 Jan;35(1):317–36.
167 Gutman DA, Holtzheimer PE, Behrens TE, Johansen-Berg H, Mayberg HS. A tractography analysis of two deep brain stimulation white matter targets for depression. Biol Psychiatry. 2009;65(4):276–82.
168 Sartorius A, Kiening KL, Kirsch P, von Gall CC, Haberkorn U, Unterberg AW, et al. Remission of major depression under deep brain stimulation of the lateral habenula in a therapy-refractory patient. Biol Psychiatry. 2010 Jan 15;67(2):e9–e11.
169 Aouizerate B, Cuny E, Bardinet E, Yelnik J, Martin-Guehl C, Rotge JY, et al. Distinct striatal targets in treating obsessive-compulsive disorder and major depression. J Neurosurg 2009 Oct;111(4):775–779.
170 Encinas JM, Hamani C, Lozano AM, Enikolopov G. Neurogenic hippocampal targets of deep brain stimulation. J Comp Neurol. 2011 Jan 1;519(1):6–20.
171 Mallet L, Polosan M, Jaafari N, Baup N, Welter ML, Fontaine D, et al. Subthalamic nucleus stimulation in severe obsessive-compulsive disorder. N Engl J Med. 2008 Nov 13;359(20): 2121–34.
172 Rauch SL, Dougherty DD, Malone D, Rezai A, Friehs G, Fischman AJ, et al. A functional neuroimaging investigation of deep brain stimulation in patients with obsessive-compulsive disorder. J Neurosurg. 2006 Apr;104(4):558–65.
173 McCracken CB, Grace AA. Nucleus accumbens deep brain stimulation produces region-specific alterations in local field potential oscillations and evoked responses in vivo. J Neurosci. 2009 Apr 22;29(16):5354–63.
174 Safadi Z, Heilbronner SR, Haber SN. Mapping the prefrontal connectivity in the internal capsule: implications for deep brain stimulation and neuroimaging. Poster presented at the annual meeting of the Society for Neuroscience, New Orleans, LA. 2012.
175 Lujan JL, Chaturvedi A, Choi KS, Holtzheimer PE, Gross RE, Mayberg HS, et al. Tractography-activation models applied to subcallosal cingulate deep brain stimulation. Brain Stimul. 2013 Sep;6(5):737–9.
176 Sheline YI, Price JL, Yan Z, Mintun MA. Resting-state functional MRI in depression unmasks increased connectivity between networks via the dorsal nexus. Proc Natl Acad Sci

U S A. [Research Support, N.I.H., Extramural]. 2010 Jun 15;107(24):11020–5.
177 Suetens K, Nuttin B, Gabriels L, Van Laere K. Differences in metabolic network modulation between capsulotomy and deep-brain stimulation for refractory obsessive-compulsive disorder. J Nucl Med. 2014 Apr 10;55(6): 951–9.
178 Steele JD, Christmas D, Eljamel MS, Matthews K. Anterior cingulotomy for major depression: clinical outcome and relationship to lesion characteristics. Biol Psychiatry. [Research Support, Non-U.S. Gov't]. 2008 Apr 1;63(7): 670–7.
179 Mantovani A, Lisanby SH, Pieraccini F, Ulivelli M, Castrogiovanni P, Rossi S. Repetitive transcranial magnetic stimulation (rTMS) in the treatment of obsessive-compulsive disorder (OCD) and Tourette's syndrome (TS). Int J Neuropsychopharmacol. 2006 Feb;9(1):95–100.
180 Padberg F, Zwanzger P, Thoma H, Kathmann N, Haag C, Greenberg BD, et al. Repetitive transcranial magnetic stimulation (rTMS) in pharmacotherapy- refractory major depression: comparative study of fast, slow and sham rTMS. Psychiatry Res. 1999;88(3):163–71.
181 Fitzgerald PB, Maller JJ, Hoy KE, Thomson R, Daskalakis ZJ. Exploring the optimal site for the localization of dorsolateral prefrontal cortex in brain stimulation experiments. Brain Stimul. 2009 Oct;2(4):234–7.
182 Feil J, Zangen A. Brain stimulation in the study and treatment of addiction. Neurosci Biobehav Rev. 2010 Mar;34(4):559–74.
183 Fregni F, Liguori P, Fecteau S, Nitsche MA, Pascual-Leone A, Boggio PS. Cortical stimulation of the prefrontal cortex with transcranial direct current stimulation reduces cue-provoked smoking craving: a randomized, sham-controlled study. J Clin Psychiatry. 2008 Jan;69(1):32–40.
184 Boggio PS, Sultani N, Fecteau S, Merabet L, Mecca T, Pascual-Leone A, et al. Prefrontal cortex modulation using transcranial DC stimulation reduces alcohol craving: a double-blind, sham-controlled study. Drug Alcohol Depend. 2008 Jan 1;92(1–3):55–60.
185 Freitas C, Fregni F, Pascual-Leone A. Meta-analysis of the effects of repetitive transcranial magnetic stimulation (rTMS) on negative and positive symptoms in schizophrenia. Schizophr Res. 2009 Mar;108(1–3):11–24.
186 George MS, Nahas Z, Lisanby SH, Schlaepfer T, Andrew Kozel FA, Greenberg BD. Transcranial Magnetic Stimulation. Neurosurg Clin N Am. 2003 Apr;14(2):283–301.
187 Fecteau S, Pascual-Leone A, Zald DH, Liguori P, Theoret H, Boggio PS, et al. Activation of prefrontal cortex by transcranial direct current stimulation reduces appetite for risk during ambiguous decision making. J Neurosci. 2007 Jun 6;27(23):6212–8.
188 Wagner T, Valero-Cabre A, Pascual-Leone A. Noninvasive human brain stimulation. Annu Rev Biomed Eng 2007;9:527–65.
189 Avery DH, Isenberg KE, Sampson SM, Janicak PG, Lisanby SH, Maixner DF, et al. Transcranial magnetic stimulation in the acute treatment of major depressive disorder: clinical response in an open-label extension trial. J Clin Psychiatry. 2008 Mar;69(3):441–51.
190 Cho SS, Strafella AP. rTMS of the left dorsolateral prefrontal cortex modulates dopamine release in the ipsilateral anterior cingulate cortex and orbitofrontal cortex. PLoS One. 2009;4(8):e6725.
191 Fox MD, Liu H, Pascual-Leone A. Identification of reproducible individualized targets for treatment of depression with TMS based on intrinsic connectivity. NeuroImage. 2012 Nov 7;66C:151–60.
192 Lehericy S, Ducros M, Van de Moortele PF, Francois C, Thivard L, Poupon C, et al. Diffusion tensor fiber tracking shows distinct corticostriatal circuits in humans. Ann Neurol. 2004 Apr;55(4):522–9.
193 Draganski B, Kherif F, Kloppel S, Cook PA, Alexander DC, Parker GJ, et al. Evidence for segregated and integrative connectivity patterns in the human Basal Ganglia. J Neurosci. 2008 Jul 9;28(28):7143–52.
194 Cohen MX, Schoene-Bake JC, Elger CE, Weber B. Connectivity-based segregation of the human striatum predicts personality characteristics. Nat Neurosci. 2009 Jan;12(1): 32–4.

CHAPTER 4

Magnetic resonance imaging in neuromodulation

Jonathan Downar[1] and Karen D. Davis[2]

[1] *University of Toronto, Toronto, Canada*

[2] *University Health Network, Toronto, Canada*

Introduction

The field of psychiatry has undergone a transformation over the last 50 years with major research efforts now focused on treatments based on neurobiology. Pharmacotherapy has been based on knowledge of neurotransmitter systems, with relatively less emphasis on neuroanatomy. However, other treatments that target the brain, such as deep brain stimulation (DBS) and transcranial magnetic stimulation (TMS), rely on detailed knowledge of brain structure, function and connectivity. Although much has been learned about basic brain function and structure from animal models, human neuroimaging plays a crucial role in establishing the neural circuitry unique to human psychiatric conditions. The last decade has seen an explosion of neuroimaging research and has provided insight into the mechanisms underlying many psychiatric conditions. These advancements not only hold promise for developing more effective therapeutic strategies but have already begun to provide some beneficial therapies. Furthermore, studies of psychiatric conditions using structural and functional neuroimaging should firmly dispel any doubts that psychiatric conditions have their underpinnings in 'real' abnormalities of brain structure and function. The traditional division between neurological and psychiatric illness thus becomes more blurred, or at least defined more concretely in terms of differing neuroanatomical substrates. This chapter will focus on magnetic resonance imaging (MRI)-based techniques (see Ref. 1) and their applications to three brain stimulation modalities: transcranial direct current stimulation (tDCS), repetitive transcranial magnetic stimulation (rTMS) and DBS.

What can MRI offer the field of psychiatry?

Crucial to any treatment that targets the brain is the understanding of brain pathology specific to a disorder. This knowledge can then guide therapeutic target selection in terms of brain location and type of therapy (e.g. to excite versus to inhibit). Mental illness is assumed to reflect dysfunction of the operations of specific brain regions and/or brain circuits. Such dysfunction could include hypo-, hyper- or aberrant activity in neurons, pathways or circuits. These functional abnormalities may reflect or drive structural deficits of brain connections and/or the grey matter within involved brain regions. Modern

Neuromodulation in Psychiatry, First Edition. Edited by Clement Hamani, Paul Holtzheimer, Andres M. Lozano and Helen Mayberg.

MRI-based techniques can be used to locate and evaluate brain abnormalities associated with psychiatric conditions. The following is an overview of the structural and functional MRI (fMRI) techniques currently being used for this purpose.

MRI measures of grey matter

There are now well-established structural MRI methods based on T1-weighted images to measure the amount of grey matter in the brain. The most popular methods are voxel-based morphometry (VBM) [2] and cortical thickness analysis (CTA) [3]. Of these two methods, VBM is by far the most commonly used. VBM involves classifying each voxel in the brain as grey matter, white matter or cerebrospinal fluid (CSF) based on its signal intensity and thereby determining grey matter volumes of structures throughout the brain. The greatest utility of VBM is for evaluation of subcortical structures. However, grey matter values obtained with VBM are relative values and not study specific, and so cannot directly be compared across studies and laboratories. Also, cortical folding complexities are not specifically considered. The approach of CTA overcomes these two limitations. In CTA, after segmenting the brain into grey matter, white matter and CSF, the pial-grey matter border and the grey /white matter border surfaces are determined. This is then used to measure the cortical thickness at each point and thus determine scalar values of cortical thickness. The advantage of CTA is that it outputs scalar values of thickness that can be compared across studies. However, CTA cannot evaluate subcortical grey matter and so it is considered a complementary method to VBM for grey matter investigations. Many studies have compared the two methods highlighting their relative utility and also factors that should be considered for clinical studies (e.g. age, sex and disease progression) [4, 5].

MRI measures of white matter and structural connectivity (DTI)

It is possible to measure white matter volume with VBM based on T1-weighed MR images. However, a much improved approach for white matter study is based on diffusion-weighted MR images. In diffusion tensor imaging (DTI), the MR acquisition is sensitive to the movement of water molecules [6] and so the dominant direction of diffusion of water along axons in the brain provides a signal that can be measured. Thus, MRI-based evaluation of white matter can be used to (a) assess the so-called 'integrity' of white matter and thus can provide evidence for disruption of axonal organization, and (b) examine white matter connections and thus can provide information pertaining to neural pathways.

Fractional anisotropy (FA) is the most commonly used diffusion-weighted MR-imaging parameter. Because it is said to reflect white matter integrity, it has been used to evaluate white matter abnormalities in a variety of patient populations. When water diffusion is unrestricted, it moves equally in all directions – a state of isotropic diffusion – and thus FA is zero. Conversely, when diffusion is completely restricted to one direction, FA = 1 [7]. Therefore, in the brain, higher FA values represent organized and directional diffusion, and reduced FA can indicate disorganization within a white matter tract. Diffusion-weighted imaging also provides three other metrics of diffusion (see Figure 4.1) [8]: radial and axial diffusivity (RD, AD) is the diffusion across and along the long axis, respectively, and mean diffusivity (MD) is the average diffusivity of all three axes of the axon. Disruption in any of these measures will impact FA and the meaning of a reduced FA can arise from different combinations of changes in AD, RD and/or MD (e.g. see Figure 4.1). There are many conditions that can alter FA (and one or more of the other metrics) such as crossing or branching of

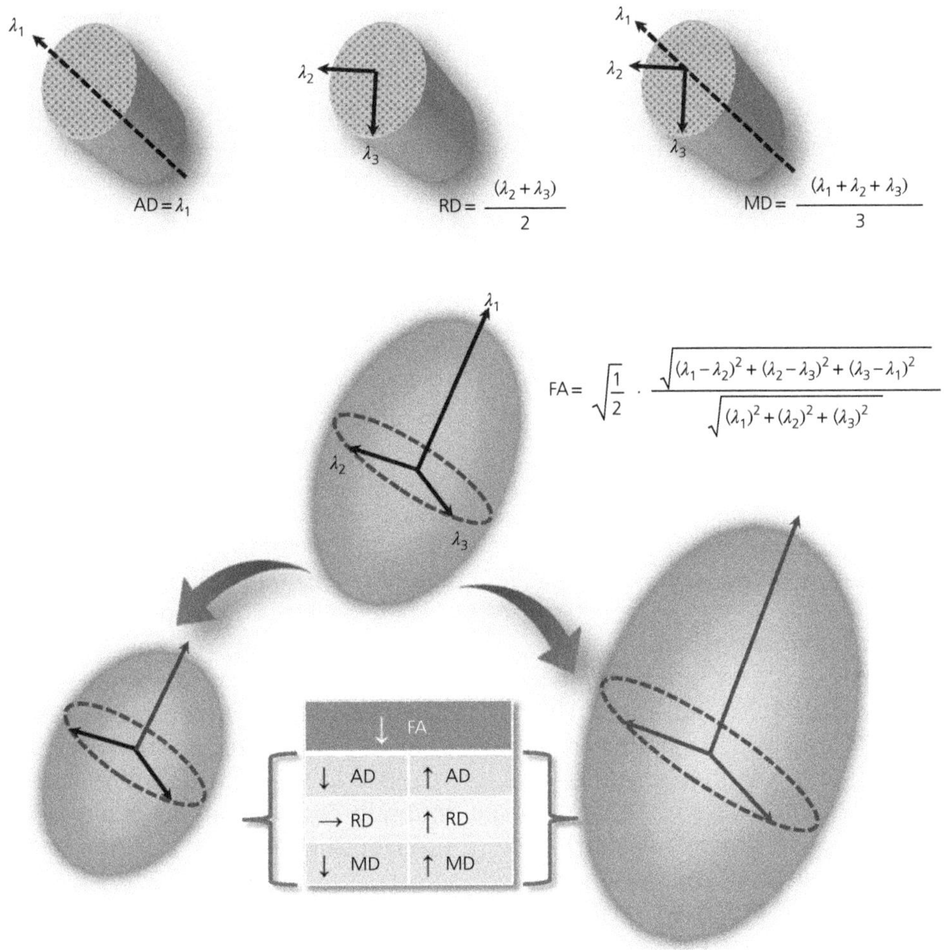

Figure 4.1 DTI metrics. Eigenvalues (λ_1, λ_2, λ_3) of the tensor model used to derive four metric: AD, RD, MD and FA are shown schematically with their formulas. Also shown in B are two different types of abnormalities that could result in reduced FA. Source: From DeDouza et al. [8]. Reproduced with permission of Wolters Kluwer Health.

axons, as well as neuroinflammation (oedema) and demyelination (see Refs. 1, 7, 9, 10).

Structural connectivity can also be evaluated using diffusion-weighted imaging and tractography methods that determine the course of white matter tracts in individual subjects. These methods can be used to examine the strength of connection between one brain area (denoted the 'seed') and other brain area(s) (denoted the target(s)) based on either FA measurements or the number of streamline samples sent out from a seed that reaches a target (for details, see Refs. 7, 10). Another approach, termed tract-based spatial statistics (TBSS), can be used to evaluate group differences in white matter FA [11]. In TBSS, FA values from all subjects within a study are transformed into a common map consisting of a thinned white matter FA 'skeleton' that represents the mean location of all subjects' major white matter tracts. Group (or individual) differences can then be determined based on deviations in FA from the mean skeleton.

MRI measures of functional activity and functional connectivity

fMRI is a non-invasive and indirect measure of neuronal activity. The metabolic needs of active neurons and synaptic activity are associated with a large increase in oxygenated blood beyond what is needed by the neurons. Thus, the most popular and nearly universal contrast used for fMRI is based on the relative proportion of oxy- to deoxy-haemoglobin in the blood, hence the term blood oxygen level dependent (BOLD) [12]. A developing alternative approach to examine neuronal activity is to measure regional cerebral blood flow (rCBF), as is performed in positron emission tomography (PET), as an indirect reflection of neuronal activity (see the following).

Functional activation within a brain region

Since first introduced in the early 1990s, the BOLD fMRI approach is now a solidly established method to examine stimulus- and task-evoked activations within a focal brain region. Such response activations are determined through a statistical comparison of the BOLD signal between two states – an active state and a control state (see Figure 4.2). Thus, conventional fMRI essentially provides a difference measure in MRI signal intensity and cannot determine ongoing activity. A typical fMRI experiment consists of alternating periods of an active state (delivery of stimuli or execution of tasks) and a control state (control stimulus or task, or simply rest). In an event-related design, the stimuli/tasks are very brief (e.g. 1–3 s), and in a block design, the stimuli/tasks are relatively long (e.g. 10–30 s). The design can also include more than one condition to study different effects and/or to control for different parameters. The determination of a so-called 'activation' essentially is a statistical search to find the voxels in the brain that show a similar pattern of signal intensity variation to that of the experimental design (e.g. period of 'condition' versus period of 'control') or an evoked percept. Before conducting the statistical analysis, a predictor function is produced by mathematically convolving the time course of the study design with a haemodynamic response function that models the slow haemodyamics of the system; typically a gamma variate function with an onset of approximately 2–3 s, peaks at approximately 6 s and last approximately 10–12 s. This predictor function is used to find brain activation related to the presence of the stimulus or task [1]. If one wants to determine brain activations that more closely represent a specific percept, the predictor function can be produced using continuous online ratings during the experiment rather than the study time course – an approach known as 'percept-related fMRI'. This approach is beyond the focus of this chapter but is reviewed and described previously (see Refs. 1, 14, 15). The statistical analysis in most fMRI studies involves evaluating a very large number of voxels and thus must include corrections for multiple comparisons to avoid type 1 errors (false positives).

Functional connectivity between brain regions

Although BOLD fMRI has long been established to examine evoked activity, until recently it was thought to be a technique that could only detect differences between states and thus required a task or stimulus. However, BOLD fMRI can now be used to study the relationship between brain areas that have synchronous activity in the absence of an overt stimulus [16]. The term 'functional connectivity' thus refers to brain areas that show temporal correlation, but the technique cannot distinguish if areas are linked through a common input or direct connection. Functional connectivity can examine brain activity during a non-task state (i.e. 'rest state') within/between networks of brain areas showing synchronous low-frequency

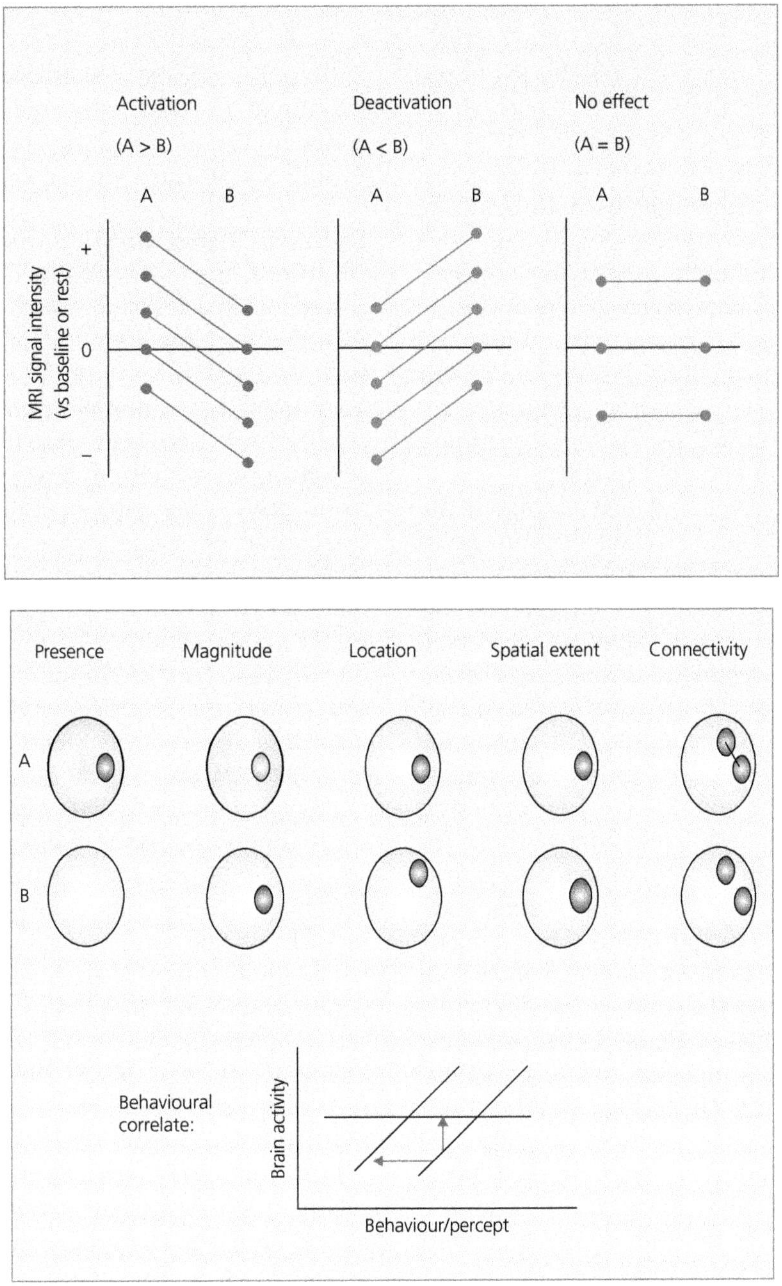

Figure 4.2 Brain activations in a conventional fMRI study. 'A' and 'B' can refer to two experimental conditions (e.g. condition of interest and a control condition) within a single fMRI session. The 'A' and 'B' can also refer to the result of the experimental paradigm in two groups of subjects (e.g. a psychiatric condition vs a healthy control group). Top: The terms 'activation', 'deactivation' and 'no effect' in patient studies are based on the relative difference between condition effects in groups A and B. However, to interpret potential pathology, it is important to consider which type of condition effects led to the A–B difference, including combinations of positive and negative activations. Bottom: Abnormal fMRI responses in patients compared to healthy control subjects can be characterized by six different types of attributes, including the magnitude, location and spatial extent of the evoked signal change, as well as functional connectivity, and correlation with a behavioural measure. Source: From Davis [13]. Reproduced with permission of Future Medicine.

fluctuations (<0.1 Hz). Such activity led to the term 'resting-state network', also known as 'intrinsically connected networks' [17, 18]. A resting-state fMRI (rs-fMRI) scan of about 5 min has been commonly used to examine functional connectivity but longer duration scans are now thought to provide superior power. Emerging data suggest a relationship between anatomical connectivity, functional activity and connectivity [19–25], and recent studies report that low-frequency electrophysiological neuronal oscillations contribute to functional connectivity [26–28].

Raichle and others [29] first identified the so-called 'default mode', a set of brain areas (including posterior cingulate cortex, precuneus, medial prefrontal cortex and lateral parietal cortex) whose activity decreased during a task (unrelated to cardiac, respiration or aliasing effects). This was proposed to represent a network of brain areas that are active at rest to monitor the internal and external environment, and attenuate when attention needs to shift for task execution, perhaps for interoception [30]. We and others also identified this and other non-task resting-state networks that are purported to serve sensorimotor, cognitive, attention, salience and visual functions [31–33]. The study of resting-state networks typically uses model-free methods, most commonly independent component analysis (ICA) and clustering analyses [32]. Model-dependent approaches can also be used, most commonly to examine seed-based functional connectivity to specifically quantify functional connectivity from one area (a seed) to another area or set of areas (i.e. targets) creating 'fingerprints' of connectivity patterns [32]. Our laboratory has used both approach to delineate resting-state networks such as the default mode and salience network [31] and functional connectivity between subregions of the cingulate cortex and insula (e.g. pain salience detectors) [34]. An emerging utility of functional connectivity is to examine abnormalities of functional connectivity associated with a disease state or the link between an individual characteristic and the functional connectivity of a resting-state networks or specific seed–target connections.

Dynamic functional connectivity

Until recently, it was assumed that functional connectivity was a static condition; that is, the relationship between activities of brain areas was thought to be fixed. Because of this assumption of temporal stationarity, functional connectivity had been based on examining synchronous activity of brain regions derived from calculating the overall inter-regional correlation over the entire course of an rs-fMRI scan, typically 5 min. This is appropriate for studying some resting-state networks under stable conditions. However, it is now known that certain conditions and tasks can alter functional connectivity and that some networks show intersubject variability [18]. In 2009, Raichle noted that functional connectivity maps could change if one examines short-time windows (for discussion, see Refs. 18, 35) and in 2010, Chang and Glover presented a new 'sliding window' technique to identify temporal variability in functional connectivity [36]. Then, in 2012, a seminal paper from Peter Bandettini's group detailed the dynamics of functional connectivity [35]. This and other recent findings have led to a re-conceptualization of functional connectivity as being capable of dynamic states [18].

Functional connectivity is determined by calculating a single correlation of the activity of one brain area (a seed) with another brain area for an entire rs-fMRI scan, typically 5–10 min. It was recently discovered that FC can fluctuate over shorter time windows of (e.g. 20–60 s). A method called the 'sliding window' has recently been introduced to study this type of functional connectivity dynamics [18, 35, 36]. In a sliding window analysis, functional connectivity is determined from the data points within a specific window of time (e.g. 20–60 s). The window is then progressively 'slid' in time, typically by 1TR (each unit of data capture in MRI is usually 2 s) and the connectivity determined for each progressive window. This creates a series of correlations that can be plotted as *Z* scores to clearly identify periods of strong positive and negative correlations and thus to 'see' dynamic functional connectivity. To quantify the dynamics of FC for an individual, a metric has been introduced: the functional connectivity variability (FCV), which is simply the SD of FC values across all sliding windows in a scan [37, 38]. This metric provides an important measure that can be used to link FC dynamics with a behavioural measure in individual subjects [37, 38]. Simultaneous fMRI and local field potentials in rats have linked FC in sliding windows as short as 10 s with electrophysiological band-limited power [39]. Furthermore, simultaneous EEG–fMRI studies in humans link dynamic fMRI fluctuations with EEG fluctuations [27, 28, 39].

Regional cerebral blood flow measured with arterial spin labelling

As described earlier, BOLD fMRI can be used to locate (1) the site of task- and stimulus-evoked activity, and (2) brain regions with intrinsic functional connectivity based on synchronous low-frequency oscillations during a non-task/non-stimulus condition. However, BOLD fMRI cannot determine the location and amount of ongoing activity within a focal region of the brain. However, another technique has been developed that can measure brain activity in a specific focal brain area related to ongoing spontaneous perceptions. Arterial spin labelling (ASL) is a non-invasive perfusion MRI technique that can produce quantitative images of rCBF that reflects neuronal activity [40]. Thus, ASL is akin to PET measures of rCBF. To produce an ASL image, a special MRI sequence magnetically 'tags' arterial blood water so that it effectively then becomes a tracer. A delay period following the tagging allows the tagged arterial blood to enter into the segment of the brain of interest to be imaged. The difference between an untagged (i.e. control image) and a tagged image provides the information to calculate perfusion and thus the rCBF. The newly developed pseudo-continuous ASL (pCASL) provides excellent spatial resolution, signal-to-noise ratio sensitivity and reliability and corresponds with ^{15}O-PET data [41]. The most exciting application of pCASL is that it can non-invasively quantify brain activity related to ongoing conditions without the need for a task or stimulus [42]. However, a limitation of ASL is that it has lower temporal resolution than BOLD imaging and so cannot detect quickly changing activity levels. Furthermore, functional connectivity studies are currently hampered by lag time that varies for spatially remote brain areas, although improved methods are being developed to account for these issues. Therefore, BOLD fMRI and ASL are complementary methods that each reveal a specific aspect of neural function related to a condition.

Detecting functional and structural MRI abnormalities

As described earlier, conventional fMRI is used to identify brain activations evoked by a stimulus or task and functional connectivity is used to detect brain areas that show synchronous low-frequency activity. However, there is no gold standard that dictates the statistical analysis that is to be used to detect abnormalities in patient groups. Therefore, in clinical studies, it is imperative to consider the myriad of study design, technical and statistical issues, including adopting a rigorous statistical approach that minimizes type 1 and type 2 errors. A fundamental issue is the methods to designate the presence of an 'activation' due to a particular experimental condition and then the determination of abnormal responses in a patient population. Figure 4.2

illustrates the various ways in which a brain area is deemed to be activated or showing a difference in patients versus healthy control subjects [13], including considerations of the signal intensity (increases and decreases), location, spatial extent and correlations to behavioural features. Similarly, abnormalities in connectivity (functional and structural) can be in the form of the strength and/or spatial distribution of connectivities.

Analysing network-level patterns in resting brain activity

As noted earlier, brain activity during tasks or in the resting state is characterized by the coordinated activation and deactivation of networks of brain regions, identifiable on fMRI. The analysis and interpretation of these networks is not necessarily straightforward. Fortunately, a toolbox of mathematical techniques known as *graph theory* is proving helpful in understanding the topology and functional roles of individual nodes within these networks, as well as the functional roles of the connections between them.

The tools of graph theory can be applied to any system characterized by 'vertices', or nodes, that are connected by 'edges' or connections. These tools are being used to understand social networks, transportation networks, electrical transmission grids, protein–protein interaction networks and, in this case, networks of neurons or brain regions. To prepare the data for analysis, the brain must first be divided into a collection of regions, which will serve as the 'nodes' of the network. These regions can be defined using standard anatomical atlases, or by selecting a catalogue of seed regions of interest *a priori* based on previous work, or by constructing atlases based on regions of homogeneous activity within the fMRI data itself. A variety of standard atlases based on either anatomical landmarks or resting-state data are available freely for download from a variety of sources; no consensus currently exists on the 'ideal' atlas for all applications, and a variety of atlases are currently in use. Once the regions are defined, the average time course of activity is extracted from each region, as in seed-based analyses described earlier. Next, the time course of each region is correlated to the time course of all other regions, to generate a 'cross-correlation matrix' of dimensions $n \times n$, where n is the total number of nodes or seed regions. This cross-correlation matrix is then used to define an 'adjacency matrix' that specifies which nodes will be considered 'connected' to one another in the graph. The usual method is to apply a minimum correlation threshold to the matrix, although 'weighted' graphs can also be constructed with stronger or weaker connections based on the strength of the correlation. The adjacency matrix then specifies which nodes are connected to which other nodes, and how strongly, and these data serve as input to the tools of graph theory.

A detailed review of graph theory as applied to neuroimaging is beyond the scope of this chapter, although several excellent overviews are available [43]. In general, three levels of analysis are possible. First, the overall topology of the network can be analysed and collapsed into a single coefficient specifying its general arrangement: for example, its 'small-worldness', which specifies a particular arrangement in which most nodes are not directly connected but can reach each other through a small number of steps. Second, the overall 'community structure' of the graph can be analysed, finding groups or 'cliques' of nodes within the network that are more tightly connected to one another and less tightly connected to other brain regions. Third, the properties of individual nodes or connections can be analysed, to determine how 'central' each node or connection is within the graph as a whole.

Because of their utility in identifying therapeutic targets and network-level effects of neuromodulation, the tools of graph theory have a variety of important potential applications in research and therapeutic use of neuromodulation. Examples include the use of connection path length to characterize the effects of tDCS on motor cortex activity [44] and the use of betweenness centrality to locate a nexus of whole-brain activity in non-responders to dorsomedial rTMS for major depression [45].

Neuromodulation in the MRI environment

The use of MRI in neuromodulation can be performed either 'offline' (before or after the neuromodulation treatment) or 'online' (during the neuromodulation treatment itself). Online MRI has a variety of potentially important uses in understanding the mechanisms of effect for neuromodulation treatments. However, the MRI environment poses a number of significant challenges to performing either invasive or non-invasive brain stimulation. Here we consider the nature of these challenges, as well as techniques that have been developed to circumvent them.

Repetitive transcranial magnetic stimulation

rTMS has been performed safely in the MRI environment since 1998 [46]; however, combining these two techniques poses several additional technical challenges. A consensus set of guidelines for combining TMS and MRI is available [47]. Ferromagnetic materials must be removed from the TMS coil to prevent traction on the device, and the stimulus generator must remain outside the MRI room. The coil must be reinforced to withstand higher mechanical stresses due to the interaction of the TMS and MRI magnetic fields. Mechanical damping is required to accommodate slight coil movements during stimulation, which can generate eddy currents and distort images. RF filters are required on the lengthened leads from the stimulator to the coil, compensatory mechanisms are required to balance leak currents through the capacitors in the TMS device, and coil recharging must be delayed until after image acquisition; significant image degradation can ensue if these measures are not adopted. Several manufacturers now offer rTMS systems in these ways to enable TMS in the MR environment.

MRI acquisition must also be modified to accommodate rTMS. Image distortion and signal loss due to susceptibility artefact can be reduced somewhat by orienting the plane of the echoplanar imaging (EPI) images parallel to the coil plane, and by oversampling in the phase encoding direction in order to displace 'ghost' images produced by phase shifts. TMS pulses themselves consist of powerful (1–2 T) magnetic fields that can severely distort the EPI images acquired during fMRI. The nature of the distortions depends on coil orientation, pulse intensity and waveform, and MRI field strength. However, a straightforward solution to avoiding image degradation is to interleave the timing of the TMS pulses and the EPI readouts so that TMS pulses are delivered between acquisition of image volumes [48], with a delay of coil recharging until after acquisition of several image volumes to avoid generating signal artefact. However, these measures do not compensate for the indirect activation of the brain in response to the auditory and somatosensory input generated by the TMS pulses; thus, suitable control conditions may be required in the experimental design.

The static B_0 field of the MRI scanner may also affect the geometry of the TMS field itself. A recent investigation found that distortions of the TMS field were greatest when the coil was located in the non-homogeneous 'fringe field' near the inner surface of the bore. With the coil fully inside the homogeneous field zone of the bore, field distortion was minor and changes in coil orientation did not lead to variations in field geometry [49]. Of note, it is also possible to use MRI to map the field geometry of a given MRI coil. By running a weak current through a non-ferromagnetic coil inside the bore, and by collecting the phase image rather than the magnitude image of a gradient echo scan, the three-dimensional (3D) coil field can be visualized directly [50]. This application may be useful in evaluating the fields associated with novel coil geometries before investigational use.

Transcranial direct current stimulation

tDCS has also been performed safely during MRI in a number of recent studies (reviewed in Ref. 51). Regarding safety, the primary concern is the possibility of excessive heating of the electrodes due to currents induced in the tDCS circuit by the RF pulses and gradient fields during active MRI. This risk can be overcome by adding resistors to the circuit close to the tDCS electrode contacts, thus limiting the induced currents.

Active tDCS may also affect the acquired structural and functional images. The electrodes themselves, when active, generate electromagnetic fields that can cause image distortion and a 3–8% loss of signal strength. B_0 field distortions and susceptibility artefact have been reported as restricted to scalp tissues rather than the brain itself [52]. Studies of tDCS artefacts during fMRI have also recently been performed, using postmortem subjects to remove the contribution of neurally induced BOLD signals [53]. These studies found that tDCS induced BOLD signal artefacts near CSF and scalp, superficial brain tissue and ventricles, with the direction of signal shift dependent on the polarity of the applied current. The magnitude of the shift was comparable to that seen with activation on a finger-tapping task.

There are two main implications to these findings. First, studies using combined tDCS-fMRI may need to adopt methods for the removal of tDCS artefacts from the acquired data. Removal could potentially exploit differences between the expected waveforms of applied tDCS and the BOLD haemodynamic responses, which have a delayed onset of 2 s and peak of 6–8 s compared to the induced neural activity. Second, the electrical fields induced by the tDCS could potentially be mapped directly using the same EPI series employed for BOLD fMRI, by using short square-wave pulses of 1–2 s duration in order to distinguish the induced field from the resultant haemodynamic responses. Such techniques could prove useful for individual-level mapping of tDCS fields.

Deep brain stimulation

The safety of performing MRI in patients with implanted deep brain stimulation (DBS) electrodes has been a subject of some controversy in the past, and some centres have considered the presence of a DBS implant as an absolute contraindication to MRI. Major safety concerns include thermocoagulation lesions due to heating of the electrode contacts when exposed to RF energy during scanning, or migration of the stimulator unit due to exposure of any ferromagnetic components to high magnetic fields. Additional concerns include induction of unintended stimulus pulses via application of the MRI gradient fields to the stimulator leads, reprogramming or damage to the electronics of the internal pulse generator (IPG) leading to implant failure or incorrect stimulation parameters, and degradation of the quality of the MRI itself.

Electrode heating issues are among the most concerning because of the possibility of a permanent thermal lesion. To quantify the effects of common MRI sequences, one group made detailed thermal and electrical measurements around the electrode tips in a phantom brain implanted with a commercially available DBS electrode set while applying common structural and functional MRI sequences (T1-weighted, EPI and fast spin echo) at 1.5 and 3.0 T [54]. For sequences with RF exposure below the common guideline SAR greater than 0.4 W/kg, heating using either T1-weighted or

EPI BOLD sequences was >0.1°C at 1.5T and >0.5°C at 3.0T, providing a 2- to 10-fold safety margin over the recommended maximum heating of brain tissue to 38°C. For comparison, a fast spin-echo sequence reaching 1.5–2.5 W/kg SAR produced heating of 1–2°C over approximately 3 min, thus exceeding the recommended temperature increase. Electrically, the induced currents from gradient switching appeared smaller than the DBS pulses themselves, with occasional slightly delayed pulses occurring approximately 1% of the time during scanning.

Empirical data on the safety of MRI with DBS were relatively lacking in the past; recently, however, a number of studies have addressed this issue via case series and literature reviews [55, 56]. In a review of >4000 MRIs performed in patients with internalized of externalized DBS electrodes, four adverse events were identified. The most serious was a permanent neurological deficit in a patient 7 months post-implant who underwent lumbar spine imaging with RF exposure exceeding 1.26 W/kg SAR (threefold higher than the 0.4 W/kg common guideline). This patient emerged from the scanner with an immediately evident deficit of movement and was later found (on MRI) to have sustained a 2–3 cm lesion with haemorrhage surrounding the electrode tip [57]. There was one less serious case of post-MRI left leg dystonia and hemiballismus following MRI, resolving after several weeks [58]. Two other cases involved failure of the IPG, with no neurological or other sequelae but requiring repeat implantation of a replacement IPG [56].

DBS manufacturers now provide guidelines for performing MRI in DBS. Common recommendations are to perform MRI only when necessary, at 1.5T, with gradients limited to <20 T/s, using a transmit/receive head coil only, limiting the SAR to >0.4 W/kg (0.1 W/kg in some cases), and without sedation if possible so that patient may report adverse sensations. It is also commonly recommended to check the lead impedance and not to proceed in the case of high impedance, which could suggest a broken lead. It is also recommended to set the IPG to the 'off' mode, while also setting the parameters to zero amplitude, bipolar pulses, with disabling of the magnetic switch.

Uses of MRI in neuromodulation

Neuroimaging and neurostimulation have enjoyed a close synergy ever since the earliest stereotaxic functional neurosurgical procedures in humans in the mid-20th century. MRI can serve at least four key roles in aiding the use of neuromodulation for clinical and research purposes:

Target selection: the identification of new stimulation targets for a given disorder based on preclinical evidence from structural and functional neuroimaging studies of the disorder itself.

Neuronavigation: the accurate placement of the invasive or non-invasive stimulator in close proximity to the stimulation target.

Mechanism investigation: characterizing the effects of the stimulation on brain structure and brain function, either 'online' during stimulation or 'offline' via pre- and post-stimulation comparisons.

Individual parameter optimization: guiding the selection of optimal stimulation parameters (both the location and the pattern of stimulation) in individuals based on brain structure or function.

The following sections focus on each of these applications in turn.

Identification of stimulation targets using structural and functional MRI

Neuromodulation, unlike other modalities of psychiatric treatment, requires knowledge of the most appropriate anatomical target for treating a given disorder. MRI has long played a key pre-clinical role in localizing the

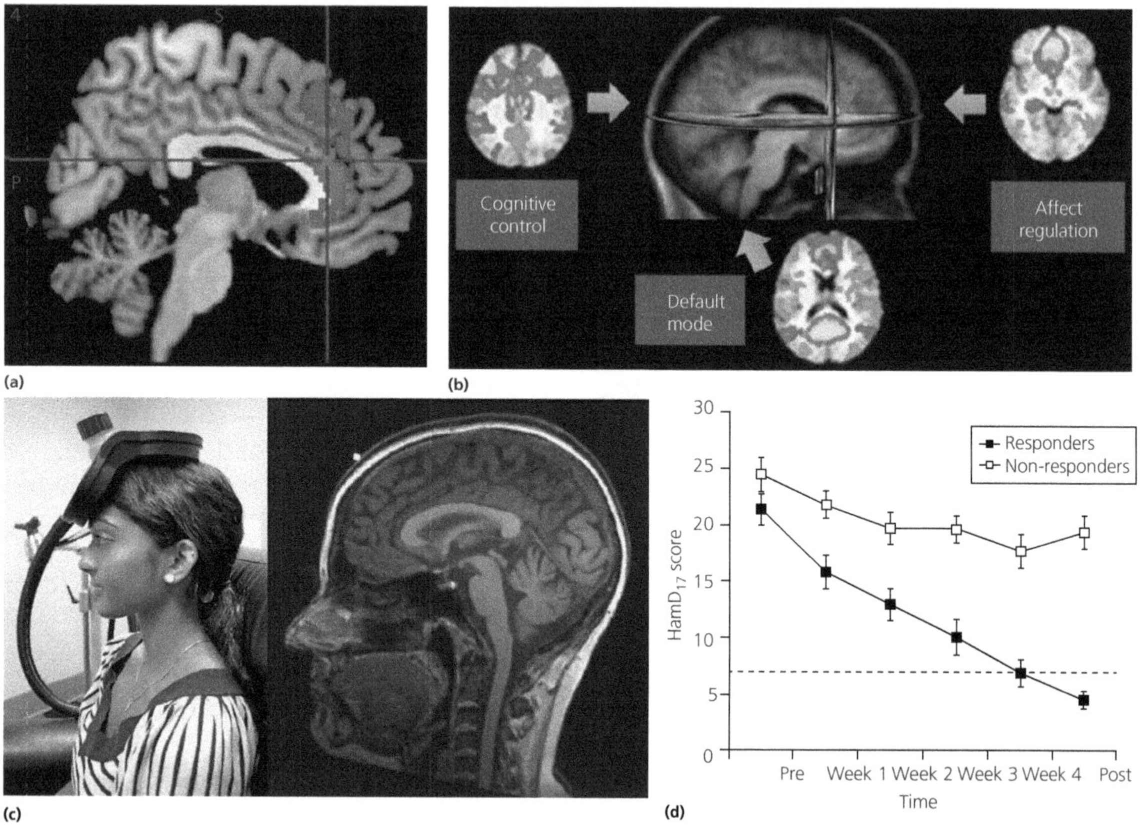

Figure 4.3 Use of MRI in preclinical identification of stimulation targets. (**a**) VBM meta-analyses identified the DMPFC as a region of consistent grey matter volume reduction in major depressive disorder. Source: From Bora et al. [59]. Reproduced with permission of Elsevier. (**b**) rs-fMRI studies also identified the DMPFC as a 'dorsal nexus' region in major depressive disorder, where networks for cognitive control, affect regulation and the 'default mode' intersected. Source: From Adapted from Sheline et al. [60]. Copyright PNAS. (**c**) These findings prompted the development of techniques for applying rTMS to the DMPFC under MRI guidance for the treatment of major depression. (**d**) As suggested by the preclinical work, rTMS of the DMPFC achieved remission in >40% of patients with major depression. Source: c and d reprinted by permission of Elsevier from Downar et al. [45]. Copyright 2013 by the Society of Biological Psychiatry. (*See insert for colour representation of the figure.*)

structural and functional pathology underlying psychiatric disorders. For this reason, one of the most important roles of MRI in neuromodulation is in the identification of potential therapeutic targets – a process akin to the preclinical work of drug discovery in the pharmaceutical realm. Here we review examples of therapeutic stimulation targets originally identified via MRI and allied neuroimaging modalities (Figure 4.3).

Repetitive transcranial magnetic stimulation

By far the most common therapeutic use of rTMS in psychiatry is in the treatment of major depression. The first trials of rTMS for depression began in the early 1990s, targeting the dorsolateral prefrontal cortex (DLPFC), most commonly on the left, but occasionally on the right, or bilaterally. Neuroimaging played a critical pre-clinical role in selecting this target during the early studies 20 years ago. Studies using functional neuroimaging, initially with PET and SPECT and later with fMRI, found the DLPFC to be hypoactive in major depression, thus providing a rationale for the first clinical trials of high-frequency rTMS as an antidepressant treatment [62, 63]. Today, the left DLPFC remains the most widely used target for rTMS in major depression.

More recently, a variety of alternative rTMS targets have been proposed for major depression, including the dorsomedial prefrontal cortex (DMPFC), ventromedial prefrontal cortex (VMPFC) and ventrolateral prefrontal cortex [61]. The rationale for these targets, as with the DLPFC in the 1990s, draws upon the convergent evidence of structural and functional neuroimaging studies of emotion regulation in depressed patients and healthy controls [64]. At least one of these targets, the DMPFC, has shown promise in the treatment of major depression in preliminary case series [65, 66].

VBM studies have also implicated the DMPFC in a variety of other psychiatric disorders characterized by intrusive thoughts and compulsive behaviours, including obsessive–compulsive disorder (OCD) [67] and post-traumatic stress disorder (PTSD) [68], and in deficits of social cognition, such as theory of mind [69]. These preclinical findings are now beginning to be translated into new rTMS treatment protocols for these disorders. For example, 1 Hz rTMS of the supplementary motor area, located in posterior DMPFC, is now being used to treat refractory OCD [70]. Likewise, deep rTMS of the DMPFC is showing promise for PTSD symptoms [71], and for social functioning in autism spectrum disorder patients [72].

Functional neuroimaging studies are also leading to new applications and targets for rTMS. For example, fMRI studies have identified regions of the superior frontal gyrus as active during nicotine craving suppression [73]. rTMS over this target showed modulatory effects on cigarette cravings in response to cues [74]. fMRI has also revealed hypoactivity in DMPFC in response to food cues in bulimia nervosa [75]. Ten hertz of rTMS of the DMPFC has shown some promise in treating this disorder in refractory patients [76]. Finally, fMRI has been helpful in locating rTMS targets for rarer disorders such as depersonalization disorder, for which 1 Hz stimulation of the overactive right temporoparietal junction is proving useful [77].

Transcranial direct current stimulation

Anatomical targets for tDCS are being identified using the same literature that is guiding past and current applications of therapeutic rTMS. For example, for trials of tDCS in major depression, the most common target has also been the DLPFC, as with rTMS [78, 79]. In another promising example, tDCS with the cathode over left temporoparietal cortex and anode over right DLPFC has been used to treat refractory auditory hallucinations in schizophrenia [80]. Encouragingly, the effects appear to be not only potent, but durable over 3 years of daily or twice-daily treatments, with minimal adverse effects. The targets of stimulation here are based, in part, on structural and functional neuroimaging studies conducted over the last 20 years on schizophrenia and the symptom of auditory hallucinations.

In another thought-provoking example, Karim and colleagues [81] recently studied the effects of tDCS on 'deceptive behaviour', or in plainer language, lying. In an experimental setting, subjects played the role of a thief, stole a wallet from a pre-arranged location, then underwent a detailed interrogation, with financial incentives for successful deception of the interrogator. Functional neuroimaging had previously implicated the anterior prefrontal cortex in deceptive behaviours [82]. Cathodal tDCS, but not anodal or sham tDCS, of this region improved subjects' facility in deception: faster reaction times in telling lies, reduced skin-conductance responses and reduced feelings of guilt during lying. Although the therapeutic applications (and ethical implications) of this finding could generate a lively debate, the example illustrates the potential for structural and functional MRI to generate new applications for tDCS, by modulating the neural infrastructure of social cognition, emotion regulation and decision-making.

Deep brain stimulation

Perhaps the canonical example of a DBS target identified directly from neuroimaging comes from the case of major depression. Through the 1990s and early 2000s, a series of neuroimaging studies identified the subcallosal cingulate cortex as consistently overactive in major depression. Furthermore, these studies showed that reducing the activity of the subcallosal cingulate was associated with treatment response across a wide variety of interventions including various pharmacotherapies, ECT and even placebo [83]. These findings led directly to the proposal that implanting DBS electrodes in the subcallosal cingulate region might be therapeutic in refractory cases of depression. The success of this approach in subsequent case series [84, 85] constitutes one of the major breakthroughs in the history of neuromodulation for psychiatric disease. Structural and functional neuroimaging studies from the research literature have also provided a rationale for targeting several other structures in major depression, including the nucleus accumbens [86], medial forebrain bundle [87] and lateral habenula [88].

Structural and functional MRI studies have also been instrumental in bringing DBS to new areas of psychiatry – for example, eating disorders such as anorexia nervosa [89]. This literature has helped to link various aspects of the underlying psychopathology (e.g. emotional dysregulation, hedonic abnormalities, rumination and distortions of body image) to specific neuroanatomical circuits and targets. The subcallosal cingulate cortex, amygdala, ventral striatum, mediodorsal thalamus, DMPFC and insula have all been identified as key regions within the pathophysiology of disordered eating. Of these, so far only the subcallosal cingulate has been targeted for DBS in anorexia nervosa, with encouraging results from a small preliminary case series [90].

Neuroimaging studies have also proved useful in identifying DBS targets for other forms of highly refractory psychiatric illness, such as OCD (reviewed in Ref. 91). Volumetric studies and fMRI studies have identified abnormalities in lateral orbitofrontal and dorsomedial regions of the prefrontal cortex, as well as associated regions of the striatum [67]. Likewise, diffusion tractography and resting-state functional connectivity studies have identified abnormal structural and functional connections along pathways through the anterior limb of the internal capsule, the inferior thalamic peduncle, and frontostriatal circuits through the nucleus accumbens and subthalamic nucleus. All these regions have been proposed or already explored as therapeutic targets for DBS in OCD, with encouraging outcomes [92–94]. The promising results for DBS in this setting are a good illustration of the potential synergies between preclinical neuroimaging and targeted neuromodulation when seeking new treatments for refractory psychiatric illness.

Neuronavigation using MRI

Transcranial magnetic stimulation

Early approaches to rTMS did not employ image guidance, instead relied on scalp landmarks or motor responses for target localization. However, some common therapeutic targets, such as the DLPFC, do not typically generate motor-evoked potentials when stimulated. In the past, heuristics such as the '5-cm rule' were commonly used: first, the scalp 'hotspot' for the abductor pollicis brevis is located, then a new spot is marked 5 cm anterior to the motor hotspot. This method is now recognized to be inadequate, missing the intended target region completely in at least one-third of cases [95]. Modified heuristics, such as a '6-cm rule', do not fully address this problem and commonly lead to the stimulation of premotor or oculomotor regions instead of the desired DLPFC target.

For these reasons, MRI-based neuronavigation is often employed to ensure accurate positioning of a TMS coil over a particular cortical location. Several manufacturers now offer frameless stereotaxic positioning systems capable of using MR images (obtained offline) to position the TMS coil over an intended target region to within an accuracy of <2 mm. MRI-based neuronavigation involves several steps. First, a T1 structural MRI volume (sometimes supplemented by a map of functional activation generated from BOLD images) is acquired before the stimulation session. Next, these images are used to generate renderings of scalp and brain surfaces in three dimensions. Upon these renderings, scalp landmarks such as the nasion or left and right preauricular areas are then marked. Next, the subject and the TMS coil are fitted with tracking markers visible to a 3D camera or positioning system. A tracker pen is then used to record the positions of the nasion, pre-auricular areas or additional scalp markers with respect to the subject's head tracker. Using this information, the neuronavigation software can then coregister the MRI to the subject's head markers. The software can then follow the movements of both the TMS coil and the subject's head in real time throughout the stimulation session using the tracking markers. Stimulation targets can be marked on the MRI using either standard stereotaxic coordinates or fMRI activation maps. The software then provides the TMS operator with visual guides to ensure that the coil is maintained at the correct location and orientation over the target site during stimulation. Accidental movements of either the coil or the subject can be detected and corrected immediately if they occur (Figure 4.4).

Modern neuronavigation systems can preprocess MRI data to be ready for use in less than 15 min, and the set-up time can be less than 5 min with an experienced operator. For this reason, MRI-based neuronavigation is appropriate for therapeutic rTMS as well as research studies, even when clinic volumes are high and patient turnover must be completed quickly. Therapeutic benefits may significant. Previous studies have found that the '5-cm anterior to motor hotspot' heuristic for positioning over the DLPFC is often too far posterior or too far dorsal, leading to treatment failure in the case of major depression [96]. MRI-based neuronavigation also achieves superior accuracy and consistency compared to the F3 or F4 EEG locations, for locating DLPFC [97]. Finally, recent studies have also identified more specific stereotaxic coordinates within the larger region of the DLPFC that yield improved responses in major depression [98]. Thus, pending improved scalp-based heuristics, MRI-guided stimulation is recommended for DLPFC stimulation in the therapeutic setting, if available.

Where cost and availability of MRI are limiting factors, or in patients with MRI contraindications, high resolution CT may be an acceptable alternative. We have found that newer 64- or 320-slice CT scans with 1-mm slice acquisitions are able to achieve sufficient resolution and tissue contrast to be used in place of MRI. Minor adjustments to the image format or to the navigation software are sometimes required. Standard stereotaxic landmarks such as the anterior and posterior commissure are slightly more difficult to identify on CT, but can be reliably located in all cases by an adequately trained technician.

Transcranial direct current stimulation

MRI-based neuronavigation is less critical for tDCS than for TMS. tDCS electrodes are relatively large, typically measuring 3–5 cm

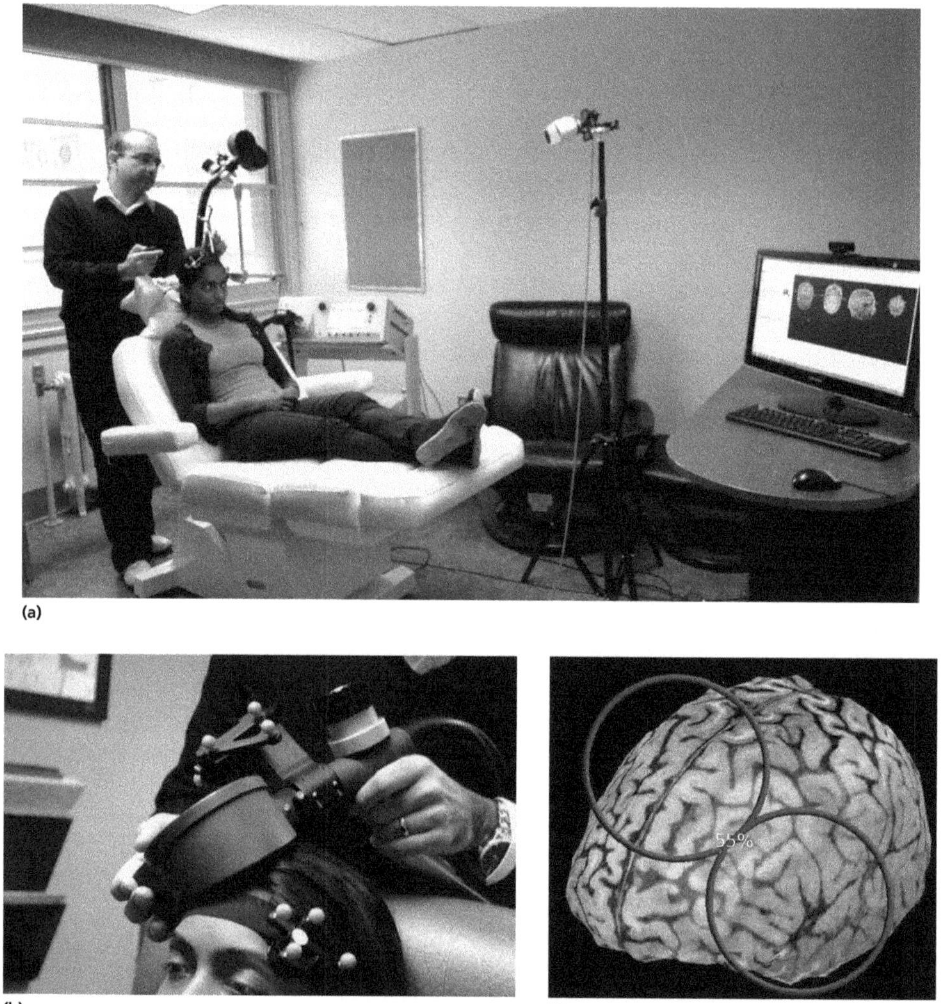

(a) (b) (c)

Figure 4.4 MRI-guided neuronavigation. (**a**) A neuronavigation suite uses a 3D position-capture camera, a pre-loaded MRI of the patient, and tracking markers on the coil and the patient's head to position the coil over the intended stimulation site during stimulation. (**b**) Tracking markers allow the camera to follow slight movements of the coil or the patient's head in real time, in order to maintain position over the target. (**c**) Neuronavigation software can establish the position of the coil vertex to an accuracy of <2 mm, and also create models of the geometry of the electrical field induced by the coil during stimulation.

along each side. For this reason, the majority of tDCS studies to date have not required image-guided approaches to electrode placement. More commonly, tDCS electrodes are placed using systems based on scalp landmarks, such as 10–20 EEG electrode positions. For example, a recent clinical trial in major depression applied tDCS to the DLPFC using the F3 and F4 scalp positions [79].

There are also situations in which tDCS must be applied to regions that are small, or regions that do not map neatly on to a standard 10–20 EEG position, or regions that are identified in individual subjects using fMRI.

In these settings, MRI-based neuronavigation methods can be used to centre the tDCS electrodes over the stimulation sites with high accuracy in individual subjects, just as with rTMS. This approach has been used, for example, to stimulate regions of the inferior parietal lobule (IPL) associated with gesture processing [99].

One key difference with tDCS versus TMS is that the inductor uses an electrical current rather than a magnetic field, and thus the stimulation may spread in complex and unpredictable ways through scalp, bone, CSF, and brain. These complexities can result in stimulation of unintended areas, and can also introduce substantial inter-individual variability in the effects of stimulation. As a result, there is now growing interest in developing neuroimaging-based methods for mapping the electrical fields induced by tDCS through the unique tissue geometries of each individual subject [100].

Methods such as finite element modelling (FEM) can be used to generate high-resolution maps of simulated current flow through the brain associated with tDCS, rTMS or DBS. These methods, however, require high-resolution images of the 3D structure of the brain. These image volumes must also be segmented into distinct tissue types to accommodate the differential electrical conductivity of scalp, bone, blood, CSF, grey matter and white matter. Furthermore, in the case of tissues that conduct electrical fields anisotropically, such as white matter tracts, the anisotropy must also be mapped for best FEM performance. Structural MRI therefore plays a critical role in individualized FEM for tDCS and other stimulation techniques.

Although still in evolution, current methods make use of a variety of structural image sequences including T1-weighted, T2-weighted and diffusion tensor images. The T1- and T2-weighted images can be used for automated, intensity-based segmentation of different tissue types. The diffusion tensor images can be used to perform seed-based or automated tractography, thereby tracing the anisotropic patterns of current flow through white matter tracts. There are now a variety of proprietary and non-proprietary automated systems for processing these structural images and generating FEM simulations of current spread for tDCS. Some make use of open-source and freely available pre-processing software [101], and are thus available for widespread use and modification in the research setting.

A promising application of automated MRI-based FEM lies in the emerging field of individualized, high-density tDCS (HD-tDCS). HD-tDCS uses a complex montage of multiple small tDCS electrodes arrayed over the scalp to achieve more focal stimulation of either superficial or deep structures within the brain [102]. One of the better-studied montages is known as 4 × 1 ring HD-tDCS. Here a small centre electrode (either anode or cathode) is placed over the desired target and then surrounded by a ring of four return electrodes of opposite polarity. The ring electrodes help to restrict the current flow to the area under the centre electrode, thus achieving more focal stimulation. With more complex montages, it may be possible to achieve maximal current flow at structures rather deep within the brain – an approach akin to 'reverse EEG', with currents being applied rather than recorded.

The success of HD-tDCS depends critically on accurate modelling of current flow within the brain tissue, and on accurate placement of the electrodes at the precise locations used during the FEM simulations. For this reason, neuroimaging is essential to the success of HD-tDCS – potentially even more so than for neuronavigated rTMS. As tDCS studies move towards more complex montages, we expect MRI-based field simulations to play an increasingly integral role in the future of non-invasive electrical brain stimulation.

Deep brain stimulation

MRI has, of course, long played an indispensable role in the stereotaxic implantation of DBS electrodes at the intended targets. MRI-compatible stereotaxic frames, the selection and specification of implantation trajectories and stereotaxic coordinates based on pre-treatment MRI, and the verification of implant positioning based on post-treatment MRI/CT are all integral steps of a DBS implantation procedure.

More recent DBS studies have begun to incorporate *in vivo* MRI-based tractography into the treatment planning process. In the setting of major depression, DT images are now beginning to be used to identify specific tracts within the white matter of the subcallosal cingulate region and the anterior limb of the internal capsule, each projecting to distinct sets of infra- and supratentorial brain regions [103]. More complex models are now beginning to incorporate other structural imaging sequences alongside DTI, to perform FEM simulations of the spread of DBS stimulation when performed at various possible locations within the general target region [104]. These tractography-activation maps, somewhat akin to the HD-tDCS methods described earlier, have the potential to allow patient-specific adjustments in the stimulation target in order to improve treatment outcomes.

Characterizing the effects of neuromodulation using MRI

Transcranial direct current stimulation

fMRI is proving useful in characterizing the effects of tDCS on cortical activity at the network level, rather than merely at the site of stimulation. The results of these studies are providing useful information on how tDCS may be used therapeutically to treat psychiatric illness.

On rs-fMRI, a 20-min session of anodal tDCS to the left DLPFC caused increases in functional connectivity form the left DLPFC to right hemisphere frontal and temporal brain regions, with decreased functional connectivity locally to other regions of the left frontal lobe [105]. Another study used the same stimulation parameters and ICA to characterize changes in the activity of resting-state networks before and after stimulation [106]. In this case, tDCS increased functional connectivity within several resting-state networks, including the default-mode network and left- and right-hemisphere frontoparietal networks. Another similar study found that bilateral stimulation of the DLPFC, regardless of polarity, increased the synchronization of the lateral frontoparietal networks under stimulation, while decreasing the synchronization of the more medially located default-mode network, which was not directly stimulated [107].

Task-related fMRI has also revealed some unexpected findings on the effects of tDCS. Classically, tDCS is expected to modulate the activity of superficial brain regions under the stimulating electrode, since current flow is typically highest at these sites. However, one recent study found much deeper activations elicited via tDCS using a non-standard montage, with the anode over VMPFC and the cathode over right DLPFC. This montage was used to stimulate reward-related regions within the VMPFC and the ventral tegmental area (VTA), the latter of which would typically be considered too deep for stimulation via tDCS. However, using a task in which subjects rated the attractiveness of faces during fMRI, the authors showed that this tDCS montage successfully increased subjects' ratings of facial attractiveness, and that the magnitude of the effect correlated with the magnitude of increases in VTA and VMPFC activity on the task. Furthermore, the magnitude of effect also correlated with the degree of increase in resting-state functional connectivity between the VMPFC region and the deeper VTA. Studies of this type illustrate that tDCS has the potential to affect deep structures within the brain, potentially through network-level effects on resting brain activity.

MRI may also prove helpful in addressing the increasingly well-recognized problem of inter-individual differences in the response to tDCS. Although anodal tDCS is classically considered excitatory (and cathodal tDCS inhibitory), more recent studies suggest that the actual effects in any given subject can vary considerably. In one recent study in motor cortex, approximately 50% of individuals showed no response to either anodal or cathodal tDCS, while the remainder showed facilitation with both kinds of stimulation [108]. Such findings have problematic implications for the therapeutic potential of tDCS in treating psychiatric illness.

Using neuroimaging methods, one recent study sought to characterize potential sources of this variability [109]. The authors in this case applied anodal tDCS over the F3 EEG site (for left DLPFC stimulation). They used performance on the three-back working memory task as a behavioural measure of effect. There was considerable variability in outcomes, with some subjects showing more working memory enhancement than others. The authors then performed FEM on each subject's brain and were able to determine that some subjects received relatively little tDCS over the DLPFC, due to inter-individual variability in the correspondence of the scalp F3 site to the Left DLPFC region active during the task. These results suggest that at least some of the variability in tDCS outcomes for DLPFC stimulation might be explained by inadequate neuronavigational methods – an issue long recognized for rTMS but previously neglected with tDCS.

Transcranial magnetic stimulation

The underlying mechanisms of rTMS have been investigated extensively over the last 20 years using a variety of methods from motor electrophysiology to EEG to pharmacological manipulations to PET imaging with a variety of metabolic and receptor-based ligands. Each of these modalities is well suited to studying rTMS effects at a different level of explanation (e.g. at the level of the receptor, the synapse, the circuit or the whole brain). fMRI is likely best suited to understanding the effects of rTMS at the circuit or whole-brain level, somewhat akin to EEG, but with the added benefit that pre-rTMS imaging can provide individualized stimulation targets based on task-based or resting-state brain activity.

As with tDCS, variability of effects and outcomes is also a problematic issue in the rTMS literature. MRI methods may therefore be helpful in better understanding this potential impediment to successful therapeutic use. One particularly revealing study [110] performed rs-fMRI to assess the activity of the default-mode network before and after two kinds of stimulation: 20 Hz rTMS, which is classically considered excitatory, and 1 Hz rTMS, which is classically considered inhibitory. Notably, the authors used the pre-treatment scan in each individual subject to localize the stimulation target, in left posterior IPL. Twenty hertz stimulation of this target decreased its functional connectivity to other nodes of the default-mode network in medial parietal and prefrontal regions – an effect consistent in direction but variable in magnitude across subjects. However, 1 Hz stimulation had widely divergent effects across subjects, enhancing functional connectivity to other default-mode nodes in some subjects but inhibiting it in others (Figure 4.5). The variable effects of 1 Hz stimulation alongside more consistent effects of 20 Hz stimulation was reminiscent of similar effects seen on motor-evoked potentials in electrophysiological studies of rTMS conducted more than a decade earlier [111]. The implication in this case is that a given rTMS protocol may exert widely different network-level effects on resting brain activity in different subjects – a potential impediment to the success of therapeutic rTMS in psychiatric disease.

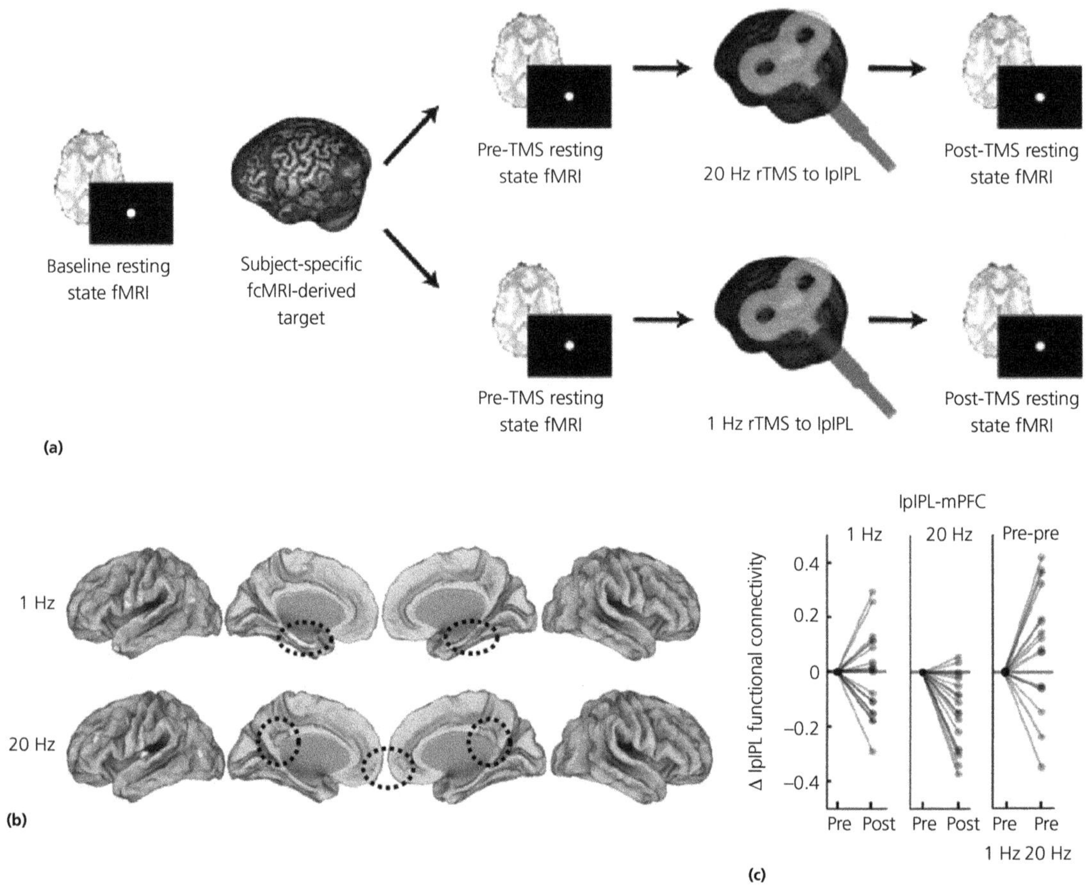

Figure 4.5 Use of MRI in characterizing effects of neuromodulation. (**a**) Eldaief et al. [110] used rs-fMRI to localize the default-mode network in individual subjects. They then applied either 1or 20 Hz rTMS to the left posterior IPL node of this network, using the peak activation coordinate in each subject. (**b**) Comparison of resting-state functional connectivity to the left posterior IPL, on fMRI scans obtained pre- and post-rTMS, revealed that 1 and 20 Hz rTMS produced distinct patterns of increases (orange) or decreases (blue) in whole-brain connectivity to the seed region, thus characterizing the effects of rTMS at the network level. (**c**) Inspection of individual subjects' changes in connectivity between two regions of the default-mode network (the IPL and the MPFC) revealed considerable inter-individual variability in both the magnitude and direction of effect for 1 Hz stimulation. Effects of 20 Hz stimulation were more consistent in direction but still variable in magnitude across subjects. Source: From Eldaidef et al. [110]. Reproduced with permission of PNAS. (*See insert for colour representation of the figure.*)

rs-fMRI is also beginning to enter use in characterizing the mechanisms by which rTMS achieves a therapeutic effect on disorders such as major depression. One recent study [112] found that 20 Hz stimulation of the left DLPFC enhanced functional connectivity between the DMPFC and subgenual cingulate cortex, which are both therapeutic targets in their own right in major depression. Furthermore, on the pre-treatment scan, responders had significantly more anti-correlated activity between subgenual cingulate cortex and medial and lateral regions of the frontopolar cortex. Following treatment, this pattern reversed, with responders achieving a positive correlation in the activity of these two regions, while non-responders showed a slight decline in functional connectivity. Changes in resting-state connectivity have also recently studied for rTMS of another target, the DMPFC, in major depression [66]. Before treatment, responders showed higher connectivity than non-responders from DMPFC to subgenual cingulate, and lower connectivity from DMPFC to striatal and thalamic regions. With successful treatment, DMPFC–thalamic connectivity increased, while DMPFC–insula connectivity decreased, as did subgenual–ventral striatal connectivity. Studies of this type may help to identify predictors and correlates of successful treatment outcome that might ultimately be used for treatment planning and parameter selection in individual patients.

MRI could also have potential uses in evaluating rTMS-induced changes in the structure of grey or white matter. The literature on rTMS-induced structural changes is fairly limited to date. However, one illustrative study [113] did use diffusion-weighted imaging sequences to examine whether the protocols used for rTMS in depression might potentially damage blood–brain barrier integrity. Apparent diffusion coefficient (ADC) scans are sensitive to even minor changes in cellular integrity, such as in ischaemic stroke – localized, measurable changes in ADC can be observed after as little as 15 min of ischaemia. In this case, the ADC imaging did not reveal any evidence that rTMS caused changes to blood–brain barrier integrity or apparent diffusion within the stimulated region.

DBS

fMRI studies in DBS have been somewhat curtailed by hesitancy over the safety of performing elective MRI in patients with implanted stimulators, as well as concerns over image quality degradation ensuing from signal artefact around the electrode itself. However, assuming that safety guidelines are followed, as reviewed earlier, fMRI can in some cases play an important post-surgical role in evaluating whether the stimulator is indeed modulating the desired pathways within the brain. In one striking illustration [114], a 36-year-old woman with medically refractory Parkinson's disease, and a past history of major depression, underwent bilateral DBS implantation in the subthalamic nucleus. Activation of the left-sided electrode elicited the usual rapid improvement in motor symptoms. However, activation of the right electrode elicited a rapid descent into acute, intense dysphoria, which the patient described as similar to a previous depressive episode but 'a thousand times worse'. Remarkably, the dysphoria also resolved rapidly with deactivation of the electrode, and the emotional state could be reproducibly elicited and abolished by activating and deactivating the electrode.

With electrodes externalized, the patient underwent fMRI using a block-design approach, with each electrode turned on and off sequentially. Stimulation via the left electrode stimulation, as expected, caused deactivations of medial motor areas such as the supplementary motor area, as well as activations in lateral premotor and motor cortex. However, stimulation of the right electrode instead deactivated medial Brodmann areas 9 and 10, anterior to the supplementary and pre-supplementary motor areas. As noted earlier, excitatory rTMS of the DMPFC has been used therapeutically to treat major depression, so the finding of acute dysphoria with deactivation of this region is consistent with the findings of other brain stimulation studies. Following fMRI, the electrode was successfully repositioned to achieve a therapeutic effect without eliciting dysphoria.

In a more recent application, fMRI was performed safely in 10 subjects with DBS electrodes implanted for Parkinson's disease [115]. Analysis of the fMRI data identified that DBS-induced activations in thalamus and insula associated with an improvement in motor symptoms. Analysis of the effective connectivity, using dynamic casual modelling, suggested that DBS reversed cortico-thalamic connections from inhibitory to excitatory, and in a reciprocal manner also reversed thalamocortical connections from inhibitory to excitatory. While preliminary, this finding illustrates the potential for fMRI to reveal mechanisms of DBS at the network level.

Optimizing individual treatment parameters using MRI

The most important future application of MRI in neuromodulation will likely be for the selection and optimization of treatment parameters in individual patients. As of this writing, there do not yet exist any widely accepted protocols for tailoring the parameters of stimulation in an individual patient based on structural or functional MRI findings. However, this is likely to change in the near future. With neuromodulation, MRI can potentially be helpful at three phases of treatment planning: diagnosis and subtyping of illness, selection of the optimal location for stimulation and selection of the optimal pattern of stimulation. Here we briefly review how MRI might contribute to each stage of treatment.

Regarding diagnosis, it is generally recognized that our current diagnostic categories encompass a heterogeneous assortment of pathologies, not all of which respond to any given form of treatment. Our current systems of subtyping (e.g. the distinction between 'atypical' and 'melancholic' depression, or even potentially between 'unipolar' and 'bipolar' depression) are also of somewhat unproven relevance to treatment decisions with neurostimulation. For example, ECT is routinely used in both unipolar and bipolar depression, DBS has been used in unipolar and bipolar depression [116] and meta-analyses of rTMS have found no difference in treatment efficacy for unipolar versus bipolar depression [117].

On the other hand, there are distinct patterns of resting-state functional connectivity that appear predictive of treatment outcome with rTMS at either the DLPFC or the DMPFC. Anhedonia and abnormal functional connectivity through ventral striatal-VMPFC reward circuits may be predictive of non-response to dorsomedial stimulation [45], while pretreatment functional connectivity to subgenual cingulate cortex [112] or within the default-mode network [118] may be predictive of response to DLPFC-rTMS.

As of this writing, rTMS responder–nonresponder differences in brain activity have been identified at the group level but not yet at the individual level. However, machine-learning methods are now being applied to rs-fMRI scans for automated classification of individual subjects as depressed or non-depressed [119] and in other diagnostic and prognostic setting in neurological and psychiatric illness [120]. It is likely that such methods will be applied successfully to outcome prediction for tDCS, rTMS and DBS in the near future, as sufficiently large datasets become available for classifier training.

Neuroimaging is also likely to play an increasingly important role in the selection of the optimal stimulation site, as has long been the case for DBS, and as is becoming the case for tDCS and for rTMS, as detailed earlier. DTI, in particular, may prove important for fine-tuning the location of stimulation using these three modalities. FEM, drawing upon structural MRI, may also prove useful. Finally, where multiple stimulation sites are potentially available (e.g. with rTMS applied to left, right or bilateral DLFPC or DMPFC), automated classifiers could eventually assume an important role in selecting the optimal treatment site based on rs-fMRI, once sufficiently large datasets become available for differential comparison of outcomes across multiple sites of stimulation.

Lastly, fMRI could also assume an important role in selecting the optimal parameters of stimulation: anodal versus cathodal in the case of tDCS, or high versus low frequency in the case of rTMS. As reviewed earlier, there is already a growing literature indicating that the effects of a given type of rTMS and tDCS are variable in both magnitude and direction across individuals. Furthermore, an incipient literature is now beginning to link this variability to pre-treatment resting-state functional connectivity patterns across the brain as a whole. The implication is that pre-treatment rs-fMRI could prove useful in predicting whether a given stimulation pattern will produce inhibition, excitation or no effect in a particular patient presenting for treatment. There is already a small body of literature on the differential effects of high- versus low-frequency rTMS in major depression, suggesting that individual subjects have opposite responses to the two types of stimulation, and that metabolic imaging using PET or SPECT can be used to predict which type of stimulation will exert a beneficial therapeutic effect [121, 122]. Given this context, it is likely that fMRI could assume a role in guiding the selection of the parameters of stimulation, as well as the site of stimulation, in the near future.

Neuromodulatory effects of MRI itself

One of the important lessons of low-intensity neuromodulation techniques such as tDCS is that even very weak electromagnetic fields can exert significant effects on neural activity, of a magnitude that is sufficient for both clinical treatment and basic research. A neglected implication of this work is that the RF fields applied to the brain during MRI itself could potentially exert measurable and clinically relevant effects on neural activity.

One of the first demonstrations of this possibility was a pair of PET studies examining the neural effects of RF emissions from the antennae of cellular telephones held in the standard position by the ear [123, 124]. The design in both cases employed cellphones placed on each side of the head, silenced, with the subject blind to which phone was active. One study [123] applied a typical GSM carrier signal of 0.5 ms bursts every 4.6 ms, while the other [124] used a more naturalistic recorded voice message. Both studies identified changes in regional cerebral glucose metabolism in the anterior temporal lobe ipsilateral to the active antenna. Of note, however, the direction of effect was opposite in the two studies, with the voice message causing enhancement and the carrier signal causing inhibition of activity. The magnitude of effect was linearly proportional to the local RF energy, and the absolute increases of approximately 7% in the latter study was comparable to that observed with rTMS (despite the 2–3 orders of magnitude difference in induced electrical field). Since the SARs associated with common MRI sequences can be more than an order of magnitude higher than those seen with cellphone use, the implication was that the RF head coil of the MRI might exert similar effects across more widespread regions of brain tissue.

A direct demonstration of MRI-induced changes in cerebral metabolism was reported around the same time [125] by injecting ^{18}fluorodeoxyglucose (FDG) tracer into subjects during either a standard EPI fMRI sequence or sham EPI with simulated scanner noise delivered via headphones. Compared to sham, active EPI induced reductions in brain metabolism of approximately 0.2–0.3%, with the reduction again being linearly proportional to the strength of the local electrical field. Spatially, the changes were least pronounced at the isocentre of the applied gradients (near the centre of the head) and greatest in the anterior, posterior, superior and inferior extrema of the brain. Thus, fMRI could *in itself* be considered as a form of spatially constrained neuromodulation.

Although the changes in metabolism with fMRI were small in absolute terms, they may still be of clinical and research significance. In a noteworthy finding [126], 40 patients with bipolar disorder entered a standard 1.5-T MRI scanner and underwent either echo-planar magnetic spectroscopy (EP-MRS) or an 'active sham' 3D spoiled gradient echo scan (SPGR) of equivalent duration. Seventy-seven percent of patients undergoing EP-MRS, but only 30% of patients undergoing 3D SPGR, showed mood improvement on the Brief Affect Scale; of unmedicated patients, 100% showed improvement with EP-MRS. The induced electrical fields, calculated to be in the order of 0.7 V/m, were comparable to those seen with tDCS but distributed over a much wider area encompassing most of the superficial regions of the cortex.

More recently, Rohan et al. [127] constructed a prototype *low-field magnetic stimulation* (LFMS) device resembling a cylindrical RF head coil without the encumbrance of an MRI scanner attached. In a randomized, double-blind, sham-controlled design, they applied 20 min to a 1-kHz oscillating field of >1 V/m (~100-fold weaker than rTMS, and comparable to tDCS) to 41 patients with bipolar disorder and 22 patients with unipolar depression. The induced electrical field was distinctly non-focal, covering most of the surface of both cortical hemispheres. Despite this non-focality, compared to sham treatment, this single session of active LFMS improved mood by about 10% of the baseline score on standard mood rating scales including the Hamilton Depression Rating Scale, the Positive and Negative Affect Schedule and a visual analogue scale for mood.

These results are certainly preliminary and will require further investigation and replication in larger samples of patients, with additional sessions of stimulation to see whether cumulative effects can be achieved. However, if robust, these observations could conceivably lead to an entirely new class of neuromodulation – one that could allow existing MRI infrastructure to be used for both imaging and intervention.

Conclusions

In summary, a wide variety of MRI sequences are available for investigation of the structure and function of the human brain *in vivo*. These sequences can be useful for 'off-line' investigations of the effects of tDCS, rTMS and DBS on brain structure and function. Most of the major neuromodulation techniques can also be performed safely 'on-line' in the MRI environment with appropriate modifications and precautions. MRI has several distinct roles in neuromodulation. These range from conducting basic research on new targets for stimulation, to ensuring accurate placement of stimulation inductors via neuronavigation, to characterizing the effects of neuromodulation on brain structure and function (including variability across individuals), to optimizing the stimulation target and sequence for each individual patient presenting for treatment. Finally, MRI itself may exert a neuromodulatory effect, and this may have the potential for translation into entirely new modalities of neuromodulation using low-intensity electromagnetic fields. Neuroimaging and neurostimulation have always been closely intertwined, and their longstanding and fruitful alliance seems destined to continue for many years to come.

Acknowledgements

Karen Davis is supported by grants from the Canadian Institutes of Health Research.

Dr Downar's research is supported by peer-reviewed funding from the Canadian Institutes of Health Research, the Ontario Brain Institute and the Klarman Family Foundation, as well as funding from the Buchan Family Foundation and the Toronto General and Western Hospital Foundation. He has also received a travel stipend from Lundbeck and in-kind support for an investigator-initiated trial from MagVenture.

References

1 Davis KD, Moayedi M. Central mechanisms of pain revealed through functional and structural MRI. J Neuroimmune Pharmacol 2013;8:518–534.

2 Ashburner J, Friston KJ. Voxel-based morphometry – the methods. Neuroimage 2000; 11:805–821.

3 Fischl B, Dale AM. Measuring the thickness of the human cerebral cortex from magnetic resonance images. Proc Natl Acad Sci U S A 2000;97:11050–11055.

4 Moayedi M, Weissman-Fogel I, Salomons TV, Crawley AP, Goldberg MB, Freeman BV, Tenenbaum HC, Davis KD. Abnormal gray matter aging in chronic pain patients. Brain Res 2012;1456:82–93.

5 Hutton C, Draganski B, Ashburner J, Weiskopf N. A comparison between voxel-based cortical thickness and voxel-based morphometry in normal aging. Neuroimage 2009;48:371–380.

6 Mori S, Zhang J. Principles of diffusion tensor imaging and its applications to basic neuroscience research. Neuron 2006;51:527–539.

7 Johansen-Berg H, Rushworth MF. Using diffusion imaging to study human connectional anatomy. Annu Rev Neurosci 2009;32: 75–94.

8 DeSouza DD, Hodaie M, Davis KD. Abnormal trigeminal nerve microstructure and brain white matter in idiopathic trigeminal neuralgia. Pain 2014;155:37–44.

9 Zatorre RJ, Fields RD, Johansen-Berg H. Plasticity in gray and white: neuroimaging changes in brain structure during learning. Nat Neurosci 2012;15:528–536.

10 Le BD, Johansen-Berg H. Diffusion MRI at 25: exploring brain tissue structure and function. Neuroimage 2012;61:324–341.

11 Smith SM, Jenkinson M, Johansen-Berg H, Rueckert D, Nichols TE, Mackay CE, Watkins KE, Ciccarelli O, Cader MZ, Matthews PM, Behrens TE. Tract-based spatial statistics: voxelwise analysis of multi-subject diffusion data. Neuroimage 2006;31:1487–1505.

12 Ogawa S, Lee TM, Kay AR, Tank DW. Brain magnetic resonance imaging with contrast dependent on blood oxygenation. Proc Natl Acad Sci U S A 1990;87:9868–9872.

13 Davis KD. Recent advances and future prospects in neuroimaging of acute and chronic pain. Future Neurol 2006;1:203–213.

14 Davis KD, Pope GE, Crawley AP, Mikulis DJ. Neural correlates of prickle sensation: a percept-related fMRI study. Nat Neurosci 2002;5: 1121–1122.

15 Kwan CL, Diamant NE, Mikulis DJ, Davis KD. Percept-related fMRI of rectal-evoked sensations in irritable bowel syndrome. Society for Neuroscience 2002.

16 Friston KJ. Functional and effective connectivity in neuroimaging: a synthesis. Hum Brain Mapp 1994;2:56–78.

17 Fox MD, Raichle ME. Spontaneous fluctuations in brain activity observed with functional magnetic resonance imaging. Nat Rev Neurosci 2007;8:700–711.

18 Hutchison RM, Womelsdorf T, Allen EA, Bandettini PA, Calhoun VD, Corbetta M, Della PS, Duyn JH, Glover GH, Gonzalez-Castillo J, Handwerker DA, Keilholz S, Kiviniemi V, Leopold DA, de PF, Sporns O, Walter M, Chang C. Dynamic functional connectivity: Promise, issues, and interpretations. Neuroimage 2013; 80:360–378.

19 Andrews-Hann JR. The brain's default network and its adaptive role in internal mentation. Neuroscientist 2012;18:251–270.

20 Greicius MD, Supekar K, Menon V, Dougherty RF. Resting-state functional connectivity reflects structural connectivity in the default mode network. Cereb Cortex 2009;19:72–78.

21 Honey CJ, Sporns O, Cammoun L, Gigandet X, Thiran JP, Meuli R, Hagmann P. Predicting human resting-state functional connectivity from structural connectivity. Proc Natl Acad Sci U S A 2009;106:2035–2040.

22 Vincent JL, Patel GH, Fox MD, Snyder AZ, Baker JT, Van E, Zempel JM, Snyder LH, Corbetta M, Raichle ME. Intrinsic functional architecture in the anaesthetized monkey brain. Nature 2007;447:83–86.

23 Mars RB, Jbabdi S, Sallet J, O'Reilly JX, Croxson PL, Olivier E, Noonan MP, Bergmann C, Mitchell AS, Baxter MG, Behrens TE, Johansen-Berg H, Tomassini V, Miller KL, Rushworth MF. Diffusion-weighted imaging tractography-based parcellation of the human parietal cortex and comparison with human and macaque

resting-state functional connectivity. J Neurosci 2011;31:4087–4100.
24 Adachi Y, Osada T, Sporns O, Watanabe T, Matsui T, Miyamoto K, Miyashita Y. Functional connectivity between anatomically unconnected areas is shaped by collective network-level effects in the macaque cortex. Cereb Cortex 2012;22:1586–1592.
25 Wang Z, Chen LM, Negyessy L, Friedman RM, Mishra A, Gore JC, Roe AW. The relationship of anatomical and functional connectivity to resting-state connectivity in primate somatosensory cortex. Neuron 2013;78:1116–1126.
26 Wang L, Saalmann YB, Pinsk MA, Arcaro MJ, Kastner S. Electrophysiological low-frequency coherence and cross-frequency coupling contribute to BOLD connectivity. Neuron 2012;76: 1010–1020.
27 Chang C, Liu Z, Chen MC, Liu X, Duyn JH. EEG correlates of time-varying BOLD functional connectivity. Neuroimage 2013;72:227–236.
28 Tagliazucchi E, von WF, Morzelewski A, Brodbeck V, Laufs H. Dynamic BOLD functional connectivity in humans and its electrophysiological correlates. Front Hum Neurosci 2012; 6:339.
29 Raichle ME, MacLeod AM, Snyder AZ, Powers WJ, Gusnard DA, Shulman GL. A default mode of brain function. Proc Natl Acad Sci U S A 2001;98:676–682.
30 Fransson P. Spontaneous low-frequency BOLD signal fluctuations: an fMRI investigation of the resting-state default mode of brain function hypothesis. Hum Brain Mapp 2005;26:15–29.
31 Weissman-Fogel I, Moayedi M, Taylor KS, Pope G, Davis KD. Cognitive and default-mode resting state networks: do male and female brains 'rest' differently? Hum Brain Mapp 2010;31:1713–1726.
32 van den Heuvel MP, Hulshoff Pol HE. Exploring the brain network: a review on resting-state fMRI functional connectivity. Eur Neuropsychopharmacol 2010;20:519–534.
33 Lee MH, Hacker CD, Snyder AZ, Corbetta M, Zhang D, Leuthardt EC, Shimony JS. Clustering of resting state networks. PLoS One 2012;7:e40370.
34 Taylor KS, Seminowicz DA, Davis KD. Two systems of resting state connectivity between the insula and cingulate cortex. Hum Brain Mapp 2009;30:2731–2745.
35 Handwerker DA, Roopchansingh V, Gonzalez-Castillo J, Bandettini PA. Periodic changes in fMRI connectivity. Neuroimage 2012;63:1712–1719.
36 Chang C, Glover GH. Time-frequency dynamics of resting-state brain connectivity measured with fMRI. Neuroimage 2010;50:81–98.
37 Kucyi A, Salomons TV, Davis KD. Mind wandering away from pain dynamically engages antinociceptive and default mode brain networks. Proc Natl Acad Sci U S A 2013;110: 18692–18697.
38 Kucyi A, Davis KD. Dynamic fluctuations in intrinsic functional connectivity within and between resting state networks. Human Brain Mapping Conference Proceedings 2013.
39 Thompson GJ, Merritt MD, Pan WJ, Magnuson ME, Grooms JK, Jaeger D, Keilholz SD. Neural correlates of time-varying functional connectivity in the rat. Neuroimage 2013;83:826–836.
40 Pan H, Epstein J, Silbersweig DA, Stern E. New and emerging imaging techniques for mapping brain circuitry. Brain Res Rev 2011;67: 226–251.
41 Wu WC, St Lawrence KS, Licht DJ, Wang DJ. Quantification issues in arterial spin labeling perfusion magnetic resonance imaging. Top Magn Reson Imaging 2010;21:65–73.
42 Tracey I, Johns E. The pain matrix: reloaded or reborn as we image tonic pain using arterial spin labelling. Pain 2010;148:359–360.
43 Bullmore E, Sporns O. Complex brain networks: graph theoretical analysis of structural and functional systems. Nat Rev Neurosci 2009; 10:186–198.
44 Polania R, Paulus W, Antal A, Nitsche MA. Introducing graph theory to track for neuroplastic alterations in the resting human brain: a transcranial direct current stimulation study. Neuroimage 2011;54:2287–2296.
45 Downar J, Geraci J, Salomons TV, Dunlop K, Wheeler S, McAndrews MP, Bakker N, Blumberger DM, Daskalakis ZJ, Kennedy SH, Flint AJ, Giacobbe P. Anhedonia and reward-circuit connectivity distinguish nonresponders from responders to dorsomedial prefrontal repetitive transcranial magnetic stimulation in major depression. Biol Psychiatry 2014;76:176–85.
46 Bohning DE, Shastri A, Nahas Z, Lorberbaum JP, Andersen SW, Dannels WR, Haxthausen EU, Vincent DJ, George MS. Echoplanar BOLD

fMRI of brain activation induced by concurrent transcranial magnetic stimulation. Invest Radiol 1998;33:336–340.
47 Siebner HR, Bergmann TO, Bestmann S, Massimini M, Johansen-Berg H, Mochizuki H, Bohning DE, Boorman ED, Groppa S, Miniussi C, Pascual-Leone A, Huber R, Taylor PC, Ilmoniemi RJ, De GL, Strafella AP, Kahkonen S, Kloppel S, Frisoni GB, George MS, Hallett M, Brandt SA, Rushworth MF, Ziemann U, Rothwell JC, Ward N, Cohen LG, Baudewig J, Paus T, Ugawa Y, Rossini PM. Consensus paper: combining transcranial stimulation with neuroimaging. Brain Stimul 2009;2:58–80.
48 Hanlon CA, Canterberry M, Taylor JJ, DeVries W, Li X, Brown TR, George MS. Probing the frontostriatal loops involved in executive and limbic processing via interleaved TMS and functional MRI at two prefrontal locations: a pilot study. PLoS One 2013;8:e67917.
49 Yau JM, Jalinous R, Cantarero GL, Desmond JE. static field influences on transcranial magnetic stimulation: considerations for TMS in the scanner environment. Brain Stimul 2014;7:388–393.
50 Bohning DE, Pecheny AP, Epstein CM, Speer AM, Vincent DJ, Dannels W, George MS. Mapping transcranial magnetic stimulation (TMS) fields in vivo with MRI. Neuroreport 1997;8:2535–2538.
51 Saiote C, Turi Z, Paulus W, Antal A. Combining functional magnetic resonance imaging with transcranial electrical stimulation. Front Hum Neurosci 2013;7:435.
52 Antal A, Polania R, Schmidt-Samoa C, Dechent P, Paulus W. Transcranial direct current stimulation over the primary motor cortex during fMRI. Neuroimage 2011;55:590–596.
53 Antal A, Bikson M, Datta A, Lafon B, Dechent P, Parra LC, Paulus W. Imaging artifacts induced by electrical stimulation during conventional fMRI of the brain. Neuroimage 2014;85 Pt 3:1040–1047.
54 Carmichael DW, Pinto S, Limousin-Dowsey P, Thobois S, Allen PJ, Lemieux L, Yousry T, Thornton JS. Functional MRI with active, fully implanted, deep brain stimulation systems: safety and experimental confounds. Neuroimage 2007;37:508–517.
55 Tagliati M, Jankovic J, Pagan F, Susatia F, Isaias IU, Okun MS. Safety of MRI in patients with implanted deep brain stimulation devices. Neuroimage 2009;47 Suppl 2:T53–T57.
56 Zrinzo L, Yoshida F, Hariz MI, Thornton J, Foltynie T, Yousry TA, Limousin P. Clinical safety of brain magnetic resonance imaging with implanted deep brain stimulation hardware: large case series and review of the literature. World Neurosurg 2011;76:164–172.
57 Henderson JM, Tkach J, Phillips M, Baker K, Shellock FG, Rezai AR. Permanent neurological deficit related to magnetic resonance imaging in a patient with implanted deep brain stimulation electrodes for Parkinson's disease: case report. Neurosurgery. 2005;57(5):E1063.
58 Spiegel J, Fuss G, Backens M, Reith W, Magnus T, Becker G, Moringlane JR, Dillmann U. Transient dystonia following magnetic resonance imaging in a patient with deep brain stimulation electrodes for the treatment of Parkinson disease. Case Rep J Neurosurg 2003;99:772–774.
59 Bora E, Fornito A, Pantelis C, Yucel M. Gray matter abnormalities in major depressive disorder: a meta-analysis of voxel based morphometry studies. J Affect Disord 2012;138:9–18.
60 Sheline YI, Price JL, Yan Z, Mintun MA. Resting-state functional MRI in depression unmasks increased connectivity between networks via the dorsal nexus. Proc Natl Acad Sci U S A 2010;107:11020–11025.
61 Downar J, Daskalakis ZJ. New targets for rTMS in depression: a review of convergent evidence. Brain Stimul 2013;6:231–240.
62 George MS, Wassermann EM, Williams WA, Callahan A, Ketter TA, Basser P, Hallett M, Post RM. Daily repetitive transcranial magnetic stimulation (rTMS) improves mood in depression. Neuroreport 1995;6:1853–1856.
63 Pascual-Leone A, Rubio B, Pallardo F, Catala MD. Rapid-rate transcranial magnetic stimulation of left dorsolateral prefrontal cortex in drug-resistant depression. Lancet 1996;348:233–237.
64 Price JL, Drevets WC. Neural circuits underlying the pathophysiology of mood disorders. Trends Cogn Sci. 2012;16(1):61–71.
65 Vanneste S, Ost J, Langguth B, De RD. TMS by double-cone coil prefrontal stimulation for medication resistant chronic depression: a case report. Neurocase 2014;20:61–68.

66 Salomons TV, Dunlop K, Kennedy SH, Flint A, Geraci J, Giacobbe P, Downar J. Resting-state cortico-thalamic-striatal connectivity predicts response to dorsomedial prefrontal rTMS in major depressive disorder. Neuropsychopharmacology 2014;39:488–498.
67 Radua J, van den Heuvel OA, Surguladze S, Mataix-Cols D. Meta-analytical comparison of voxel-based morphometry studies in obsessive-compulsive disorder vs other anxiety disorders. Arch Gen Psychiatry 2010;67:701–711.
68 Kuhn S, Gallinat J. Gray matter correlates of posttraumatic stress disorder: a quantitative meta-analysis. Biol Psychiatry 2013;73:70–74.
69 Hirao K, Miyata J, Fujiwara H, Yamada M, Namiki C, Shimizu M, Sawamoto N, Fukuyama H, Hayashi T, Murai T. Theory of mind and frontal lobe pathology in schizophrenia: a voxel-based morphometry study. Schizophr Res 2008;105:165–174.
70 Mantovani A, Simpson HB, Fallon BA, Rossi S, Lisanby SH. Randomized sham-controlled trial of repetitive transcranial magnetic stimulation in treatment-resistant obsessive-compulsive disorder. Int J Neuropsychopharmacol 2010;13:217–227.
71 Isserles M, Shalev AY, Roth Y, Peri T, Kutz I, Zlotnick E, Zangen A. Effectiveness of deep transcranial magnetic stimulation combined with a brief exposure procedure in post-traumatic stress disorder – a pilot study. Brain Stimul 2013;6:377–383.
72 Enticott PG, Fitzgibbon BM, Kennedy HA, Arnold SL, Elliot D, Peachey A, Zangen A, Fitzgerald PB. A double-blind, randomized trial of deep repetitive transcranial magnetic stimulation (rTMS) for autism spectrum disorder. Brain Stimul 2014;7:206–211.
73 McClernon FJ, Hiott FB, Huettel SA, Rose JE. Abstinence-induced changes in self-report craving correlate with event-related FMRI responses to smoking cues. Neuropsychopharmacology 2005;30:1940–1947.
74 Rose JE, McClernon FJ, Froeliger B, Behm FM, Preud'homme X, Krystal AD. Repetitive transcranial magnetic stimulation of the superior frontal gyrus modulates craving for cigarettes. Biol Psychiatry 2011;70:794–799.
75 Joos AA, Saum B, Zeeck A, Perlov E, Glauche V, Hartmann A, Freyer T, Sandholz A, Unterbrink T, van Elst LT, Tuscher O. Frontocingular dysfunction in bulimia nervosa when confronted with disease-specific stimuli. Eur Eat Disord Rev 2011;19:447–453.
76 Downar J, Sankar A, Giacobbe P, Woodside B, Colton P. Unanticipated rapid remission of refractory bulimia nervosa, during high-dose repetitive transcranial magnetic stimulation of the dorsomedial prefrontal cortex: a case report. Front Psychiatry 2012;3:30.
77 Mantovani A, Simeon D, Urban N, Bulow P, Allart A, Lisanby S. Temporo-parietal junction stimulation in the treatment of depersonalization disorder. Psychiatry Res 2011;186:138–140.
78 Loo CK, Alonzo A, Martin D, Mitchell PB, Galvez V, Sachdev P. Transcranial direct current stimulation for depression: 3-week, randomised, sham-controlled trial. Br J Psychiatry 2012; 200:52–59.
79 Brunoni AR, Valiengo L, Baccaro A, Zanao TA, de Oliveira JF, Goulart A, Boggio PS, Lotufo PA, Bensenor IM, Fregni F. The sertraline vs. electrical current therapy for treating depression clinical study: results from a factorial, randomized, controlled trial. JAMA Psychiatry 2013;70:383–391.
80 Andrade C. Transcranial direct current stimulation for refractory auditory hallucinations in schizophrenia. J Clin Psychiatry 2013;74:e1054–e1058.
81 Karim AA, Schneider M, Lotze M, Veit R, Sauseng P, Braun C, Birbaumer N. The truth about lying: inhibition of the anterior prefrontal cortex improves deceptive behavior. Cereb Cortex 2010;20:205–213.
82 Ganis G, Kosslyn SM, Stose S, Thompson WL, Yurgelun-Todd DA. Neural correlates of different types of deception: an fMRI investigation. Cereb Cortex 2003;13:830–836.
83 Ressler KJ, Mayberg HS. Targeting abnormal neural circuits in mood and anxiety disorders: from the laboratory to the clinic. Nat Neurosci 2007;10:1116–1124.
84 Mayberg HS, Lozano AM, Voon V, McNeely HE, Seminowicz D, Hamani C, Schwalb JM, Kennedy SH. Deep brain stimulation for treatment-resistant depression. Neuron 2005; 45:651–660.
85 Kennedy SH, Giacobbe P, Rizvi SJ, Placenza FM, Nishikawa Y, Mayberg HS, Lozano AM. Deep brain stimulation for treatment-resistant dep-

CHAPTER 5

Nuclear medicine in neuromodulation

Alexandra M. Rodman[1] and Darin D. Dougherty[2]
[1]*Harvard University, Cambridge, USA*
[2]*Massachusetts General Hospital, Boston, USA*

Introduction

In the first half of the 20th century, neuromodulation interventions such as psychosurgery and electroconvulsive shock therapy were sometimes administered in an excessive and indiscriminant fashion (e.g. Walter Freeman's frontal lobotomies), with poor outcomes, a high risk for mortality and low regard for patient rights [14]. More recently, however, neuromodulation techniques, which include both invasive targeted psychosurgery and non-invasive stimulation techniques, have gained approbation as they have proven to be a useful treatment for intractable (i.e. treatment resistant) psychiatric disorders, such as major depressive disorder (MDD) and obsessive–compulsive disorder (OCD). Patients with these disorders are the most common candidates for neuromodulation, as approximately 20% of patients do not respond to conventional treatments. Moreover, the better-established pathophysiology of these disorders enhances the ability to target specific regions for neuromodulation. Common neuromodulatory treatments for psychiatric disorders include electroconvulsive therapy (ECT), transcranial magnetic stimulation (TMS), transcranial direct current stimulation (tDCS), vagus nerve stimulation (VNS), ablative procedures (i.e. refined and targeted lesion surgeries) and deep brain stimulation (DBS).

Positron emission tomography (PET) emerged early on as a functional neuroimaging technique suitable for measuring the effects of neuromodulation. PET is particularly amenable to the imaging of individuals with neurotherapeutic implants (e.g. DBS and VNS) because the acquisition of images relies upon gamma ray signalling and is not susceptible to disruptions in electrical or magnetic fields. Currently, there are three leading experimental designs that utilize PET imaging in the study of neuromodulation. First, PET has been used to examine abnormalities in neuronal functioning in specific neuropsychiatric disorders in order to determine suitable targets for treatment. Second, studies have acquired images pre- and post-intervention to assess the mechanisms of action or change for a given treatment. Lastly, and perhaps most clinically useful, a small number of studies have used PET to determine neural patterns of activation that predict treatment response (Figure 5.1).

The discovery of biological predictors based on neuroimaging phenotypes in combination with clinical phenotypes would be a profound clinical tool and could eventually allow for individually tailored treatment plans. Currently, behavioural characteristics that have been useful in predicting response to conventional treatments (e.g. psychotropic medication and

Neuromodulation in Psychiatry, First Edition. Edited by Clement Hamani, Paul Holtzheimer, Andres M. Lozano and Helen Mayberg.

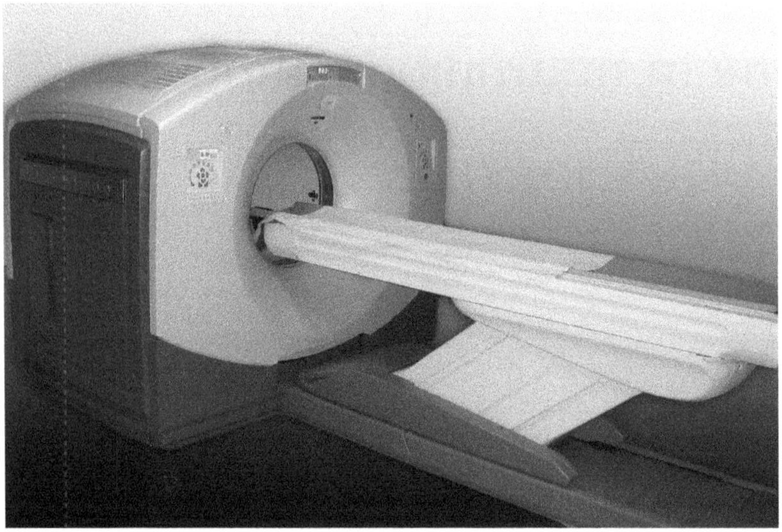

Figure 5.1 Photograph of a PET/CT machine developed by General Electric.

behavioural therapy) are limited to patients with low-to-moderate severity of psychiatric symptoms. Neuroimaging could provide insights that assist in diagnosis and indicate probabilistic outcomes to treatment options. This is especially of value to candidates for neuromodulation interventions, which are not without its associated risks, burdens and costs.

Currently, the use of PET imaging tools to predict treatment response for psychiatric disorders in the context of research studies has primarily been limited to conventional treatments such as behavioural and psychopharmacological treatment. In a seminal study by Mayberg and colleagues, authors showed that, when compared to healthy controls, depressed patients with hypermetabolism in the pregenual anterior cingulate cortex (ACC) predicts favourable treatment response to antidepressants, while hypometabolism in this region predicts non-response [28]. Another study found that lower metabolism in the midbrain predicted MDD remission as well as percentage of symptom reduction following 12 weeks of antidepressant treatment [32]. PET research can also be used to predict treatment outcome based on the strength of connectivity along pathways implicated in MDD. Investigators used structural equation modelling to identify pathways that predict response to different treatment types. While cingulo-subcortical pathways distinguished responders from non-responders across treatment types, limbic-cortical pathways to and from the subgenual cingulate selectively identified pharmacological treatment responders and a medial prefronto-orbitofrontal pathway selectively identified cognitive behavioural therapy (CBT) responders [46]. Similar studies have been conducted to predict outcome in the treatment of OCD. While hypermetabolism in the orbitofrontal regions predicts favourable outcomes in response to behavioural therapy, hypometabolism in this region predicts response to pharmacological intervention, namely selective serotonin reuptake inhibitors (SSRIs; [52, 7, 39]). This dichotomy highlights the potential for neuroimaging to guide treatment course decisions in a clinical setting. Although OCD and MDD respond to similar treatments, the mechanisms of change are believed to be distinct. In an SSRI treatment study that examined the disorders head-to-head, responders with MDD had lower pre-treatment metabolism in the amygdala and thalamus, whereas those with OCD had higher pre-treatment metabolism in the right caudate nucleus [44]. These predictor studies also serve to clarify the pathophysiology of psychiatric disorders and the underlying processes that result from treatment interventions [29].

However, neuroimaging can cost upwards of $2000, while conventional treatments are of relatively low cost. Therefore, the utilization of neuroimaging to determine a suitable behavioural or pharmacological treatment regimen in clinical practice may not be feasible. Neuromodulatory treatments, on the other hand, are extremely costly and intended only for the severely ill. DBS, VNS and ablative procedures can cost upwards of $100000 and confer the standard risks associated with neurosurgery. Even non-invasive techniques, such as TMS, tDCS and ECT are burdensome, as they require frequent treatment sessions that amount to a substantial sum of time and resources. Although the success of neuromodulation for intractable mental illness is promising, not all patients who receive these treatments exhibit a positive clinical response. Therefore, there is a major impetus to distinguish potential responders of specific neuromodulatory treatments and refine patient selection. As discussed, neuroimaging techniques may be able to elucidate neural correlates of treatment response and guide clinical decisions in ways that symptom profiles alone cannot. First, we will introduce basic principles and function of PET imaging. This will provide a framework from which we will discuss the role of PET in neuromodulation for psychiatric disorders.

Basic principles of PET

PET is a relatively non-invasive neuroimaging technique that measures various aspects of brain function. Using quantitative analysis, PET imaging allows scientists to measure biological processes such as blood flow, oxygen utilization, glucose metabolism and neurochemistry. This technique is based on the detection of radioactive decay emitted from body tissue after a small dose of radioactive tracer is injected into a peripheral vein. Commonly used radiotracers, or nuclides, are 11-carbon (^{11}C), 15-oxygen (^{15}O), 18-flourine (^{18}F) and 13-nitrogen (^{13}N). As carbon, oxygen, hydrogen (^{18}F substitutes an existing hydrogen atom) and nitrogen are the building blocks of all organic molecules, these nuclides can be easily incorporated into a molecule of choice and are particularly useful for the study of biological processes.

These unstable, radioactive nuclides possess an excess of protons and, as such, emit a positively charged atomic particle called a positron in order to return to a stable state. The positron subsequently collides with a negatively charged electron resulting in an annihilation event, whereby the mass of the two particles is converted to energy in the form of two gamma photons. As these photons travel in exactly opposite directions from each other, the PET camera is able to detect these gamma photons, or gamma rays, and determine the point of collision (Figure 5.2).

Gamma ray detection

Following the positron–electron annihilation event, the resulting gamma rays are detected by using the PET camera, which is shaped like a ring. The camera uses a series of crystalline scintillation detectors to capture the gamma rays and convert them into light. Photomultiplier tubes then convert the light into data that are recorded by the PET camera computer.

In practice, an individual is injected (intravenously) with a radiopharmaceutical and placed inside the ring of the PET camera. According to its properties, the radiopharmaceutical, from which gamma rays are emitted, is distributed throughout the different tissues of the body. Because the gamma rays project in opposite directions (180°) from the site of the collision, it is presumed that annihilation event occurred at some point along a hypothetical line that connects opposing sides of

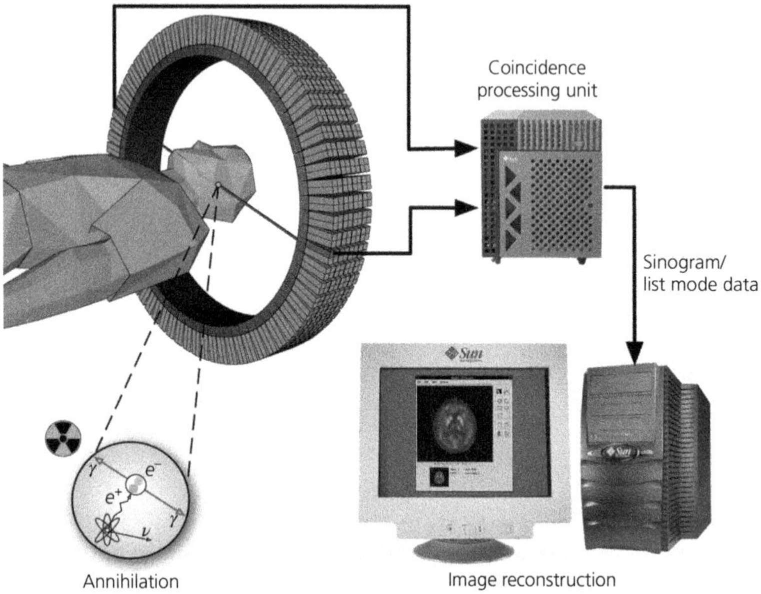

Figure 5.2 Illustration of gamma ray camera.

the PET camera. Therefore, detectors on opposite sides of the camera ring are coupled to form a coincidence circuit. Sophisticated computer algorithms are then used to calculate the location of all the coincidence events to create tomographic images of the biological tissue. This allows us to visualize relative concentrations of radioactive decay in different regions of the body.

What can PET measure?

PET can measure regional cerebral blood flow (rCBF) and glucose metabolism in the brain, which acts as an indirect measure of neuronal activity. Blood flow is typically measured by using ^{15}O compounds, which has a short half-life of 2 min. ^{18}F-Fluorodeoxyglucose (FDG) is used to measure glucose metabolism. ^{18}F-FDG is phosphorylated through the same pathway as glucose, but is unable to move beyond this metabolic step and becomes trapped in the neuron. This is referred to as FDG uptake and serves as a marker of metabolic activity (Figure 5.3).

PET can also be used to investigate different aspects of neurotransmitter functioning. Radiopharmaceuticals can be synthesized to specifically target a variety of processes such as neurotransmitter function, pre- and post-synaptic receptor densities, along with transporter and reuptake mechanisms. Recent advances in radiopharmaceutical synthesis allow scientists to examine more complex processes such as protein synthesis, DNA replication, second-messenger systems and gene expression (e.g. mRNA transcription).

Radiopharmaceuticals

Molecules involved in any biological process can be coupled with a radionuclide to create a radiopharmaceutical. For instance, H_2O and CO_2 are molecules that can be labelled with ^{15}O as a marker of blood flow, as water and carbon dioxide are molecules that are commonly transported by blood. Likewise, by labelling fluorodeoxyglucose with ^{18}F, we can measure glucose metabolism. Both blood flow and glucose metabolism serve as an indirect measure of neuronal activity. A number of radiopharmaceuticals can also be synthesized to bind to different types of neuroreceptors (see Table 5.1). By acquiring PET images sequentially, or over time, studies can examine the dynamic

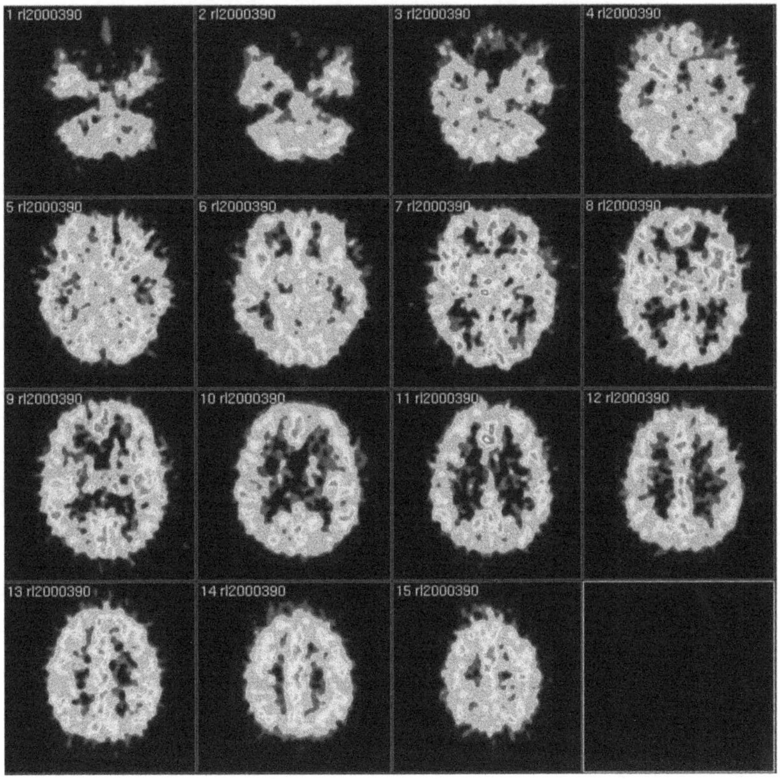

Figure 5.3 Axial view of a FDG-PET images.

Table 5.1 Common radioligands used in PET are provided.

Nuclide	Half-life (min)	Decay product	Radioligands	Target
^{11}C	20.4	^{11}B	[^{11}C] methylphenidate	DAT reuptake
			[^{11}C] raclopride	D_2 receptor
			[^{11}C] diprenorphine	Opioid receptor
			[^{11}C] DASB	5-HTT
^{13}N	9.98	^{13}C	[^{13}N] ammonia	
^{15}O	2.03	^{15}N	[^{15}O] water	rCBF
			[^{15}O] oxygen	rCBV
			[^{15}O] carbon dioxide	rCBF
^{18}F	109.8	^{18}O	[^{18}F] fluorodeoxyglucose	Glucose metabolism
			[^{18}F] FDOPA	DA synthesis
			[^{18}F] Fallypride	D_2 receptor

Common radioligands used in PET are provided.
DA, dopamine; DAT, dopamine transporter; DOPA, dihydroxyphenylalanine; rCBF, regional cerebral blood flow.

biological processes that follow the injection of the radiopharmaceutical. Specifically, the characterization of regional uptake and washout of a given radiopharmaceutical allows for the quantification of biological processes.

While the synthesis of a radiopharmaceutical is highly powerful in understanding basic mechanistic properties of the body, there are several important considerations related to its synthesis. First, the integration of a radionuclide with a biological molecule must not alter the functional properties (biological or biochemical) of the biological molecule of interest. This would confound the biological process being studied. Second, when synthesizing a radiopharmaceutical for a receptor study, it must have a high affinity for the target receptor. This ensures that the target process is sufficiently observed and all available receptors will be occupied. For instance, in order to characterize dopaminergic receptor density in the striatum, the radiopharmaceutical must be designed to have a high affinity for D_2 receptors (dopaminergic receptors commonly found in the striatum). Third, the radiopharmaceutical must be highly selective for the biological process of interest. In the case of a receptor study, the radiopharmaceutical must have a much higher affinity for the target receptor than any other neuroreceptor (i.e. a radiopharmaceutical designed to characterize dopaminergic function as described earlier must have a much higher affinity for striatal D_2 receptors than any other neuroreceptors, such as glutamatergic receptors or even dopaminergic D_1 autoreceptors). Fourth, in order to maximize signal in the relevant regions of interest, radiopharmaceuticals must bind to relevant target sites and clear through an organism's system fairly quickly. Fifth, the radiopharmaceutical must be lipophilic and able to cross the blood–brain barrier. Sixth, the radiopharmaceutical must have no physiological effect on the organism. Due to the incredible sensitivity of PET, studies typically use 'tracer' doses, which are rarely physiologically activating. Lastly, the integration of the radionuclide with the biological molecule must occur rapidly because of radionuclide decay.

Clinical research applications

PET studies of neurobiological function have played an important role in understanding the underpinnings of mental illness and mechanisms of change in treatment. Some experimental designs that have been used to study clinical populations include resting-state studies and activation paradigm studies. The simplest approach is a resting-state paradigm, whereby participants undergo a PET scan while 'at rest' in the scanner. Typically, participants are instructed to passively view a fixation cross on a projector screen. There is no explicit cognitive task involved. These studies usually involve the radiopharmaceutical ^{18}F-FDG due to its long half-life, but studies assessing neurochemical function at 'baseline' (e.g. receptor density) also use ^{11}C radiopharmaceuticals. These resting-state studies are useful for comparing general brain functioning between groups (e.g. psychiatric population vs. control population). However, this experimental approach is limited because resting-state brain activation is likely reflective of multiple cognitive and affective processes. The clinical application of resting-state studies in psychiatry is also limited in that individual differences are not easily detectable.

Another powerful tool is the use of PET imaging to assess brain function during task-elicited processing. This approach can uncover differences associated with task-induced neural activation that is not detectable at rest. These data could also be collected in both clinical and healthy populations and convey meaningful difference in task-induced brain functioning. Radiopharmaceuticals with a shorter half-life that can quickly dissipate from the body, such as ^{15}O, allow investigators to examine an individual under multiple conditions, one after the other. In this way, researchers can examine whether differences are present during resting state or task-elicited functioning. This approach has been useful in investigating neural processing during states relevant to psychiatric disorders. Some of these conditions include tasks that require executive functioning, affective regulation during mood induction, and symptom provocation and capture studies, all of which examine activation associated with symptom-related functioning compared to baseline.

PET has also been critical in measuring the effects of treatment. One experimental design involves the acquisition of baseline neural functioning before treatment. These pre-treatment experimental designs may include resting-state paradigms or may involve a number of cognitive tasks to examine task-induced activation. After subjects have completed treatment, analyses can determine whether neural functioning pre-treatment is correlated with, or predictive of, treatment outcome. Subjects may be analysed by comparing responders to non-responders or by using a continuous outcome variable. In addition, researchers can collect functional imaging scans before and after treatment. Similar to the baseline-predictor paradigm, subjects will have a pre-treatment scan. However, the addition of a post-treatment scan allows researchers to determine whether the treatment effects were related to detectable changes in brain function. This approach provides insight into the mechanisms of action for a given treatment. Moreover, PET imaging allows for unique access to *in vivo* brain activation during stimulation (e.g. DBS or TMS) in order to assess the acute mechanistic changes associated with various treatments.

Pathophysiology of psychiatric illness

Utilizing these techniques, PET studies have played an important role in establishing the pathophysiology of psychiatric disorders. It has contributed to the understanding of both neuroanatomical and neurochemical functioning underlying mental illness during rest and task-elicited cognitive states. We focus here on MDD and OCD due to their relatively well-established pathophysiology and high candidacy for neurosurgical intervention.

Major depressive disorder

Symptoms of the MDD include depressed mood, loss of interest in pleasurable activities, increased irritability, guilt and hopelessness, sleep and appetite disturbances, cognitive impairment and lack of motivation. It can lead to crippling impairment of daily functioning, with 30% of depressed individuals classified as severely depressed. A substantial proportion of individuals with MDD, in the range of 40–60%, are resistant to conventional treatments (e.g. SSRIs or psychotherapy; [16]).

Functional imaging studies have demonstrated that depression is not the result of a single aberrant brain region or neurotransmitter system. Rather, it is the dysfunctional interactions between specific brain regions that underlie depression [27]. Dysfunction within the dorsal neocortex, including the prefrontal cortex (PFC), the dorsal ACC and the premotor cortex, may contribute to the psychomotor and cognitive disturbances seen in depression [11]. This cognitive component projects to the striatum and is regulated via a feedback loop through the thalamus. Ventral brain region abnormalities are seen in the subgenual anterior cingulate (i.e. Brodmann's area 25), the orbitofrontal cortex (OFC) and limbic structures such as the amygdala and nucleus accumbens (NAcc). Aberrant signalling in these ventral brain regions likely gives rise to the negative emotional experience of depression (e.g. anhedonia and sadness; [15]). This component also loops through the striatum and thalamus. Finally, other abnormalities are seen in the hypothalamic–pituitary–adrenal axis, hippocampus and pregenual anterior cingulum. The pregenual anterior cingulum is thought to regulate the dorsal and ventral components. Dysfunction of this entire network gives rise to the exaggerated autonomic and endocrine response to stress in depression [43].

Importantly, depression is not merely a result of one or more of these pathways not functioning properly, but also a failure of compensatory mechanisms to maintain homeostasis when the organism is under duress. Depressive patients have also shown cognitive inflexibility or lack of adaptive behaviour in response to environmental stressors. Dysfunction in pathways that promote neuronal plasticity may contribute to these symptoms.

Obsessive–compulsive disorder

OCD is a relatively common disorder that is characterized by recurrent, intrusive thoughts or impulses (i.e. obsessions) followed by repetitive behaviours or rituals (i.e. compulsions). While individuals with OCD may acknowledge that their thoughts and behaviours are unreasonable, their symptoms cause marked impairment in daily functioning. First-line treatments such as SSRIs and exposure and response prevention therapy are highly effective for the majority of patients with OCD. Still, over 20% of OCD patients suffer from treatment-resistant OCD and a subset of these patients may be eligible for novel treatments such as neuromodulation [16].

As with depression, the symptoms of OCD are not the result of dysfunction within a singular brain region or neurotransmitter system, but rather they are the result of faulty dysfunction between many regions that form a circuit. Functional imaging studies in the last few decades have contributed to the identification of a primary network of dysfunction in OCD: the cortico-striatothalamocortical circuit (CSTC) termed the ventral cognitive network. As first postulated in the mid-1980s, there are several, parallel CSTC circuits that have specialized trajectories connecting an area of the PFC to a striatal region, then through the thalamus and back to the original cortical region [2, 17]. Depending on their specific projection regions, these networks subserve distinct functions. These include the sensorimotor circuit, the affective circuit, the dorsal cognitive circuit and the ventral cognitive circuit. The ventral cognitive circuit projects from the anterior lateral OFC through the striatum and regulates context monitoring and response inhibition. The dysregulation of this ventral cognitive circuit and adjacent structures has consistently been implicated in the underlying mechanism of OCD [13].

Within the ventral cognitive network is the corticothalamic pathway, which runs from the thalamus to the OFC through the anterior limb of the internal capsule, a white matter tract connecting these nodes of the network. This corticothalamic pathway is excitatory and is regulated by the corticostriatothalamic pathway running from the OFC through the striatum to the thalamus [13]. OCD symptoms are believed to arise when the corticostriatothalamic pathway does not adequately regulate (i.e. inhibit) the corticothalamic pathway. Thus, any treatment intervention that either enhances input from the corticostriatothalamic pathway or disrupts communication along the corticothalamic pathway may stabilize the ventral cognitive network and alleviate the symptoms of OCD [47]. These notions have been supported by more recent PET studies examining OCD-related function.

Resting-state studies have found hyperactivity in the CSTC circuit in patients with OCD as compared to healthy controls. In particular, these studies found increased rCBF in the OFC, ACC, caudate nucleus and thalamus [40]. During symptom provocation studies, the hyperactivation in this network is exacerbated [40]. Moreover, treatment studies examining the effects of psychotropic medication, behavioural therapy and psychosurgery found attenuation in network activity following successful reduction in symptoms [4, 38].

Neuromodulation

PET studies examining brain function in individuals with MDD and OCD have contributed to the circuit-based model of pathophysiology. With these insights, psychiatrists have partnered with neurologists and neurosurgeons to devise suitable targets, elucidate mechanisms of action and determine response predictors for neuromodulation.

Electroconvulsive therapy

ECT is a non-invasive neuromodulatory treatment option for individuals with depression who do not respond to conventional treatments. Treatment involves the placement of unilateral or bilateral electrodes along the frontotemporal region (i.e. across the forehead and on the temples). While the patient is under general anaesthesia, an electrical current induces a mild, general seizure. Unilateral ECT involves less risk for transient cognitive impairments than bilateral ECT, but bilateral treatment is more efficacious in symptom reduction. While the mechanisms of ECT are largely unknown, this brief seizure of 20 s or less seems to alter brain functioning and ameliorate psychiatric symptoms.

Originally developed for schizophrenia, ECT has been a treatment option for several decades, although modern applications use lower and safer dosages that have far fewer cognitive side effects than previous applications. Patient selection has also been refined, with depression as a primary indication for ECT treatment (schizophrenia remains a secondary indication). ECT for depression has persisted as one of the most effective and fast-acting treatments for intractable depression. Clinical trials have estimated that the response rate is approximately 60% (e.g. [20]), which is highly significant considering patients receiving ECT have usually not achieved response to pharmacological or behavioural intervention. Although there are a few retrospective studies that mention a reduction in OCD symptoms following ECT, there are no controlled studies to date that support this claim. Thus, ECT is not a recommended treatment for OCD.

Mechanistic changes

There have been a number of PET studies that examined functional and neurochemical changes in the brain associated with ECT treatment for depression. The most consistent findings show that ECT leads to a global decrease in activation, with particularly notable decreases in the frontoparietal regions [55, 33, 18, 53, 51] and temporal cortex [33, 51]. This decrease in neural activation appears to be correlated with a reduction in depressive symptoms [18]. Decreases have also been demonstrated in the anterior and posterior cingulate cortex [33, 53]. Although another study found that ECT led to increased activation in the subgenual cingulate, this study examined a sample of MDD patients with psychotic features, which may constitute a different pathophysiological mechanism [31]. Subcortical regions such as the striatum and amygdala have shown increased metabolic activity following ECT [18, 51]. Interestingly, while all of the previous studies examined changes in brain function following ECT (post-treatment scan occurred in the range of days to weeks after the last ECT session), one PET study examining activation during ECT stimulation found increased global metabolism, including frontoparietal and subcortical areas [53, 1]. In general, it appears that treatment with ECT results in decreased activity in wide swaths of cortical regions (although activity may be increased in these regions during the actual administration of ECT), perhaps with concurrent increases in activity in subcortical regions.

A number of studies have also examined neurochemical changes associated with ECT. As the primary pharmacological treatment for depression (SSRI) impacts the serotonergic system, a few studies have examined the effect of ECT on serotonin. One study found that ECT led to an increase in serotonin release (decreased binding) in the subgenual cingulate, OFC, amygdala, hippocampus and amygdala ([23]. However, [41]) another study showed a global reduction in 5-HT receptors, especially in the parahippocampus and medial PFC [56]. In this study, the reduction in serotonin (5-HT) receptors was correlated with the decrease in depressive symptoms. Because dopaminergic systems have also been implicated in the pathophysiology of depression, a study examined dopamine receptor binding in depressed patients following ECT treatment. Following successful treatment, depressed patients showed decreased dopamine receptor binding in the right rostral anterior cingulate. Of note, no differences were detected between depressed patients and controls before treatment [42].

Transcranial magnetic stimulation and transcranial direct current stimulation

TMS is a non-invasive technique that delivers stimulation to a target area of the brain. Stimulation is produced by passing a strong, brief electrical current through an insulated coil of wire, creating a transient magnetic field. When the TMS device is placed over the scalp, a secondary current is created in the brain that is capable of either hyperpolarizing (i.e. inhibiting) or depolarizing (i.e. exciting) neurons. The frequency, duration of stimulation, shape of the coil and strength of the magnetic field contribute to the effects of the stimulation, including whether it activates or suppresses cortical regions.

A similar method of stimulation is tDCS, which is also non-invasive. This device delivers a weak direct current to the target brain region through two electrodes placed on the scalp. One of the electrodes is an active electrode and is positioned directly over the target brain region. The second electrode is a reference electrode that is typically positioned over the contralateral (i.e. opposite side) supraorbital region or on another part of the body. tDCS delivers current and induces sustained changes in the neural membrane electrical potential using either cathodal or anodal stimulation. Cathodal tDCS results in hyperpolarization (i.e. inhibition) of neurons, whereas anodal tDCS results in depolarization (i.e. excitation) of neurons.

Some key differences between these two techniques include the ostensible mechanism of action, whereby TMS is more of a direct neurostimulator and tDCS is an indirect neuromodulator. In experimental practice, TMS tends to be favoured for its spatial and temporal resolution and well-established protocols. tDCS, on the other hand, is advantageous because it is possible to keep on/off conditions indistinguishable, allowing for better controlled studies (e.g. double-blind or sham-controlled). tDCS is also less cumbersome, which enables simultaneous use of behavioural tasks. Ultimately, both approaches can lead to long-term effects on cortical excitability that may translate to observable changes in behaviour. Of course, these properties have led to the application of TMS and tDCS in clinical research studies. Unfortunately, there have not been any PET studies to date that examine functional properties of tDCS in psychiatric illness.

Similar to ECT, TMS is primarily used in the treatment of depression and is not yet recommended for treatment of OCD. For this reason, PET studies that examine TMS and its effect on brain function have been limited to depression.

Functional targets

Excitatory TMS for major depression is typically localized over the left dorsolateral PFC (DLPFC) while inhibitory TMS for major depression is typically localized over the right DLPFC. Some researchers have examined the utility of targeting the most hypometabolic prefrontal region as informed by PET. Investigators compared symptom reduction in left PET-guided targets, right PET-guided targets, standard left DLPFC and sham conditions. Results indicated that the left PET-guided and standard targeting conditions led to significantly better treatment response as compared to right PET-guided and sham. However, left PET-guided did not outperform the standard protocol for target localization [35, 19].

Mechanistic changes

PET studies have also been used to discern the effect of TMS treatment on the brain. Changes in brain function among individuals who respond to TMS have demonstrated inconsistent results. A study by Baeken and colleagues [3] examined metabolic changes associated with TMS in treatment responders. Using FDG-PET, investigators found that responders had increased metabolic activity in the ACC following treatment [3]. A subsequent study examining responders also implicated the cingulate cortex, noting increased metabolism in the middle cingulum, as well as the somatosensory and precuneus regions [25]. Investigators also observed TMS-induced metabolic decreases in the left fusiform gyrus and the left middle temporal cortex. This same group sought to extend these findings in a larger sample and found that, following TMS, responders demonstrated decreased metabolism in the subgenual anterior cingulate, a brain region often implicated in depression. Decreases were also found in the parahippocampus, thalamus, midbrain, posterior cingulate cortex, basal ganglia, thalamus, cerebellum and occipital cortex. Non-responders did not show any changes in metabolism following TMS. Of note, all changes reported here were recorded 1–4 months post TMS treatment, suggesting that TMS has long-lasting effects on brain metabolism [24].

Some studies have investigated whether TMS alters neurochemical functioning in the dopaminergic system. Kuroda and colleagues [21, 22] have examined both pre-and post-synaptic functions, using L-B-^{11}C-DOPA and ^{11}C-raclopride, respectively. These studies suggest that TMS does not seem to alter dopaminergic function. While this finding suggests that dopamine may not be directly involved in the mechanism of action in TMS, it cannot be ruled out completely. An earlier study by Strafella and colleagues [49] found increased release of dopamine in the caudate nucleus following TMS. In addition, these studies may have been limited in the ability to detect these changes due to the inclusion of both responders and non-responders in this analysis, as well as the low statistical power with less than 10 subjects.

Given that TMS can function as an excitatory (>1 Hz) or inhibitory (<1 Hz) neuromodulator, one study examined blood flow changes associated with these parameters in depression. Investigators used $^{15}O\text{-}H_2O$ PET to measure changes in blood flow following low- (1 Hz) and high-frequency (20 Hz) TMS delivered over the left DLPFC. Low-frequency TMS resulted in decreased blood flow, namely in small areas of the right PFC, left medial temporal cortex, left basal ganglia and left amygdala. Meanwhile, high-frequency TMS resulted in increases in blood flow in the PFC, left cingulate gyrus and left amygdala. In this sample ($n=10$), significant responses (symptom reduction of at least 50%) were not observed in either the low- or high-frequency phases. However, the moderate changes in symptoms following the two TMS conditions were inversely related, such that individuals who improved with one frequency tended to worsen with the other [48].

Predictors

Some studies have utilized PET to examine baseline metabolic activity that predicts treatment outcome following TMS. When comparing responders to non-responders, higher baseline metabolic activity in the DLPFC and ACC was associated with favourable outcome [3]. Others have found that successful TMS treatment is predicted by higher metabolic function in the medial PFC and rostral ACC and lower metabolic function in the parahippocampus at baseline. In addition, improvement in depression correlated with baseline metabolism in the rostral ACC [25]. Interestingly, one group showed that non-responders demonstrated lower baseline metabolism in the left OFC and higher metabolism in the amygdala. These regions were negatively correlated in non-responders and positively correlated in responders, while healthy subjects did not demonstrate any relationship [36]. Overall, while baseline symptom severity did not differentiate responders, lessened dysfunction along the networks implicated in depression predicted more favourable outcome.

Vagus nerve stimulation

VNS was originally approved by the United States Food and Drug Administration (FDA) for the treatment for intractable epilepsy in the mid-1990s. Interestingly, dramatic antidepressant effects were observed following treatment with VNS in epilepsy patients, independent of reduction in epileptic symptoms. Therefore, clinical trials of VNS for patients with treatment-resistant depression were initiated and VNS was approved by the FDA for the treatment of intractable depression in the mid-2000s. Clinical trials have shown that VNS as an adjunctive therapy can improve response rates in treatment-resistant depression from 14 to 32% after 2 years [5]. While there have been some cases of successful VNS treatment for intractable OCD, there have not been controlled trials to support the use of VNS for OCD.

VNS delivers a small electrical pulse through an implanted electrode attached to the left vagus nerve. The vagus nerve has been found to have projections to the PFC, amygdala, cingulate cortex and indirect connections to the serotonergic and noradrenergic systems via the locus coeruleus. Therefore, VNS may have detectable effects on brain function.

Mechanistic changes

Studies utilizing PET imaging have examined the effects of VNS for treatment-resistant depression. Immediately following VNS stimulation, reductions in cerebral blood flow were seen in the bilateral OFC and left inferior temporal lobe [8]. The same group examined long-term effects (3–12 months) of successful treatment and found decreased metabolism in the right DLPFC and rostral cingulate [10]. Another group found reductions in regional blood flow to the ventral medial PFC following chronic VNS treatment, which is a brain region that extends to the subgenual cingulate [37].

Predictors

One study examined whether pre-treatment patterns of metabolic activity predicted response to VNS. Conway and colleagues examined metabolic markers that distinguish responders in a sample of 15 intractably depressed patients. Results indicated that pre-treatment hypometabolism in the anterior insula predicted later response to VNS and correlated with symptom reduction. In addition, a negative correlation was found between hypometabolism in the anterior insula and hypermetabolism in the OFC, such that the magnitude of the inverse relationship predicted the per cent reduction in depressive symptoms [9]. The same research group also examined whether acute VNS effects (i.e. intraoperative, immediately following implant) predict long-term outcomes in patients with depression. Results showed that VNS-induced increase in rCBF in the dorsal ACC predicted symptoms reduction after 12 months of chronic VNS activation [8].

Ablative procedures

Focal ablative surgeries for the treatment of refractory OCD or MDD have been used since the 1960s. These procedures are typically carried out using either stereotactic craniotomy and thermocoagulation or Gamma

Knife radiosurgery for targeted ablation. The stereotactic method involves the fastening of a frame to the head before surgery and the use of MRI anatomical images to help neurosurgeons visualize the brain in a three-dimensional space. The brain is then mapped onto a specific coordinate system that allows for precision and minimal tissue disturbance when reaching deep subcortical structures. The four ablative psychosurgical procedures performed today for the treatment of OCD and MDD are anterior cingulotomy, anterior capsulotomy, subcaudate tractotomy and limbic leucotomy.

Anterior cingulotomy targets fibres of the cingulum adjacent to the ACC, while anterior capsulotomy and subcaudate tractotomy disrupt frontothalamic fibres. A limbic leucotomy is a multi-site procedure that combines the anterior cingulotomy and subcaudate tractotomy. Ablative surgeries are utilized for severe cases of various neuropsychiatric disorders. The primary psychiatric indications are depression and OCD with a response rate of 40–60%.

Mechanisms

One study used PET to examine changes in brain function following anterior capsulotomy in eight patients with intractable depression. Investigators compared these patients to eight matched healthy controls to determine baseline pathophysiology. Surprisingly, rather than the canonical hypometabolism often seen in depressed populations, these patients showed hypermetabolism in the PFC, ACC and striatum. Furthermore, anterior capsulotomy seemed to normalize some of these disturbances, even 6 months after surgery. Compared to baseline, patients exhibited decreased metabolism in the ACC extending to the OFC. The magnitude of decreased metabolism in the ACC was positively correlated with symptom reduction. In addition, metabolic increases were observed in the precentral gyrus, the left inferior parietal lobule and bilateral superior temporal gyrus [57].

Predictors

Two studies have examined baseline brain functioning as a possible predictor of treatment outcome. The first study examined pre-treatment metabolic activity that distinguished responders and non-responders in the treatment of OCD with anterior cingulotomy. Findings indicated that resting metabolic activity in the right posterior cingulate cortex was significantly correlated with reduction in OCD symptoms [38]. In a study for intractable depression, investigators similarly assessed whether pre-treatment brain function predicted treatment response to anterior cingulotomy. Results suggested that greater metabolism in the subgenual cingulate cortex and the left thalamus significantly correlated with improvement in depressive symptoms following treatment [12].

Deep brain stimulation

DBS for psychiatric treatment has become an alternative to ablative procedures as a result of the careful patient selection procedures that ensure patients have exhausted all other treatment options, the remarkable outcomes in the treatment of movement disorders, and the adjustable and reversible nature of the treatment. DBS first arose as a treatment option for psychiatric disorders in the late 1990s. Originally developed for the treatment of Parkinson's disease, DBS involves the implant of electrodes in targeted areas of the brain that are controlled by a neurostimulator pack typically placed subcutaneously below the clavicle. Using stereotactic methods, the electrodes are directed to the target site through small burr holes in the skull. Following implantation, a trained psychiatrist adjusts the parameters. Adjustments can include use of different electrode contacts along with modification in electrical current polarity (+/−), intensity (voltage), pulse width and frequency (Hz). In the treatment of intractable OCD and

MDD, several DBS targets have been studied, including the ventral capsule/ventral striatum (VC/VS), NAcc and subgenual cingulum.

Functional targets

PET studies examining brain function at rest have been used to determine suitable target options for DBS. Mayberg and colleagues [30] observed hypermetabolism in the subgenual cingulum in six patients with treatment refractory depression. This area was subsequently chosen as a target for DBS, in an effort to attenuate activation in the region. Stimulation of the white matter tracts adjacent to the subgenual cingulate resulted in a dramatic and sustained reduction of symptoms in four of six patients. Antidepressant effects were associated with attenuation in rCBF at the target site, as well as changes in downstream limbic and cortical sites. These findings were supported and expanded upon in a study by Lozano and colleagues [26] examined as follows.

Mechanistic changes

Several studies have examined changes in brain function that accompany treatment using DBS. As mentioned before, PET is an ideal neuroimaging technique, as the quality of the images is not disrupted by electrical or magnetic disturbances. The earliest studies examined the effect of NAcc DBS on brain function in patients with OCD. The first ever only acquired $^{15}OH_2O$ PET imaging of one patient with NAcc DBS and found that chronic stimulation to the left shell of the NAcc resulted in a decrease in blood flow to the left DLPFC and rostral putamen, but led to increases in the right DLPFC and cingulate cortex [50]. In another study targeting the NAcc with DBS for depression, Schlaepfer and colleagues [45] measured changes in metabolism following 1 week of chronic stimulation. Findings included an increase in metabolic activity in the bilateral ventral striatum, DLPFC, dorsal medial PFC, cingulate cortex and amygdala. In addition, decreases were observed in the ventral medial PFC, ventral lateral PFC, dorsal caudate nucleus and thalamus. The most recent study examining the effects of DBS in the NAcc included a group of patients with intractable depression. However, the electrodes used in this study had four contacts each spaced 1.5 mm apart. While the first contact was embedded in the shell of the NAcc, the others were located in the core region of the NAcc, the ventral internal capsule and the medial internal capsule. DBS in this extended target region resulted in decreased metabolic activity in OFC, the subgenual cingulate cortex, the posterior cingulate cortex, the thalamus and caudate nucleus. Responders tended to have decreased metabolism in the amygdala as compared to the non-responders receiving DBS [6].

PET studies have also been conducted for DBS at the VC/VS target. The first study examining DBS in the anterior limb of the internal capsule captured FDG-PET in three patients with OCD. After 3 months of stimulation, patients showed decreased metabolism in the frontal cortex [34]. Van Laere and colleagues [54] examined chronic treatment effects for six patients with OCD, DBS-induced effects included a further decrease in prefrontal metabolic activity, namely, the subgenual anterior cingulate, the right DLPFC and the right anterior insula. Symptom reduction was inversely related to decreases in metabolic activity in the ventral striatum, amygdala and left hippocampus. These findings were captured between 3 and 20 months after implant. Others have examined acute effects of DBS at the VC/VS target in patients with OCD. Rauch and colleagues [40] compared high-frequency (185 Hz) stimulation to low-frequency (15 Hz) and 'off' control conditions immediately after implant. High-frequency activation induced increased blood flow in the OFC, subgenual cingulate and posterior cingulate cortex, striatum, globus pallidus and thalamus, whereas low and off conditions produced no detectable changes in blood flow.

Others have examined the effects of DBS in cingulate cortex. Mayberg and colleagues [30] assessed changes in blood flow following subgenual cingulate DBS in patients with intractable depression. Of the six patients, three responded favourably after 3 months of stimulation. Findings indicated that subgenual stimulation led to decreases in blood flow in the subgenual cingulate and adjacent OFC. Long-term responders at 12 months showed additional decreases in the hypothalamus, anterior insula and medial PFC along with increases in the DLPFC, dorsal ACC, posterior cingulate cortex, premotor and parietal regions. These increases brought prefrontal CBF in depressed patients up to the level seen in healthy controls [30]. Lozano and colleagues [26] measured metabolic changes following DBS of the subcollosal cingulate gyrus in patients with depression. Significant decreases in metabolism were noted in the OFC, medial PFC and insula, while increases were observed in the lateral PFC, parietal, anterior midcingulate and posterior cingulate cortex. The medial PFC and OFC decreases were the earliest changes that emerged at 3 months followed by changes in the remaining regions at 6 months.

Predictor studies

Few studies have examined baseline regional metabolism as a predictor of treatment outcome. Mayberg and colleagues examined pre-treatment rCBF for patterns of activation that distinguished responders to DBS of the subgenual for depression. Investigators found that responders had less severe hypoactivity in the PFC and also exhibited hyperactivation in the medial PFC [30]. The Belgian group [54] acquired preoperative FDG-PET images in a group of six OCD patients undergoing DBS in the VC/VS target. They found that increased metabolic activity in the subgenual cingulate predicted favourable outcome following DBS treatment.

Discussion

As outlined in this chapter, PET imaging is a particularly useful tool that can be used to study the immediate and long-term effects of neuromodulation. The results from many PET studies discussed in this chapter suggest that this technique can reveal neuropathophysiology of psychiatric disorder and provide insights into the mechanisms of action associated with neuromodulatory treatments. Most importantly, PET imaging has been used to uncover patterns of functional and neurochemical dysfunction that may predict response to specific treatment approaches. Given that many interventions using neuromodulation come with considerable costs and risks, it is important to continue investigating neuroimaging biomarkers that predict likelihood of favourable response or, as important, nonresponse. Although the studies reviewed demonstrate promising strides towards this application, the data are preliminary and limited in their instantiation due to small sample sizes and lack of replication. Future research should seek to better understand mechanisms of action following neuromodulation on a functional and neurochemical level, as well as the predictive value of pretreatment neuropathophysiology.

References

1 Ackermann, R. F., Engel, J., & Baxter, L. (1986). Positron emission tomography and autoradiographic studies of glucose utilization following electroconvulsive seizures in humans and rats. Annals of the New York Academy of Sciences, 462(1), 263–269.
2 Alexander, G. E., DeLong, M. R., & Strick, P. L. (1986). Parallel organization of functionally segregated circuits linking basal ganglia and cortex. Annual Review of Neuroscience, 9, 357–381.
3 Baeken, C., De Raedt, R., Van Hove, C., Clerinx, P., De Mey, J., & Bossuyt, A. (2009). HF-rTMS treatment in medication-resistant melancholic

depression: results from (18) FDG-PET brain imaging. CNS spectrums, 14(8), 439–448.
4 Baxter Jr, L. R., Thompson, J. M., Schwartz, J. M., Guze, B. H., Phelps, M. E., Mazziotta, J. C., Selin, C. E., Moss, L. (1987). Trazodone treatment response in obsessive-compulsive disorder–correlated with shifts in glucose metabolism in the caudate nuclei. Psychopathology, 20 (Suppl. 1), 114–122.
5 Berry, S. M., Broglio, K., Bunker, M., Jayewardene, A., Olin, B., & Rush, A. J. (2013). A patient-level meta-analysis of studies evaluating vagus nerve stimulation therapy for treatment-resistant depression. Medical Devices, 6, 17–35.
6 Bewernick, B. H., Hurlemann, R., Matusch, A., Kayser, S., Grubert, C., Hadrysiewicz, B., Axmacher, N., Lemke, M., Cooper-Mahkorn, D., Cohen, M. X., Brockann, H., Lenartz, D., Sturm, V., & Schlaepfer, T. E. (2010). Nucleus accumbens deep brain stimulation decreases ratings of depression and anxiety in treatment-resistant depression. Biological Psychiatry, 67(2), 110–116.
7 Brody, A. L., Saxena, S., Schwartz, J. M., Stoessel, P. W., Maidment, K., Phelps, M. E., & Baxter Jr, L. R. (1998). FDG-PET predictors of response to behavioral therapy and pharmacotherapy in obsessive compulsive disorder. Psychiatry Research: Neuroimaging, 84(1), 1–6.
8 Conway, C. R., Sheline, Y. I., Chibnall, J. T., Bucholz, R. D., Price, J. L., Gangwani, S., & Mintun, M. A. (2012a). Brain blood-flow change with acute vagus nerve stimulation in treatment-refractory major depressive disorder. Brain stimulation, 5(2), 163–171.
9 Conway, C. R., Chibnall, J. T., Gangwani, S., Mintun, M. A., Price, J. L., Hershey, T., Giuffra, L. A., Bucholz, R. D., Christensen, J. J., & Sheline, Y. I. (2012b). Pretreatment cerebral metabolic activity correlates with antidepressant efficacy of vagus nerve stimulation in treatment-resistant major depression: A potential marker for response?. Journal of affective disorders, 139(3), 283–290.
10 Conway, C. R., Chibnall, J. T., Gebara, M. A., Price, J. L., Snyder, A. Z., Mintun, M. A., Craig, A. D., Cornell, M. E., Perantie, D. C., Giuffra, L. A., Bucholz, R. D., & Sheline, Y. I. (2013). Association of Cerebral Metabolic Activity Changes with Vagus Nerve Stimulation Antidepressant Response in Treatment-Resistant Depression. Brain stimulation, 6(5), 788–797.
11 Deckersbach, T., Dougherty, D. D., & Rauch, S. L. (2006). Functional imaging of mood and anxiety disorders. Journal of Neuroimaging, 16(1), 1–10.
12 Dougherty, D. D., Weiss, A. P., Cosgrove, G. R., Alpert, N. M., Cassem, E. H., Nierenberg, A. A., Price, B. H., Mayberg, H. S., Fischman, A. J., & Rauch, S. L. (2003). Cerebral metabolic correlates as potential predictors of response to anterior cingulotomy for treatment of major depression. Journal of Neurosurgery, 99(6), 1010–1017.
13 Dougherty, D. D., Rauch, S. L., Greenberg, B. D. (2010). Pathophysiology of obsessive-compulsive disorder. In: Textbook of Anxiety Disorders (2nd Edition). Stein D, Hollander E, Rothbaum B (Eds.), American Psychiatric Publishing, Inc., Washington DC, 287–310.
14 El-Hai, J. (2005). The lobotomist: a maverick medical genius and his tragic quest to rid the world of mental illness. John Wiley & Sons, Inc, Hoboken, NJ.
15 Evans, K. C., Dougherty, D. D., Pollack, M. H., & Rauch, S. L. (2006). Using neuroimaging to predict treatment response in mood and anxiety disorders. Annals of Clinical Psychiatry, 18(1), 33–42.
16 Greenberg, B. D., Price, L. H., Rauch, S. L., Friehs, G., Noren, G., Malone, D., Carpenter, L. L., Rezai, A. R.,& Rasmussen, S. A. (2003). Neurosurgery for intractable obsessive-compulsive disorder and depression: critical issues. Neurosurgery Clinics of North America, 14(2), 199–212.
17 Haber SN, Calzavara R. The cortico-basal ganglia integrative network: the role of the thalamus. Brain Research Bulletin, 78(2–3), 69–74 (2009).
18 Henry, M. E., Schmidt, M. E., Matochik, J. A., Stoddard, E. P., & Potter, W. Z. (2001). The effects of ECT on brain glucose: a pilot FDG PET study. The journal of ECT, 17(1), 33–40.
19 Herwig, U., Lampe, Y., Juengling, F. D., Wunderlich, A., Walter, H., Spitzer, M., & Schönfeldt-Lecuona,

C. (2003). Add-on rTMS for treatment of depression: a pilot study using stereotaxic coil-navigation according to PET data. Journal of psychiatric research, 37(4), 267–275.

20 Kellner, C. H., Knapp, R., Husain, M. M., Rasmussen, K., Sampson, S., Cullum, M., McClintock, S. M., Tobias, K. G., Martino, C., Meuller, M., Bailine, S. H., Fink, M., & Petrides, G. (2010). Bifrontal, bitemporal and right unilateral electrode placement in ECT: randomised trial. The British Journal of Psychiatry, 196(3), 226–234.

21 Kuroda, Y., Motohashi, N., Ito, H., Ito, S., Takano, A., Nishikawa, T., & Suhara, T. (2006). Effects of repetitive transcranial magnetic stimulation on [11C]raclopride binding and cognitive function in patients with depression. Journal of Affective Disorders, 95(1–3), 35–42.

22 Kuroda, Y., Motohashi, N., Ito, H., Ito, S., Takano, A., Nishikawa, T., & Suhara, T. (2010). Chronic repetitive transcranial magnetic stimulation failed to change dopamine synthesis rate: preliminary L-[β-11C]DOPA positron emission tomography study in patients with depression. Psychiatry and Clinical Neurosciences 64(6), 659–662.

23 Lanzenberger, R., Baldinger, P., Hahn, A., Ungersboeck, J., Mitterhauser, M., Winkler, D., Micskei, Z, Stein, P., Karanikas, G., Wadsak, W., Kasper, S., & Frey, R. (2013). Global decrease of serotonin-1A receptor binding after electroconvulsive therapy in major depression measured by PET. Molecular psychiatry, 18(1), 93–100.

24 Li, C. T., Chen, L. F., Tu, P. C., Wang, S. J., Chen, M. H., Su, T. P., & Hsieh, J. C. (2013). Impaired prefronto-thalamic functional connectivity as a key feature of treatment-resistant depression: a combined MEG, PET and rTMS Study. PLoS one, 8(8), e70089.

25 Li, C. T., Wang, S. J., Hirvonen, J., Hsieh, J. C., Bai, Y. M., Hong, C. J., Liou, Y. J., & Su, T. P. (2010). Antidepressant mechanism of add-on repetitive transcranial magnetic stimulation in medication-resistant depression using cerebral glucose metabolism. Journal of affective disorders, 127(1), 219–229.

26 Lozano, A. M., Mayberg, H. S., Giacobbe, P., Hamani, C., Craddock, R. C., & Kennedy, S. H. (2008). Subcallosal cingulate gyrus deep brain stimulation for treatment-resistant depression. Biological psychiatry, 64(6), 461–467.

27 Mayberg, H. S. (1997). Limbic-cortical dysregulation: a proposed model of depression. The Journal of neuropsychiatry and clinical neurosciences, 9(3):471–481

28 Mayberg, H. S., Brannan, S. K., Mahurin, R. K., Jerabek, P. A., Brickman, J. S., Tekell, J. L., Silva, A. J., McGinnis, S., Glass, T. G., Martin, C. C., & Fox, P. T. (1997). Cingulate function in depression: a potential predictor of treatment response. Neuroreport, 8(4), 1057–1061.

29 Mayberg, H. S. (2003). Modulating dysfunctional limbic-cortical circuits in depression: towards development of brain-based algorithms for diagnosis and optimised treatment. British medical bulletin, 65(1), 193–207.

30 Mayberg, H. S., Lozano, A. M., Voon, V., McNeely, H. E., Seminowicz, D., Hamani, C., Schwalb, J. M., & Kennedy, S. H. (2005). Deep brain stimulation for treatment-resistant depression. Neuron, 45(5), 651–660.

31 McCormick, L. M., Ponto, L. L. B., Pierson, R. K., Johnson, H. J., Magnotta, V., & Brumm, M. C. (2007). Metabolic correlates of antidepressant and antipsychotic response in patients with psychotic depression undergoing electroconvulsive therapy. The journal of ECT, 23(4), 265–273.

32 Milak, M. S., Parsey, R. V., Lee, L., Oquendo, M. A., Olvet, D. M., Eipper, F., Malone, K., & Mann, J. J. (2009). Pretreatment regional brain glucose uptake in the midbrain on PET may predict remission from a major depressive episode after three months of treatment. Psychiatry Research: Neuroimaging, 173(1), 63–70.

33 Nobler, M. S., Oquendo, M. A., Kegeles, L. S., Malone, K. M., Campbell, C., Sackeim, H. A., & Mann, J. J. (2001). Decreased regional brain metabolism after ECT. American Journal of Psychiatry, 158(2), 305–308.

34 Nuttin, B. J., Gabriëls, L. A., Cosyns, P. R., Meyerson, B. A., Andréewitch, S., Sunaert, S. G., Maes, A. D., Dupont, P. J., Gybels, J. M., Gielen, F., & Demeulemeester, H. G. (2003). Long-term electrical capsular stimulation in patients with obsessive-compulsive disorder. Neurosurgery, 52(6), 1263–1274.

35 Paillère Martinot, M. L., Galinowski, A., Ringuenet, D., Gallarda, T., Lefaucheur, J. P., Bellivier, F., Picq,

C., Bruguiere, P., Mangin, I. F., Riviere, D., Willer, J. C., Falissard, B., Leboyer, M., Olie, J. P., Artiges, E., & Martinot, J. L. (2010). Influence of prefrontal target region on the efficacy of repetitive transcranial magnetic stimulation in patients with medication-resistant depression: a [18F]-fluorodeoxyglucose PET and MRI study. The International Journal of Neuropsychopharmacology, 13(01), 45–59.

36 Paillère Martinot, M. L., Martinot, J. L., Ringuenet, D., Galinowski, A., Gallarda, T., Bellivier, F., Lefaucheur, J. P., Lemaitre, H., & Artiges, E. (2011). Baseline brain metabolism in resistant depression and response to transcranial magnetic stimulation. The International Journal of Neuropsychopharmacology 36(13), 2710–2719.

37 Pardo, J. V., Sheikh, S. A., Schwindt, G. C., Lee, J. T., Kuskowski, M. A., Surerus, C., Lewis S. M., Abuzzahab, F. S., Adson, D. E., & Rittberg, B. R. (2008). Chronic vagus nerve stimulation for treatment-resistant depression decreases resting ventromedial prefrontal glucose metabolism. Neuroimage, 42(2), 879–889.

38 Rauch, S. L., Dougherty, D. D., Cosgrove, G. R., Cassem, E. H., Alpert, N. M., Price, B. H., Nierenberg, A. A., Mayberg, H. S., Baer, L., Jenike, M. A., & Fischman, A. J. (2001). Cerebral metabolic correlates as potential predictors of response to anterior cingulotomy for obsessive compulsive disorder. Biological psychiatry, 50(9), 659–667.

39 Rauch, S. L., Shin, L. M., Dougherty, D. D., Alpert, N. M., Fischman, A. J., & Jenike, M. A. (2002). Predictors of fluvoxamine response in contamination-related obsessive compulsive disorder: a PET symptom provocation study. Neuropsychopharmacology, 27(5), 782–791.

40 Rauch, S. L., Dougherty, D. D., Malone, D., Rezai, A., Friehs, G., Fischman, A. J., Alpert, N. M., Haber, S. N., Stypulkowski, P. H., Rise, M. T., Rasmussen, S. A., & Greenberg, B. D. (2006). A functional neuroimaging investigation of deep brain stimulation in patients with obsessive-compulsive disorder. Journal of neurosurgery, 104(4), 558–565.

41 Saijo, T., Takano, A., Suhara, T., Arakawa, R., Okumura, M., Ichimiya, T., Ito, H., & Okubo, Y. (2010a). Effect of electroconvulsive therapy on 5-HT1A receptor binding in patients with depression: a PET study with [11C] WAY 100635. The International Journal of Neuropsychopharmacology, 13(06), 785–791.

42 Saijo, T., Takano, A., Suhara, T., Arakawa, R., Okumura, M., Ichimiya, T., Ito, H., & Okubo, Y. (2010b). Electroconvulsive therapy decreases dopamine D_2receptor binding in the anterior cingulate in patients with depression: a controlled study using positron emission tomography with radioligand [^{11}C] FLB 457. The Journal of clinical psychiatry, 71(6), 793–799.

43 Sapolsky, R. M. (2000). Glucocorticoids and hippocampal atrophy in neuropsychiatric disorders. Archives of general psychiatry, 57(10), 925–935.

44 Saxena, S., Brody, A. L., Ho, M. L., Zohrabi, N., Maidment, K. M., & Baxter, L. R. (2003). Differential brain metabolic predictors of response to paroxetine in obsessive-compulsive disorder versus major depression. American Journal of Psychiatry, 160(3), 522–532.

45 Schlaepfer, T. E., Cohen, M. X., Frick, C., Kosel, M., Brodesser, D., Axmacher, N., Joe, A. Y., Kreft, M., Lenartz, D., & Sturm, V. (2008). Deep brain stimulation to reward circuitry alleviates anhedonia in refractory major depression. Neuropsychopharmacology, 33(2), 368–377.

46 Seminowicz, D. A., Mayberg, H. S., McIntosh, A. R., Goldapple, K., Kennedy, S., Segal, Z., & Rafi-Tari, S. (2004). Limbic–frontal circuitry in major depression: a path modeling metanalysis. Neuroimage, 22(1), 409–418.

47 Shah, D. B., Pesiridou, A., Baltuch, G. H., Malone, D. A., & O'Reardon, J. P. (2008). Functional neurosurgery in the treatment of severe obsessive compulsive disorder and major depression: overview of disease circuits and therapeutic targeting for the clinician. Psychiatry (Edgmont), 5(9), 24.

48 Speer, A. M., Kimbrell, T. A., Wassermann, E. M., Repella, J., Willis, M. W., Herscovitch, P., & Post, R. M. (2000). Opposite effects of high and low frequency rTMS on regional brain activity in depressed patients. Biological Psychiatry 48(12), 1133–1141.

49 Strafella, A. P., Paus, T., Barrett, J., & Dagher, A. (2001). Repetitive transcranial magnetic stimulation of the human prefrontal cortex induces dopamine release in the caudate nucleus. The Journal of neuroscience: the official journal of the Society for Neuroscience, 21(15), RC157–RC157.

50 Sturm, V., Lenartz, D., Koulousakis, A., Treuer, H., Herholz, K., Klein, J. C., & Klosterkötter, J. (2003). The nucleus accumbens: a target for deep brain stimulation in obsessive–compulsive-and anxiety-disorders. Journal of chemical neuroanatomy, 26(4), 293–299.

51 Suwa, T., Namiki, C., Takaya, S., Oshita, A., Ishizu, K., Fukuyama, H., Suga, H., & Murai, T. (2012). Corticolimbic balance shift of regional glucose metabolism in depressed patients treated with ECT. Journal of affective disorders, 136(3), 1039–1046.

52 Swedo, S. E., Schapiro, M. B., Grady, C. L., Cheslow, D. L., Leonard, H. L., Kumar, A., Fiedland, R., Rapoport, S. I., & Rapoport, J. L. (1989). Cerebral glucose metabolism in childhood-onset obsessive-compulsive disorder. Archives of general psychiatry, 46(6), 518.

53 Takano, H., Motohashi, N., Uema, T., Ogawa, K., Ohnishi, T., Nishikawa, M., Kashima, H., & Matsuda, H. (2007). Changes in regional cerebral blood flow during acute electroconvulsive therapy in patients with depression Positron emission tomographic study. The British Journal of Psychiatry, 190(1), 63–68.

54 Van Laere, K., Nuttin, B., Gabriels, L., Dupont, P., Rasmussen, S., Greenberg, B. D., & Cosyns, P. (2006). Metabolic imaging of anterior capsular stimulation in refractory obsessive-compulsive disorder: a key role for the subgenual anterior cingulate and ventral striatum. Journal of Nuclear Medicine, 47(5), 740–747.

55 Yatham, L. N., Clark, C. C., & Zis, A. P. (2000). A preliminary study of the effects of electroconvulsive therapy on regional brain glucose metabolism in patients with major depression. The journal of ECT, 16(2), 171–176.

56 Yatham, L. N., Liddle, P. F., Lam, R. W., Zis, A. P., Stoessl, A. J., Sossi, V., Adam, M. J., & Ruth, T. J. (2010). Effect of electroconvulsive therapy on brain 5-HT2 receptors in major depression. The British Journal of Psychiatry, 196(6), 474–479.

57 Zuo, C., Ma, Y., Sun, B., Peng, S., Zhang, H., Eidelberg, D., & Guan, Y. (2013). Metabolic imaging of bilateral anterior capsulotomy in refractory obsessive compulsive disorder: an FDG PET study. Journal of Cerebral Blood Flow & Metabolism, 33(6), 880–887.

CHAPTER 6

Basic principles of deep brain and cortical stimulation

Caio Matias[1], Scott Lempka[1,2] and Andre Machado[1]
[1]*Cleveland Clinic Neurological Institute, Cleveland, USA*
[2]*Louis Stokes Cleveland VA Medical Center, Cleveland, USA*

Electrical stimulation of the nervous system is utilized to modify neuronal activity and alleviate symptoms of neurological or behavioural disorders. There are multiple applications of electrical stimulation, ranging from peripheral functional electrical stimulation for post-spinal cord injury paralysis [1–3] to deep brain stimulation for movement disorders [4–6] and emerging indications [7]. Since the introduction of deep brain stimulation and spinal cord stimulation, neurostimulation technologies have rapidly advanced over the past decades. While some principles of electrical stimulation are very well established, some of the mechanisms underlying the benefits and side effects of stimulation remain the topic of lively academic debate. This chapter focuses on the basic principles of deep brain and cortical stimulation.

The electrode

An electrode is an electrical conductor that forms the interface between stimulation systems and the nervous system. The electrode at which electron removal occurs towards the tissue is defined as cathode, while the electrode at which electron gain occurs is defined as anode. Voltage is the electromotive force that drives electrical charges and is measured in volts (V). Electrons flow from the cathode (negative pole) to the anode (positive pole); thus a conventional current (flow of positive charges) takes place in the opposite direction and is measured in amperes (A). The opposing force to the flow of electrons through a conductor is called resistance or impedance and is measured in ohms (Ω). The relationship among these concepts is defined by Ohm's law:

$$I = \frac{V}{Z}$$

where I is current, V is voltage and Z is resistance or impedance. A greater impedance demands higher voltage to deliver the same current.

Electrical charges are mediated in the brain by ions such as sodium (Na^+), potassium (K^+) and chloride (Cl^-). Ion concentration differences between the extracellular and intracellular spaces leads to a voltage difference across the cell membrane. At rest, a cell typically has a membrane voltage (inside potential – outside potential) of about −70 mV [8]. An increase in the membrane voltage, or depolarization, results from the influx of positive charges, such as Na^+ ions. A more depolarized membrane is closer to reaching the threshold for an

Neuromodulation in Psychiatry, First Edition. Edited by Clement Hamani, Paul Holtzheimer, Andres M. Lozano and Helen Mayberg.

action potential. Conversely, hyperpolarization is a decrease (more negative) in the membrane potential that often happens due to the efflux of K^+ ions or the influx of Cl^- ions and represents a decrease in cell excitability.

Effects of electrical stimulation on tissue

Voltage-gated sodium and potassium channels

Voltage-gated sodium (Na_v) and potassium (K_v) channels consist of transmembrane proteins that span the cell membrane. When open, these proteins allow ions to flow across the membrane. The opening and closing of these ion channels are largely determined by the cell membrane potential. At rest, a majority of both Na_v and K_v channels are closed. However, if the cell membrane is depolarized (e.g. by electrical stimulation), a number of Na_v and K_v channels begin to open. Na_v channels open more rapidly than K_v channels and allow for further membrane depolarization due to the influx of Na^+ ions along their concentration gradient (i.e. higher concentration of Na^+ ions outside the cell). After a short period of time, Na_v channels begin to close due to inactivation while K_v channels remain open. The decrease in Na^+ influx and the continued efflux of K^+ out of the cell (higher concentration of K^+ inside the cell) lead to repolarization of the membrane potential and an eventual return to rest.

Action potentials

Within a myelinated axon, the nodes of Ranvier contain a high concentration of Na_v channels. When a node is sufficiently depolarized, a large number of Na_v channels open within a short period of time and allow for a large influx of Na^+ ions. This influx of Na^+ ions is part of a process, called an action potential, which is characterized by a rapid increase in the membrane potential from negative (approximately −70 mV) to positive voltages (approximately +20 mV). This localized influx of Na^+ ions creates an intracellular potential difference between the particular node of Ranvier and adjacent nodes. The positive charges move to the next adjacent node and depolarize the membrane, activating the voltage-gated channels and generating another action potential. This process of action potential propagation from one node to the next (a.k.a. saltatory conduction) continues to the terminal end of the axon where eventually a neurotransmitter is released.

For axons near a stimulation electrode, a cathode delivers negative charges into the tissue that counter positive charges outside the membrane and cause the negative charges inside the axons to move away from the membrane. This movement of negative charges is equivalent to positive charges flowing from inside the axon across the cell membrane towards the extracellular space. Therefore, a cathodic pulse has the effect of driving a positive current from the inside of the axon to the outside, with a bulk of the current travelling through the node of Ranvier closest to the stimulating electrode. The opposite currents of positive ions travelling from the extracellular space into the axons occur at adjacent nodes of Ranvier. The magnitude of the inward current flowing through these flanking nodes is significantly lower than the outward current travelling through the node closest to the stimulating electrode. These current paths are described in Figure 6.1 (see Ref. [8]).

Current flowing from inside of the axon to the extracellular space at the node of Ranvier closest to the stimulating electrode increases or depolarizes the membrane voltage. As described above, this depolarization can cause Na_v channels in this patch of membrane to open and may lead to subsequent action potential generation. If the depolarization is insufficient to open enough Na_v channels, then an action potential is not generated and this stimulus is considered to be subthreshold.

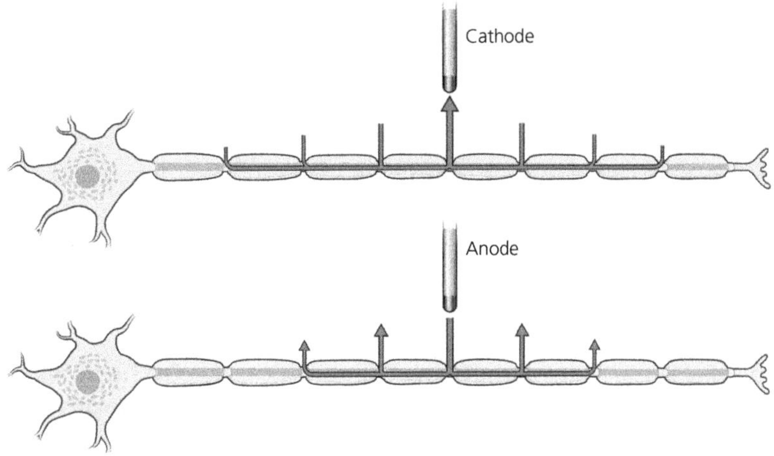

Figure 6.1 Current flow under cathodic and anodic stimulation. Under cathodic stimulation, the highest currents flow outward through the closest nodes of Ranvier, while under anodic stimulation, the opposite process occurs. Source: Illustration by David Schumick, BS, CMI. Reprinted with the permission of the Cleveland Clinic Center for Medical Art & Photography. Copyright 2014. (*See insert for colour representation of the figure.*)

If an anodic stimulus is applied, the current flow through the respective nodes of Ranvier are reversed [8]. Positive ions flow from the extracellular space into the axon through the nodes closest to the stimulating electrode and decrease or hyperpolarize the membrane voltage. However, at flanking nodes, positive currents flow out of the axon and produce depolarizations that may lead to an action potential. These outward currents are distributed over several distant nodes instead of a single node as is with the case of a cathodic pulse. Because these outward depolarizing currents are distributed over many nodes, a stronger stimulation is necessary to open enough Na_v channels to generate an action potential. Therefore, cathodic pulses require lower amplitudes to generate action potentials relative to anodic pulses.

Neuron

Generation of action potentials also depends on whether the stimulus is delivered close to the axon, cell body, or dendrites [9]. Cathodic pulses applied away from the cell body generate action potentials at the node of Ranvier located closest to the electrode. However, when the stimulus is applied near the cell body, action potentials are initiated at the first node of the axon distal to the soma. Cathodic pulses applied near the dendrites can cause membrane hyperpolarization in the soma and axon, so action potentials are not generated during the stimulus. Anodic pulses applied distant to the cell body generate action potentials on the two nodes adjacent to the axon node closest to the stimulating electrode. During anodic stimulation near the cell body, action potentials are not initiated at the node closest to the soma as with cathodic stimulation, but at the second node closest to the soma. However, if the electrode is positioned over the dendrites, then anodic pulses generate action potentials at the node closest to the soma.

Distance to electrode

The current needed to generate an action potential is directly proportional to the distance from the stimulating electrode [10].

$$i = kr^2$$

where i = threshold current, k = constant and r = distance from the electrode. Increasing the distance between an axon and the stimulating electrode raises the threshold current to initiate an action potential. Therefore, axons closer to the electrode are more affected by an electrical stimulus than distant cells.

Strength-duration relationship

At a given distance from the stimulating electrode, the relationship between the current amplitude and stimulus duration (i.e. pulse width) necessary to generate an action potential is described by the following equation (Figure 6.2):

$$I_{\text{th}} = I_{\text{rh}}\left(1 + \frac{T_{\text{ch}}}{\text{PW}}\right)$$

where I_{th} = current threshold, I_{rh} = rheobase current, T_{ch} = chronaxie and PW = pulse width. Rheobase current is defined as the lowest current necessary to generate an action potential (i.e. infinite stimulus duration). Chronaxie is the pulse duration required for the generation of an action potential when current amplitude is twice the rheobase current. When the current amplitude is decreased, the duration (pulse width) must be increased to produce the same effect. If the current amplitude is below the rheobase, the stimulus will never be able to activate the neural element, even for an infinite stimulus duration. Large myelinated axons have the shortest chronaxies (~30–200 μs) and are thus more easily activated by electrical stimulation relative to other neural elements. Smaller diameter axons have chronaxies approximately 200–700 μs, and cell bodies and dendrites have much larger chronaxies (~1–10 ms) [11, 12].

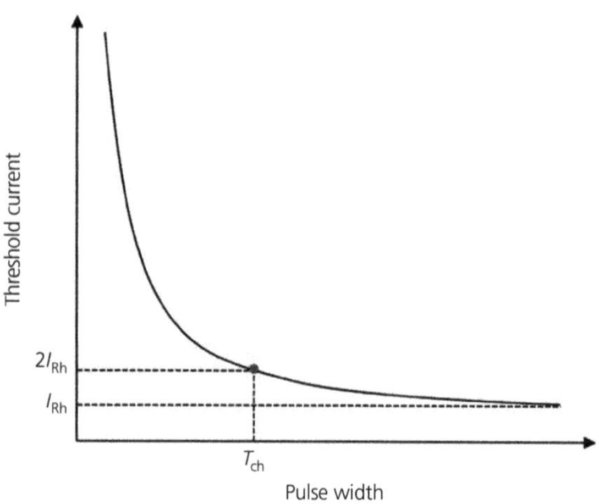

Figure 6.2 Strength-duration relationship. Rheobase (I_{Rh}) is the lowest current necessary to generate an action potential (i.e. infinite stimulus duration). Chronaxie (I_{Ch}) is the pulse duration (pulse width) required for the generation of an action potential when current amplitude is twice the rheobase current. The current required to stimulate a neural element decreases as pulse width increases.

Orthodromical and antidromical propagation

Physiological action potentials propagate in the orthodromic direction from the cell body towards the axon terminals. Antidromic propagation refers to the opposite direction, towards the soma. When electrical stimulation is applied to an axon, action potentials are propagated in both directions. Orthodromic propagation may evoke neurotransmitter release that results in excitation or inhibition of downstream neurons [13, 14]. The effects of antidromic propagation are more complex. Antidromic action potentials do not necessarily invade the soma and activate the afferent neurons. This phenomenon depends on two factors: first, the diameter and myelination of the axon, and second, the geometric ratio between axon and soma diameters. Action potentials may also propagate into axonal collaterals, changing direction from antidromic to orthodromic and eventually activating synaptic transmission. Finally, antidromic action potentials may collide with spontaneous orthodromic action potentials (physiological or stimulated) and prevent them from modulating downstream neurons [15].

Stimulation configuration

Stimulation parameters and electrode configurations can be selected in such a fashion as to improve the efficacy of stimulation and reduce undesirable side effects. Efficacy can be improved by increasing the number of axons excited by the stimulus; however, limiting excitation of fibres can reduce side effects.

Cathode-anode configuration

The initial step is to define the active contacts in the electrode. In a monopolar configuration, one (or more) contact is set as the cathode and the pulse generator case is set as the anode. From an electrical standpoint, the anode is considered to be at an infinite distance away from the cathode, thus the stimulation comes only from the cathode and the configuration is considered to be monopolar. In bipolar configuration, two contacts (or more) of the electrode are activated, one as cathode and the other as anode. Charges flow from the cathode to the anode in a bipolar configuration, whereas in monopolar configuration, charges flow out in all directions. Therefore, monopolar stimulation produces a more radial electrical field, whereas bipolar stimulation creates a narrower electrical field with a maximal effect near the cathode (Figure 6.3). Monopolar stimulation is often preferred because it can activate a larger volume of tissue with less battery consumption. However, if current spreads to adjacent structures, side effects may be elicited [16, 17].

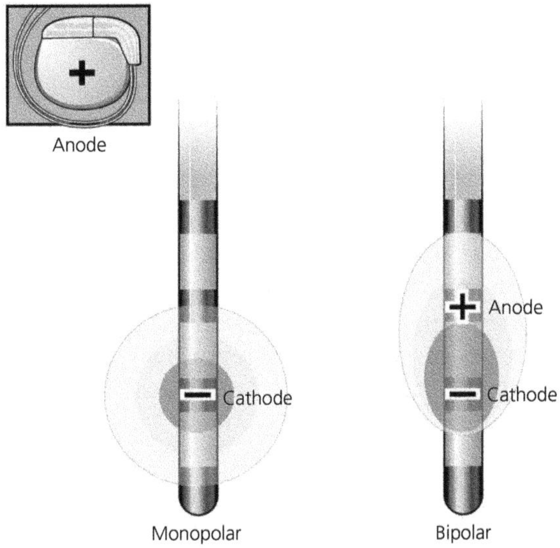

Figure 6.3 Schematic representation of the electrical field generated by different cathode–anode configurations. Monopolar configuration: one (or more) contact is set as the cathode and the pulse generator case is set as the anode. Bipolar stimulation: two contacts (or more) are activated, one as cathode and the other as anode. Source: Illustration by David Schumick, BS, CMI. Reprinted with the permission of the Cleveland Clinic Center for Medical Art & Photography. Copyright 2014. (*See insert for colour representation of the figure.*)

Commercially available neurostimulation systems may be constant current or constant voltage. In constant current systems, the practitioner sets the desired current intensity, typically in milliamps (mA), and the device will adjust the voltage according to the impedance fluctuations to maintain the set current level (see Ohm's law, above). In constant voltage devices, the practitioner sets a given voltage amplitude and the output current of the stimulator depends on the electrode impedance. Therefore, the electrical current travelling through the target neural tissue can vary over time due to fluctuations in the electrode impedance [8, 18]. Impedance fluctuations may produce significant variability in the currents 'seen' by the target neural tissue that may affect stimulation efficacy and potentially require parameter adjustment [19].

Charge and charge density

Charges are carried by electrons in the stimulation system, whereas ions (e.g. Na^+) are the carriers in the neural tissue. As a cathodic current is applied to the electrode, negative charges build up on the metal side while positive charges move to the interface on the tissue side. In most standard clinical pulses, it is believed that charge carriers do not move across the interface. However, the movement of ions produces a current, defined as capacitive (non-Faradaic) current. If the current continues to be applied, more negative charges build up at the electrode, to a point where actual electron transfer to the tissue may occur, through a chemical reaction (Faradaic current). This results in reduction and oxidation, which can be toxic to the surrounding tissue and can lead to electrode corrosion. Therefore, by limiting the charge density, that is the amount of charge at the electrode–tissue interface for a given electrode surface area, tissue and electrode damage can be avoided.

Shannon proposed a model of neuronal damage based on data reported by several investigators [20]. This model uses charge, that is current amplitude multiplied by the stimulus pulse width, and charge densities to predict safe levels of stimulation. Based on this model, charge densities less than $30\,\mu C/cm^2$ are considered to be safe [21]. Currently available deep brain stimulation (DBS) systems provide a warning if the parameter combination may produce charge densities above this limit. However, substantial neuronal loss adjacent to the stimulating electrode has been described despite the use of common parameters [22]. Thus, other factors may also be involved in tissue/electrode damage. Charge distribution across the electrode is non-uniform and although mean charge density may be below the recommended limit, the peak charge density may exceed it. Frequency may also play a role that is not accounted for, as some of the studies used by the Shannon model used stimulation frequencies below the typical range (≥130 Hz) employed in DBS [23].

One way to limit charge density is to use charge-balanced biphasic pulses. A biphasic pulse consists of a cathodic and an anodic phase. For example, a cathode cumulates negative charges during the first (cathodic) phase and discharges them during the second (anodic) phase. Thus, the electrode–tissue interface remains in the same chemical condition prior to the pulse. Another way to prevent damage is to use materials with a high charge-carrying capacity. Several neurostimulation systems use electrodes made of a platinum-iridium alloy, which allows a large amount of current to be passed before Faradaic reactions occur and therefore helps prevent tissue and electrode damage.

Amplitude versus pulse width

Stimulation parameters such as amplitude and pulse width also affect the activation of neural elements. Increasing the current or voltage creates a stronger electric field that can activate axons that are farther away from the electrode as well as smaller diameter axons near the electrode that were not activated at lower amplitudes. Increasing the pulse width can also activate additional axons. As the pulse width is increased, more charge is delivered to the tissue, and thus an axon is more likely to be activated. The current required to stimulate a neural element decreases as pulse width increases (Figure 6.2).

Deep brain stimulation – specific concerns

Although this chapter is about psychiatry, we will describe a few sentences on movement disorders to explain how DBS evolved. Surgery for movement was initially performed through ablative procedures (e.g. pallidotomy, thalamotomy). Symptoms such as tremor, rigidity and bradykinesia could be effectively managed by creating lesions in specific neural targets such as the pars interna of the globus pallidus and the ventral intermedius nucleus of the thalamus [24, 25]. Electrical stimulation was used to refine target localization during these procedures. The observation that symptoms were improved during stimulation led to the advent of deep brain stimulation [26]. Even though DBS carries disadvantages related to the permanent implantation and long-term management of implantable hardware, it has several advantages over lesioning procedures including reversibility and adjustability. For these reasons, DBS has become the tool of choice for managing movement disorders and is also preferred over lesions by many investigators conducting studies on treatment-refractory psychiatric disorders. Of note, DBS has not completely replaced ablative procedures, which are still performed at several centres worldwide.

Despite the proven safety and efficacy of DBS, the specific mechanisms underlying its effects on the neural elements have not been fully determined. DBS may be used at different frequencies resulting in different brain effects. While high frequency stimulation (>100 Hz) improves tremor, bradykinesia and rigidity, stimulation with less than 50 Hz is usually less effective or ineffective [27, 28]. Furthermore, symptoms such as tremor can even be worsened by low-frequency stimulation in patients with essential tremor or Parkinson's disease [27, 29]. Most of what we will describe next is related to stimulation at frequencies around 100 Hz or at high frequencies. Several explanations have been proposed such as a local inhibitory action, modulation of synaptic transmission and network jamming [13, 26, 30]. It is important to note that these theories are not necessarily mutually exclusive and the effects of DBS may stem from a combination of them. The hypothesis of a local inhibitory action was originated from the observation that high-frequency stimulation and surgical lesion produced similar clinical effects [26]. A possible explanation is that high-frequency stimulation produces a transient blockade of voltage-gated currents [31], thus precluding action potential generation and a subsequent reduction in the output of the stimulated area. The modulation of synaptic transmission theory [32] states that DBS activates afferent fibres close to the electrode, resulting in release of neurotransmitters at the stimulated site. Local neuronal activity is decreased if an inhibitory neurotransmitter (e.g. GABA) is released [13], while increased activity is observed with the release of an excitatory neurotransmitter (e.g. glutamate) [14]. However, another possible mechanism is that stimulation produces the continuous release of neurotransmitters that eventually leads to neurotransmitter depletion [33]. As a consequence, transmission would be blocked through that particular pathway. Under pathological conditions, brain circuits have abnormal firing patterns with increased synchronization and rhythmic oscillations that may be responsible for producing symptoms [30]. The neural jamming hypothesis states that DBS replaces these patterns with a tonic high-frequency output. This new pattern is also abnormal, but downstream neural networks are unable to recognize it, resulting in an informational lesion.

Cortical stimulation

Motor cortical stimulation was pioneered for the management of central post-stroke pain by Tsubokawa and colleagues [34]. Human studies following initial in vivo electrophysiological models suggested that cathodic stimulation of the motor cortex could inhibit pathological thalamic hyperactivity. To date, cortical stimulation has been clinically utilized less frequently relative to deep brain stimulation almost exclusively for the treatment of pain [35]. However, recent studies have investigated the effects of cortical stimulation on motor recovery after stroke [36–38] and depression [39].

Several factors can influence the outcome of cortical stimulation. For example, the electrical conductivity of cerebrospinal fluid (CSF) is much higher than the electrical conductivity of neural tissue. The thickness of CSF layer between the electrode and the brain is critical for stimulation efficacy. When the electrodes are placed epidurally (the most common technique for chronically implanted cortical neuromodulation systems), around 60% of the total current dissipates laterally through the CSF before entering the cortex. Thicker CSF layers increase current dissipation and reduce

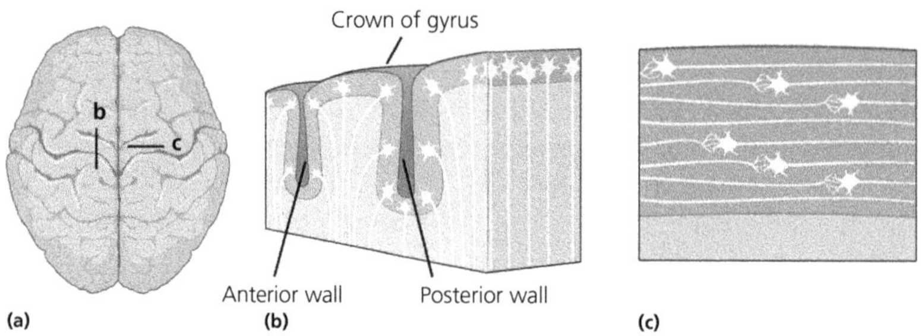

Figure 6.4 Orientation of cortical neural fibres in relation to the cortical surface. (**a**) Superior view of the cerebrum showing sulci and gyri. (**b**) Perpendicular and oblique fibres (e.g. cortico-spinal fibres, cortico-thalamic fibres). (**c**) Parallel fibres (e.g. cortico-cortical fibres). Source: Illustration by David Schumick, BS, CMI. Reprinted with the permission of the Cleveland Clinic Center for Medical Art & Photography. Copyright 2014.

the effective depth of stimulation [40]. Thinner CSF layers allow the current to penetrate deeper into the cortex and white matter.

Cortical neural fibres can be parallel or perpendicular to the cortical surface. Parallel fibres include collateral and cortico-cortical connections. Perpendicular and oblique fibres include ascending (e.g. thalamo-cortical) and descending pathways (e.g. cortico-spinal, cortico-thalamic) and can be further divided into three types: (i) perpendicular to the crown of the gyrus, (ii) perpendicular to the lip of the sulcus and (iii) perpendicular to the wall of the sulcus (Figure 6.4). Due to tissue inhomogeneity, the electrodes positioned over the gyral crowns or over the sulci result in different electrical field penetrations, influencing the fibers that will be activated. Moreover, the stimulus polarity (cathodic or anodic) influences the fibre excitation thresholds [41]. When cortical electrodes are positioned over a gyrus, the electrical field concentrates on the crown and spreads symmetrically to the anterior and posterior walls. Because stimulation charges are thought to concentrate more near the fibres that are parallel to the electrode, cortico-cortical fibres are more likely to be activated by cathodic stimulation, while corticofugal fibres are more excitable by anodic stimulation [41]. When the electrode is positioned over a sulcus, the electrical field penetrates deeper into the neural tissue, but spreads asymmetrically to the gyrus walls. In this scenario, parallel fibres are also more easily activated by cathodic stimulation. However, fibres pointing at the lip of the sulcus become more excitable by anodic stimulation [41].

Cortical stimulation is often performed with electrodes manufactured (and labelled) for dorsal column stimulation. These circular electrodes are flat, insulated on one side and have a wider spacing between contacts than DBS electrodes. Bipolar stimulation with contacts at least 10 mm apart allows minor overlap between cathodic and anodic electrical fields. Consequently, both poles can be considered as virtual monopoles [40]. As cathodic and anodic stimulation can recruit different types of cortical fibres, bipolar configurations may be preferred [42].

References

1 Barbeau H, Ladouceur M, Mirbagheri MM, Kearney RE. The effect of locomotor training combined with functional electrical stimulation in chronic spinal cord injured subjects: walking and reflex studies. Brain Research. Brain Research Reviews. 2002; 40(1–3):274–91.

2 Ladouceur M, Barbeau H. Functional electrical stimulation-assisted walking for persons with

incomplete spinal injuries: changes in the kinematics and physiological cost of overground walking. Scandinavian Journal of Rehabilitation Medicine. 2000; 32(2):72–9.
3 Ladouceur M, Barbeau H. Functional electrical stimulation-assisted walking for persons with incomplete spinal injuries: longitudinal changes in maximal overground walking speed. Scandinavian Journal of Rehabilitation Medicine. 2000; 32(1):28–36.
4 Benabid AL, Pollak P, Gao D, Hoffmann D, Limousin P, Gay E, *et al.* Chronic electrical stimulation of the ventralis intermedius nucleus of the thalamus as a treatment of movement disorders. Journal of Neurosurgery. 1996; 84(2): 203–14.
5 Krack P, Batir A, Van Blercom N, Chabardes S, Fraix V, Ardouin C, *et al.* Five-year follow-up of bilateral stimulation of the subthalamic nucleus in advanced Parkinson's disease. The New England Journal of Medicine. 2003; 349(20): 1925–34.
6 Follett KA, Weaver FM, Stern M, Hur K, Harris CL, Luo P, *et al.* Pallidal versus subthalamic deep-brain stimulation for Parkinson's disease. The New England Journal of Medicine. 2010; 362(22):2077–91.
7 Hariz M, Blomstedt P, Zrinzo L. Future of brain stimulation: new targets, new indications, new technology. Movement Disorders. 2013; 28(13): 1784–92.
8 Mortimer JT, Bahdra N. Fundamentals of Electrical Stimulation. In: Krames E, Peckham P, Rezai AR, editors. Neuromodulation. Volume 1 Amsterdam: Elsevier; 2009. pp. 109–21.
9 McIntyre CC, Grill WM. Excitation of central nervous system neurons by nonuniform electric fields. Biophysical Journal. 1999; 76(2): 878–88.
10 Stoney SD, Jr., Thompson WD, Asanuma H. Excitation of pyramidal tract cells by intracortical microstimulation: effective extent of stimulating current. Journal of Neurophysiology. 1968; 31(5):659–69.
11 Ranck JB, Jr. Which elements are excited in electrical stimulation of mammalian central nervous system: a review. Brain Research. 1975; 98(3):417–40.
12 Laxton AW, Dostrovsky JO, Lozano AM. Stimulation Physiology in Function Neurosurgery. In: Lozano AM, Gildenberg PL, Tasker RR, editors. Textbook of Stereotactic and Functional Neurosurgery Berlin: Springer; 2009. pp. 1383–99.
13 Dostrovsky JO, Levy R, Wu JP, Hutchison WD, Tasker RR, Lozano AM. Microstimulation-induced inhibition of neuronal firing in human globus pallidus. Journal of Neurophysiology. 2000; 84(1):570–4.
14 Lee KH, Chang SY, Roberts DW, Kim U. Neurotransmitter release from high-frequency stimulation of the subthalamic nucleus. Journal of Neurosurgery. 2004; 101(3):511–7.
15 Carron R, Chaillet A, Filipchuk A, Pasillas-Lepine W, Hammond C. Closing the loop of deep brain stimulation. Frontiers in Systems Neuroscience. 2013; 7:112.
16 Volkmann J, Moro E, Pahwa R. Basic algorithms for the programming of deep brain stimulation in Parkinson's disease. Movement Disorders. 2006; 21(Suppl 14):S284–9.
17 Montgomery E. Deep Brain Stimulaiton Programming: Principles and Practice. Oxford: Oxford University Press, Inc.; 2010.
18 Merrill DR, Bikson M, Jefferys JG. Electrical stimulation of excitable tissue: design of efficacious and safe protocols. Journal of Neuroscience Methods. 2005; 141(2):171–98.
19 Lempka SF, Johnson MD, Miocinovic S, Vitek JL, McIntyre CC. Current-controlled deep brain stimulation reduces in vivo voltage fluctuations observed during voltage-controlled stimulation. Clinical Neurophysiology. 2010; 121(12):2128–33.
20 Shannon RV. A model of safe levels for electrical stimulation. IEEE Transactions on Bio-Medical Engineering. 1992; 39(4):424–6.
21 Kuncel AM, Grill WM. Selection of stimulus parameters for deep brain stimulation. Clinical Neurophysiology. 2004; 115(11):2431–41.
22 Henderson J, Rodriguez M, O'Sullivan D, Pell M, Fung V, Benabid AL, *et al.* Partial lesion of thalamic ventral intermediate nucleus after chronic high-frequency stimulation. Movement Disorders. 2004; 19(6):709–11.
23 Grill WM. Signal Considerations for Chronically Implanted Electrodes for Brain Interfacing. In: Reichert WM, editor. Indwelling Neural Implants: Strategies for Contending with the In Vivo Environment Boca Raton: CRC Press; 2008. pp. 41–61.

24 Laitinen LV, Bergenheim AT, Hariz MI. Leksell's posteroventral pallidotomy in the treatment of Parkinson's disease. Journal of Neurosurgery. 1992; 76(1):53–61.
25 Jankovic J, Cardoso F, Grossman RG, Hamilton WJ. Outcome after stereotactic thalamotomy for parkinsonian, essential, and other types of tremor. Neurosurgery. 1995; 37(4):680–6.
26 Benabid AL, Pollak P, Louveau A, Henry S, de Rougemont J. Combined (thalamotomy and stimulation) stereotactic surgery of the VIM thalamic nucleus for bilateral Parkinson disease. Applied Neurophysiology. 1987; 50(1–6):344–6.
27 Rizzone M, Lanotte M, Bergamasco B, Tavella A, Torre E, Faccani G, *et al.* Deep brain stimulation of the subthalamic nucleus in Parkinson's disease: effects of variation in stimulation parameters. Journal of Neurology, Neurosurgery and Psychiatry. 2001; 71(2):215–9.
28 Moro E, Esselink RJ, Xie J, Hommel M, Benabid AL, Pollak P. The impact on Parkinson's disease of electrical parameter settings in STN stimulation. Neurology. 2002; 59(5):706–13.
29 Kuncel AM, Cooper SE, Wolgamuth BR, Grill WM. Amplitude- and frequency-dependent changes in neuronal regularity parallel changes in tremor with thalamic deep brain stimulation. IEEE Transactions on Neural Systems and Rehabilitation Engineering. 2007; 15(2):190–7.
30 Montgomery EB, Jr., Baker KB. Mechanisms of deep brain stimulation and future technical developments. Neurological Research. 2000; 22(3):259–66.
31 Beurrier C, Bioulac B, Audin J, Hammond C. High-frequency stimulation produces a transient blockade of voltage-gated currents in subthalamic neurons. Journal of Neurophysiology. 2001; 85(4):1351–6.
32 Vitek JL. Mechanisms of deep brain stimulation: excitation or inhibition. Movement Disorders. 2002; 17(Suppl 3):S69–72.
33 Lozano AM, Mahant N. Deep brain stimulation surgery for Parkinson's disease: mechanisms and consequences. Parkinsonism & Related Disorders. 2004; 10(Suppl 1):S49–57.
34 Tsubokawa T, Katayama Y, Yamamoto T, Hirayama T, Koyama S. Chronic motor cortex stimulation for the treatment of central pain. Acta Neurochirurgica Supplementum. 1991; 52:137–9.
35 Machado A, Azmi H, Rezai AR. Motor cortex stimulation for refractory benign pain. Clinical Neurosurgery. 2007; 54:70–7.
36 Plow EB, Carey JR, Nudo RJ, Pascual-Leone A. Invasive cortical stimulation to promote recovery of function after stroke: a critical appraisal. Stroke. 2009; 40(5):1926–31.
37 Brown JA, Lutsep HL, Weinand M, Cramer SC. Motor cortex stimulation for the enhancement of recovery from stroke: a prospective, multicenter safety study. Neurosurgery. 2008; 62(Suppl 2): 853–62.
38 Levy R, Ruland S, Weinand M, Lowry D, Dafer R, Bakay R. Cortical stimulation for the rehabilitation of patients with hemiparetic stroke: a multicenter feasibility study of safety and efficacy. Journal of Neurosurgery. 2008; 108(4): 707–14.
39 Kopell BH, Halverson J, Butson CR, Dickinson M, Bobholz J, Harsch H, *et al.* Epidural cortical stimulation of the left dorsolateral prefrontal cortex for refractory major depressive disorder. Neurosurgery. 2011; 69(5):1015–29.
40 Manola L, Roelofsen BH, Holsheimer J, Marani E, Geelen J. Modelling motor cortex stimulation for chronic pain control: electrical potential field, activating functions and responses of simple nerve fibre models. Medical & Biological Engineering & Computing. 2005; 43(3): 335–43.
41 Manola L, Holsheimer J, Veltink P, Buitenweg JR. Anodal vs cathodal stimulation of motor cortex: a modeling study. Clinical Neurophysiology. 2007; 118(2):464–74.
42 Nguyen JP, Lefaucheur JP, Decq P, Uchiyama T, Carpentier A, Fontaine D, *et al.* Chronic motor cortex stimulation in the treatment of central and neuropathic pain. Correlations between clinical, electrophysiological and anatomical data. Pain. 1999; 82(3):245–51.

CHAPTER 7

Electrophysiology in neuromodulation: Current concepts of the mechanisms of action of electrical and magnetic cortical stimulation

Jean-Pascal Lefaucheur
Paris Est Créteil University, Créteil, France

There are several ways of stimulating the cerebral cortex in humans for therapeutic purposes, that is neuromodulation therapy. First, invasive and non-invasive (transcranial) methods must be distinguished [1]. Regarding invasive methods, the goal is to place electrodes over a cortical region via a surgical intervention, either epidurally or subdurally. Epidural approach is often preferred because the risk for adverse events (e.g. haemorrhage or epilepsy) is less [2]. Next, there are different patterns of stimulation, based on an open-loop (without internal control) or a closed-loop design, in which stimulation is delivered as a function of neuronal activities recorded and analysed online [3]. Regarding non-invasive methods, magnetic and electrical stimulation must be distinguished [1]. Magnetic stimulation is currently the most often used technique for therapeutic neuromodulation. Transcranial magnetic stimulation (TMS) is based on the scientific principle of electromagnetic induction discovered by Faraday in 1831. The first magnetic stimulator designed to stimulate the human brain transcranially was proposed by Barker et al. [4], providing the prerequisite for subsequent clinical use of TMS. Briefly, TMS consists in the passage of a high-intensity current pulse of several thousand amperes flowing through a coil of wire, which, in turn, generates a brief magnetic pulse with field strengths up to several Teslas and lasting for about 100 μs. If the coil is placed on the head of a subject, the magnetic field is able to pass through the skull bone without being affected and is able to induce an electric field when entering the brain. The intensity of this induced current is sufficient to generate action potentials and to activate neural networks in the cortex safely and painlessly. To modulate brain function at a clinical, therapeutic level, it is necessary to deliver prolonged trains of TMS pulses in daily sessions of cortical stimulation for several days or weeks. This approach is called repetitive TMS (rTMS), of which clinical indications have been recently reviewed [5]. Regarding transcranial electrical stimulation, there is a variety of current patterns that are able to modulate neural activities in the cortex [6], and the most currently developed technique is transcranial direct current stimulation (tDCS) [7]. However, in contrast to invasive

Neuromodulation in Psychiatry, First Edition. Edited by Clement Hamani, Paul Holtzheimer, Andres M. Lozano and Helen Mayberg.

cortical stimulation and rTMS, the intensity of the current flow induced into the brain by tDCS is very low (1 or 2 mA are delivered over the scalp), insufficient to generate action potentials. Thus, tDCS modulates resting membrane potential of the axons in the direction of excitatory depolarization or inhibitory hyperpolarization.

However, whatever be the type of neurostimulation protocol applied, a key point is that the strength-duration relationship of membrane properties makes fibres of passage more excitable than local cell bodies at the stimulation site [8, 9]. Therefore, one key feature of therapeutic brain stimulation is that axons are more prone to be activated than cell bodies, with respect to their spatial orientation and diameter [10]. For example, when using a figure-of-eight coil, the net effect of TMS depends on the position and orientation of the coil over a gyrus or a sulcus and the direction of the current induced in the brain. When applied to the motor cortex, a monophasic pulse delivered by a figure-of-eight coil oriented perpendicular to the interhemispheric midline (latero-medial direction) directly activates the pyramidal tract, evoking mostly 'direct' corticospinal volleys waves (D-waves) [11]. In contrast, when the handle of a figure-of-eight coil is oriented parallel to the interhemispheric midline (postero-anterior direction), motor cortex TMS activates the pyramidal tract only indirectly, through the recruitment of cortical interneurons. At the spinal level, this is demonstrated by the recording of a succession of 'indirect' descending volleys (I-waves), showing the activation of various interneuronal circuits [12–16]. These observations may be relevant for stimulation applied outside the motor cortex, at least in the neocortex [17].

The intensity of stimulation also frankly impacts on the effects of cortical stimulation, because the induced electric field spreads and goes deeper into the brain according to intensity increase, which is able to recruit additional neural networks. For example, when TMS is applied to the motor cortex at high intensity using a figure-of-eight coil, D-waves arising from the axonal hillock of pyramidal cells can be elicited in addition to I-waves, even if the coil has postero-anterior orientation [15]. Therefore, in rTMS practice, the 'dose' of stimulation is usually standardized according to a percent of the resting motor threshold (RMT), determined in each individual. However, RMT measurement is subject to many sources of variability, in particular according to the method used [18–21], and primarily assesses the excitability of the motor cortex. Correlation may be lacking between RMT and excitability threshold in other cortical areas, such as the visual cortex [22], and interindividual intensity calibration for rTMS outside the motor cortex continues to be a challenge.

Although cortical stimulation may generate local activation, the stimulation is at the origin of biological effects that are not only local but also occur at a distance from the stimulation site via the activated networks. Depending on the intrinsic properties and the geometrical orientation of fibres within the stimulated cortical region, the axons recruited by cortical stimulation can be short fibres of intracortical interneurons, as well as afferent or efferent fibres connected with distant structures. Thus, axonal excitation can give rise to both orthodromic and antidromic volleys [23–26]. Orthodromic volleys induce post-synaptic excitation or inhibition in cortical or subcortical targets, whereas antidromic volleys reach the neural structures from which efferents arise.

The distant action of cortical stimulation was demonstrated by many functional imaging studies. For example, premotor cortex stimulation modulates functional activities in the contralateral dorsolateral prefrontal cortex (DLPFC), supplementary motor area, primary somatosensory, motor cingulate and inferior temporal cortices, as well as in subcortical structures such as the caudate nucleus and cerebellum [27]. A number of studies have also evidenced the influence of cortical stimulation over the basal ganglia, including the effect on dopamine release, especially following the stimulation of the primary motor cortex (M1) or the DLPFC [28–33]. In pain control, for example, epidural stimulation of M1 can also modulate non-motor neurotransmission systems, such as endogenous opioid secretion [34]. This effect is produced in deep brain structures, such as the periaqueductal grey matter and anterior cingulum [35], similar to what was observed following rTMS delivered over the DLPFC [36, 37]. However, even if the site of stimulation is not the site of action, it must be precisely determined to allow between-study comparability and session repeatability. This goal is achieved by using navigation systems dedicated for rTMS practice [38–40] or by performing a precise pre- and intra-operative mapping before implanting cortical electrodes in case of surgical procedure [41].

Beside these 'spatial' considerations, the 'temporal' relationship between clinical changes and stimulation time needs to be carefully assessed, because it can provide valuable information on the underlying cellular mechanisms of the action of neurostimulation. On one hand, there are acute or short-lasting neural changes occurring during the stimulation and resulting from stimulus-locked activation, inhibition, or modification of oscillatory activities in cortico-subcortical networks [42]. Thus, the frequency- and pattern-dependent therapeutic effects of rTMS could arise, at least in part, from an interaction with functional connectivity, synchronization and some altered oscillations involving cortical and subcortical networks [43]. Similar connectional effects have been observed in the application of tDCS, according to stimulation polarity [44, 45].

In any case, stimulation frequency is more often put forward to explain the direction of cortical excitability changes or the clinical effects that are induced by rTMS [46, 47]. From the results obtained in different studies based on motor evoked potential (MEP) measurement in healthy subjects, some form of consensus appeared to consider low-frequency (LF) rTMS (1 Hz or less), consisting of continuous trains of single pulses, as 'inhibitory' [48], and high-frequency (HF) rTMS (5 Hz and higher), consisting of bursts of stimuli that usually last for 5–10 s and are separated by pauses of 20–50 s, as 'excitatory' [49]. In most therapeutic trials, the total duration of rTMS sessions is about 20 min. Functional or clinical effects increases with the number of stimuli delivered and may persist for minutes to hours or even days beyond the rTMS session [48, 50–52]. These after-effects are closely reminiscent of the phenomena of long-term depression (LTD) of synaptic transmission for LF rTMS and long-term potentiation (LTP) for HF rTMS [48, 53, 54], as obtained in the hippocampus or cerebellum following electrical stimulations performed in animal experiments [55, 56]. Notwithstanding these striking similarities between rTMS effects and experimental data on long-term synaptic plasticity, Ziemann and other authors [57–59] have underscored that such a hypothesis was based only on indirect arguments and common output effects.

Besides the conventional LF/HF rTMS protocols, several new TMS paradigms have been developed, aimed at modifying cortical excitability and eventually producing therapeutic effects [1]. One of the most developed protocols is 'theta burst stimulation' (TBS), which usually consists of short bursts of three low-intensity pulses with inner high frequency (50 Hz, within the gamma range) that are delivered at 5 Hz (within the theta range). When delivered to the motor cortex of healthy subjects, the continuous application of TBS (cTBS) results in MEP inhibition [60], whereas the intermittent application of TBS (iTBS) results in MEP facilitation [61]. Excitatory effects build up within 1 s, whereas inhibitory effects occur with a delay of several seconds.

The concept of functional antagonism between 'inhibitory' LF rTMS/cTBS and 'excitatory' HF rTMS/iTBS is appealing, but not entirely satisfying, since it has been shown that both HF and LF rTMS may have mixed excitatory and inhibitory effects [62], while several studies reported similar effects produced by cTBS and iTBS [63–65]. Even when the effect on the motor cortex appears specific, doubling the duration of stimulation, for example, can reverse the outcome from inhibition to excitation and vice versa [66]. The underlying mechanisms of 'excitatory' versus 'inhibitory' aspects of rTMS paradigms should also be taken as relative, because MEP increase after 'excitatory' HF rTMS might be in fact the result of a decrease of gamma-aminobutyric acid (GABA)-mediated intracortical inhibition (hence, inhibition of inhibition), rather than a direct enhancement of motor cortex excitability [57, 67, 68]. Conversely, LF rTMS can enhance the net inhibitory corticospinal control, probably via GABA-B transmission, since this protocol lengthens corticospinal silent period duration, as observed in healthy subjects [69–71] and in patients with movement disorders [72–74]. In fact, it should be considered that the effects of the various TMS protocols suppressing or enhancing cortical excitability are not homogeneous and may result from targeting and modulating different cortical circuits [75]. For example, LF rTMS can selectively suppress the excitability of circuits producing late I-waves, while cTBS reduces the excitability of circuits generating instead the early I-waves [75]. On the other hand, it has been recently demonstrated [76] that the 'excitatory' vs. 'inhibitory' effects of iTBS vs. cTBS on MEP size was highly variable between individuals, depending on the differences in the interneuronal cortical networks that are preferentially recruited by the TMS pulse. This study also showed that, at a given site of stimulation, different populations of cortical interneurons are more easily activated at different times in the TMS train. This may explain why an rTMS train delivered at 5 Hz over M1 can either increase or decrease cortical excitability according to a continuous or intermittent pattern [77]. Thus, a comparison between studies using different protocols, even those considered equally 'excitatory' or 'inhibitory', should be made with caution, in particular, regarding TBS.

On the other hand, there are delayed and long-lasting effects depending on the frequency, polarity or pattern of stimulation that are considered to be governed by plastic synaptic changes. For example, the analgesic effects produced by motor cortex stimulation in patients with chronic pain are delayed but prolonged for hours or days after the stimulation period [78]. This could relate to time-consuming neurochemical or neuroendocrine processes, expression of secondary messengers and synaptic plasticity [79]. In particular, calcium-dependent synaptic plasticity of glutamatergic neurons is thought to play a key role in the mechanism of action of tDCS, since blockade of *N*-methyl D-aspartate (NMDA) receptors or calcium channels abolishes or diminishes tDCS effects [80, 81]. Glutamatergic plasticity can be further promoted by a reduction of GABA activity, which was observed after tDCS, regardless of stimulation polarity [82].

Synaptic plasticity depends on firing rate, spike timing and temporal and spatial summations of the inputs arriving at the presynaptic level. Whether a synapse is strengthened or weakened by presynaptic activity also depends upon the level of activity in the postsynaptic neuron. The processes leading to depression of synaptic transmission are more effective when postsynaptic activity is high. Conversely, potentiation of synaptic transmission is more likely when postsynaptic activity is low. This is known as the 'Bienenstock-Cooper-Munro (BCM) model' [83]. Generally speaking, a previous neuronal activity modulates the capacity for subsequent plastic changes. This has been termed 'metaplasticity' [84]. All these phenomena could help in stabilizing neuronal networks and therefore contribute to 'homeostatic plasticity' [85].

Accordingly, priming cortical stimulation aimed at modulating the initial state of cortical excitability could influence the subsequent effects of a cortical stimulation protocol on this excitability. The priming stimulation can have no detectable effects per se on synaptic transmission. There are several reports of efficacious priming protocols in the literature: subthreshold 6 Hz-rTMS was found to reinforce the depression of motor responses induced by suprathreshold 1 Hz-rTMS subsequently applied to the motor cortex [86]; the priming effect of iTBS was assessed on a subsequent 1 Hz-rTMS session delivered to temporoparietal language areas during an auditory word-detection task [87]; the analgesic effects of 'conventional' 10 Hz-rTMS delivered to M1 was found to be enhanced by TBS priming, at least using iTBS [65]; a former session of tDCS was found to enhance or reverse the effects of 1 Hz- or 5 Hz-rTMS depending on stimulation polarity [88, 89] and so on. Priming cortical stimulation is surely a potent way of improving the efficacy of various non-invasive cortical stimulation techniques in clinical practice.

Thus, the level of cortical excitability at baseline, before the stimulation, is an important source of inter- and intra-individual variability of cortical stimulation effects [25]. A study showed that rTMS effects on intracortical inhibition depended more on baseline individual values than on stimulation frequency [70]: subjects with less inhibition before rTMS tended to have an increased inhibition post-rTMS (and vice versa). A similar observation was made in patients with chronic pain, in whom 'facilitatory' HF rTMS of M1 increased intracortical inhibition, which is defective at baseline [90]. The impact of disease-related plasticity should be considered at the origin of pre-existing homeostatic changes resulting in a variability of biological or clinical effects produced by apparently identical rTMS protocols. For example, DLPFC stimulation produces differential effects on mood between healthy subjects and depressive patients according to the side of the stimulated hemisphere [91, 92].

Many other factors may also explain a large variability in the clinical response to cortical stimulation. These mechanisms include genetic factors [93, 94], gender or hormonal factors [95], attentional capacities [96], or inter-individual differences in the anatomy of the brain and possible shift of cortical areas of interest. Image-guided navigation systems can now be used to limit this latter source of variation by including individual morphological or functional brain imaging data. Nevertheless, it can be difficult to know whether the failure of a protocol of cortical stimulation to produce a clinical effect in a given study is related to an intrinsic therapeutic inefficacy of the protocol or to the inclusion of non-responders to this protocol arising from the usually large inter-individual variability of effects.

In pathological conditions, concomitant medication also represents a source of enhanced inter-individual variability in the efficacy of cortical stimulation therapy, because it produces major changes in brain excitability. For example, amphetamines can suppress the long-lasting plastic changes induced by rTMS delivered to the motor cortex [97]. The duration of drug administration and drug plasma levels are also influential. For example, low- and high-plasma valproate levels lead to opposite effects of 1 Hz-rTMS on corticospinal excitability in patients with juvenile myoclonic epilepsy [98]. Conversely, in some applications, medication might be also a prerequisite before considering the therapeutic potential of cortical stimulation. For example, the functional interaction between premotor and primary motor cortical areas is defective in untreated patients with Parkinson's disease and needs to be restored by dopaminergic medication before considering rTMS efficacy on parkinsonian motor symptoms [99, 100].

Other interventions are able to prolong, reinforce or reverse the effects produced by cortical stimulation, especially related to synaptic and connectivity changes. These interventions include peripheral sensory stimulation [101], transient sensory deafferentation [102], constraint-induced movements [103], practice [104] and learning [105, 106]. Conversely, cortical stimulation may be applied to promote the effects of other therapies. For example, rTMS of the left DLPFC was found to accelerate the onset of action and to augment the response to antidepressant drugs [107]. Cortical stimulation can also increase the response to physical therapy in stroke patients, improving practice-dependent plasticity and rehabilitative training [108–110].

In addition, because cortical stimulation affects the whole axon, this may result in non-synaptic or excitatory effects, rather related to changes of conformation and function of various axonal molecules exposed to the electromagnetic field, for example, involved in membrane structure, cytoskeleton or axonal transport [111]. These changes may also occur in the non-neuronal cells that present in this field, such as glial, endothelial and inflammatory cells. This may have an impact on the underlying inflammatory or degenerative causal mechanisms of various brain disorders, thus playing a role in the resulting effect of cortical stimulation on the course of the disease. Electromagnetic fields are also known to be able to promote axonal regeneration and neurite outgrowth [112–115]. These aspects of the cellular mechanisms of the action of neuromodulation are clearly less well characterized than the effects on the firing pattern of axons, synaptic plasticity or brain network connectivity, but they are worth to be further investigated, especially regarding the therapeutic effects of neuromodulation therapies in the long term.

Finally, another potential mechanism of action of cortical stimulation deals with neuroprotection. Cortical stimulation is not only able to increase the expression and release of neuroprotective substances within the brain, but it is also able to promote neuroprotection by reducing neural cell degeneration caused due to excitotoxic processes. Excitotoxicity includes cellular and synaptic phenomena. 'Cellular' excitotoxicity relates to membrane depolarization and intra-axonal Na^+ overload in the context of ischaemia or energetic resource failure. This results in increased Ca^{2+} influx and neural cell death or apoptosis [116]. Increased Ca^{2+} influx may also result from an excessive synaptic activation of the NMDA-type glutamate receptors ('synaptic' excitotoxicity) [117]. In brain injury, such as stroke, NMDA-mediated excitotoxicity leads to a vicious circle of autodestructive events, including glutamate release by the lysed cells and cell membrane depolarization. The reduction of glutamatergic excitotoxicity by 'inhibitory' procedures of cortical stimulation may also be valuable in neurodegenerative disorders, such as amyotrophic lateral sclerosis [118, 119], in which NMDA-mediated excitotoxicity is largely involved in motoneuron loss [120]. Indeed, various methods of 'inhibitory' cortical stimulation might be proposed for neuroprotection purpose, including tDCS, well beyond the sole change of neuronal excitability. Whether these procedures could be equally effective, and in which pathological condition they can be applied, remains to be further studied.

To conclude, any neurological or psychiatric disorder that includes primary or secondary cortical dysfunction could be theoretically a good indication for cortical stimulation therapy. We must keep in mind that cortical stimulation impacts primarily the excitability of neuronal networks. Therefore, one key point is to determine how excitability changes relate to 'activation' and 'inhibition' and of which networks. Overall, cortical stimulation can be used to reactivate hypoactive structures or to inhibit overactive structures. This concept underlies the application of rTMS in stroke, that is to restore the balance of activation between both the hemispheres using either HF rTMS to reactivate the affected hemisphere [121] or LF rTMS to reduce the deleterious influence of the contralateral homologous cortical territory [122]. In depression, functional improvement may equally result from the activation of the left DLPFC by HF rTMS [123] or the inhibition of the right DLPFC by LF rTMS [124]. However, as mentioned above, caution should be exercised before generalizing this simplistic dichotomous view of rTMS. Cortical stimulation may also impact diseases by enhancing the processes of cortical reorganization or by modulating synchronized or oscillatory activities in cortico-subcortical networks. The resulting changes can last beyond the time of stimulation, mostly due to processes of synaptic plasticity, but other potential effects could only last during the time of stimulation. Considering the variety of applicable methods, the primary challenge is to find the optimal strategy of brain stimulation for each disease condition, or more precisely for each type of clinical symptom.

References

1 Lefaucheur JP. Methods of therapeutic cortical stimulation. Neurophysiol Clin 2009;39:1–14.
2 Nguyen JP, Lefaucheur JP, Decq P, Uchiyama T, Carpentier A, Fontaine D, et al. Chronic motor cortex stimulation in the treatment of central and neuropathic pain. Correlations between clinical, electrophysiological and anatomical data. Pain 1999;82:245–51.
3 Beuter A, Lefaucheur JP, Modolo J. Closed-loop cortical neuromodulation in Parkinson's disease: an alternative to deep brain stimulation? Clin Neurophysiol 2014;125:874–85.
4 Barker A, Freeston I, Jalinous R, Jarrat J. Non invasive magnetic stimulation of the human motor cortex. Lancet 1985;2:1106–7.
5 Lefaucheur JP, André-Obadia N, Antal A, Ayache SS, Baeken C, Benninger DH, et al. Evidence-based guidelines on the therapeutic use of repetitive transcranial magnetic stimulation (rTMS). Clin Neurophysiol 2014;125: 2150–206.
6 Guleyupoglu B, Schestatsky P, Edwards D, Fregni F, Bikson M. Classification of methods in transcranial electrical stimulation (tES) and evolving strategy from historical approaches to contemporary innovations. J Neurosci Methods 2013;219:297–311.
7 Nitsche MA, Paulus W. Transcranial direct current stimulation – update 2011. Restor Neurol Neurosci 2011;29:463–92.
8 Nowak LG, Bullier J. Axons, but not cell bodies, are activated by electrical stimulation in cortical gray matter. I. Evidence from chronaxie measurements. Exp Brain Res 1998;118:477–88.
9 McIntyre CC, Grill WM. Extracellular stimulation of central neurons: influence of stimulus waveform and frequency on neuronal output. J Neurophysiol 2002;88:1592–604.
10 Lefaucheur JP. Principles of therapeutic use of transcranial and epidural cortical stimulation. Clin Neurophysiol 2008;119:2179–84.
11 Di Lazzaro V, Oliviero A, Pilato F, Mazzone P, Insola A, Ranieri F, et al. Corticospinal volleys evoked by transcranial stimulation of the brain in conscious humans. Neurol Res 2003;25:143–50.
12 Kaneko K, Kawai S, Fuchigami Y, Morita H, Ofuji A. The effect of current direction induced by transcranial magnetic stimulation on the corticospinal excitability in human brain. Electroencephalogr Clin Neurophysiol 1996;101:478–82.
13 Nakamura H, Kitagawa H, Kawaguchi Y, Tsuji H. Direct and indirect activation of human corticospinal neurons by transcranial magnetic and electrical stimulation. Neurosci Lett 1996;210:45–8.
14 Sakai K, Ugawa Y, Terao Y, Hanajima R, Furubayashi T, Kanazawa I. Preferential activation of different I waves by transcranial magnetic stimulation with a figure-of-eight-shaped coil. Exp Brain Res 1997;113:24–32.
15 Di Lazzaro V, Oliviero A, Profice P, Saturno E, Pilato F, Insola A, et al. Comparison of descending volleys evoked by transcranial magnetic and electric stimulation in conscious humans. Electroencephalogr Clin Neurophysiol 1998; 109:397–401.

16 Di Lazzaro V, Oliviero A, Pilato F, Saturno E, Dileone M, Mazzone P, et al. The physiological basis of transcranial motor cortex stimulation in conscious humans. Clin Neurophysiol 2004a;115:255–66.
17 Amassian VE, Stewart M. Motor cortical and other cortical interneuronal networks that generate very high frequency waves. Suppl Clin Neurophysiol 2003;56:119–42.
18 Rossini PM, Barker AT, Berardelli A, Caramia MD, Caruso G, Cracco RQ, et al. Non-invasive electrical and magnetic stimulation of the brain, spinal cord and roots: basic principles and procedures for routine clinical application. Report of an IFCN committee. Electroencephalogr Clin Neurophysiol 1994;91:79–92.
19 Awiszus F. TMS and threshold hunting. Suppl Clin Neurophysiol 2003;56:13–23.
20 Hanajima R, Wang R, Nakatani-Enomoto S, Hamada M, Terao Y, Furubayashi T, et al. Comparison of different methods for estimating motor threshold with transcranial magnetic stimulation. Clin Neurophysiol 2007;118:2120–2.
21 Silbert BI, Patterson HI, Pevcic DD, Windnagel KA, Thickbroom GW. A comparison of relative-frequency and threshold-hunting methods to determine stimulus intensity in transcranial magnetic stimulation. Clin Neurophysiol 2013;124:708–12.
22 Antal A, Kincses TZ, Nitsche MA, Bartfai O, Paulus W. Excitability changes induced in the human primary visual cortex by transcranial direct current stimulation: direct electrophysiological evidence. Invest Ophthalmol Vis Sci 2004;45:702–7.
23 Fox P, Ingham R, George MS, Mayberg H, Ingham J, Roby J, et al. Imaging human intracerebral connectivity by PET during TMS. Neuroreport 1997;8:2787–91.
24 Siebner HR, Bergmann TO, Bestmann S, Massimini M, Johansen-Berg H, Mochizuki H, et al. Consensus paper: combining transcranial stimulation with neuroimaging. Brain Stimul 2009;2:58–80.
25 Di Lazzaro V, Dileone M, Pilato F, Capone F, Musumeci G, Ranieri F, et al. Modulation of motor cortex neuronal networks by rTMS: comparison of local and remote effects of six different protocols of stimulation. J Neurophysiol 2011;105:2150–6.
26 Lefaucheur JP. Neurophysiology of cortical stimulation. Int Rev Neurobiol 2012;107:57–85.
27 Bestmann S, Baudewig J, Siebner HR, Rothwell JC, Frahm J. BOLD MRI responses to repetitive TMS over human dorsal premotor cortex. Neuroimage 2005;28:22–9.
28 Keck ME, Sillaber I, Ebner K, Welt T, Toschi N, Kaehler ST, et al. Acute transcranial magnetic stimulation of frontal brain regions selectively modulates the release of vasopressin, biogenic amines and amino acids in the rat brain. Eur J Neurosci 2000;12:3713–20.
29 Keck M, Welt T, Muller M, Erhardt A, Ohl F, Toschi N, et al. Repetitive transcranial magnetic stimulation increases the release of dopamine in the mesolimbic and mesostriatal system. Neuropharmacology 2002;43:101–9.
30 Strafella AP, Paus T, Barrett J, Dagher A. Repetitive transcranial magnetic stimulation of the human prefrontal cortex induces dopamine release in the caudate nucleus. J Neurosci 2001;21:RC157.
31 Strafella AP, Paus T, Fraraccio M, Dagher A. Striatal dopamine release induced by repetitive transcranial magnetic stimulation of the human motor cortex. Brain 2003;126:2609–15.
32 Ohnishi T, Hayashi T, Okabe S, Nonaka I, Matsuda H, Iida H, et al. Enodgenous dopamine release induced by repetitive transcranial magnetic stimulation over the primary motor cortex: an (11C) Raclopride positron emission tomography study in anesthetized macaque monkeys. Biol Psychiatry 2004;55:484–9.
33 Kim JY, Chung EJ, Lee WY, Shin HY, Lee GH, Choe YS, et al. Therapeutic effect of repetitive transcranial magnetic stimulation in Parkinson's disease: analysis of (11C) raclopride PET study. Mov Disord 2008;23:207–11.
34 de Andrade DC, Mhalla A, Adam F, Texeira MJ, Bouhassira D. Neuropharmacological basis of rTMS-induced analgesia: the role of endogenous opioids. Pain 2011;152:320–6.
35 Maarrawi J, Peyron R, Mertens P, Costes N, Magnin M, Sindou M, et al. Motor cortex stimulation for pain control induces changes in the endogenous opioid system. Neurology 2007;69:827–34.
36 Taylor JJ, Borckardt JJ, George MS. Endogenous opioids mediate left dorsolateral prefrontal cortex rTMS-induced analgesia. Pain 2012;153:1219–25.

37 Taylor JJ, Borckardt JJ, Canterberry M, Li X, Hanlon CA, Brown TR, et al. Naloxone-reversible modulation of pain circuitry by left prefrontal rTMS. Neuropsychopharmacology 2013;38:1189–97.
38 Ahdab R, Ayache SS, Brugieres P, Goujon C, Lefaucheur JP. Comparison of 'standard' and 'navigated' procedures of TMS coil positioning over motor, premotor and prefrontal targets in patients with chronic pain and depression. Neurophysiol Clin 2010;40:27–36.
39 Lefaucheur JP. Why image-guided navigation becomes essential in the practice of transcranial magnetic stimulation. Neurophysiol Clin 2010;40:1–5.
40 Ruohonen J, Karhu J. Navigated transcranial magnetic stimulation. Neurophysiol Clin 2010; 40:7–17.
41 Lefaucheur JP, de Andrade DC. Intraoperative neurophysiologic mapping of the central cortical region for epidural electrode placement in the treatment of neuropathic pain by motor cortex stimulation. Brain Stimul 2009;2: 138–48.
42 Houzé B, Bradley C, Magnin M, Garcia-Larrea L. Changes in sensory hand representation and pain thresholds induced by motor cortex stimulation in humans. Cereb Cortex 2013; 23:2667–76.
43 Fuggetta G, Noh NA. A neurophysiological insight into the potential link between transcranial magnetic stimulation, thalamocortical dysrhythmia and neuropsychiatric disorders. Exp Neurol 2013;245:87–95.
44 Marshall L, Molle M, Hallschmid M, Born J. Transcranial direct current stimulation during sleep improves declarative memory. J Neurosci 2004;24:9985–92.
45 Polanía R, Paulus W, Nitsche MA. Modulating cortico-striatal and thalamo-cortical functional connectivity with transcranial direct current stimulation. Hum Brain Mapp 2012;33:2499–508.
46 Lefaucheur JP, Drouot X, Keravel Y, Nguyen JP. Pain relief induced by repetitive transcranial magnetic stimulation of precentral cortex. Neuroreport 2001a;12:2963–5.
47 Fitzgerald PB, Benitez J, de Castella A, Daskalakis ZJ, Brown TL, Kulkarni J. A randomized, controlled trial of sequential bilateral repetitive transcranial magnetic stimulation for treatment-resistant depression. Am J Psychiatry 2006;163:88–94.
48 Chen R, Classen J, Gerloff C, Celnik P, Wassermann EM, Hallett M, et al. Depression of motor cortex excitability by low-frequency transcranial magnetic stimulation. Neurology 1997;48:1398–403.
49 Pascual-Leone A, Valls-Sole J, Wassermann EM, Hallett M. Responses to rapid-rate transcranial magnetic stimulation of the human motor cortex. Brain 1994b;117:847–58.
50 Maeda F, Keenan J, Tormos J, Topka H, Pascual-Leone A. Modulation of corticospinal excitability by repetitive transcranial magnetic stimulation. Clin Neurophysiol 2000;111:800–5.
51 Touge T, Gerschlager W, Brown P, Rothwell JC. Are the after-effects of low-frequency rTMS on motor cortex excitability due to changes in the efficacy of cortical synapses? Clin Neurophysiol 2001;112:2138–45.
52 Gangitano M, Valero-Cabre A, Tormos JM, Mottaghy FM, Romero JR, Pascual-Leone A. Modulation of input-output curves by low and high frequency repetitive transcranial magnetic stimulation of the motor cortex. Clin Neurophysiol 2002;113:1249–57.
53 Pascual-Leone A, Tormos JM, Keenan J, Tarazona F, Canete C, Catala MD. Study and modulation of human cortical excitability with transcranial magnetic stimulation. J Clin Neurophysiol 1998;15:333–43.
54 Post RM, Kimbrell TA, McCann UD, Dunn RT, Osuch EA, Speer AM, et al. Repetitive transcranial magnetic stimulation as a neuropsychiatric tool: present status and future potential. J ECT 1999;15:39–59.
55 Bliss TV, Lomo T. Long-lasting potentiation of synaptic transmission in the dentate area of the anaesthetized rabbit following stimulation of the perforant path. J Physiol 1973;232: 331–56.
56 Malenka RC. Postsynaptic factors control the duration of synaptic enhancement in area CA1 of the hippocampus. Neuron 1991;6:53–60.
57 Ziemann U. TMS induced plasticity in human cortex. Rev Neurosci 2004;15:253–66.
58 Cooke SF, Bliss TV. Plasticity in the human central nervous system. Brain 2006;129:1659–73.
59 Ziemann U, Paulus W, Nitsche MA, Pascual-Leone A, Byblow WD, Berardelli A, et al.

Consensus: motor cortex plasticity protocols. Brain Stimul 2008;1:164–82.
60 Goldsworthy MR, Pitcher JB, Ridding MC. A comparison of two different continuous theta burst stimulation paradigms applied to the human primary motor cortex. Clin Neurophysiol 2012;123:2256–63.
61 Huang YZ, Edwards MJ, Rounis E, Bhatia KP, Rothwell JC. Theta burst stimulation of the human motor cortex. Neuron 2005;45:201–6.
62 Houdayer E, Degardin A, Cassim F, Bocquillon P, Derambure P, Devanne H. The effects of low- and high-frequency repetitive TMS on the input/output properties of the human corticospinal pathway. Exp Brain Res 2008;187: 207–17.
63 Koch G, Brusa L, Caltagirone C, Peppe A, Oliveri M, Stanzione P, et al. rTMS of supplementary motor area modulates therapy-induced dyskinesias in Parkinson disease. Neurology 2005;65:623–5.
64 Poreisz C, Antal A, Boros K, Brepohl N, Csifcsák G, Paulus W. Attenuation of N2 amplitude of laser-evoked potentials by theta burst stimulation of primary somatosensory cortex. Exp Brain Res 2008;185:611–21.
65 Lefaucheur JP, Ayache SS, Sorel M, Farhat WH, Zouari HG, Ciampi de Andrade D, et al. Analgesic effects of repetitive transcranial magnetic stimulation of the motor cortex in neuropathic pain: influence of theta burst stimulation priming. Eur J Pain 2012;16:1403–13.
66 Gamboa OL, Antal A, Moliadze V, Paulus W. Simply longer is not better: reversal of theta burst after-effect with prolonged stimulation. Exp Brain Res 2010;204:181–7.
67 Wu T, Sommer M, Tergau F, Paulus W. Lasting influence of repetitive transcranial magnetic stimulation on intracortical excitability in human subjects. Neurosci Lett 2000;287: 37–40.
68 Di Lazzaro V, Oliviero A, Saturno E, Pilato F, Insola A, Mazzone P, et al. The effect on corticospinal volleys of reversing the direction of current induced in the motor cortex by transcranial magnetic stimulation. Exp Brain Res 2001;138:268–73.
69 Cincotta M, Borgheresi A, Gambetti C, Balestrieri F, Rossi L, Zaccara G, et al. Suprathreshold 0.3 Hz repetitive TMS prolongs the cortical silent period: potential implications for therapeutic trials in epilepsy. Clin Neurophysiol 2003;114: 1827–33.
70 Daskalakis ZJ, Möller B, Christensen BK, Fitzgerald PB, Gunraj C, Chen R. The effects of repetitive transcranial magnetic stimulation on cortical inhibition in healthy human subjects. Exp Brain Res 2006;174:403–12.
71 Eichhammer P, Kleinjung T, Landgrebe M, Hajak G, Langguth B. TMS for treatment of chronic tinnitus: neurobiological effects. Prog Brain Res 2007;166:369–75.
72 Murase N, Rothwell JC, Kaji R, Urushihara R, Nakamura K, Murayama N, et al. Subthreshold low-frequency repetitive transcranial magnetic stimulation over the premotor cortex modulates writer's cramp. Brain 2005;128:104–15.
73 Borich M, Arora S, Kimberley TJ. Lasting effects of repeated rTMS application in focal hand dystonia. Restor Neurol Neurosci 2009;27:55–65.
74 Filipović SR, Rothwell JC, Bhatia K. Slow (1 Hz) repetitive transcranial magnetic stimulation (rTMS) induces a sustained change in cortical excitability in patients with Parkinson's disease. Clin Neurophysiol 2010;121:1129–37.
75 Di Lazzaro V, Profice P, Pilato F, Dileone M, Oliviero A, Ziemann U. The effects of motor cortex rTMS on corticospinal descending activity. Clin Neurophysiol 2010;121:464–73.
76 Hamada M, Murase N, Hasan A, Balaratnam M, Rothwell JC. The role of interneuron networks in driving human motor cortical plasticity. Cereb Cortex 2013;23:1593–605.
77 Rothkegel H, Sommer M, Paulus W. Breaks during 5 Hz rTMS are essential for facilitatory after effects. Clin Neurophysiol 2010;121:426–30.
78 Lefaucheur JP, Drouot X, Nguyen JP. Interventional neurophysiology for pain control: duration of pain relief following repetitive transcranial magnetic stimulation of the motor cortex. Neurophysiol Clin 2001b;31:247–52.
79 Padberg F, Goldstein-Muller B, Zwanzger P, Moller HJ. Prefrontal cortex stimulation as antidepressant treatment: mode of action and clinical effectiveness of rTMS. Suppl Clin Neurophysiol 2003;56:406–32.
80 Liebetanz D, Nitsche MA, Tergau F, Paulus W. Pharmacological approach to the mechanisms

of transcranial DC-stimulation-induced after-effects of human motor cortex excitability. Brain 2001;125:2238–47.
81 Nitsche MA, Fricke K, Henschke U, Schlitterlau A, Liebetanz D, Lang N, et al. Pharmacological modulation of cortical excitability shifts induced by transcranial direct current stimulation in humans. J Physiol (London) 2003;553: 293–301.
82 Stagg CJ, Best JG, Stephenson MC, O'Shea J, Wylezinska M, Kincses ZT, et al. Polarity-sensitive modulation of cortical neurotransmitters by transcranial stimulation. J Neurosci 2009;29:5202–6.
83 Bienenstock EL, Cooper LN, Munro PW. Theory for the development of neuron selectivity: orientation specificity and binocular interaction in visual cortex. J Neurosci 1982;2:32–48.
84 Abraham WC, Tate WP. Metaplasticity: a new vista across the field of synaptic plasticity. Prog Neurobiol 1997;52:303–23.
85 Turrigiano GG, Nelson SB. Homeostatic plasticity in the developing nervous system. Nat Rev Neurosci 2004;5:97–107.
86 Iyer MB, Schleper N, Wassermann EM. Priming stimulation enhances the depressant effect of low-frequency repetitive transcranial magnetic stimulation. J Neurosci 2003;23:10867–72.
87 Andoh J, Artiges E, Pallier C, Rivière D, Mangin JF, Paillère-Martinot ML, et al. Priming frequencies of transcranial magnetic stimulation over Wernicke's area modulate word detection. Cereb Cortex 2008;18:210–6.
88 Lang N, Siebner HR, Ernst D, Nitsche MA, Paulus W, Lemon RN, et al. Preconditioning with transcranial direct current stimulation sensitizes the motor cortex to rapid-rate transcranial magnetic stimulation and controls the direction of after-effects. Biol Psychiatry 2004;56:634–9.
89 Siebner HR, Lang N, Rizzo V, Nitsche MA, Paulus W, Lemon RN, et al. Preconditioning of low-frequency repetitive transcranial magnetic stimulation with transcranial direct current stimulation: evidence for homeostatic plasticity in the human motor cortex. J Neurosci 2004;24:3379–85.
90 Lefaucheur JP, Drouot X, Menard-Lefaucheur I, Keravel Y, Nguyen JP. Motor cortex rTMS restores defective intracortical inhibition in chronic neuropathic pain. Neurology 2006;67: 1568–74.
91 George MS, Wassermann EM, Williams WA, Steppel J, Pascual-Leone A, Basser P, et al. Changes in mood and hormone levels after rapid-rate transcranial magnetic stimulation (rTMS) of the prefrontal cortex. J Neuropsychiatry Clin Neurosci 1996;8:172–80.
92 Pascual-Leone A, Catala MD, Pascual-Leone PA. Lateralized effect of rapid-rate transcranial magnetic stimulation of the prefrontal cortex on mood. Neurology 1996;46:499–502.
93 Edwards MJ, Huang YZ, Mir P, Rothwell JC, Bhatia KP. Abnormalities in motor cortical plasticity differentiate manifesting and non-manifesting DYT1 carriers. Mov Disord 2006;21:2181–6.
94 Kleim JA, Chan S, Pringle E, Schallert K, Procaccio V, Jimenez R, et al. BDNF val66met polymorphism is associated with modified experience-dependent plasticity in human motor cortex. Nat Neurosci 2006;9:735–7.
95 Inghilleri M, Conte A, Curra A, Frasca V, Lorenzano C, Berardelli A. Ovarian hormones and cortical excitability. An rTMS study in humans. Clin Neurophysiol 2004;115: 1063–8.
96 Stefan K, Wycislo M, Classen, J. Modulation of associative human motor cortical plasticity by attention. J Neurophysiol 2004:92:66–72.
97 Ziemann U, Tam A, Butefisch C, Cohen LG. Dual modulating effects of amphetamine on neuronal excitability and stimulation-induced plasticity in human motor cortex. Clin Neurophysiol 2002;113:1308–15.
98 Fregni F, Boggio PS, Valle AC, Otachi P, Thut G, Rigonatti SP, et al. Homeostatic effects of plasma valproate levels on corticospinal excitability changes induced by 1Hz rTMS in patients with juvenile myoclonic epilepsy. Clin Neurophysiol 2006;117:1217–27.
99 Buhmann C, Gorsler A, Baumer T, Hidding U, Demiralay C, Hinkelmann K, et al. Abnormal excitability of premotor-motor connections in de novo Parkinson's disease. Brain 2004;127:2732–46.
100 Mir P, Matsunaga K, Gilio F, Quinn NP, Siebner HR, Rothwell JC. Dopaminergic drugs restore

facilitatory premotor-motor interactions in Parkinson disease. Neurology 2005;64:1906–12.
101 Conforto AB, Kaelin-Lang A, Cohen LG. Increase in hand muscle strength of stroke patients after somatosensory stimulation. Ann Neurol 2002;51:122–5.
102 Ziemann U, Hallett M, Cohen LG. Mechanisms of deafferentation-induced plasticity in human motor cortex. J Neurosci 1998;18:7000–7.
103 Liepert J. Motor cortex excitability in stroke before and after constraint-induced movement therapy. Cogn Behav Neurol 2006;19:41–7.
104 Pascual-Leone A, Nguyet D, Cohen LG, Brasil-Neto JP, Cammarota A, Hallett M. Modulation of muscle responses evoked by transcranial magnetic stimulation during the acquisition of new fine motor skills. J Neurophysiol 1995;74: 1037–45.
105 Pascual-Leone A, Grafman J, Hallett M. Modulation of cortical motor output maps during development of implicit and explicit knowledge. Science 1994a;263:1287–9.
106 Ziemann U, Ilic TV, Pauli C, Meintzschel F, Ruge D. Learning modifies subsequent induction of long-term potentiation-like and long-term depression-like plasticity in human motor cortex. J Neurosci 2004;24:1666–72.
107 Rumi DO, Gattaz WF, Rigonatti SP, Rosa MA, Fregni F, Rosa MO, et al. Transcranial magnetic stimulation accelerates the antidepressant effect of amitriptyline in severe depression: a double-blind placebo-controlled study. Biol Psychiatry 2005;57:162–6.
108 Ayache SS, Farhat WH, Zouari HG, Hosseini H, Mylius V, Lefaucheur JP. Stroke rehabilitation using noninvasive cortical stimulation: motor deficit. Expert Rev Neurother 2012;12: 949–72.
109 Brown JA, Lutsep HL, Weinand M, Cramer SC. Motor cortex stimulation for the enhancement of recovery from stroke: a prospective, multicenter safety study. Neurosurgery 2006;58:464–73.
110 Kim YH, You SH, Ko MH, Park JW, Lee KH, Jang SH, et al. Repetitive transcranial magnetic stimulation-induced corticomotor excitability and associated motor skill acquisition in chronic stroke. Stroke 2006; 37:1471–6.
111 Jefferys JG. Nonsynaptic modulation of neuronal activity in the brain: electric currents and extracellular ions. Physiol Rev 1995;75: 689–723.
112 Macias MY, Battocletti JH, Sutton CH, Pintar FA, Maiman DJ. Directed and enhanced neurite growth with pulsed magnetic field stimulation. Bioelectromagnetics 2000;21:272–86.
113 De Pedro JA, Pérez-Caballer AJ, Dominguez J, Collía F, Blanco J, Salvado M. Pulsed electromagnetic fields induce peripheral nerve regeneration and endplate enzymatic changes. Bioelectromagnetics 2005;26:20–7.
114 Wood M, Willits RK. Short-duration, DC electrical stimulation increases chick embryo DRG neurite outgrowth. Bioelectromagnetics 2006;27:328–31.
115 Koppes AN, Seggio AM, Thompson DM. Neurite outgrowth is significantly increased by the simultaneous presentation of Schwann cells and moderate exogenous electric fields. J Neural Eng 2011;8:046023.
116 Lipton SA, Nicotera P. Calcium, free radicals and excitotoxins in neuronal apoptosis. Cell Calcium 1998:23:165–71.
117 Lipton SA, Rosenberg PA. Excitatory amino acids as a final common pathway for neurologic disorders. N Engl J Med 1994;30:613–22.
118 Di Lazzaro V, Oliviero A, Saturno E, Pilato F, Dileone M, Sabatelli M, et al. Motor cortex stimulation for amyotrophic lateral sclerosis: time for a therapeutic trial? Clin Neurophysiol 2004b;115:1479–85.
119 Di Lazzaro V, Dileone M, Pilato F, Profice P, Ranieri F, Musumeci G, et al. Repetitive transcranial magnetic stimulation for ALS: a preliminary controlled study. Neurosci Lett 2006;408:135–40.
120 Van Damme P, Dewil M, Robberecht W, Van Den Bosch L. Excitotoxicity and amyotrophic lateral sclerosis. Neurodegener Dis 2005;2: 147–59.
121 Khedr EM, Ahmed MA, Fathy N, Rothwell JC. Therapeutic trial of repetitive transcranial magnetic stimulation after acute ischemic stroke. Neurology 2005;65:466–8.
122 Mansur CG, Fregni F, Boggio PS, Riberto M, Gallucci-Neto J, Santos CM, et al. A sham stimulation-controlled trial of rTMS of the

unaffected hemisphere in stroke patients. Neurology 2005;64:1802–4.

123 George MS, Wassermann EM, Williams WA, Callahan A, Ketter TA, Basser P, et al. Daily repetitive transcranial magnetic stimulation (rTMS) improves mood in depression. NeuroReport 1995;6:1853–6.

124 Klein E, Kreinin I, Chistyakov A, Koren D, Mecz L, Marmur S, et al. Therapeutic efficacy of right prefrontal slow repetitive transcranial magnetic stimulation in major depression: a double-blind controlled study. Arch Gen Psychiatry 1999;56:315–20.

CHAPTER 8

Transcranial magnetic stimulation: Introduction and technical aspects

Yiftach Roth, Gaby S. Pell and Abraham Zangen
Ben Gurion University, Beer Sheva, Israel

Background

Historical background

The notion of non-invasive and indirect brain stimulation using a time-varying magnetic field gradually evolved during the 19th century, following the discovery of electromagnetic induction in 1831 by Faraday [1, 2]. In 1855, Foucault discovered the eddy currents, which are induced in a conductive medium when exposed to a time-varying magnetic field. It was soon realized that this principle might be utilized to stimulate neuronal tissue. The first known attempt to induce magnetic brain stimulation was by d'Arsonval [3], who applied an alternating current to a coil surrounding the head and induced phosphenes, vertigo and syncope. In the following years, several researchers [4–8] induced visual sensations by alternating currents at various frequencies in large coils located near the head. In 1959, Kolin and colleagues [9] gave the first demonstration of a magnetic stimulation of a nerve when they stimulated a frog sciatic nerve and induced muscle contractions. In 1965, Bickford and Freming induced magnetic stimulation of peripheral nerves in animals and human subjects [10].

Transcranial magnetic stimulation (TMS) emerged in 1985, when Barker and colleagues at the University of Sheffield in the U.K. achieved non-invasive and painless stimulation of human motor cortex using a stimulator consisting of a capacitor discharging into a stimulating coil placed on the scalp [11]. The TMS technique represented a novel research tool for studying the functionality, morphology and connectivity of various cortical regions, especially the motor cortex [12]. By the early 1990s, further development of magnetic stimulators expanded the range of stimulus frequency, allowing rapid-rate TMS (rTMS) at frequencies of up to 30 Hz [13–15]. Several studies demonstrated that application of rTMS to the motor cortex could produce several minutes of persistent increased [15] or decreased corticospinal excitability [16–18]. Generally, two principal rTMS modalities have been applied in intervention studies: Low-frequency rTMS (<3 Hz), which is proposed to reduce cortical excitability, and high-frequency rTMS (≥5 Hz), which is proposed to increase cortical excitability [19]. Since the 1990s, there has been a rapidly growing interest in the potential of rTMS to modulate excitability of various brain regions, and to treat various neurological and psychiatric disorders [20–22].

Neuromodulation in Psychiatry, First Edition. Edited by Clement Hamani, Paul Holtzheimer, Andres M. Lozano and Helen Mayberg.

Physical principles of TMS

TMS is a technique for non-invasive stimulation of neuronal structures. Magnetic pulses are administered by passing a strong current through an electromagnetic coil placed upon the scalp that induces an electric field and, therefore, current in the underlying cortical tissue. The TMS technique is based on the law of electromagnetic induction discovered by Michael Faraday in 1831. Faraday's set of experiments constituted a key milestone of electromagnetism and also a masterpiece of empirical science in general. Faraday was surprised and disappointed to discover that a constant current in a conductor had no effect on a nearby conductor. Yet, he noticed that upon switching on or off the primary current in the first conductor, there was an induced current in the secondary wire. He pursued this line of research and discovered that an *alternating* – but not a constant – electric current in one conductor, induces currents in the opposite direction in nearby conductors. This law of induction was termed Faraday's law and was generalized as one of the four fundamental equations of classical electromagnetism, the Maxwell equations:

$$\vec{\nabla} \times \vec{E} = -\frac{d\vec{B}}{dt} \qquad (8.1)$$

where $\vec{E}$ is the induced primary electric field, $\vec{B}$ is magnetic field and t is time. Basically, this law states that a changing magnetic field produces an electric field. Any electric current in a conductor induces a magnetic field around it.

Any electric field in a conductive medium generates electric currents. Hence, when an alternating current is passed in a coil, currents, known as eddy currents, will be induced in a nearby conductive medium. If the electromagnetic coil is placed near a human head, an electric field is induced in the brain tissue. At high enough intensity, the electric field can be sufficient to cause membrane depolarization in neuronal structures, initiation of action potential and hence neuronal activation. The basics of the neuronal response to the TMS pulse are described in the next sections.

Neuronal activation

Mechanisms that activate a neuron when stimulated

Electromagnetic fields can induce excitation of neurons without the need for mechanical contact. The basic mechanism of neural activation induced by implanted electrodes in the brain or by direct electrical or magnetic stimulation relies on forcing free charges (ions) in intra- and extra-cellular spaces to move coherently by an electric field. Outward-directed trans-membrane currents will trigger an action potential if above a certain threshold. Depolarization or hyperpolarization is induced in cell membranes that interrupt current progress and eventually neural action potential is triggered by depolarization of the axon membrane [23]. It should be noted that TMS does not activate solely the target area but also the tissues around and above it and, indirectly, the distant interconnected sites in the brain [24].

In general, several excitation mechanisms may be involved in the process of neuronal activation by TMS. Straight long axons are stimulated at the strongest point of the electric field gradient along the axon [25–28]. This seems to be the dominant mechanism in long peripheral nerves [29]. In contrast, in cortical excitation, it was found that it is the peak of the macroscopic applied electric field rather than its first spatial derivative that effectively controls the location of excitation [30]. This apparent contradiction is resolved when accounting for the finding that curved axons are preferably stimulated at the bends, where effective electric field gradient is maximal [27, 29, 31–33], while short axons are most easily stimulated at their ends [23]. For a nerve with a series of bends, a complex pattern of zones of hyperpolarization and depolarization is expected [34].

Indeed, most neural structures in the brain have complex geometry including bend points, terminations and branches. Recent modelling studies imply that cortical excitation is predominantly induced by TMS at the bends of corticocortical or corticospinal fibres, at nerve endings or at constrictions near the surface of the brain [35–38], although the complex shapes of neurons make predictions of precise excitation sites difficult. In all situations, trans-membrane current must be outward for excitation to occur.

Volume-conductor inhomogeneities introduce another complexity. The strongest discontinuity occurs at the brain–bone boundaries, where charge accumulation leads to a reduction in the amplitude of the electric field induced in the brain and changes its spatial distribution [39–44]. Other important boundaries are the cerebrospinal fluid (CSF)–grey matter and the grey matter–white matter (GM–WM) interfaces. Thereby, a distinction must be made between the electric field's primary and secondary components [45], the latter arising from abrupt changes in the electric field at brain boundaries. Recent modelling studies indicate that the brain tissue heterogeneity and anisotropy can significantly affect the electric field distribution, the location of stimulation sites [35, 37, 38, 46–49] and the threshold of neuronal stimulation [36]. Moreover, there is a jump in the intensity of the electric field component perpendicular to the boundary at a CSF–brain tissue or a GM–WM interface, due to the differences in electric conductivity. This may introduce an independent mechanism for membrane depolarization and action potential [35, 48, 49]. Hence, three distinct mechanisms can be defined by which the TMS pulse may lead to membrane depolarization in the brain: (i) The peak electric field induced at axon terminations, bend points and branching points, (ii) the discontinuity in the electric field at a tissue interface and (iii) the gradient of the electric field along the fibre.

The membrane space constant, λ, is another important parameter that governs location of the excitation site [50, 51]. The axon length with respect to λ and the coil orientation [33], as well as the coil position, and current polarity with respect to a bend or termination site dictate the primary source of influence and hence the excitation site [35–38, 52]. Thus, in the cortex, stimulation may preferably occur where the induced electric field is perpendicular to CSF–GM or GM–WM interfaces [36–38].

When a single TMS pulse is administered over the primary motor cortex (M1) at gradually increasing intensities of stimulation, an increasing number of descending, epidurally recordable corticospinal volleys are induced [12, 53, 54]. This is followed by a period of electromyography (EMG) silence (the cortical silent period (CSP)) in a tonically contracted muscle (see Table 8.2). Indirect waves known as I-waves are preferentially observed in the descending volleys for postero-anterior-directed induced current and appear with a periodicity of approximately 1.5 ms (i.e. a discharge frequency of ~667 Hz). These waves reflect the interaction of different levels of trans-synaptic activation of pyramidal tract neurons (PTNs) via excitatory glutamatergic interneurons with oscillatory properties [55]. The initial wave, the I1-wave, is believed to be induced by monosynaptic excitatory connections between P2/P3 excitatory cells (i.e. pyramidal neurons of cortical layers II and III) and P5 cells, whereas the later I-waves are driven by connections of these cortical elements to GABAergic inhibitory interneurons [56]. Direct or D-waves reflecting direct stimulation of the PTN close to the cell body are only induced at higher stimulus intensities. This can be contrasted with transcranial electric stimulation for which D-waves are preferentially evoked. The spatio-temporal summation of I-waves at the cortico-motoneuronal synapses in the spinal cord will trigger an action potential in the spinal motoneuron if at a sufficient integrated level, which leads ultimately to the generation of a motor-evoked potential (MEP) in the target muscle [57]. The pattern of descending volleys is sensitive to pulse shape and polarity as well as pulse timings and pulse protocol [55, 58]. Based on a computer model of the coil and a heterogeneous, isotropic cortical sulcus, the complexity of the situation was demonstrated with observation of an array of potential excitation sites that depended on the interaction of coil orientation with the underlying tissue geometry and heterogeneity [35].

Cable equation

In order to gain a basic understanding of the interaction between the TMS pulse and the neural tissue, a simplistic model of an axon can be used. A long, straight axon stimulated by a figure-8 TMS coil will be initially considered (Figure 8.1). A changing current $I(t)$ is passed through the coil. The axon is located beneath the central segment of the coil. A longitudinal current $\vec{i}_1(t)$ is induced in the axon in an opposite direction. At this stage, an assumption will be made that the axon is straight and very long compared to the coil dimensions. This assumption is much more realistic for peripheral nerves than for cortical neuronal structures. Yet, for the sake of clarity, this simplistic case will be considered first, and, in the next two sections, cases will be described that are more relevant for cortical stimulation.

The transmembrane potential

The neural parameter that is most relevant for the initiation of an action potential is the transmembrane potential. In neurons, there exists an inherent difference in the electric potential between the intracellular and the extracellular media (Figure 8.2). This results from the differences in ion concentrations between the two media and from the presence of macromolecules (such as proteins) in the intracellular space, which are partially charged. Thus, at a baseline state, there is an excess of positive sodium (Na^+) and negative chlorine (Cl^-) ions in the extracellular medium. On the other hand, there is an excess of potassium (K^+) ions in the intracellular medium. The overall effect of all these concentrations is that at baseline, the intracellular potential is more negative than the extracellular one, and hence, the transmembrane potential V_m is approximately −70 mV.

An action potential occurs when the transmembrane potential is depolarized below a threshold value. The main stages of an action potential are shown in Figure 8.3.

A detailed description of the action potential stages is beyond the scope of this Chapter and the focus will therefore be on the most important condition for action potential initiation. When V_m is depolarized (i.e. becomes less negative) above a certain critical value (−60 mV in the example of Figure 8.3), an action potential is initiated. In order to understand how V_m is affected, the passive cable

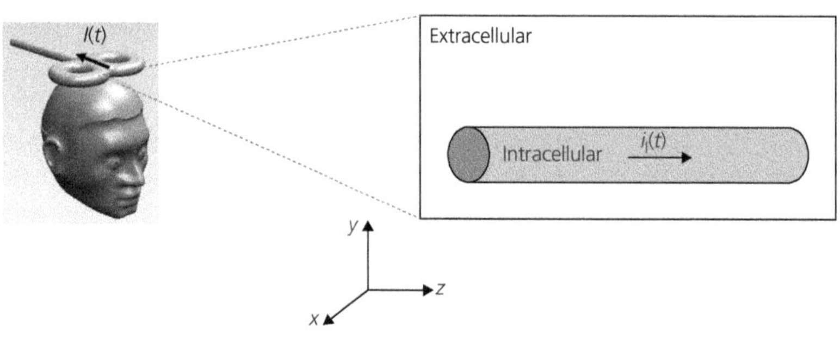

Figure 8.1 A sketch of a figure-8 TMS coil (left) activating a long, straight axon (right). The axon is beneath the central segment of the coil. A changing current $I(t)$ is passed through the coil in the $-z$ direction, inducing an electric field in the underlying axon. This induces a longitudinal current $\vec{i}_1(t)$ in the opposite direction ($+z$) in the axon.

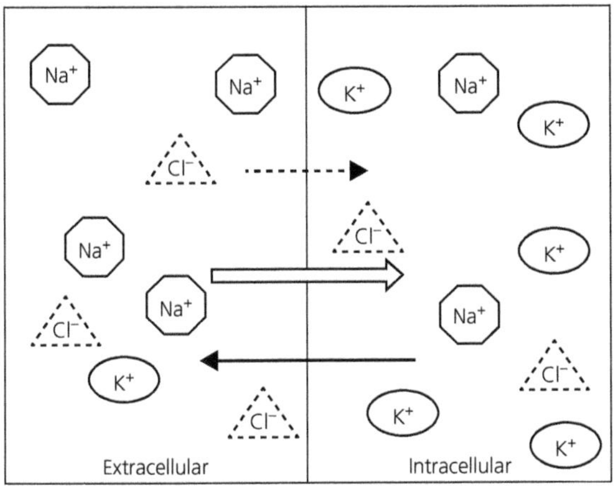

Transmembrane potential ΔV_m = intracellular – extracellular potential = –70 mV

Figure 8.2 An illustration of the differences in ion concentrations between the intracellular cytoplasm of a neuron or a nerve fibre and the extracellular space.

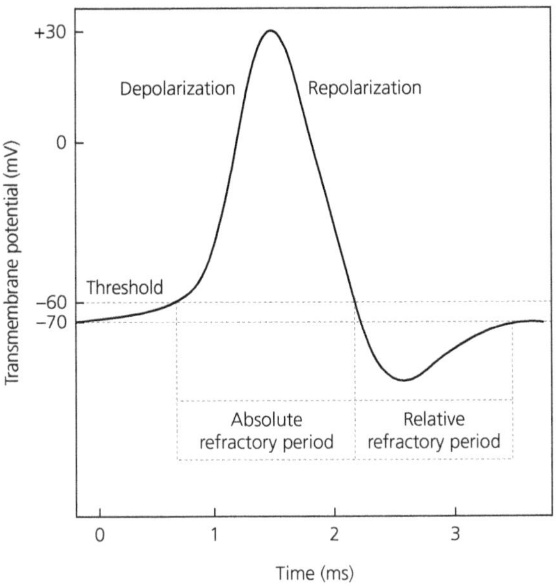

Figure 8.3 An illustration of the action potential. The transmembrane potential, V_m, is plotted as a function of time in ms. When V_m is depolarized below a critical value (–60 mV in this example), a positive-feedback process of ion channel opening and current influx is initiated, and an action potential is produced. The action potential then propagates from the initiation point in both directions along the axon.

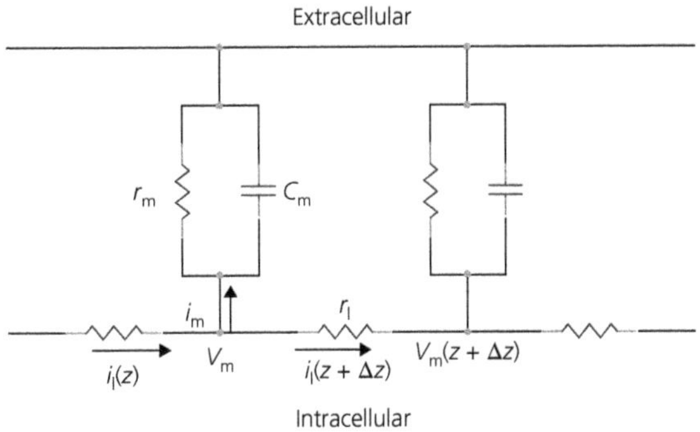

Figure 8.4 A passive cable model for an axon. The membrane segment is represented by a resistance, r_m, and a capacitance, C_m. The axon is modelled by a longitudinal resistance per unit length, r_L in the intracellular medium. The membrane current per unit length is $\vec{i}_m(z)$ and the longitudinal intracellular current is $\vec{i}_l(z)$, where z is the spatial variable along the axon longitudinal axis. The transmembrane potential is $V_m(z)$.

model for an axon will be used [28, 59, 60]. The model is shown in Figure 8.4.

The axon is modelled by a longitudinal resistance per unit length, r_l, in the intracellular medium.

Addition of the TMS effect to the cable equation: long straight axons

The effect of initiating a TMS pulse over the axon will now be considered. The magnetic pulse induces an electric field, E_z, along the axon.

The gradient of the induced electric field along the axon (z axis in our case) is the crucial factor in the modulation of V_m in case of long, straight axons. The effect of the electromagnetic induction on the axon is illustrated in Figure 8.5.

At point **a** in Figure 8.5, there is a positive gradient of the induced electric field $\vec{E}_Z$. Higher electric field induces higher current intensity. Hence, the current to the right of point **a**, $\vec{i}_l(z+\Delta z)$, is higher than the current to the left of point **a**, $\vec{i}_l(z)$.

Kirchoff's law states that at any junction, the sum of incoming currents is equal to the

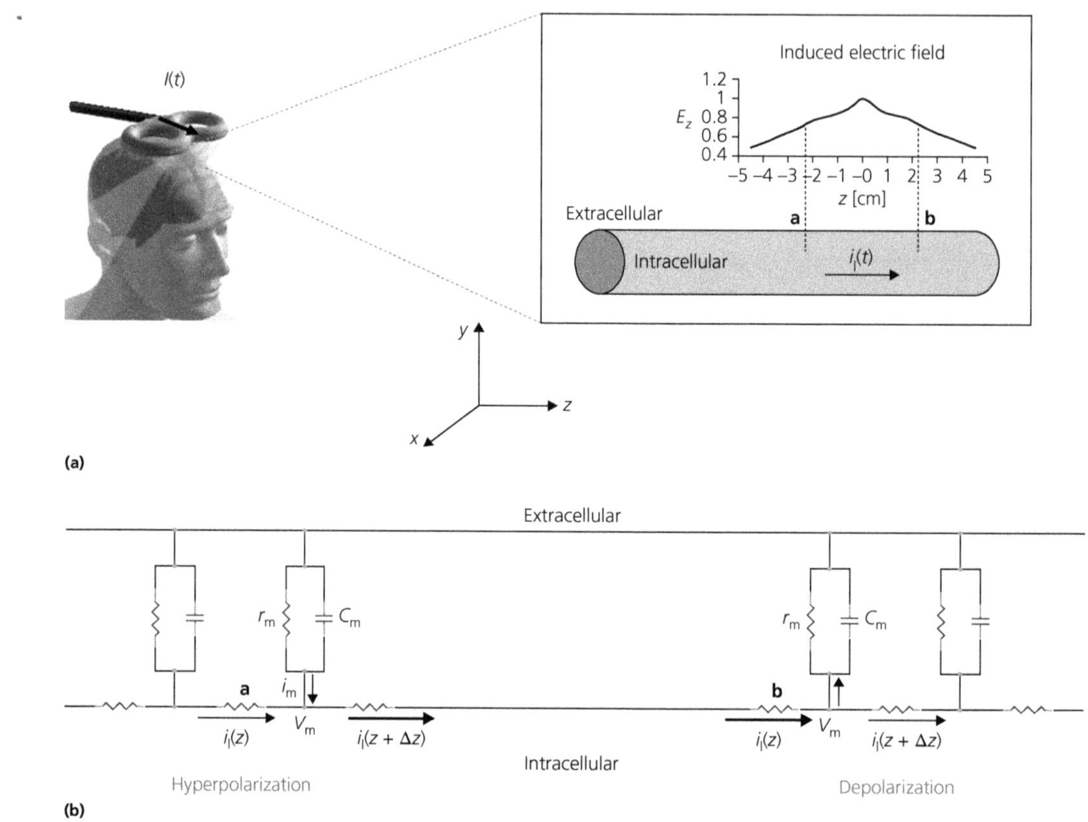

Figure 8.5 An illustration of the effect of a TMS pulse on a long, straight axon. (**a**) The normalized electric field induced along the axon. At points **a** and **b**, the electric field gradients along the z axis are maximally positive and negative, respectively. (**b**) The passive cable model for this case. At point **a**, the membrane current $\vec{i}_m$ flows inward leading to membrane hyperpolarization, while at point **b**, $\vec{i}_m$ flows outward leading to membrane depolarization and initiation of an action potential.

sum of outgoing currents. Hence, there must be a membrane current $\vec{i}_m$ directed inward into the intracellular space. This current leads to membrane hyperpolarization. In contrast, at point **b** in Figure 8.5, the membrane current $\vec{i}_m$ is directed outward and membrane depolarization occurs. Hence, in this case, an action potential may be initiated at point **b**. In case the coil is turned to the opposite direction (i.e. in the $+z$ direction in Figure 8.5), the sites of hyperpolarization and depolarization will be exchanged. Hence, in that case, depolarization and possible action potential initiation may occur at point **a**. Thus far, only the spatial properties of the induced electric field at a certain point in time have been considered. In section 'Circuits of OCD, depression, schizophrenia, and addiction', temporal issues dictated by the dynamic pulse shape will be incorporated, and it will be seen that the depolarization/hyperpolarization scheme of each site may vary with time.

The main conclusion of this derivation is that the most important parameter for initiation of action potential in a case of a long, straight nerve fibre is the gradient of the induced electric field along the nerve axis. In the next sections, few different neuronal structures will be discussed.

Long and curved axons

The effect of electromagnetic induction on a long curved axon is illustrated in Figure 8.6. Due to the axon curvature, the spatial derivative of the effective electric field along the axon is maximal at this point, and this is the key factor affecting the neural response.

In this case, the intracellular axial current going downward is much smaller than the current going to the left, resulting in a membrane current, $\vec{i}_{m,}$ flowing outward from the intracellular space. This directed current flow leads to membrane depolarization.

In case the coil current is in the opposite direction, the induced intracellular current, $\vec{i}_{ax}$,

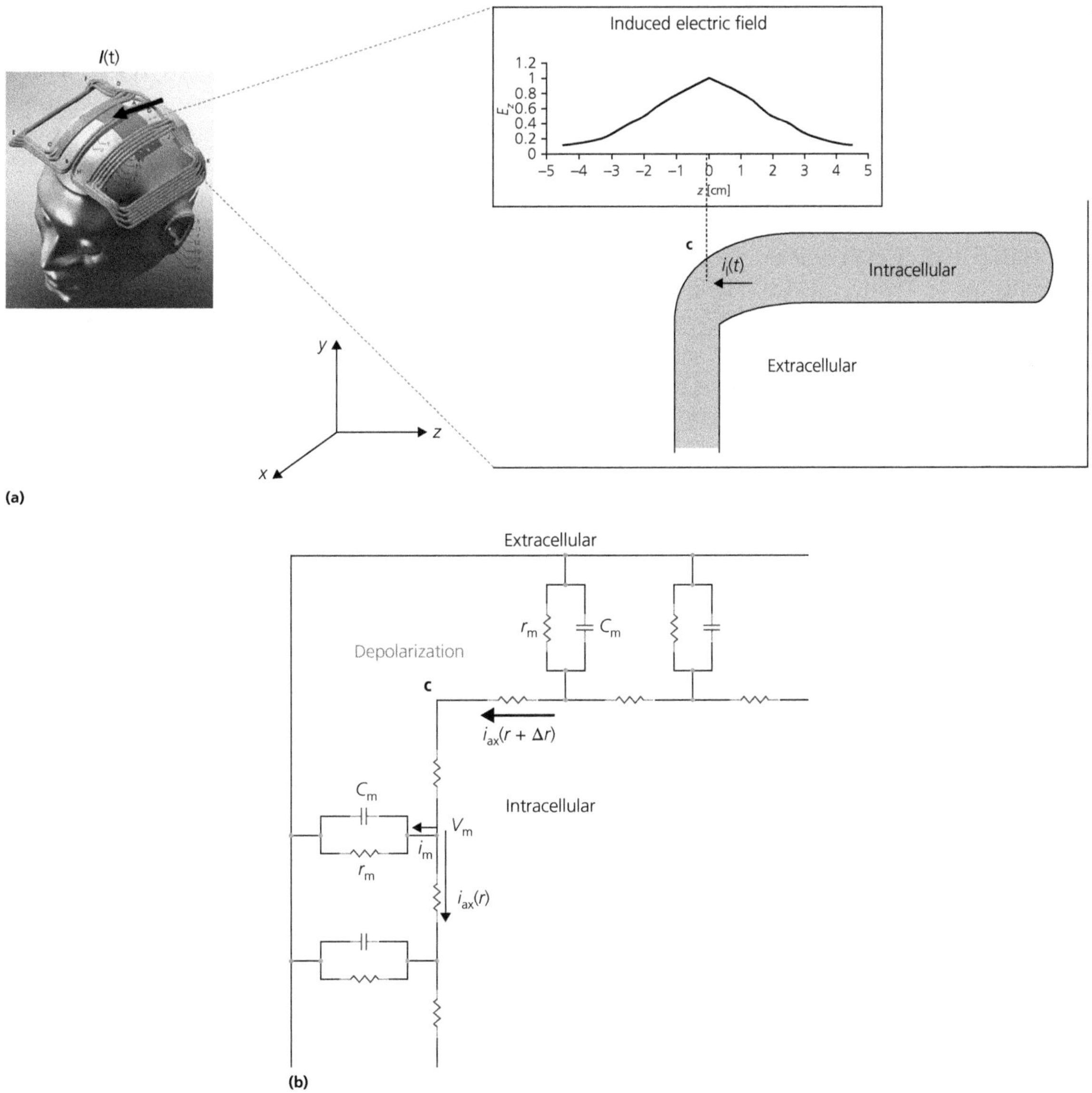

Figure 8.6 An illustration of the effect of a TMS pulse on a long, curved axon. (**a**) The normalized electric field induced along the z axis. (**b**) The passive cable model for this case.

will flow to the right, hence a membrane current, $\vec{i}_{m}$, will flow inward and a membrane hyperpolarization will occur. It can be concluded that in the case of a curved fibre, the most important parameters for initiation of action potential are the intensity and direction of the induced electric field itself, and not its gradient, at the bend point. At the bend point, the electric field gradient *along the fibre tract* is maximal. Hence, the bend points are especially prone for initiation of action potentials by TMS. This conclusion will be generalized in the next section where the practical case of brain stimulation by TMS will be discussed.

Nerve terminals and constrictions

As demonstrated in the previous section, a location of maximal effective electric field derivative will exist for an induced electric field along the axon at points where the axon terminates or bends away from the field. Short convoluted neurons are common in the cortex [30, 35–38] where neuronal paths are short compared to the spatial extent of the field. Hence, there are numerous points of bends, terminations or branchings of nerve fibres. These points are the most likely sites for stimulation.

Hence, when TMS of brain neuronal structures is discussed, as opposed to long peripheral nerves, the following assertions may be made:

1 The intensity of the induced electric field itself, and not its derivative, is the key factor for stimulation.

2 The electric field orientation relative to the neuronal structure is important. The lowest threshold for activation occurs where the induced field is parallel to the neuronal structure.

3 The direction along the nerve axis is crucial. As was demonstrated above, for a certain direction, a membrane depolarization will occur at the bend point, which above a critical value may lead to neural stimulation. On the other hand, the opposite direction will lead to membrane hyperpolarization and will reduce the chance for stimulation.

TMS electronics

TMS circuit design

The goal of the TMS circuit is to create a brief current pulse in a stimulating coil. This current pulse can induce an electric field in an adjacent tissue, thus leading to neuronal activation. The TMS stimulation circuit consists of a high-voltage power supply that charges a capacitor or a bank of capacitors, which are then rapidly discharged via a fast electronic switch into the TMS coil, to create the briefly changing magnetic field pulse. A typical circuit is shown in Figure 8.7, where low-voltage AC is transformed into high-voltage DC, which charges the capacitor. A crucial component is the fast switch, which has to pass very high current of very short duration of 50–250 μs.

The stimulator also includes a control unit that operates the switch and enables the operator to programme and determine the operation parameters. The discharge circuit is basically an RCL circuit, characterized by *R*, the resistance; *C*, the capacitance; and *L*, the inductance. The capacitance, *C*, is a characteristic of the capacitor that reflects how much electrical energy it can store in the form of an electric charge. The inductance, *L*, is a property that determines how much voltage is required to change the current in the circuit.

In the TMS circuit, the main contributor to inductance is the stimulating coil, although there may be an additional inductance of the leads and other components. The resistance *R* determines the amount of energy dissipated as heat, and its main contribution is from the TMS coil. During a pulse, the TMS circuit must sustain high peak currents and voltages for short cycle times. Typical ranges of circuit parameters and pulse widths are shown in Table 8.1.

The first TMS stimulators produced monophasic pulses of current, in which the current flows in a single direction. The current rises for approximately 50–100 μs during which the action potentials can be initiated if the

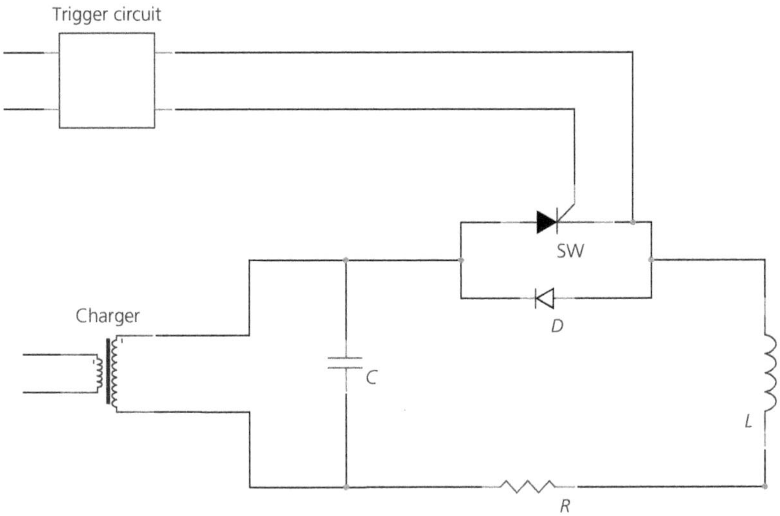

Figure 8.7 A schematic TMS circuit for biphasic pulses. An AC–DC transformer charges the capacitor *C* to a certain voltage V_C. A controlled switch, SW, enables the capacitor to discharge via the coil, *L*. The switch gate is controlled by a trigger circuit. A diode, *D*, is connected in parallel to the switch in order to enable current flow in the opposite direction and capacitor recharging. The total resistance in the discharge circuit is *R*.

Table 8.1 Typical ranges of parameters in a TMS circuit.

Property	Typical range
Peak voltage	0.5–3 kV
Peak current	2–10 kA
Pulse width	60–1000 μs
Inductance *L*	10–30 μH
Capacitance *C*	10–250 μF
Resistance *R*	20–80 mΩ

conditions are right. Following this initial 'active' phase, the current slowly returns to baseline over several 100 μsl; however, the pulse can be largely considered as inactive at this stage. These relatively simple pulses are ideal for neurophysiological studies in which unidirectional current changes are preferred. However, the pulses are very inefficient for repetitive pulsing, since all the energy is lost in the circuit resistance and the capacitor has to be charged each time from zero voltage. The most common pulse used for today's TMS stimulators is therefore with a biphasic shape, where the current flows in both directions and the pulse is terminated after a single sinusoidal cycle. A substantial portion of the voltage is returned to the capacitor at the end of each cycle, enabling more rapid pulsing. However, these pulses are not ideal for neurophysiological experiments since both phases will induce transmembrane currents of different directions, which may preferentially excite different neuronal populations or different sites in the same population leading to unpredictable experimental variability. Representative monophasic and biphasic pulses are shown in Figure 8.9.

A scheme of a basic TMS circuit for biphasic pulses is shown in Figure 8.7.

What are the most favourable values of *L*, *C* and the pulse duration? This question leads us to discuss the temporal characteristics of the neuronal response to the TMS pulse. The neuronal response depends not only on the electric field magnitude but also on the pulse duration. As the pulse duration is extended, the electric field required to reach neuronal threshold, E_{thr}, becomes smaller. The dependence of E_{thr} on pulse duration is given by the strength–duration curve [61].

The biological parameters determining neural response are the threshold at infinite duration, termed the rheobase (β, measured in V/m), and the duration at which the threshold is twice the rheobase, termed the chronaxie (γ, in μs), which is related to the time constant of the neuronal membrane. The chronaxie and rheobase depend on many biological and experimental factors, such as whether the nerves are myelinated or not (hence peripheral and cortical parameters are different) and other factors. It can be shown that the strength–duration curve is equivalent to the requirement that the transmembrane potential, V_m, is depolarized to the threshold value. Figure 8.8 shows an example of a strength–duration curve [62].

The duration of a TMS pulse can be extended in two ways, by increasing the capacitance C or by increasing the coil inductance L.

It can be shown that increasing the capacitance, C, leads to increased energy consumption, on the one hand, but lessens the required capacitor voltage and the current swing, on the other hand. Both of these effects enable the use of cheaper circuit elements and the simplification of the circuit design. Hence, all these conflicting considerations must be accounted for when choosing the optimized circuit capacitor. Regarding the inductance, L, it can be shown that both energy consumption and capacitor voltage increase with increasing L. In addition, increased inductance is usually related to increased number of windings and to increased coil resistance. Both the resistance and the pulse duration are associated with energy dissipation and heating rate in the stimulating coil (these issues will be discussed in Sections 4.6 and 4.7). All these reasons point to the need to minimize the circuit inductance. On the other hand, very small L values lead to very high rate of current change $\partial I / \partial t$ in the circuit, which may require expensive and bulky circuit elements such as the switch. Hence, optimization must be carried out. In practice, most TMS coil inductances are in the range between 10 and 20 μH.

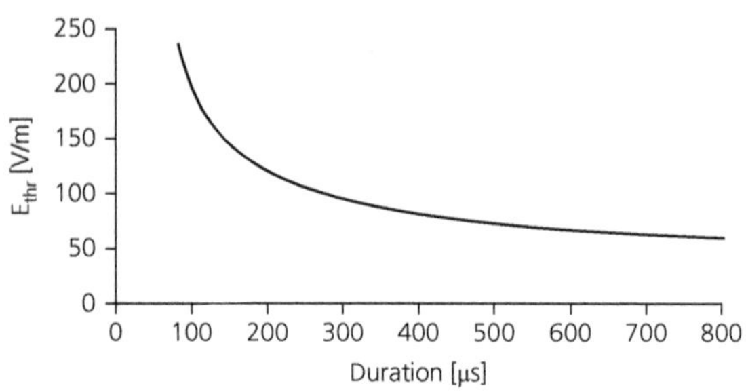

Figure 8.8 A strength–duration curve of the minimal electric field required to reach the threshold for neuronal activation, E_{thr}, in units of V/m, as a function of the pulse duration in μs [62]. Source: From Roth *et al.* [62]. Reproduced with permission from S. Karger AG.

Pulse waveforms and sequences of pulses

As discussed above, the most widely used pulse shapes in TMS are monophasic and biphasic pulses. Another possibility is a polyphasic pulse, where, unlike a biphasic pulse, the oscillation is not terminated after a single cycle, but the signal alternates for many cycles until its amplitude is almost zero. This waveform is less favourable since the energy is dissipated completely and does not return to the capacitor, and the second and later cycles have lower amplitude and hence are less effective than the first cycle. Hence, polyphasic pulses are rarely used. Half-sine waves have also been implemented and are an option on the MagPro advanced stimulator (MagVenture Inc, Denmark). These pulses are composed essentially of the first lobe of a biphasic pulse [63]. Their directionality has been assessed and shares similar characteristics as that of a monophasic pulse, although their use for rTMS has not been investigated [64].

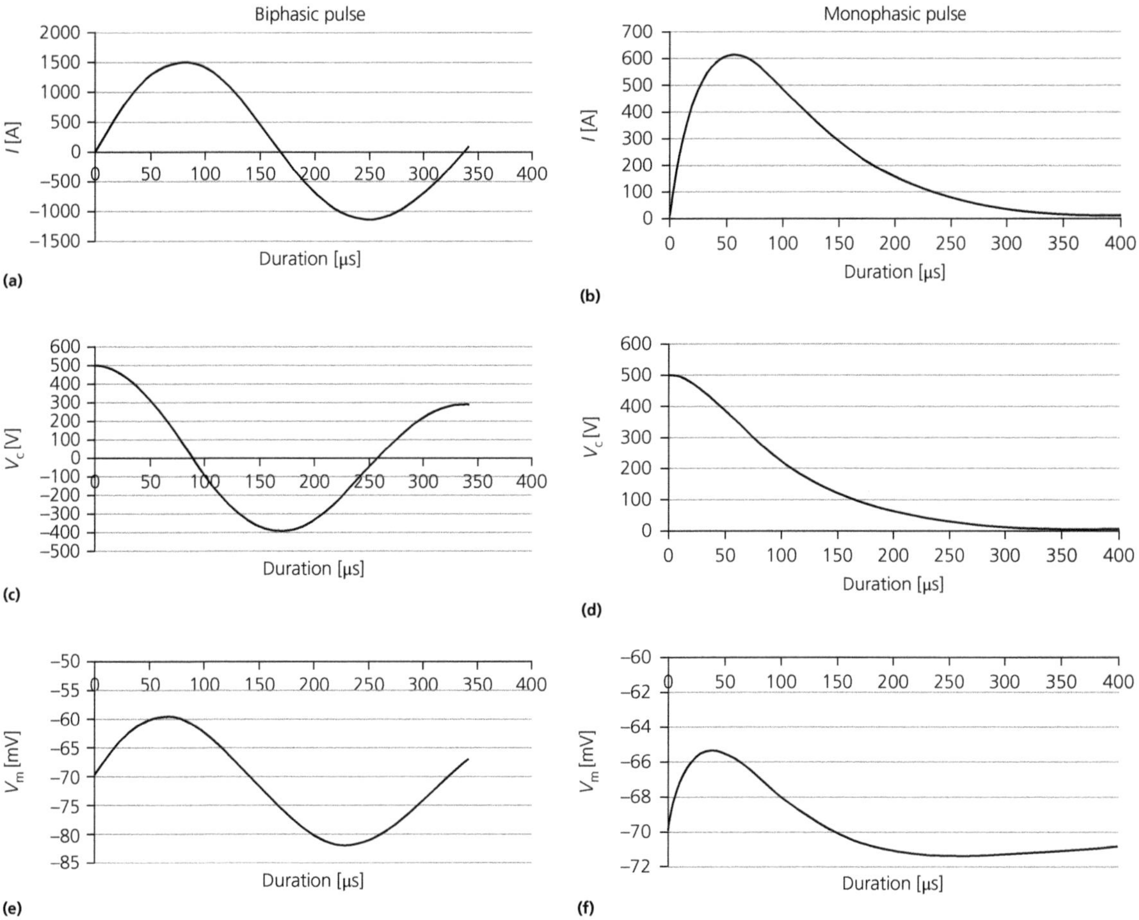

Figure 8.9 Typical pulse waveforms. (**a**) Biphasic coil current. (**b**) Monophasic coil current. (**c**) Capacitor voltage, V_C, for a biphasic pulse. The voltage changes polarity and is recharged to about 60% of its initial value at the end of the pulse. (**d**) The capacitor voltage, V_C, for a monophasic pulse. The voltage decays to close to zero at the end of the pulse. (**e**) The transmembrane potential, V_m, during a biphasic current pulse. There are phases of depolarization and hyperpolarization, with the second phase leading to larger swing in V_m. (**f**). The transmembrane potential, V_m, during a monophasic current pulse. Only the first phase leads to a significant modulation of V_m.

A novel TMS stimulator design has been described that enables one to control the pulse width, to terminate the current at a desired time point, thereby reducing energy consumption and heating losses [65]. Various other pulse shapes may be developed in future TMS stimulators. The characteristics of typical biphasic and monophasic pulses are shown in Figure 8.9, for $C = 180\,\mu F$, $L = 16\,\mu H$ and $R = 50\,m\Omega$. The derivation of the transmembrane potential follows solution of the cable equation [66].

As can be seen in Figure 8.9e, at each neuronal site, both depolarization and hyperpolarization occur during a biphasic pulse. In the example of Figure 8.9e, depolarization occurs first, followed by subsequent hyperpolarization. This situation will be reversed at other locations. Neuronal activation will usually occur only at a depolarization site. Since the change in V_m is larger during the second phase, the threshold for neuronal activation would be lower if the current polarity is reversed in this case. This demonstrates the current polarity dependence of TMS effect on motor activation, as observed in many studies. A broad variety of TMS pulse schemes are used in clinical and investigational protocols. The most important modes of operation are classified below:

1 *Single pulses:* Single TMS pulses are used mainly for diagnostic, follow-up and neurophysiological research purposes. In addition, single pulses to the motor cortex are used to determine the stimulation intensity required to reach the threshold for a motor response. This motor threshold (MT) may vary significantly across subjects and even in individual subjects across different excitability states, hence the TMS treatment is usually calibrated based on the individual MT.
2 *Paired pulses:* In this method, a conditioning stimulus (CS) and a test stimulus (TS) are delivered through the same or different coils. The TMS coil locations, pulse amplitudes, pulse polarities and inter-stimulus interval (ISI) are adjusted so as to be sensitized to particular aspects of the excitatory and inhibitory neuronal network of interest. Paired-pulse schemes are usually used for neurophysiological research, although clinical applications have been described (for review, see Ref. 67). Table 8.2 summarizes the range of different paired-pulse experiments.
3 *Repetitive TMS (rTMS):* most investigational and clinical protocols use repetitive TMS where multiple TMS pulses are delivered at a pre-defined frequency.

   An rTMS sequence is characterized by several parameters, listed in Table 8.3, with typical ranges. All or most of these parameters are user-controllable in most current TMS stimulators.

   A typical rTMS scheme is shown in Figure 8.10.

   By convention, sequences with frequencies above 5 Hz are considered high frequency and those with frequencies of 1 Hz and below are considered low frequency. The distinction between these protocols relates to different patterns of modulation of excitability, which shares similarities with the induction of synaptic plasticity. This will be discussed in the section 'White Matter Pathways'.
4 *Theta bursts:* An example of a 'patterned' protocol with variable ISIs, this sequence is based on the naturally occurring theta rhythm (5 Hz) of the hippocampus [68]. In a typical sequence, a three-pulse burst at 50 Hz (ISI = 20 ms) is repeated every 200 ms (i.e., at 5 Hz, which is the theta frequency). There are two common excitability-modulating implementations of the sequence both utilizing sub-threshold TMS pulses (commonly, 80% of resting motor threshold): continuous TBS (cTBS), which normally consists of 40 s of continuous pulse trains, and intermittent theta burst stimulation (iTBS), composed of 2 s trains of bursts separated by 10 s. Interestingly, these two sequences induce opposite effects on the neuronal excitability – iTBS tends to increase the excitability, while cTBS decreases it. In iTBS, the inter-train interval and the number of trains determine the total session time and the number of pulses, which is typically 600. An example of an iTBS sequence is shown in Figure. 8.11.

The relationship of rTMS and synaptic plasticity

Synaptic plasticity is the ability of synapses to strengthen or weaken over time in response to increases or decreases in their activity. On the synaptic level, this may occur via alteration of the number of receptors on the synapse and the quantity of neurotransmitters released into the synapse. On the biochemical level, a complex cascade of changes has been

Table 8.2 Summary of the most common paired-pulse experiments.

Technique	Effect on excitability	ISI	Amplitudes	Location of coils	Proposed mechanism	*Main reference* and notes
Single-coil experiments						
SICI	Inhibition	1–6 ms with two phases at 1 ms and 2.5 ms	CS: sub-threshold (70–80%) TS: supra-threshold	CS: M1 TS: M1 (same location)	$GABA_A$ receptor	[104] Short ISI phase may be due to axonal refractoriness. CS: ~70% RMT optimal (U-curve) TS↑: Stronger inhibition. Relatively insensitive to CS pulse direction
ICF	Facilitation	6–25 ms	CS: sub-threshold (70–80%) TS: supra-threshold	CS: M1 TS: M1 (same location)	Glutamergic-NMDA receptor	[104] CS↑, TS↓: stronger facilitation. Sensitive to CS pulse direction.
SICF	Facilitation	1.0–1.5 ms or multiples thereof (~3.0,4.5 ms)	CS: at-threshold or supra-threshold TS: at-threshold or sub-threshold	CS: M1 TS: M1 (same location)	Interneuronal chains involved in I-wave generation	[107, 113] For repeated application with ITI = 5 s (known as iTMS), sustained cortical facilitation occurs (plasticity) with no changes in I-wave intensity
LICI	Inhibition	50–200 ms	CS: supra-threshold TS: just-above-threshold	CS: M1 TS: M1 (same location)	$GABA_B$ receptor	[111] TS↑: weaker inhibition

(continued)

Table 8.2 (Continued)

Technique	Effect on excitability	ISI	Amplitudes	Location of coils	Proposed mechanism	*Main reference* and notes
Dual coil experiments						
Double coil experiment	Inhibition or facilitation	1–25 ms	CS: variable	CS: Area of cortex that is believed to be connected to M1 or V1 (ipsi- or contra-lateral)	Causal cortico-spinal interactions. Structural and functional connectivity.	[100]
			T2: supra-threshold	TS: M1 or V1		*CS regions tested include SMA, S1 & parietal areas* For example, with CS on ipsilateral PMd, ISI=6 ms: For CS: 80% AMT -> inhibition; For CS: 120% AMT-> facilitation. Sensitive to CS pulse direction.
IHI/IHF	Inhibition or facilitation	F: 4–5 ms	I: CS: just-below-threshold	Homologous areas of M1 on opposite hemispheres	Transcallosal projections. $GABA_B$ receptor	[102, 103]
		I: >7 ms (commonly 10 ms)	I: TS: just-above-threshold			IHF usually uses voluntary contraction of muscle ipsilateral to conditioning site.
			F: CS: supra-threshold			IHI: two phases (early: ISI=8–10 ms, and late: ~40 ms).
			F: TS: supra-threshold			TS↑: weaker inhibition Sensitive to CS and TS pulse direction.
CBI	Inhibition	5–7 ms	CS: 95% of pyramidal tract AMT	CS: *Contralateral* cerebellar hemisphere		[109]
				TS: M1		Debate if cerebellar or corticospinal origin [110]
Related techniques						
SAI/LAI	Inhibition	SAI: 10–20 ms	CS: supra-perceptual-threshold	CS: Electrical peripheral nerve stimulation	SAI: GABAergic-mediated, Ach influence	[105, 108]
		LAI: 200 ms	TS: supra-threshold	TS: Contralateral M1	LAI: Cortical and sub-cortical origin	Techniques used to study sensorimotor interactions.

PAS	Inhibition or facilitation	F: 25 ms (PAS+)	See SAI/LAI	CS: Electrical peripheral nerve (usually median nerve)	STDP plasticity	[106]
		I: 10 ms (PAS-)		TS: Contralateral M1		Plasticity-modulation with SAI-like stimulations repeated at low frequency (~0.1 Hz). Sensitive to TMS pulse direction
CSP	Inhibition (EMG silence)	N/A	Supra-threshold	M1	Early phase (<50 ms): Spinal	[112] TMS pulse applied to contralateral hemisphere during voluntary contraction of target muscle results in suppression of EMG activity for ~100 ms. Early and late phases.
					Late phase (>50 ms): $GABA_B$ receptor	Sensitive to TMS pulse direction. Reciprocal relationship with SICI
iCSP	Inhibition (EMG silence)	N/A	Supra-threshold	M1	Transcallosal project	[103] Corresponding suppression of EMG (duration ~35 ms) following TMS pulse to ipsilateral hemisphere during voluntary contraction of target muscle. Sensitive to TMS pulse direction.

Notes

The cortical silent period is included since its inhibitory action is believed to be similar to that of some of the paired-pulse experiments. For references and an overview of paired-pulse experiments, see Refs. 67, 99, 105. Pulse amplitudes are relative to RMT unless otherwise stated.

AMT, active motor threshold; CBI, cerebellar brain inhibition; CS, conditioning stimulus; CSP, cortical silent period; F, facilitation; I, inhibition; ICF, intracortical facilitation; iCSP, ipsilateral cortical silent period; IHI, inter-hemispheric inhibition; LAI, long-latency afferent inhibition; LICI, long-interval cortical inhibition; M1, primary motor cortex; N/A, non-applicable; PAS, paired associative stimulation; PMd, dorsal premotor cortex; RMT, resting motor threshold; S1, primary somatosensory cortex; SAI, short-latency afferent inhibition; SICF, short-interval intracortical facilitation; SICI, short-interval cortical inhibition; SMA, supplementary motor cortex; STDP, spike-timing-dependent plasticity; TS, test stimulus; V1, primary visual cortex.

implicated driven by post-synaptic calcium release. Long-term potentiation (LTP) and long-term depression (LTD) are the two most common types of long-lasting changes in synaptic plasticity observed; these are believed to form the basis of memory and learning.

Table 8.3 Typical ranges of repetitive TMS sequence parameters.

Parameter	Typical range
Frequency	1–25 Hz
Train duration	1–10 s
Inter-train interval (ITI)	10–40 s
Number of trains	10–60
Total number of pulses	400–3000

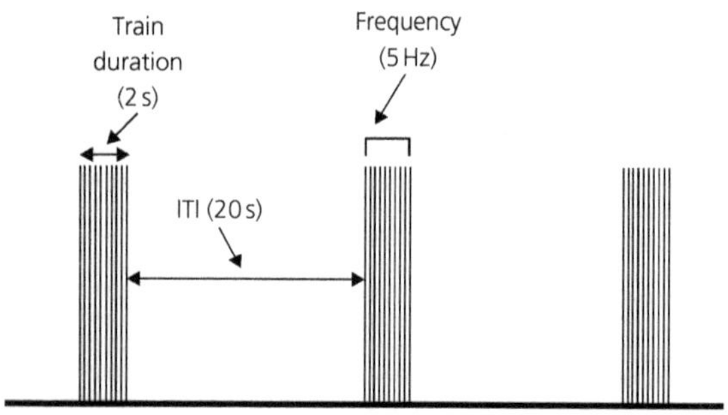

Figure 8.10 Typical rTMS pattern. In this example, the frequency is 5 Hz, the train duration is 2 s and ITI is 20 s. The total number of trains in a session is typically 40–60, leading to 400–600 pulses delivered in a session time of 15–22 min.

Repetitive TMS is able to change and modulate activity beyond the stimulation period. The question is by which mechanism rTMS influences the brain. It is appealing to link the influence of rTMS on the brain to LTP-like and LTD-like effects and therefore its mechanism to that of synaptic plasticity. This question is of fundamental importance to understanding the basic mechanism of rTMS. There is no doubt that rTMS-induced excitability modulation and LTP/LTD synaptic plasticity share common characteristics especially in their general methods of induction and in their expression as changes in neuronal excitability. Most obviously, rTMS appears to closely resemble the frequency-dependence of tetanic stimulation, the most common induction method of LTP and LTD. Moreover, rTMS exhibits other similar characteristics, which include metaplasticity (where a previous history of activity determines the current level of plasticity) with the influence of baseline cortical excitability levels; Priming, where a preceding period of brain stimulation modifies the level of excitability modulation attained by subsequent stimulation [69] and sensitivity to pulse trains shaped by the theta frequency. However, there are also fundamental differences between the magnitude and scale of some of the defining characteristics of the methods. For more information, see the reviews of Refs. 70–72.

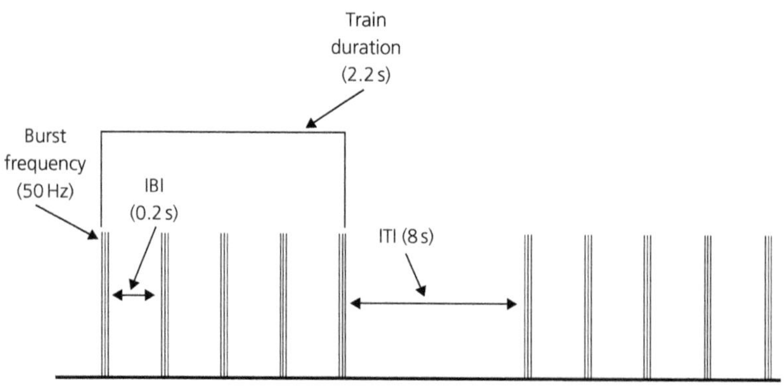

Figure 8.11 Typical iTBS scheme. Each burst includes three pulses at a 50 Hz frequency. The inter-burst interval (IBI) is 0.2 s, the train duration is 2.2 s (i.e. 10 bursts per train) and the ITI is 8 s. Total number of trains in a session is typically 20, leading to total number of 600 pulses.

Coil design and construction

Types of TMS coils

The TMS coil controls the distribution and strength of the stimulation field and therefore plays a crucial role in the characteristics of TMS. The most important trade-off in their design is the interplay between depth and focality.

The original coil designs were circular due to their ease of design and simple construction. Several studies are still being performed with these coils of various sizes. In these coils, the stimulation field follows the circular profile and therefore forms a non-focal annulus under the coil potentially stimulating a disparate area under the coil surface. These coils thereby allow stimulation of a relatively large cortical volume including deeper brain regions but at the expense of focality. Therefore, these coils are typically used for diagnostic purposes such as measurement of conduction velocities to various spinal cord levels and detection of lesions, cortical atrophy and other neuromorphological changes, for which the finer control of stimulation location is not required.

The most commonly used coil in TMS studies is the figure-8 coil, sometimes referred to as a double-D or butterfly coil, with adjacent circular coils with opposing current flow. This shape allows relatively focal stimulation of superficial layers of the cortex beneath the central portion of the coil where the two coils meet, at the expense of depth profile. Neuronal fibres that are oriented parallel to the central segment of the coil are the most likely to be affected by the stimulation [50, 71, 73]. The coil angle on the scalp surface is controlled by the direction of the coil handle, and the orientation for optimal stimulation of the hand representation of M1 is such that the induced current is directed approximately 45° medial to the antero-posterior plane [74]. At this orientation, the induced field is perpendicular to the cortical surface within the sulcal depth so that stimulation will preferentially occur in the sulcal wall where the neuronal axes are lying parallel to the field [75].

Several TMS stimulators and coils are shown in Figure 8.12, including Magstim Rapid^2 stimulator and 70 mm figure-8 coil (Magstim, Whitland, Wales, UK), MagVenture MagPro stimulator and C-B60 Butterfly coil (MagVenture, Farum, Denmark) and Brainsway Deep TMS system and H1 coil (Brainsway, Jerusalem, Israel).

Coil elements that are not tangential to the scalp induce accumulation of charge on the surface and reduce coil effectiveness [39, 41, 76]. Thus, angled coil designs based on the fundamental figure-8 shape but which use less than 180° between the wings are more tangential to the scalp and hence more efficient [77]. However, a planar design is the most popular because it is well suited for fine localization over most of the scalp.

The typical double-cone coil is formed by two large adjacent circular wings at an angle of approximately 95° so that the wiring of both wings is tangential to the head. This large coil induces a stronger and less focal electric field relative to a figure-8 coil [78] and allows direct stimulation of deeper brain regions, but is more likely to produce a certain level of discomfort especially when at higher intensities (needed to stimulate deeper brain regions). A variety of other coil designs exist, each exhibiting different aspects of the depth-focality trade-off. These include coils that emphasize focality performance such as the slinky coil with multiple loops joined together at one edge forming a helical coil on a half torus [79] and the planar clover-leaf design with four adjacent circular loops [80]. Other coils emphasize depth performance. These include the H-coil, which will be described in the next section. Other theoretical designs for deep stimulation include the stretched C-core coil [81, 82] and the circular crown coil [82]. All of these coils are based on common design principles essential for effective deep brain TMS [62, 83, 84] and exhibit a significantly slower decay rate of the electric field with

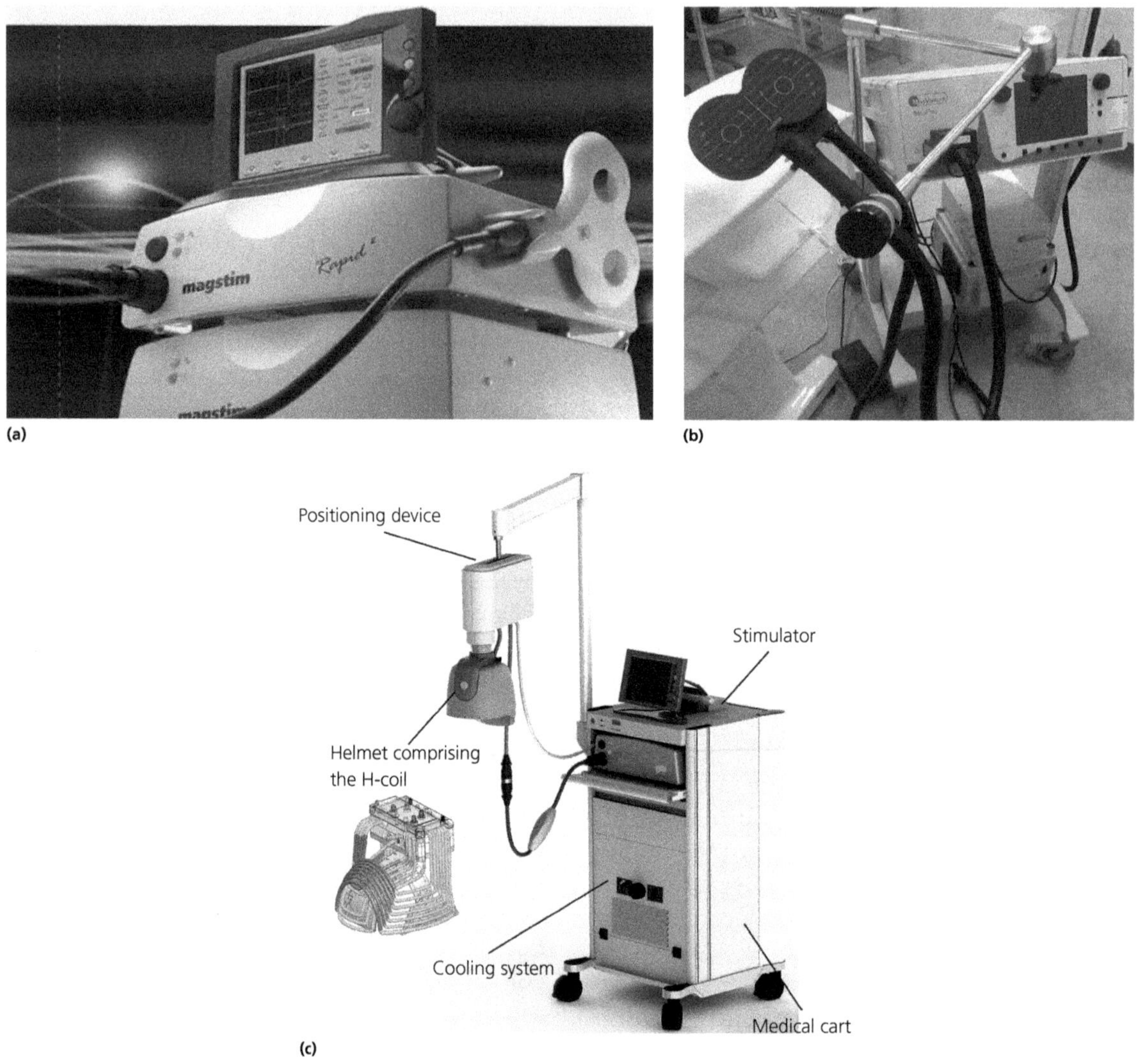

Figure 8.12 Images of TMS devices and coils. (**a**) Magstim Rapid² stimulator and 70 mm figure-8 coil. (**b**) MagVenture MagPro stimulator and C-B60 Butterfly coil. (**c**) Brainsway deep TMS system and H1 coil. (*See insert for colour representation of the figure.*)

distance, although the stimulated area is less focal. Various metrics related to coil performance in ideal spherical models have been devised to characterize coil designs based on their depth-focality performance [85], although the situation in the human head is always going to be considerably more complex [86].

Maps of electric field distribution produced in the brain by several TMS coils are shown in Figure 8.13, based on measurements in a phantom head model filled with physiological saline solution.

Each map is calibrated based on the relevant treatment protocol. In Figure 8.13a are shown maps of the figure-8 coil and the H1 coil, which are designed to stimulate structures in the left prefrontal cortex, with an intensity of 120% of the hand motor threshold (MT), which is the minimal stimulator power output required to evoke motor response from hand muscles when the coil is placed over the hand motor cortex. Routinely, the MT is determined for each subject and the treatment session is applied with the calibrated intensity.

In Figure 8.13b and c are shown maps of the 90 mm circular coil (Magstim, Whitland, Wales, UK) and the Deep TMS H7 coil (Brainsway, Jerusalem, Israel), with an intensity of 100% of the leg MT. The leg motor representation lies more medial and deeper than the hand representation (about 3 cm compared to 1.5 cm). In occasions where medial structures are the target regions for stimulation, such as the anterior cingulate cortex in the case of the H7 coil, the stimulation intensity is calibrated based on the leg MT.

Effectiveness and safety of the stimulation procedure can be compromised by overheating of the coil during the multiple pulses delivered during the rTMS procedure. Water, oil and air cooling methods have been implanted

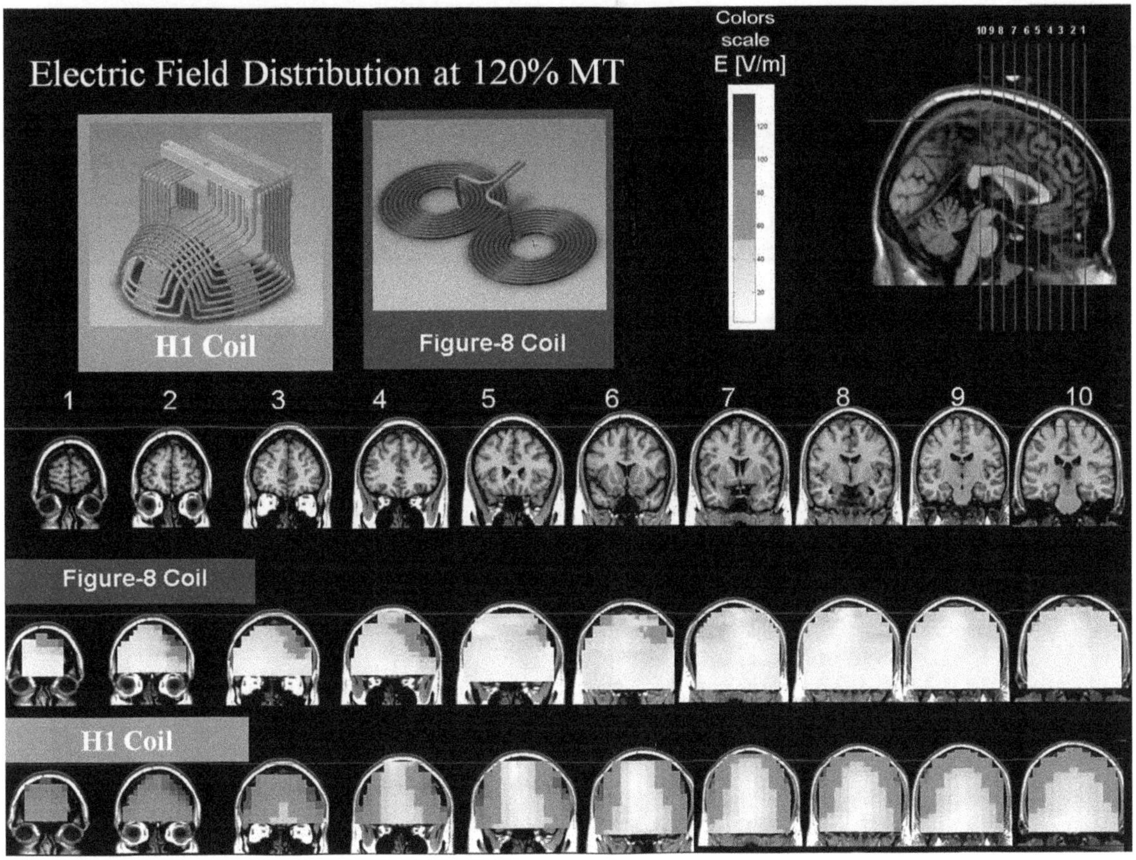

(a)

Figure 8.13 Coloured field maps indicating the electrical field absolute magnitude in each pixel over coronal slices 1 cm apart. The red pixels indicate field magnitude above the threshold for neuronal activation, which was set to 100 V/m. (**a**) Maps for a figure-8 coil and deep TMS H1 coil. The field maps are adjusted for stimulator power output level required to obtain 120% of the hand motor threshold for each coil, at a depth of 1.5 cm. (**b** and **c**) Maps for the 90 mm circular coil (**b**) and the deep TMS H7 coil (**c**). The field maps are adjusted for stimulator power output level required to obtain 100% of the leg motor threshold for each coil, at a depth of 3 cm. (*See insert for colour representation of the figure.*)

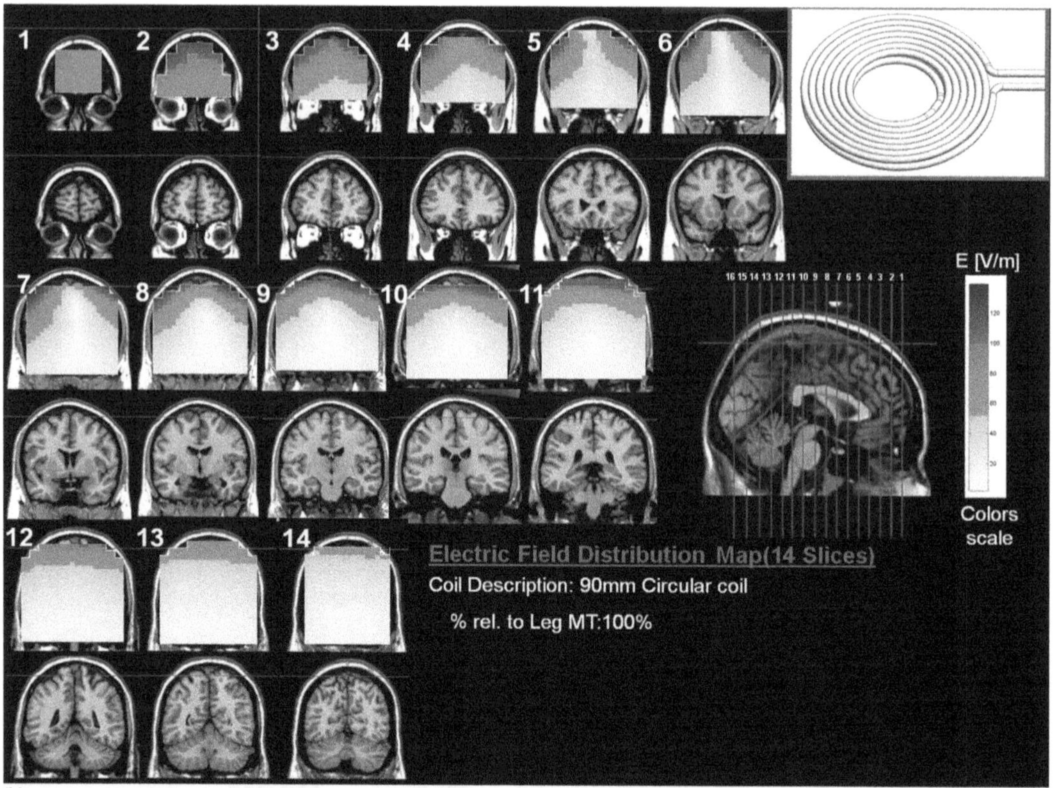

(b)

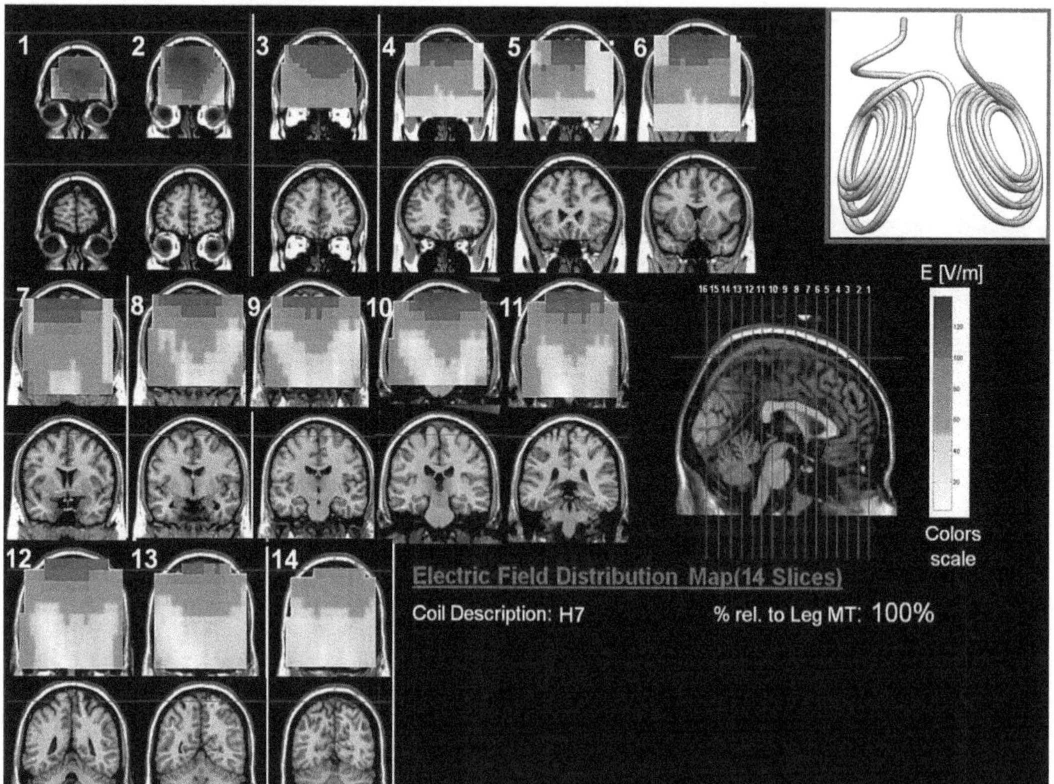

(c)

Figure 8.13 (Continued)

to overcome this serious challenge. A figure-8 coil with a reduced resistance has been designed [87], achieving improved thermal characteristics. Ferromagnetic cores can serve as heat sinks, and coils with ferromagnetic cores have been developed, resulting in significant reduction in heat generation and power consumption [88]. The use of such iron-core coils, using a relatively high intensity (120% of MT) and frequency (10 Hz, 4 s trains), was demonstrated in a large multicentre study evaluating its antidepressant effects [89]. Specialized coils for operation within the magnetic resonance imaging (MRI) scanner have also been devised typically based on figure-8 designs and are available commercially. These coils are obviously devoid of any iron-containing components and are also often optimized for mechanical damping, eddy current, power line filtering and leakage current performance.

Targeting deep neuronal structures

Until several years ago, the capacity of TMS to elicit neuronal responses has been limited to superficial structures. The coils used for TMS (such as circular or figure-8 coils) induce stimulation in cortical regions mainly only superficially under the windings of the coil. The intensity of the electric field drops dramatically deeper in the brain as a function of the distance from the coil [39–41, 90]. Therefore, to stimulate deep brain regions with such coils, a very high intensity would be needed, which is not feasible with standard magnetic stimulators. Moreover, the intensity needed to stimulate deeper brain regions effectively would stimulate superficial muscles and nerves at a level that might lead to facial and scalp pain and cervical muscle contractions and increase the likelihood of inducing a seizure [62].

The difficulty of efficiently activating deep neuronal structures using TMS emerges from physical properties of the brain, and from physical and physiological aspects of the interaction of a TMS system with the human brain. As shown by Heller and Van Hulsteyn [91], the three-dimensional maximum of the electric field intensity will always be located at the brain surface, for any configuration or superposition of TMS coils. However, both the TMS coils and the stimulator may be optimized for effective stimulation of deeper brain regions.

Coil designs for stimulation of deeper brain areas have been proposed and evaluated, which are termed as H-coils [62, 83, 84]. The safety of stimulation with these coils and their effects on cognition have been carefully assessed using stimulation at relatively high intensity (120% of MT) and frequency (20 Hz) [92]. In addition, several clinical studies have shown promising effects of these coils in psychiatric disorders [93, 94]. The H1 coil was recently cleared by the Food and Drug Administration for the treatment of major depression disorder, based on a large multicentre trial [95].

The design of deep TMS coils follows the goals:

a High enough electric field intensity in the desired deep brain region that will surpass the threshold for neuronal activation
b High percentage of electric field in the desired deep brain region relative to the maximal intensity in the cortex
c Minimal adverse effects such as pain, motor activation and activation of facial muscles.

The design principles essential for effective stimulation of deeper brain regions include the following [83, 84, 62]:

1 Summation of electric impulses: The induced electric field in the desired deep brain regions is obtained by optimal summation of electric fields, induced by several coil elements with common direction, in different locations around the skull. The principle of summation may be applied in several ways [62].
2 Minimization of non-tangential components: Coil elements that are non-tangential to the surface induce accumulation of surface

charge, which leads to the cancellation of the perpendicular component of the directly induced field at all points within the tissue, and usually to the reduction of the electric field in all other directions. In order to reduce accumulation of electrostatic charge, non-tangential elements in the coils are minimized, especially around the stimulation target. Therefore, these coils always include a flexible base complementary to the human head. The part of the coil close to the head (i.e. the base) must be optimally complementary to the human skull at the desired region.

3 Proper orientation of stimulating coil elements: Coils must be oriented such that they will produce a considerable field in a desired direction tangential to the surface, which should also be the preferable direction to activate the neuronal structures under consideration.

4 Remote location of return paths: The wires leading currents in a direction opposite to the preferred direction (i.e. the return paths) should be located far from the base and the desired brain region. This enables a higher absolute electric field in the desired brain region.

A comparison of the electric field profile along a line going from the coil surface into the centre of a realistic phantom head model is shown in Figure 8.14 for five different TMS coils: a commercial figure-8 coil (70-mm diameter of each wing), a commercial double cone coil (120-mm diameter of each wing, with an opening angle of 95°), large and small custom circular coils (with diameters of 160 and 55 mm, respectively) and a version of the H-coil that was used in a previous study [84]. The electric field distribution was measured in a realistic model of the human head ($x \times y \times z = 15 \times 13 \times 18$ cm, where x, y and z are postero-anterior, right-left and inferior-superior axes, respectively) filled with physiological saline solution.

A sketch of the H-coil version is shown in Figure 8.14a. The electric field amplitudes for all the coils were calculated along a line going downward (z axis in Figure 8.14a) with coordinates of $x,y = (0,3)$, that is 3 cm laterally to the midline. For the figure-8 coil and the double cone coil, the line started at the coil centre. For the two circular coils, the line started at the coil edge. For the H-coil, the line started at the centre of elements A–B (Figure 8.14a). From the plot in Figure 8.14b, it can be seen that the H-coil has the most favourable field profile (i.e. field attenuation to 66% at a distance of 4 cm). Among the rest of the coils, the large circular coil has the slowest rate of field decay with distance (i.e. field attenuation to 52% at a distance of 4 cm). Yet, the circular coil induces a non-specific effect over a complete cortical ring underneath the coil windings. The other three coils present a much weaker depth penetration with a strong attenuation of the electric field with depth (i.e. field attenuation to 29–37% at a distance of 4 cm). The field amplitude produced by the double cone coil at any distance is much larger than the figure-8 coil. Yet, the rate of decay of the field with distance from the coil is similar between the two coils. This demonstrates that the coil size is not the only factor affecting the efficiency in activating deeper brain regions, and the principles detailed previously must be accounted for.

Electrical safety and technical considerations

During a TMS pulse, peak currents of the order of several kA are delivered through the stimulating coil, and the capacitor voltage may be 2–3 kV. The coil windings and leads must have an electrical insulation rated far above the maximal voltage at 100% of the stimulator power output. The coil windings insulation must prevent any risk of electric shock to the patient or the operator, as well as any short circuit between the coil windings or any electrical arcing between the coil and any of the surrounding facilities All TMS devices must comply with international standards

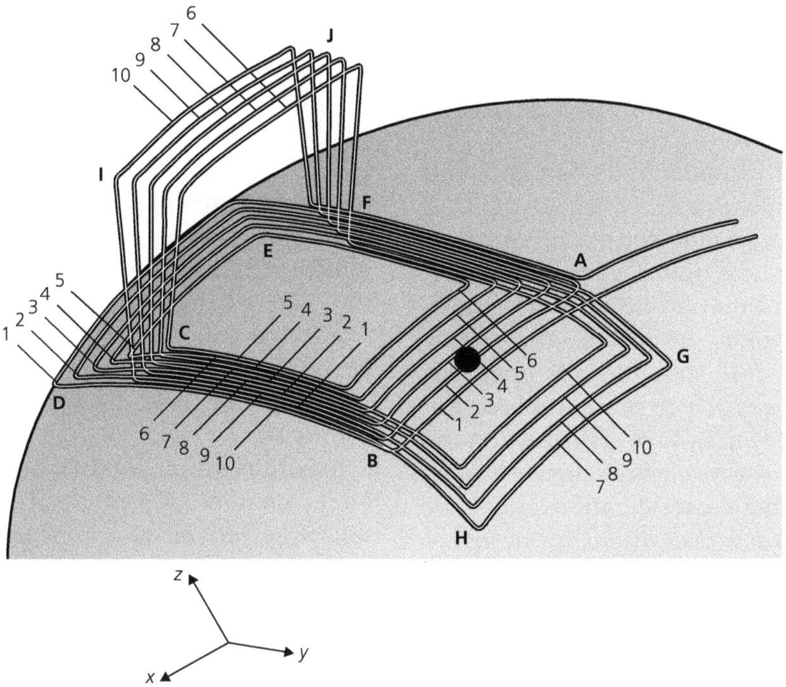

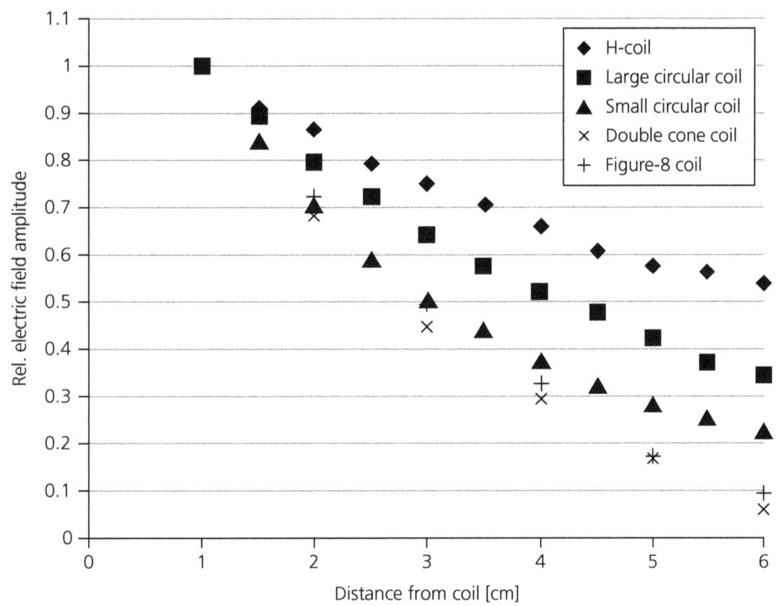

Figure 8.14 (**a**) A sketch of the H-coil version used in this comparison. (**b**) Plots of the electric field amplitude induced by several TMS coils, as a function of distance from the coil, normalized to the amplitude at 1 cm distance. The electric field was calculated in a phantom head model filled with a saline solution with physiological concentration. The coils are an H-coil version (diamonds), a large circular coil with 160 mm average diameter (squares), a small circular coil with 55 mm average diameter (triangles), a commercial figure-8 coil having 70 mm diameter of each wing and a commercial double-cone coil with 120 mm diameter of each wing.

such as IEC 60601. Safety regulations, guidelines and recommendations for TMS studies are summarized in consensus papers [96, 97].

Energy consumption

In a typical TMS stimulator, a charger circuit transforms the network AC voltage to high DC voltage on the capacitor. Hence, the maximal energy consumption occurs during charging. Typical charging times are from tens to hundreds of milliseconds. In general, the energy consumption of TMS stimulators is often not uniform with peaks of high power and current consumption. This may have an impact on the network and nearby electric devices, such as flickering. These considerations must be accounted for in the TMS stimulator design.

The actual power consumption during a train of pulses may be significantly reduced in a biphasic pulse device due to capacitor recharging at the end of each pulse. The TMS coil configuration has a tremendous effect on the efficacy of neuronal activation. Thus, to obtain a certain neurological effect, an optimized coil would enable to achieve the goal with significantly lower energy consumption.

Coil heating

During repetitive TMS operation, a large amount of heat may be produced in the stimulating coil (see section 'Types of TMS coils'). The most widely used cooling systems are based on streaming cooled air. Water is an effective coolant because of its high specific heat. Yet, water-based systems must cope with the need to prevent any accidental contact between the water and the high-voltage circuitry of the TMS coil and stimulator.

Reduction in coil heating and in energy consumption may be achieved by one or more of the following methods:

a Reducing coil (and lead) resistance, by increasing the wire cross section and reducing the number of windings N. Yet, N also affects the coil inductance and the induced electric field. Hence, each of these factors has to be optimized, accounting for these conflicting considerations.

b Shortening the pulse duration, by reducing either the coil inductance L or the capacitance C.

Mechanical strength

The high currents flowing in the TMS coil induce significant mechanical forces between the coil elements. Each current element is affected by a Lorentz force, which is proportional to the product of the current and the magnetic field from all the other coil elements.

Regarding the dependence of the mechanical forces on the coil's physical dimensions, the following general assertions can be stated:

a The forces would in general be stronger for coils with smaller dimensions.

b Shorter elements would be exposed to stronger forces.

The design of any TMS coil should account for the mechanical forces and strains and include casings and mechanical elements that should guarantee the coil's mechanical stability under the most extreme conditions. For TMS coils operating inside an MRI scanner, there are additional Lorentz forces due to the interactions between the currents in the coil elements and the MRI scanner's high steady magnetic field. Hence, such coils have to be designed to sustain even stronger mechanical forces.

Acoustic artefact

The mechanical forces produced during operation lead to rapid vibrations of the coil elements. This in turn produces a broadband acoustic artefact, which may exceed 140 dB of sound pressure level [98]. The strength and quality of the mechanical packing and casing of the coil elements may significantly reduce the audible artefact. In any case, the use of hearing protection is recommended for all individuals receiving TMS stimulation or those being in the vicinity.

Summary

TMS is a powerful technique of non-invasive neurostimulation that offers a window into the workings of the brain as well as providing a new way of treating neuropsychiatric diseases. Its mechanism of action is intrinsically linked to the ability of magnetic fields and the associated electric fields to stimulate and modulate neuronal populations. In order to optimize the use of the technique, consideration must be made of these underlying mechanisms as well as of the sources of variability in its operation including stimulator, coil and pulse protocol design.

References

1 Faraday, M. 1831. Effects on the production of electricity from magnetism. In Michael Faraday, ed. Willliams L.P. New York: Basic Books (Chapman Hall), 1965: 531 pp.
2 Faraday, M. (1839, 1844). Experimental Researches in Electricity, vols. i and ii. London: Richard and John Edward Taylor.
3 d'Arsonval, A. 1896. Dispositifs pour la mesure des courants alternatifs detoutes frequences. CR Soc Biol (Paris). 2: 450–1.
4 Beer, B. 1902. Ueber das Auftraten einer objective Lichtempfindung in magnetischen Felde. Klin Wochenschr. 15: 108–9.
5 Thompson, S.P. 1910. A physiological effect of an alternating magnetic field. Proc R Soc Lond Biol B 82: 396–9.
6 Dunlap, K. 1911. Visual sensations from the alternating magnetic field. Science. 33: 68–71.
7 Magnuson, C.E., Stevens, H.C. 1911. Visual sensations caused by the changes in the strength of a magnetic field. Am J Physiol. 29: 124–36.
8 Magnuson, C.E., Stevens, H.C. 1914. Visual sensations created by a magnetic field. Philos Mag. 28: 188–207.
9 Kolin, A., Brill, N.Q., Broberg, P.J., 1959. Stimulation of irritable tissues by means of an alternating magnetic field. Proc Soc Exp Biol Med. 102: 251–3.
10 Bickford, R.G., Freming, B.D. 1965. Neural stimulation by pulsed magnetic fields in animals and man. Digest of the 6th International Conference on Medical Electronics and Biological Engineering, Tokyo, paper 7–6.
11 Barker, A.T., Jalinous, R., Freeston, I.L. 1985. Non-invasive magnetic stimulation of human motor cortex. Lancet. 1: 1106–7.
12 Terao, Y., Ugawa, Y. 2002. Basic mechanisms of TMS. J Clin Neurophysiol. 19: 322–43.
13 Pascual-Leone, A., Gates, J.R., Dhuna, A. 1991. Induction of speech arrest and counting errors with rapid-rate transcranial magnetic stimulation. Neurology. 41: 697–702.
14 Dhuna, A., Gates, J., Pascual-Leone, A. 1991. Transcranial magnetic stimulation in patients with epilepsy. Neurology. 41: 1067–71.
15 Pascual-Leone, A., Vall-Sole, J., Wassermann, E.M. *et al.* 1994. Responses to rapid-rate transcranial magnetic stimulation of the human motor cortex. Brain. 117: 847–58.
16 Chen, R., Classen, J., Gerloff, C., *et al.* 1997. Depression of motor cortex excitability by low-frequency transcranial magnetic stimulation. Neurology. 48: 1398–403.
17 Wassermann, E.M., Cohen, L.G., Flitman, S.S. *et al.* 1996a. Seizures in healthy people with repeated 'safe' trains of transcranial magnetic stimuli. Lancet. 347: 825–6.
18 Wassermann, E.M., Grafman, J., Berry, C. *et al.* 1996b. Use and safety of a new repetitive transcranial magnetic stimulator. Electroencephalogr Clin Neurophysiol. 101: 412–7.
19 Padberg, F.G., Pogarell, N., Moller, H.J., Fregni, F. 2007. Efficacy and safety of prefrontal repetitive transcranial magnetic stimulation in affective disorders. In Advances in Biological Psychiatry, ed. Marcolin, M.A., Padberg, F. Vol. 23. Basal: Karger.
20 Wassermann, E.M., Lisanby, S.H. 2001. Therapeutic application of repetitive transcranial magnetic stimulation: a review. Clin Neurophysiol. 112:1367–77.
21 Rossini, P.M., Rossi, S. 2007. Transcranial magnetic stimulation: diagnostic, therapeutic and research potential. Neurology. 68: 484–8.
22 Ridding, M.C., Rothwell, J.C. 2007. Is there a future for therapeutic use of transcranial magnetic stimulation? Nat Rev Neurosci. 8: 559–67.
23 Ruohonen, J. 2003. Background physics for magnetic stimulation. Suppl Clin Neurophysiol. 56: 3–12.

24 Keck, M.E. 2007. Repetitive transcranial magnetic stimulation effects in vitro and in animal models. In Transcranial Brain Stimulation for Treatment of Psychiatric Disorders, ed. Marcolin, M.A., Padberg, F. Vol. 23. Basel: Karger.
25 Katz, B. 1939. Nerve excitation by high-frequency alternating current. J Physiol Lond. 96: 202–24.
26 Rattay, F. 1986. Analysis of models for external stimulation of axons. IEEE Trans Biomed Eng. 33: 974–7.
27 Reilly, J.P. 1989. Peripheral nerve stimulation by induced electric currents: exposure to time-varying magnetic fields. Med Biol Eng Comput. 27: 101–10.
28 Roth, B.J., Basser, P.J. 1990. A model of the stimulation of a nerve fiber by electromagnetic induction. IEEE Trans Biomed Eng. 37: 588–97.
29 Maccabee, P.J., Amassian, V.E., Eberle, L.P., Cracco, R.Q. 1993. Magnetic coil stimulation of straight and bent amphibian and mammalian peripheral nerve in vitro: locus of excitation. J Physiol. 460: 201–19.
30 Thielscher, A., Kammer, T. 2002. Linking physics with physiology in TMS: a sphere field model to determine the cortical stimulation site in TMS. Neuroimage. 17: 1117–30.
31 Tranchina, D., Nicholson, C. 1986. A model for the polarization of neurons by extrinsically applied electric fields. Biophys J. 50: 1139–56.
32 Amassian, V.E., Eberle, L., Maccabee, P.J., Cracco, R.Q. 1992. Modelling magnetic coil excitation of human cerebral cortex with a peripheral nerve immersed in a brainshaped volume conductor: the significance of fiber bending in excitation. Electroencephalogr Clin Neurophysiol. 85: 291–301.
33 Nagarajan, S.S. Durand, D.M., Warman, E.N. 1993. Effects of induced electric fields on finite neuronal structures: a simulation study. IEEE Trans Biomed Eng. 40: 1175–88.
34 Iles, J.F. 2005. Simple models of stimulation of neurones in the brain by electric fields. Prog Biophys Mol Biol. 87: 17–31.
35 Silva, S., Basser, P.J., Miranda, P.C. 2008. Elucidating the mechanisms and loci of neuronal excitation by transcranial magnetic stimulation using a finite element model of a cortical sulcus. Clin Neurophysiol. 119: 2405–13.
36 Salvador, R., Silva, S., Basser, P.J., Miranda, P.C. 2011. Determining which mechanisms lead to activation in the motor cortex: a modeling study of transcranial magnetic stimulation using realistic stimulus waveforms and sulcal geometry. Clin Neurophysiol. 122: 748–58.
37 Thielscher, A., Opitz, A., Windhoff, M. 2011. Impact of the gyral geometry on the electric field induced by transcranial magnetic stimulation. Neuroimage. 54: 234–43.
38 Opitz, A., Windhoff, M., Heidemann, R.M., *et al.* 2011. How the brain tissue shapes the electric field induced by transcranial magnetic stimulation. Neuroimage. 58: 849–59.
39 Tofts, P.S. 1990. The distribution of induced currents in magnetic stimulation of the nervous system. Phys Med Biol 35: 1119–28.
40 Tofts, P.S., Branston, N.M. 1991. The measurement of electric field, and the influence of surface charge, in magnetic stimulation. Electroencephalogr Clin Neurophysiol. 81: 238–9.
41 Eaton, H. 1992. Electric field induced in a spherical volume conductor from arbitrary coils: application to magnetic stimulation and MEG. Med Biol Eng Comput. 30: 433–40.
42 Roth, B.J., Saypol, J.M., Hallett, M., Cohen, L.G. 1991a. A theoretical calculation of the electric field induced in the cortex during magnetic stimulation. Electroencephalogr Clin Neurophysiol. 81: 47–56.
43 Roth, B.J., Cohen, L.G., Hallett, M. 1991b. The electric field induced during magnetic stimulation. Electroencephalogr Clin Neurophysiol Suppl. 43: 268–78.
44 Maccabee, P.J. Amassian, V.E., Eberle, L.P. *et al.* 1991. Measurement of the electric field induced into inhomogeneous volume conductors by magnetic coils: Application to human spinal neurogeometry. Electroencephalogr Clin Neurophysiol. 81: 224–37.
45 Nagarajan, S.S., Durand, D.M. 1996. A generalized cable equation for magnetic stimulation of axons. IEEE Trans Biomed Eng. 43: 304–12.
46 Kobayashi, M., Ueno, S., Kurokawa, T. 1997. Importance of soft tissue inhomogeneity in magnetic peripheral nerve stimulation. Electroencephalogr Clin Neurophysiol. 105: 406–13.
47 Liu, R., Ueno, S. 2000. Calculating the activation function of nerve excitation in inhomogeneous

volume conductor during magnetic stimulation using the finite element method. IEEE Trans Magn. 36: 1796–9.

48 Miranda, P.C., Hallett, M., Basser, P.J. 2003. The electric field induced in the brain by magnetic stimulation: a 3-D finite-element analysis of the effect of tissue heterogeneity and anisotropy. IEEE Trans Biomed Eng. 50: 1074–85.

49 Miranda, P.C., Correia, L., Salvador, R., Basser, P.J. 2007. Tissue heterogeneity as a mechanism for localized neural stimulation by applied electric fields. Phys Med Biol. 52: 5603–17.

50 Basser, P.J., Roth, B.J. 1991. Stimulation of a myelinated nerve axon by electromagnetic induction. Med Biol Eng Comput. 29: 261–8.

51 Roth, B.J. 1994. Mechanisms for electrical stimulation of excitable tissue. Crit Rev Biomed Eng. 22: 253–305.

52 Nagarajan, S.S., Durand, D.M., Hsuing-Hsu, K. 1997. Mapping location of excitation during magnetic stimulation: effects of coil position. Ann Biomed Eng. 25: 112–25.

53 Rothwell, J.C., Thompson, P.D., Day, B.L. *et al.* 1991. Stimulation of the human motor cortex through the scalp. Exp Physiol. 76: 159–200.

54 Ziemann, U., Rothwell, J.C. 2000. I-waves in motor cortex. J Clin Neurophysiol. 17: 397–405.

55 Di Lazzaro, V., Profice, P., Pilato, F., *et al.* 2010. The effects of motor cortex rTMS on corticospinal descending activity. Clin Neurophysiol. 121(4):464–73.

56 Di Lazzaro, V., Profice, P., Ranieri, F., *et al.* 2012. I-wave origin and modulation. Brain Stimul. 5(4):512–25.

57 Groppa, S., Oliviero, A., Eisen, A., *et al.* 2012. A practical guide to diagnostic transcranial magnetic stimulation: report of an IFCN committee. Clin Neurophysiol. 123(5):858–82.

58 Di Lazzaro, V., Oliviero, A., Pilato, F., *et al.* 2004. The physiological basis of transcranial motor cortex stimulation in conscious humans. Clin Neurophysiol. 115(2):255–66.

59 Hodgkin, A.L., Rushton, W.A.H. 1946. The electrical constants of a crustacean nerve fiber. Proc R Soc Lond E. 133: 444–79.

60 Lorente de No, R. 1947. A Study of Nerve Physiology, Studies Rockefeller Institute and Medical Research vol. 131–132. Rockefeller Institute: New York.

61 Bourland, J.D., Nyenhuis, J.A., Noe, W.A, *et al.* 1996. Motor and sensory strength-duration curves for MRI gradient fields. Proc Int Soc Magn Reson Med 4th Scientific Meeting and Exhibit, New York, p. 1724.

62 Roth, Y., Padberg, F., Zangen, A. 2007. Transcranial magnetic stimulation of deep brain regions: Principles and methods. In Transcranial Stimulation As Treatment in Mental Disorders, ed. Marcolin, M., Padberg, F. Advances in Biological Psychiatry vol. 23. Switzerland: Karger Publishers Zürich, pp. 204–24.

63 Sommer, M., Alfaro, A., Rummel, M., *et al.* 2006. Half sine, monophasic and biphasic transcranial magnetic stimulation of the human motor cortex. Clin Neurophysiol. 117: 833–44.

64 Jung, N.H., Delvendahl, I., Pechmann, A., *et al.* 2012. Transcranial magnetic stimulation with a half-sine wave pulse elicits direction-specific effects in human motor cortex. BMC Neurosci. 13: 139.

65 Peterchev, A.V., Jalinous, R., Lisanby, S.H. 2008. A transcranial magnetic stimulator inducing near-rectangular pulses with controllable pulse width (cTMS). IEEE Trans Biomed Eng. 55: 257–66.

66 Roth, Y., Levkovitz, Y., Pell, G.S., *et al.* 2014. Safety and characterization of a novel multichannel TMS stimulator. Brain Stimul. 7: 194–205.

67 Reis, J., Swayne, O.B., Vandermeeren, Y., *et al.* 2008. Contribution of transcranial magnetic stimulation to the understanding of cortical mechanisms involved in motor control. J Physiol. 586(2): 325–51.

68 Bland, B.H. 1986. The physiology and pharmacology of hippocampal formation theta rhythms. Prog Neurobiol. 26: 1–54.

69 Iyer, M.B., Schleper, N., Wassermann, E.M., 2003. Priming stimulation enhances the depressant effect of low-frequency repetitive transcranial magnetic stimulation. J Neurosci. 23: 10867–72.

70 Hoogendam, J.M., Ramakers, G.M., Di Lazzaro, V. 2010. Physiology of repetitive transcranial magnetic stimulation of the human brain. Brain Stimul. 3(2):95–118.

71 Pell, G.S., Roth, Y., Zangen, A. 2011. Modulation of cortical excitability induced by repetitive transcranial magnetic stimulation: influence of

timing and geometrical parameters and underlying mechanisms. Prog Neurobiol. 93: 59–98.
72 Ridding, M.C., Ziemann, U. 2010. Determinants of the induction of cortical plasticity by non-invasive brain stimulation in healthy subjects. J Physiol. 588(Pt 13): 2291–304.
73 Chen, R., Yung, D., Li, J.Y. 2003. Organization of ipsilateral excitatory and inhibitory pathways in the human motor cortex. J Neurophysiol. 89: 1256–64.
74 Mills, K.R., Boniface, S.J., Schubert, M. 1992. Magnetic brain stimulation with a double coil: the importance of coil orientation. Electroencephalogr Clin Neurophysiol. 85(1): 17–21.
75 Fox, P.T., Narayana, S., Tandon, N., Sandoval, H., *et al.* 2004. Column-based model of electric field excitation of cerebral cortex. Hum Brain Mapp. 22(1):1–14.
76 Branston, N.M. Tofts, P.S. 1991. Analysis of the distribution of currents induced by a changing magnetic field in a volume conductor. Phys Med Biol. 36: 161–8.
77 Thielscher, A., Kammer, T. 2004. Electric field properties of two commercial figure-8 coils in TMS: calculation of focality and efficiency. Clin Neurophysiol. 115: 1697–708.
78 Lontis, E.R., Voigt, M., Struijk, J.J. 2006, Focality assessment in transcranial magnetic stimulation with double and cone coils. J Clin Neurophysiol. 23: 462–71.
79 Ren, C., Tarjan, P.P., Popović, D.B. 1995. A novel electric design for electromagnetic stimulation – the Slinky coil. IEEE Trans Biomed Eng. 42(9): 918–25.
80 Roth, B.J., Maccabee, P.J., Eberle, L.P. *et al.* 1994. In vitro evaluation of a 4-leaf coil design for magnetic stimulation of peripheral nerve. Electroencephalogr Clin Neurophysiol. 93(1): 68–74.
81 Davey, K.R., Riehl, M.E. 2006. Suppressing the surface field during transcranial magnetic stimulation. IEEE Trans Biomed Eng. 53: 190–4.
82 Deng, Z.D. Peterchev, A. Lisanby, S.H. 2008. Coil design considerations for deep-brain transcranial magnetic stimulation (dTMS). Conf Proc IEEE Eng Med Biol Soc. 2008: 5675–9.
83 Roth, Y., Zangen, A., Hallett, M. 2002. A coil design for transcranial magnetic stimulation of deep brain regions. J Clin Neurophysiol. 19: 361–70.
84 Zangen, A., Roth, Y., Voller, B., Hallett, M. 2005. Transcranial magnetic stimulation of deep brain regions: evidence for efficacy of the H-coil. Clin Neurophysiol. 116: 775–9.
85 Deng, Z.D., Lisanby, S.H., Peterchev, A.V. 2013. Electric field depth-focality tradeoff in transcranial magnetic stimulation: simulation comparison of 50 coil designs. Brain Stimul. 6(1): 1–13.
86 Roth, Y., Pell, G.S., Zangen, A. 2013. Commentary on: Deng *et al.* Electric field depth-focality tradeoff in transcranial magnetic stimulation: simulation comparison of 50 coil designs. Brain Stimul. 6(1): 14–5.
87 Weyh, T., Wendicke, K., Mentschel, C. *et al.* 2005. Marked differences in the thermal characteristics of figure-of-eight shaped coils used for repetitive transcranial magnetic stimulation. Clin Neurophysiol. 116: 1477–86.
88 Epstein, C.M., Davey, K.R. 2002. Iron-core coils for transcranial magnetic stimulation. J Clin Neurophysiol. 19: 376–81.
89 O'Reardon, J., Solvason, B., Janicak, P. *et al.* 2007. Efficacy and safety of transcranial magnetic stimulation in the acute treatment of major depression: a multi-site randomized controlled trial. Biol Psychiatry. 62: 1208–16.
90 Maccabee, P.J., Eberle, L., Amassian, V.E. *et al.* 1990. Spatial distribution of the electric field induced in volume by round and figure '8' magnetic coils: relevance to activation of sensory nerve fibers. Electroencephalogr Clin Neurophysiol. 76: 131–41.
91 Heller, L., van Hulsteyn, D.B. 1992. Brain stimulation using electromagnetic sources: theoretical aspects. Biophys J 63: 129–38.
92 Levkovitz, Y., Roth, Y., Harel, E.V. *et al.* 2007. A randomized controlled feasibility and safety study of deep transcranial magnetic stimulation. Clin Neurophysiol. 118: 2730–44.
93 Levkovitz, Y., Harel, E.V., Roth, Y. *et al.* 2009. Deep transcranial magnetic stimulation of the prefrontal cortex – Effectiveness in major depression. Brain Stimul. 2: 188–200.
94 Harel, E.V., Zangen, A., Roth, Y., *et al.* 2011. H-coil repetitive transcranial magnetic stimulation for the treatment of bipolar depression: an add-on, safety and feasibility study. World J Biol Psychiatry. 12: 119–26.

95 Levkovitz, Y., Isserles, M., Padberg, F., *et al.* 2015. Efficacy and safety of deep transcranial magnetic stimulation for major depression: a prospective multicenter randomized controlled trial. World Psychiatry. 14(1): 64–73.
96 Wassermann, E.M. 1998. Risk and safety of repetitive transcranial magnetic stimulation: report and suggested guidelines from the International Workshop on the Safety of Repetitive Transcranial Magnetic Stimulation, June 5–7, 1996. Electroencephalogr Clin Neurophysiol. 108: 1–16.
97 Rossi, S., Hallett, M., Rossini, P.M. *et al.* 2009. Safety, ethical considerations, and application guidelines for the use of transcranial magnetic stimulation in clinical practice and research. Clin Neurophysiol. 120: 2008–39.
98 Counter, S.A., Borg, E. 1992. Analysis of the coil generated impulse noise in extracranial magnetic stimulation. Electroencephalogr Clin Neurophysiol. 85: 280–8.
99 Chen, R. 2000. Studies of human motor physiology with transcranial magnetic stimulation. Muscle Nerve Suppl. 9: S26–32.
100 Civardi, C., Cantello, R., Asselman, P., Rothwell, J.C. 2001. Transcranial magnetic stimulation can be used to test connections to primary motor areas from frontal and medial cortex in humans. Neuroimage. 14(6): 1444–53.
101 Daskalakis, Z.J., Paradiso, G.O., Christensen, B.K., *et al.* 2004. Exploring the connectivity between the cerebellum and motor cortex in humans. J Physiol. 557(Pt 2): 689–700.
102 Daskalakis, Z.J., Christensen, B.K., Chen, R., *et al.* 2002. Evidence for impaired cortical inhibition in schizophrenia using transcranial magnetic stimulation. Arch Gen Psychiatry. 59(4): 347–54.
103 Ferbert, A., Priori, A., Rothwell, J.C., *et al.* 1992. Interhemispheric inhibition of the human motor cortex. J Physiol. 453:525–46.
104 Kujirai, T., Caramia, M.D., Rothwell, J.C., *et al.* 1993. Corticocortical inhibition in human motor cortex. J Physiol. 471: 501–19.
105 Sailer, A., Molnar, G.F., Cunic, D.I., Chen, R. 2002. Effects of peripheral sensory input on cortical inhibition in humans. J Physiol. 544(Pt 2): 617–29.
106 Stefan, K., Kunesch, E., Cohen, L.G., *et al.* 2000. Induction of plasticity in the human motor cortex by paired associative stimulation. Brain. 123(Pt 3): 572–84.
107 Tokimura, H., Ridding, M.C., Tokimura, Y., *et al.* 1996. Short latency facilitation between pairs of threshold magnetic stimuli applied to human motor cortex. Electroencephalogr Clin Neurophysiol. 101(4):263–72.
108 Tokimura, H., Di Lazzaro, V., Tokimura, Y., *et al.* 2000. Short latency inhibition of human hand motor cortex by somatosensory input from the hand. J Physiol. 523(Pt 2): 503–13.
109 Ugawa, Y., Uesaka, Y., Terao, Y., *et al.* 1995. Magnetic stimulation over the cerebellum in humans. Ann Neurol. 37(6): 703–13.
110 Ugawa Y. 2009. Can we see the cerebellar activation effect by TMS over the back of the head? Clin Neurophysiol. 120(12): 2006–7.
111 Valls-Solé, J., Pascual-Leone, A., Wassermann, E.M., Hallett, M. 1992. Human motor evoked responses to paired transcranial magnetic stimuli. Electroencephalogr Clin Neurophysiol. 85(6): 355–64.
112 Wilson, S.A., Lockwood, R.J., Thickbroom, G.W., Mastaglia, F.L. 1993. The muscle silent period following transcranial magnetic cortical stimulation. J Neurol Sci. 114(2):216–22.
113 Ziemann, U., Tergau, F., Wassermann, E.M., *et al.* 1998. Demonstration of facilitatory I wave interaction in the human motor cortex by paired transcranial magnetic stimulation. J Physiol. 15: 511.

CHAPTER 9

Magnetic stimulation for depression: Subconvulsive and convulsive approaches

Andrada D. Neacsiu[1] and Sarah Hollingsworth Lisanby[1,2]

[1]*Duke University School of Medicine, Durham, USA*

[2]*Duke University School of Arts and Sciences, Durham, USA*

Introduction

Despite the availability of antidepressant medications and validated psychotherapies, treatment-resistant depression remains an important clinical problem and a source of considerable suffering and disability worldwide. Electroconvulsive therapy (ECT) is the most effective and rapidly acting treatment we have today for severe treatment-resistant depression, but its current cognitive side effect profile limits its clinical utility [1]. Developing treatment modalities that possess the powerful efficacy of ECT but without the attendant side effects would represent a major advance in depression care. Modern ECT involves the application of a tetanic train of electrical pulses under anaesthesia and the induction of a seizure. Is it the tetanic train of electrical pulses, or the seizure, or both, that is/are responsible for its efficacy? The same question may be asked about the side effects as well as the mechanisms underlying those that are incompletely understood [2]. Magnetic stimulation allows the uncoupling of these factors so that we may begin to address the question of how ECT, the most potent available antidepressant, works (Fig. 9.1).

Rapidly alternating magnetic fields induce electrical eddy currents in the brain. When administered in pulse trains at levels below the threshold for seizure induction, this is called repetitive transcranial magnetic stimulation (rTMS). When administered at levels above the threshold for seizure induction in a patient under anaesthesia, this is termed as magnetic seizure therapy (MST). In both cases, magnetic stimulation induces tetanic trains of electrical pulses in the brain in a far more focal fashion than is possible with conventional ECT.

TMS was recently cleared by the US Food and Drug Administration (FDA) as a treatment for depression, based on reproducible evidence of antidepressant efficacy and safety [3, 4]. MST is under investigation as an experimental treatment for depression. Contrasting these interventions in their efficacy and side effects allows us to examine the relative roles of the induced electric field and seizure in the efficacy and adverse effects of ECT.

This chapter reviews the body of evidence for the subconvulsive and convulsive approaches using magnetic stimulation for the treatment of depression and discusses the implications of these findings for our understanding of depression and the mechanisms of action of magnetic treatments for depression.

Neuromodulation in Psychiatry, First Edition. Edited by Clement Hamani, Paul Holtzheimer, Andres M. Lozano and Helen Mayberg.

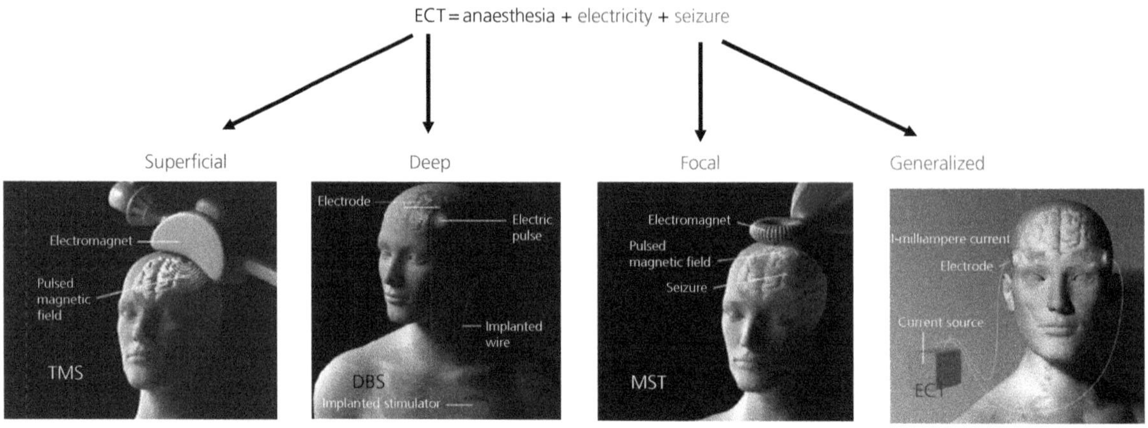

Figure 9.1 Conceptual schema for studying the independent contributions of pulsed electric fields and seizure induction in the therapeutic efficacy of ECT. Contrasting these tools in their neurobiological and clinical effects may shed light on the unparalleled efficacy of ECT and point towards the development of safer alternatives.

Definitions and regulatory status

Transcranial magnetic stimulation (TMS)

Definition of TMS

TMS applies rapidly alternating magnetic fields to the scalp using an electromagnetic coil to induce electrical currents in the brain.

Key characteristics of TMS

TMS is a non-invasive tool used to induce neuromodulation of targeted circuitry to study and treat neuropsychiatric disorders. It does not require anaesthesia and can be given at levels below the threshold for inducing a seizure. The local effect of eddy current induction results in neuronal depolarization that, in turn, activates distributed networks connected to the stimulated site trans-synaptically. The short-lived effects of acute application of TMS are useful for mapping brain function and determining brain–behaviour relationships. The lasting effects of repeated application are useful for therapeutic purposes.

In contrast to ECT (Fig. 9.2), TMS does not require anaesthesia, can be given at subconvulsive levels, is indicated for depression (but not psychotic or catatonic subtypes) and is administered in an office-based setting rather than an ECT suite or recovery room setting. The intended use of TMS is limited to adults with unipolar depression, while ECT has an extraordinarily broad therapeutic spectrum including bipolar depression, mania, psychotic depression, catatonia and medication-resistant schizophrenia. ECT is also helpful in a number of neurological conditions including status epilepticus, neuroleptic malignant syndrome, Parkinson's disease and self-injurious behaviours in autism.

Regulatory status of TMS

The FDA identified a generic type of TMS devices as: 'A transcranial magnetic stimulation system is a device intended for the treatment of major depressive disorder (MDD) that non-invasively delivers repetitive pulsed magnetic fields of sufficient magnitude to induce neural action potentials in the patient's cerebral cortex to treat the symptoms of MDD without inducing seizure.' [21 CFR 882.5805] At the time of writing this chapter, two TMS devices were cleared by the FDA for the treatment of depression, which are Neuronetics and Brainsway (Table 9.1 and Fig. 9.3). Both

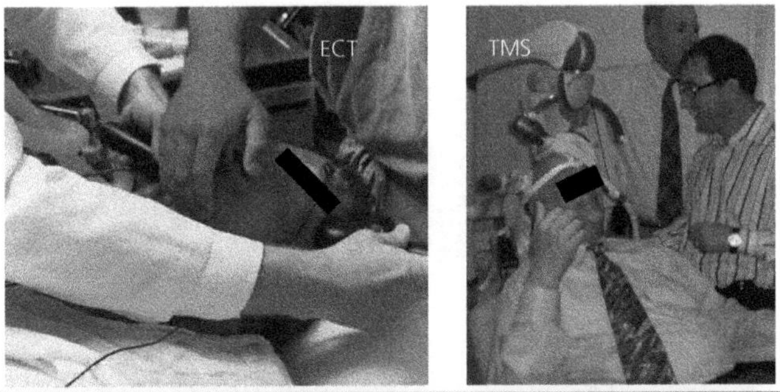

Comparison	ECT	TMS
Anaesthesia?	Yes	No
Seizure?	Yes	No*
Intended population	Severe depression, psychotic subtype	Moderate depression
Setting	ECT suite	Office

Figure 9.2 Comparison of ECT and TMS. In contrast to ECT, TMS does not require anaesthesia, can be given at subconvulsive levels, is not indicated for psychotic or catatonic subtypes of depression and does not need to be given in an ECT suite or recovery room setting. *TMS does carry a risk of seizure at dosages in excess of safety guidelines. (*See insert for color representation of the figure.*)

Table 9.1 Comparison of TMS devices Approved by the FDA for depression treatment.

	Neuronetics	**Brainsway**
Coil		
Design	Figure 8	H-coil
Focality	Focal	Non-focal
Core	Iron	Air
Stimulation parameters		
Percent of motor threshold	120	120
Frequency (Hz)	10	18
Train duration (s)	4	2
Inter-train interval (s)	26	20
Number of trains	75	55
Pulses per session	3000	1980
Treatment session duration (min)	37.5	20.2
Sessions per week	5	5
Treatment schedule	5/week × 6 weeks	5/week × 4 weeks, 2/week × 12 weeks
Intended use	Treatment of major depressive disorder in adult patients who have failed to receive satisfactory improvement from prior antidepressant medication in the current episode	Treatment of depressive episodes in adults suffering from major depressive disorder who failed to achieve satisfactory improvement from previous antidepressant medication in the current episode
FDA clearance status	Original 510K Clearance: K083538, 16 December 2008. Revised 510K Clearance: K133408, 28 March 2014	K122288, 1/7/2013

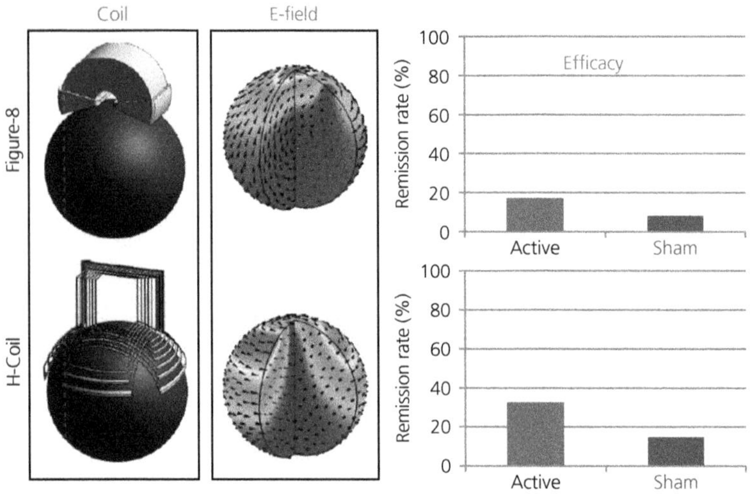

Figure 9.3 TMS coils approved by the FDA for the treatment of depression. Top row: Neuronetics iron-core figure-8 coil. Bottom row: Brainsway H-coil. Left column depicts finite element model of each coil, overlaid on a five concentric spherical model of the head. Middle column: E-field simulation. Right column: efficacy of active and sham TMS from the pivotal trial leading to FDA approval. Source: Adapted from Deng *et al.* [5] and O'Reardon *et al.* [3] and FDA 510K 122288. (*See insert for color representation of the figure.*)

are classified as Class II devices, and both are considered to be of the generic type of transcranial magnetic stimulation systems.

The first TMS device to be approved for depression [Neuronetics] was originally indicated for 'the treatment of major depressive disorder in adult patients who have failed to achieve satisfactory improvement from one prior antidepressant medication at or above the minimal effective dose and duration in the current episode.' [K083538, 16 December 2008]. This limitation to patients who have failed one medication was based upon the study by Lisanby *et al.* [4], which demonstrated that active TMS differed significantly from sham only for those patients who had failed to respond to a single antidepressant medication, while those with more resistant depression did not show a difference between active and sham.

A new 510K ruling has revised the indication for the Neuronetics device to be used for the 'treatment of major depressive disorder in adult patients who have failed to receive satisfactory improvement from prior antidepressant medication in the current episode.' [510K 133408, 28 March 2014]. This label expansion was an FDA ruling based on a pooled analysis of the original industry-sponsored pivotal trial with a separately conducted NIMH-funded trial (OPT-TMS), which used different sham methods.

The second TMS device to receive clearance for depression was the Brainsway device [K122288, cleared 1 June 2013], which was found by the FDA to be substantially equivalent to the Neuronetics device, also Class II, and labelled for the following intended use: 'treatment of depressive episodes in adults suffering from major depressive disorder who failed to achieve satisfactory improvement from previous antidepressant medication in the current episode'.

Off-label use of legally marketed TMS devices is allowed under the FDA Practice of Medicine Provision [Section 906, Federal Food, Drug and Cosmetic Act]. According to this provision, a practitioner is allowed to use a legally marketed device for an unapproved (off-label) use if all of the following three criteria apply: (a) it is used to treat a disease or condition, (b) it is used within a legitimate practitioner–patient relationship and (c) there is no advertising or promotion of the off-label use by the practitioner or the manufacturer. In some cases, Institutional Review Board (IRB) approval may be required.

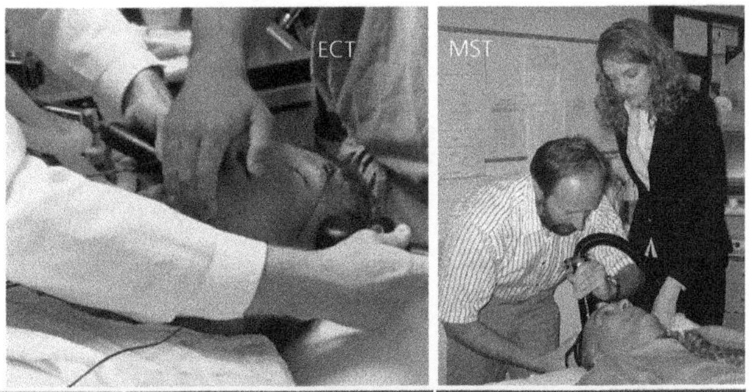

Comparison	ECT	MST
Means of induction	Electrical	Magnetic
Scalp preparation?	Yes	No
Tissue impedance?	Yes	No
Site of stimulation	Diffuse	Focal

Figure 9.4 Comparison of ECT and MST. In contrast to ECT, MST uses electromagnetic induction to trigger the seizure. Scalp preparation is not required as no electricity is applied directly to the scalp. Magnetic induction is not affected by tissue impedance from the scalp or skull. MST is relatively more focal than ECT. (*See insert for color representation of the figure.*)

Magnetic seizure therapy (MST)

Definition of MST

MST refers to the induction of seizures using rTMS under anaesthesia for the treatment of depression [6–8].

Key characteristics

The aim of MST is to retain the superior efficacy of ECT and reduce its side effects through the enhanced focality offered by magnetic induction. The ability to induce seizures with enhanced control over the site of stimulation enables studies to evaluate the relationships between the spatial distribution of the induced electric field, the subsequent seizure and the clinical outcomes. This can inform the mechanisms of action of convulsive therapy, which is especially relevant considering the superior efficacy of ECT compared with medications and compared with subconvulsive TMS.

In contrast to ECT (Figs. 9.4 and 9.5), MST induces the seizure using transcranially applied magnetic fields. Because no electrical current is applied directly to the scalp, preparation of the scalp to reduce impedance is not required. The magnetic fields are not affected by tissue impedance, permitting enhanced control over focality in comparison with ECT.

The intended use of MST is meant to mirror the broad therapeutic spectrum of ECT, including psychotic subtype of depression, depression in bipolar disorder, etc.

Regulatory status of MST

At the time of writing this chapter, MST was not approved by the FDA. Two manufacturers are currently making investigational devices that may be used to perform MST, which are Magstim and MagVenture (Table 9.2). A variety of coils have been evaluated for seizure induction, but the most efficient appear to be the large round coil and the double-cone or twin-coil (Fig. 9.5).

Comparing and contrasting actions of TMS, MST and ECT

Figure 9.6 compares and contrasts the actions of TMS, MST and ECT with respect to magnetic fields, electrical fields, neuronal depolarization and seizure initiation.

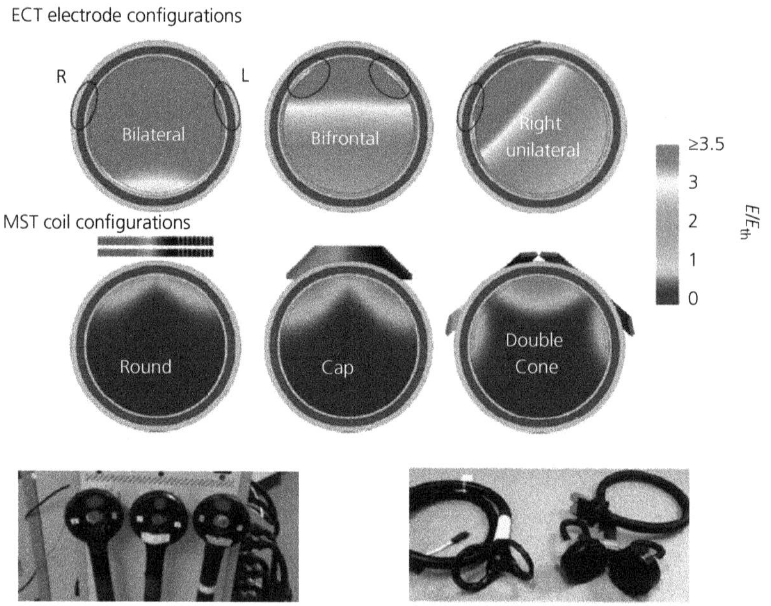

Figure 9.5 Finite element modelling of electric field strength induced in a five-concentric spherical model of the head by ECT (top row) and MST (bottom row) configurations. Adapted from Deng *et al.* [9]. Photo insert on left shows MagStim Theta Round coil switcher box allowing rapid coil swapping between trains. Photo insert on right shows Magstim Double Cone coil for MST on left and MagVenture Twin-Coil on right. Both deliver a field distribution similar to the double-cone configuration. (*See insert for color representation of the figure.*)

Table 9.2 Comparison of investigational MST devices.

	MagStim	MagVenture
Coil		
Design	Round/double cone	Twin-coil
Focality	Non-focal/focal	Focal
Core	Air	Air
Stimulation parameters		
Percent of maximal stimulator output	100%	100%
Frequency (Hz)	Up to 100	Up to 240
Train duration (s)	Up to 10	Up to 30
Number of trains	1	1
Sessions per week	3	2 or 3
Treatment schedule	3/week × 3–4 weeks	3/week × 3–4 weeks
Intended use	Adults with major depressive episodes referred for ECT	Adults with major depressive episodes referred for ECT

Magnetic field (TMS and MST only)

TMS and MST share the application of a magnetic field and induction of an electrical current in the cortex, while ECT involves the direct application of an electrical field to the scalp. Avoiding the impedance of the scalp and skull improves the focal precision of TMS and MST relative to ECT. TMS and MST induce the same strength magnetic pulses, but in the case of MST, higher frequencies and train durations are used to induce the seizure.

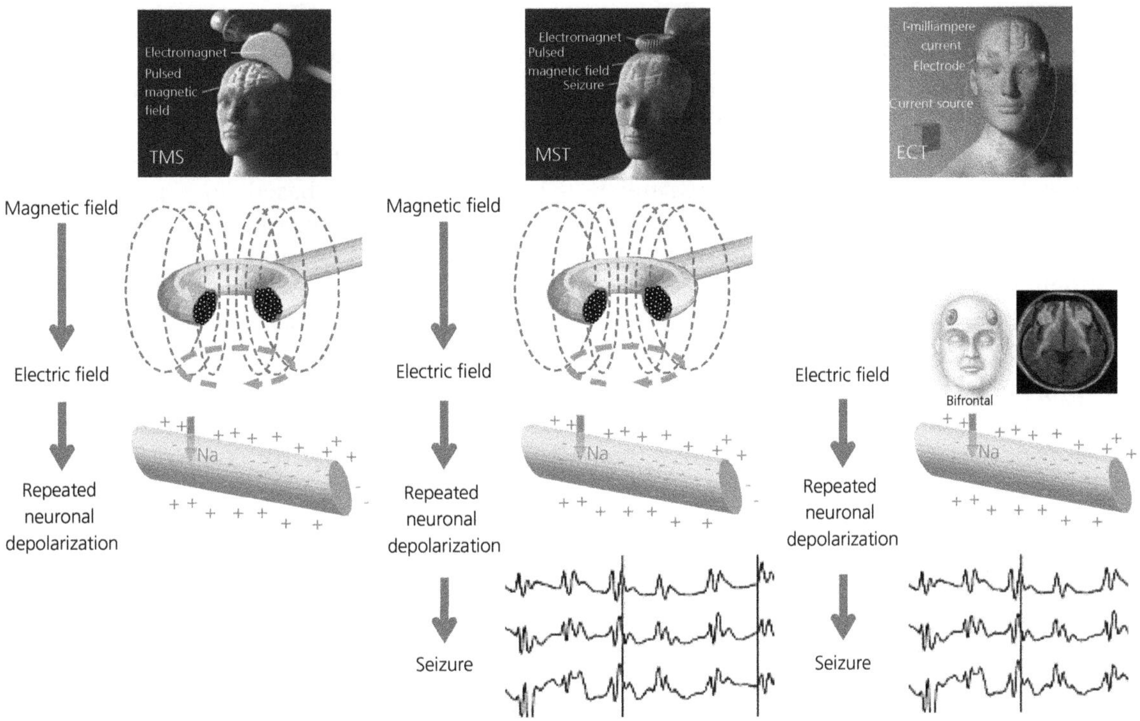

Figure 9.6 Comparative mechanisms of TMS, MST and ECT. TMS and MST share the application of a magnetic field. TMS, MST and ECT all involve the repeated application of an electric field, which induces repeated neuronal depolarization. In the case of MST and ECT, this results in deliberate seizure induction. TMS can induce a seizure at sufficiently high dosage, and this is a known potential side effect. (*See insert for color representation of the figure.*)

Magnetic induction carries the advantages of being non-invasive and possessing excellent spatial resolution. Disadvantages include being confined to superficial cortex (only a disadvantage if the therapeutic target is deep). While deeper penetrating coils address this limitation, there remains a depth-focality trade-off such that deeper coils are always intrinsically less focal [10].

Electric field (TMS, MST and ECT)

TMS, MST and ECT all involve an electric field in the brain, but the magnetic and electrical approaches differ in the field strength, directionality and focality of the electric field. The resulting induced electrical current with ECT has radial components (with electric field direction radiating towards the centre of the brain), while with both TMS and MST, the direction of the induced electrical current is tangential to the surface of the scalp.

The strength of the electrical current induced in the brain with TMS and MST is far weaker and more focal than that induced by ECT. In vivo recordings and computational modelling of the induced field strengths demonstrate that E-field exposure to deep brain structures, such as the hippocampus, is robust with ECT, while TMS and MST provide relative sparing of hippocampus and other deep brain structures from the induced electric field [11, 12, 9].

Neuronal depolarization (TMS, MST and ECT)

TMS, MST and ECT all involve the repeated depolarization of neuronal populations, induced by the repeated application of electrical fields. The spatial extent of the neuronal effects is dramatically different between the magnetic and electrical approaches, due to the enhanced focality of TMS/MST in comparison to ECT. The repeated induction of neuronal depolarization through repeated electrical pulses has the potential to induce neuroplasticity, similar to the mechanisms of long-term potentiation (LTP) and long-term depression (LTD).

Whether neuroplasticity related to the tetanic train delivered with ECT is important for clinical outcome apart from its seizure-inducing property is presently not known. The availability of a tool to induce seizures without exposing deep regions of the brain to repeated electrical pulses and neuronal depolarization (as we now have with MST) provides the potential to answer this mechanistic question.

Seizure (MST and ECT only)

Both MST and ECT induce seizures, but they differ in their strength and spatial extent [13, 14]. TMS can also induce seizures when used outside of the safety guidelines, or when applied to individuals with seizure risk factors [15, 16]. ECT-induced seizures are more robust, have stronger ictal power and stronger post-ictal suppression and are more generalized across the brain than those induced by MST [11, 13, 14]. Neuroplastic effects of seizures have been well described and include mossy fibre sprouting as well as cellular proliferation.

Subconvulsive TMS for depression treatment

Repetitive transcranial magnetic stimulation (rTMS)

Clinical trial evidence

Since its introduction in 1985 [17], more than 6300 studies have been conducted on rTMS that have examined its therapeutic effects on depression. By 2007, research on this topic significantly advanced our knowledge about the optimal parameters needed to obtain therapeutic effects, increasing the meta-analytic effect sizes from small (0.35) in early studies to moderate (0.55–0.76) in later studies [18, 19].

The approval of rTMS for depression by the FDA in 2008 was based on a pivotal multicentre, industry-sponsored, randomized controlled trial (RCT), where rTMS or sham TMS was administered to 301 medication-free patients who met the criteria for MDD [3]. The treatment was administered using the Neurostar rTMS device (Neuronetics, Inc.) that uses a figure-8 coil and delivers pulses that reach a depth of 1.5 cm. Treatment involved daily 37.5-min sessions (5/week) for 4–6 weeks. rTMS was administered over the left DLPFC, identified by moving the TMS coil 5 cm anterior to the motor threshold (MT) location [20]. Administration parameters were: 120% MT, 10 pulses/s, 4s train and 26s inter-train interval. After 6 weeks, the active rTMS group was twice more likely to have achieved remission from depression than the sham group (16% vs. 7%), based on interview but not self-reported data, a difference corresponding to a small effect size (d = 0.34) [3]. There was also a significant between-group difference in improving the quality of life and functional status at the end of treatment and at a 6-month follow-up favouring rTMS [21]. There were few adverse events (scalp discomfort, mild increase in suicidality), and no serious adverse events (e.g. death, seizures) [3]. Despite some limitations (e.g. not reporting inter-rater reliability on assessment measures, not presenting longitudinal effect sizes), this study provided compelling evidence that rTMS has therapeutic antidepressant effects for treatment-resistant adults with MDD. In particular, patients who are early in the course of their treatment resistance seemed to benefit the most from rTMS [4].

Industry-independent studies using the FDA-approved specifications also obtained similar results. George *et al.* [22] conducted an NIMH-sponsored study on 190 treatment-resistant adults with MDD. With a high retention rate (88%), they found that rTMS was almost three times more likely to lead to remission when compared with sham TMS (14% vs. 5%), a difference corresponding to a moderate effect size (both interview and self-reported data). When compared with the O'Reardon trial [3], this federally supported study addressed the measurement limitations of the industry trial and showed significant improvements much earlier (by week 3 as opposed to week 6). Nevertheless, the authors recommended that a longer treatment course should be used if patients do not remit by the end of a 3-week course [22]. In the second phase of their trial (uncontrolled, open-label, $N = 141$), increasing the treatment to up to 6 additional weeks resulted in 31% of those who did not remit by week 3 to fully remit [23]. Furthermore, those who had failed fewer courses of treatment tended to have a higher probability to improve [22].

Mantovani *et al.* [24] recently published a follow-up of this study on the durability effects of rTMS. Of the 32 patients who remitted in the original study, completed the TMS taper and were available 3 months later for follow-up, 91% were classified to be in remission based on a depression interview, 6% as partial responders and 3% as relapsed [24]. Given that prior studies with longer term follow-up (>4 weeks) provide mixed evidence for the durability of rTMS [25], this finding by Mantovani *et al.* [24] clarifies that the therapeutic effects of TMS are durable in about 50% of responders.

Efficacy trials were followed by several community trials demonstrating the effectiveness of the on-label use of rTMS in clinical practice. One noteworthy example is the study conducted by Carpenter *et al.* [26] who followed 307 real-world patients receiving Neurostar rTMS in community settings. Treatment length varied for this sample ($M = 28.3$, $SD = 10.1$); nevertheless, 58% of the participants improved and 37% remitted based on the treating clinician's rated global severity index (CGI-S) [26]. Response and remission were similar when examining self-reported findings (56% and 29%, respectively). Significant improvements were also found in the self-reported quality of life and functioning [27]. Severity of prior treatment resistance did not moderate these findings, a result different from what was found in efficacy trials. One seizure was reported in this study [26].

Similar effectiveness findings emerged from a naturalistic study in an academic setting. Data from 100 treatment-resistant depressed patients treated with the FDA-approved rTMS protocol suggested that 51% improved and 25% remitted after 6 weeks of treatment, as measured by CGI-S [28]. About 50% of these patients entered a 6-month maintenance rTMS treatment: 62% of them maintained their responder status by the end of this period [28]. Given that these participants had failed on average 3.4 medications before starting rTMS, these results strongly support that both efficacy and effectiveness trials show promise for rTMS as a treatment for treatment-resistant depression.

Meta-analyses

In addition to these pivotal trials, several meta-analyses have been conducted that summarize current findings of the efficacy and effectiveness of rTMS for treatment-resistant depression. Dell'osso *et al.* [29] conducted a meta-review of 15 meta-analytic studies of rTMS for depression published between 2001 and 2011. Initial meta-analyses found mixed results, with some supporting the efficacy of rTMS, while others contesting it. More recent meta-analytic studies are consistent in their findings that rTMS administered for at least 3 weeks has therapeutic effects for depression. Reported effect sizes varied from .39 to .76 and, in general, the severity of depression was reduced by more than 30% from pre- to post-treatment [29]. Other noteworthy findings are that (1) ECT tends to have significantly higher acute efficacy when compared with rTMS [19], (2) left high-frequency (HF)-rTMS produces comparable results to right low-frequency (LF)-rTMS [30] and (3) antidepressant effects are maintained for at least 1–2 weeks following treatment [25].

More recent meta-analyses continue to support the efficacy of rTMS [31, 32], although the clinical relevance continues to be contested [33]. Berlim *et al.* [31] summarize data from 29 RCTs that included more than 1300 subjects with MDD. Participants treated with HF-rTMS were 3.3 times more likely to have a clinically significant response to treatment when compared with participants treated with sham TMS. In the summarized trials, 18.6% in HF-rTMS and 5% in sham TMS remitted from depression. Dropout rates were low in both treatments (~7.5%). There were no differences in efficacy when TMS was used alone and when it was administered in conjunction with medication. The authors did not find any significant stimulation parameter to predict outcome. Effect sizes were not given [31].

A different meta-analysis [32] included nine trials (425 subjects) and examined the differences between rTMS and ECT. For psychotic depression, ECT is acceptable and more effective than rTMS in the short term. In non-psychotic depression, both rTMS and ECT appear to be equally effective. More studies are needed to examine and compare the long-term effects and problems that can arise from both ECT and rTMS [32].

By examining 63 studies for comparing rTMS and sham TMS (a total of 3236 participants) published up to January 2014, Lepping and colleagues [33] transformed primary outcome findings into CGI scores in order to assess clinical significance across the trials. They concluded that although rTMS has a clear antidepressant efficacy (i.e. 35%–45% reduction in depression severity), the strong placebo effect seen in TMS RCTs (i.e. 22–25% reduction in depression severity) lends a CGI improvement of 0.5 points for non-refractory depression and 0.75 for treatment-resistant depression, which corresponds to minimal clinical improvement [33]. Therefore, the authors question the clinical relevance of rTMS above and beyond placebo.

In addition to examining the effects on non-medicated depressed subjects, meta-analyses partially support rTMS as an efficient method to augment response to psychotropic medications. For example, Berlim, van den Eyde and Daskalakis [34] reviewed six RCTs including 392 depressed subjects where rTMS was combined with an antidepressant treatment. A significant effect of rTMS when compared with sham TMS was found when analysing the response rates (OR = 2.5), but not remission rates. High heterogeneity in the study designs may have led to the lack of a finding for remission; therefore, the authors argue that additional research on this topic is highly needed [34].

An additional important finding emerged through a recent meta-analysis that showed similar antidepressant effects, but fewer side effects, when using LF-rTMS over the right DLPFC when compared with HF-rTMS over the left DLPFC [35]. By reviewing eight RCTS with a total of 249 patients (123 stimulated with HF-rTMS and 126 stimulated with LF-rTMS), the authors found similar response rates for the two methods (43.1% and 42.8%, respectively). Nevertheless, LF-rTMS patients reported fewer headaches and lower likelihood for seizures, although these safety findings were primarily based on two of the RCTs included [35]. Therefore, LF-rTMS may have a slight advantage, although much more investigation is needed. (For a recent review on LF-rTMS findings alone, see Berlim, van den Eynde and Daskalakis [36].)

A few additional RCTs have been published since the most recent meta-analyses. A pilot trial examined the feasibility, acceptability and preliminary efficacy of HF-rTMS to left DLPFC (120% MT, 10 Hz, 5 s train, 10 s inter-train,

30 min) or sham TMS administered three times daily for 3 days (54,000 pulses) to 41 highly suicidal military inpatients [37]. The trial indicated that the course of treatment was feasible and safe. There was a non-significant trend for a faster decrease in suicidality during the first day of active TMS; nevertheless, both active and sham TMS led to similar reductions in suicidality (15.4 vs. 15.3 points decrease in the Beck Scale of Suicidal Ideation). The authors concluded that the potential for a rapid anti-suicidal effect during a 1-day rTMS course warrants further investigation [37].

Krstic *et al.* [38] randomly assigned 19 women with treatment-resistant depression who were on stable antidepressants to 10 sessions of either LF-rTMS (110% of the MT, 3000 pulses) or sham stimulation over the right DLPFC. All participants were also partially sleep deprived once a week during the treatment. Only participants in the active group responded, showing a 50% reduction in depression severity by the end of treatment. Of the 11 responders, 50% remitted by the end of the treatment and more than 50% continued to show partial remission 12 and 24 weeks later. Four participants maintained remission by the 6-month follow-up. These participants were found to have a Val66Val homozygous genotype, which is showing promise as a genetic marker that may indicate who may be more likely to benefit from rTMS [38].

Speer and colleagues [39] attempted to gather additional information about the parameters of rTMS stimulation. They conducted a 3-week RCT on 24 depressed patients who received stimulation over the left DLPFC and who were randomized to sham, 20-Hz rTMS or 1-Hz rTMS. Participants in both active conditions reported significant improvement compared to the participants in the sham condition, supporting that 10-Hz stimulation may not be the only configuration with antidepressant effects [39].

One study attempted to assess whether stimulation of specific portions of the DLPFC led to differential treatment responses [40]. Fifteen depressed patients were randomly assigned to receive 10 sessions of LF stimulation of either Brodmann area 9 or 46. There were no significant differences in treatment response in the two groups. Participants in both conditions experienced a decrease in depression corresponding to a moderate effect size [40].

Going forward, Wang *et al.* [41] describes the protocol of an ongoing RCT aimed towards relapse prevention of depression. This Chinese multi-centre trial will include 540 adults with MDD. The design involves an open-label flexible dose treatment of venlafaxine for 8 weeks (lead in) followed by 6 weeks (stabilization). Pharmacotherapy responders will be randomly assigned to rTMS, sham TMS or no TMS for a 12-month relapse prevention treatment [41]. Results from this study are not yet available, but will provide interesting insight into an innovative way to use TMS treatment as an augmentation of medication with the goal to maintain remission from MDD.

Approaches to enhance efficacy

Despite the significant advancements made in TMS research, the efficacy of the intervention when compared with sham remains modest. Several reasons have been proposed as potential obstacles to increasing the efficacy: infrequent use of bilateral stimulation, use of the 5-cm rule to identify the DLPFC, insufficient number of sessions to achieve the therapeutic effect and inadequate intensity [42]. However, research studies that examined these limitations refuted some of these hypotheses. For example, intensity does not appear to play a role in TMS response [43], although this parameter merits further study given the fact that intensity controls the degree of focality and spatial extent of stimulation. Furthermore, bilateral stimulation may not increase efficacy of rTMS. Slotema *et al.* [19] found right-sided LF-TMS to have the highest efficacy (d = 0.82), when compared with left-sided

HF-TMS ($d = 0.53$) or bilateral TMS ($d = 0.47$). In addition, recent meta-analyses found similar efficacy for right and left TMS [35] and for bilateral and unilateral TMS [44]. These findings strongly support that stimulation of the right, left or bilateral DLPFC leads to comparable results, with right DLPFC stimulation possibly having a slight advantage, as well as enhanced safety, given its lower seizure risk compared with high frequency.

The number of sessions, however, does seem to be an important parameter of efficacy. While a single session of HF-TMS was not found to alter mood [45], 3 weeks of daily sessions do lead to measurable benefit [29]. Adding maintenance rTMS sessions following the acute course led to a relapse rate of 38% by 20 weeks post-treatment, less than half the rate of relapse (82%) in participants who did not undergo maintenance treatment [46]. In the maintenance phase, participants were tapered as follows: three sessions in week 1, two sessions in weeks 2–3, one session in weeks 3–4, one session every other week in weeks 5–12 and one session per month in weeks 13–20 [46].

An additional parameter that supports for the impeding efficacy of rTMS treatments is the use of the 5-cm rule. Studies have shown that the 5-cm technique used in the Neurostar rTMS trial [3] frequently misses the DLPFC [47, 48], and studies employing imaging-guided rTMS have potential to significantly improve treatment efficacy [49].

Research findings have also determined several moderators that significantly affect response to rTMS. Meeting criteria for MDD with psychotic features, having long episodes of depression, having prefrontal atrophy (as in the case of geriatric depression, although see Lisanby *et al.* [4] for a contesting result), having failed several courses of treatment [50] and having high baseline anhedonia [51] may lead to reduced likelihood for a positive response. Moderators of a favourable response are: (a) early response to rTMS [52], (b) Val-Met polymorphism on the BDNF gene [53] and (c) preserved hedonic function [51].

Limited effectiveness may also relate to the fact that DLPFC rTMS addresses some, but not all, of the problems associated with depression. For example, despite the demonstrated changes in connectivity in brain networks with abnormal function, rTMS-treated subjects continue to show hypoconnectivity in the central executive network (CEN), an area involved in decision-making [54]. In addition, rTMS fails to downregulate the hypothalamic-pituitary-adrenocortical (HPA) system. Even after following a successful course of rTMS, the HPA system remains overactive [55]. Moreover, findings suggest that some subtypes of depression (i.e. with unaltered reward circuitry) may be more responsive to TMS than others (i.e. with disrupted reward circuitry) [51]. Taken together, these findings provide insight into some core problems for depression that may not be successfully addressed with DLPFC rTMS alone or that may contribute to relapse after rTMS. Therefore, to improve treatment efficacy, more research is needed to elucidate the mechanisms and identify the augmentation strategies (i.e. simultaneous cognitive behavioural therapy or pharmacotherapy).

Other promising directions

Future studies should further assess the effectiveness of stimulation in other populations and across the life cycle. For example, depression is also a serious problem for adolescents in need of more effective treatments. In a case series, Yang *et al.* [56] present data from six adolescents who received 3 weeks of HF-rTMS. Objective and subjective assessments of depression response supported the preliminary efficacy of rTMS in adolescents. This support adds to a recently completed review [57] that also supported the safety and efficacy of this treatment for depression in adolescents.

Regarding geriatric depression, early reports with TMS were negative [58]. It has been hypothesized that age-related anatomical atrophy (resulting in increased coil-to-cortex distance) may explain this. Computational modelling shows that brain atrophy significantly reduces the stimulated brain volume with TMS (Fig. 9.7 and see [59]). Nahas reported that brain activation response to TMS reduced with increasing coil-to-cortex distance [60]. There may also be age-related physiological changes affecting the ability to acquire TMS-induced plastic changes, as suggested by in vivo studies with TMS-induced LTP in aged rodents [61]. More recently Jorge *et al.* conducted a study of 92 medication-free patients with vascular depression with 10 Hz rTMS to the left DLPFC and found significant antidepressant effects with 1800 pulses per treatment course (while 1200 did not differ from sham) [62]. The response was negatively correlated with age and reduced frontal grey matter volume.

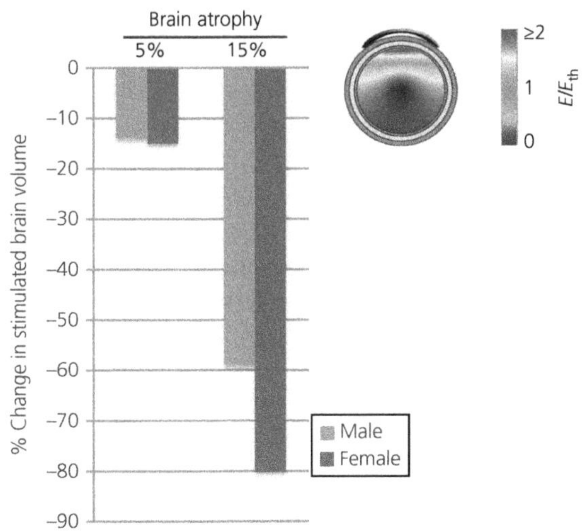

Figure 9.7 Impact of age-related atrophy on the volume of brain stimulated with TMS. Inset – Electric field relative to neuronal activation threshold from a simulation in a five concentric spherical model. Adapted from Deng *et al.* [59].

New directions for technology development include optimizing the targeting spatially (through innovations in coil design as exemplified by deep TMS, below), image guidance to inform targeting and combining TMS with psychotherapy as well as psychopharmacology in a target fashion.

Deep transcranial magnetic stimulation (dTMS)

The term deep TMS (dTMS) refers to the various attempts to optimize the depth of penetration through novel coil designs. dTMS has the potential to increase efficacy if therapeutic targets are too deep to be directly stimulated with conventional coils. While dTMS coils can penetrate more deeply, they remain subject to the same depth/focality trade-off that applies to all coils (Table 9.3). Specifically, the deeper the penetration, the less focal it will be [10]. In 2002, Roth, Zangen and Hallett [63] introduced the H-coil, designed for deeper and broader brain stimulation [64] than the conventional figure-8 coil used for rTMS. This novel approach began to gain growing support as an alternative treatment for depression, although limited research has been conducted thus far with direct comparison of dTMS with rTMS. Levkovitz *et al.* [65] administered 20 Hz of dTMS using the H-coil to the PFC (110 or 120% MT, 42s trains, 20s inter-train intervals,

Table 9.3 The depth/focality trade-off dictates that with non-invasive modalities, stimulation is focal and superficial, or deep and non-focal, but not focal and deep (unless an invasive surgical approach is used, as in the case of deep brain stimulation).

	Focal	Deep	Non-invasive
DBS	Yes	Yes	No
TMS	Yes	No	Yes
dTMS	No	Yes	Yes

1680 pulses, 15 min sessions) for 4 weeks to 65 treatment-resistant depressed patients. They tested three types of H-coils (H1, H2, H1-L) and two stimulation intensities and found a significant improvement in depression severity from pre- to post-treatment following high (120% MT) but not low (110% MT) stimulation. Clinical response was sustained at a 3-month follow-up. H1 and H1-L coils led to the highest remission rates (88% and 83%, respectively); the H2 coil resulted in a low remission rate (33%). No serious adverse events occurred during the study [65]. Their findings support a 120% MT stimulation intensity and the use of an H1 or H1-L coil.

Deng, Lisanby and Petrchev [66] discuss the benefits and disadvantages of several types of dTMS coils, including the H-coil and other coils for dTMS. They conclude that the double-cone coil is the most energy efficient and offers the best balance between stimulated volume and superficial field strength. They also introduced a novel coil design for dTMS, the Crown Coil, which can achieve deeper penetration than the H-coil. Low-field magnetic stimulation is another approach to dTMS using week oscillatory fields originally delivered during echoplanar imaging with fMRI, which is showing promise in early work [67].

Two additional studies in 2011 provided more support for dTMS for depression [68, 69]. Both studies assessed the effects of 20 dTMS stimulation sessions to the PFC (20 Hz) for 4 weeks. Isserles *et al.* [68] assessed the use of an H1 coil and the study included 4 weeks of weekly maintenance stimulation in addition to 4 weeks of acute stimulation. dTMS was administered as an add-on to antidepressants for 57 patients with major depression. By the end of the acute phase, 46% improved and 28% remitted from depression. Levkovitz *et al.* [69] studied the effects of acute dTMS administered to non-medicated depressed participants on apathy and depression. According to their findings, 30% of 54 adult participants scored in a non-clinical range on the HAM-D apathy subscale by the end of the study. In addition, baseline apathy was a moderator of treatment response for depression. Although the use of the same scale for both depression and apathy constructs is a limitation of this study that warrants replication, these results (similar to those of Downar *et al.* [51]) suggest that non-anhedonic/apathetic subtypes of depression may be more responsive to brain stimulation.

In 2013, the FDA approved dTMS (Brainsway H-Coil) as a safe and effective treatment for patients with treatment-resistant depression. Approval was based on a large-scale industry-sponsored trial conducted at 20 sites with 229 depressed patients (121 in sham and 108 in dTMS) who did not have any psychotic features and who had failed between one and four courses of medication or were intolerant to at least two antidepressants. The trial involved 4 weeks of acute treatment (daily sessions) and 12 weeks of maintenance treatment (twice-weekly sessions). Completer analyses (including 181 patients) found a remission rate of 33% in the active and 15% in the sham group. In addition, 38% improved but did not remit in the active condition when compared with sham-treated patients of whom 21% improved significantly. Results were maintained at a 16-week follow-up. The adverse events reported were significantly different in the active group when compared with the sham-stimulated group. These adverse effects were pain in the jaw (10% of cases) and discomfort and pain in the application site (19% and 25% of cases). More than 35% in both conditions reported headaches, and one seizure was reported (http://www.accessdata.fda.gov/cdrh_docs/pdf12/K122288.pdf). This trial is currently under peer review.

No additional RCTs could be found that examined the effects of dTMS; nevertheless, several other investigations provide important insight into the utility and mechanisms of dTMS. For example, recent data support dTMS as a safe and feasible maintenance treatment for 29 MDD patients following 4 weeks of acute rTMS [70]. Kaplan– Meier probability analyses suggested that 81% reported some improvements in depression and 71% remitted from depression after 18 weeks of maintenance dTMS. No adverse events were reported and the procedure was well tolerated [70]. An additional recent finding provides a potential moderator of dTMS treatment efficacy. In this study, higher baseline level of agreeableness and conscientiousness was correlated with treatment response and extraversion with remission from depression [71].

Several case reports point towards potential interesting future avenues for dTMS research. Vanneste, Ost, Langguth & De Rider [72] presented a case report of using a double-cone coil TMS (dccTMS) placed over the supplementary motor area aimed to target the ACC using HF stimulation (10 Hz, 2000 stimuli/session) for 10 sessions. They found a significant reduction in depression (27% on the BDI-II; 40% on HADS-depression) and anxiety (33% on HADS-anxiety). They also found changes in the resting state function of the ACC in comparison to a matched normative control group [72]. Other case reports examine the use of dTMS in other subtypes of depression. For example, Bersani *et al.* [73] examined a case of treatment-resistant bipolar depression treated with dTMS. Treatment included 20 daily consecutive sessions and six bi-weekly maintenance sessions. They found significant improvements in depression severity, a response that was maintained at 6 months. Another example is a series of three case studies where dysthymia and comorbid alcohol dependence were targeted in a residential setting via augmenting pharmacotherapy with dTMS (20 min HF sessions for 28 days) [74]. A significant response (that led to reduction in the psychotropic medication administered) could be seen after 10 dTMS sessions [74]. Harvey *et al.* [75] also targeted comorbidity in a case report. In one female patient with treatment-resistant depression, a standard course of dTMS resulted in a 46% reduction in both depression and anxiety severity after 4 weeks of acute treatment, gains that were maintained 1 month later. Increased cognitive performance following treatment was also noted [75]. Taken together, these findings support promising new avenues of investigation, especially in the area of comorbid disorders, which may increase the severity of the clinical presentation of those who have treatment-resistant depression.

Safety

Several studies support that TMS is a safe treatment for treatment-resistant depression with few side effects. Thus far, two meta-analyses have focused on safety findings. Machii and colleagues [76] reviewed studies where rTMS was applied in non-motor areas. They found across studies that the most common side effect was headaches, which occurred in about 23% of all patients included. More recent studies confirm this result. Serious side effects are rare; more frequently, rTMS leads to minor side effects such as headaches, local pain, neck pain, discomfort during stimulation or transient hearing changes can occur [15].

There are concerns with brain stimulation about the potential of seizures. In the meta-analysis cited above [76], there were two reports of seizures, and both occurred when high-frequency (higher than 10 Hz) rTMS was utilized. A different meta-analysis [77] did not report any seizures. Thus, rTMS frequencies above 10 Hz may increase the risk for seizures. Nevertheless, a recent pilot study has shown that a single short, low-intensity burst of rTMS at 50 Hz is safe and does not lead to seizures [78]. For dTMS, the trial that led to FDA approval reported one seizure. According to the report, the seizure occurred in one subject who drank a bottle of wine the night before stimulation. Therefore, caution is warranted in administering dTMS after drinking binges.

Additional side effects to be considered when using this treatment are hearing loss, manic and psychotic symptoms and vasodepressor syncope [29, 76, 79]. For example, left side rTMS led to induced psychotic symptoms in four cases [76]. It is important to highlight that unlike ECT, rTMS treatment does not lead to neurocognitive or memory impairments and may even lead to improvements in neurocognitive functioning [65, 75].

Method of motor threshold assessment

A key driver of safety is intensity relative to motor threshold (MT). Therefore, the accuracy of the MT is paramount. The Neuronetics trial for rTMS [3] led to FDA approval of stimulating the DLPFC at the intensity of 100% of the determined MT. In the supporting trial, MTs were determined using consistent visual confirmation of activity in a target resting muscle [80]. A different approach is using electromyography (EMG) to identify the lowest threshold of intensity for which muscle activity can be determined [81]. To clarify whether both methods are comparable in the resultant intensity of stimulation, Westin *et al.* [82] compared both methods in 20 healthy subjects. Visually established MTs tended to be on average 11.3% higher (range: 0–27.8) than EMG MTs. There are several concerns therefore with using visually established MTs: (1) more than 50% of subjects may be given doses that are above the safety parameters, (2) they may cause more discomfort, (3) they interfere with standardization and render the established parameters of safety unclear and (4) they may reduce the focality of stimulation and therefore lead to less efficacy of the treatment. Therefore, the authors urge researchers and clinicians to consistently use EMG in determining the MTs [82].

Mechanisms of antidepressant action

Recently, there have been significant research efforts aimed towards a better understanding the mechanisms of action behind rTMS. A number of patho-aetiological mechanisms have been proposed to underlie depression, including disordered neurochemistry and the functioning of distributed networks of cortico-limbic regions. Psychopharmacology has been designed to target neurotransmitter systems implicated in depression with considerable success, but systemically administered medications are not regionally specific. Focal neuromodulation has the unique ability to target brain regions involved in depression and as such adds a degree of spatial specificity, which is not possible with systemic application of pharmacotherapy. This feature lends itself well to an experimental medicine approach to inform treatment development by several possible approaches, such as directly engaging targets for focal induction of plasticity, restoration of connectivity in specific circuits and focal modulation of oscillatory actions.

Plasticity

Recent work with TMS using the paired associative stimulation (PAS) paradigm provides new support for the hypothesized deficit in plasticity in depression [83]. Therefore, it is appealing to use TMS as a tool to restore plasticity in a focal fashion. Indeed, unlike implanted stimulators, transcranially applied magnetic fields are administered intermittently; thus for clinical benefit to be realized, they must exert a lasting change in cortical activity that outlives the period of direct stimulation. The mechanism by which repeated stimulation induces lasting change in cortical function is considered to be a form of plasticity, which has been likened to LTP and LTD [84].

Several studies suggest that 1 Hz rTMS exerts inhibitory effects on cortical excitability that persist beyond the end of the stimulation train, although there is considerable inter-individual variation in this effect. Recent work with controllable pulse TMS (cTMS) suggests that the inhibitory effects of 1 Hz can be deepened and prolonged through the use of more optimized pulse waveform and the use of predominantly unidirectional pulse trains [85–87]. In addition, continuous theta burst (cTBS) has been reported to deepen the inhibitory effects [88]. The TBS technology was built upon findings regarding burst patterns of stimulation that are more effective in inducing LTP and LTD in animal models. These burst patterns are more effective at creating long-lasting plasticity changes of the targeted circuit. Plewnia *et al.* [89] conducted a preliminary RCT for assessing the feasibility and preliminary efficacy of 6 weeks (30 sessions) of bilateral TBS when compared with sham stimulation of the DLPFC in 32 patients with MDD. The stimulation parameters were 80% of the MT, two trains of 600 pulses applied in bursts of three stimuli at 50Hz given every 200 ms, intermittent stimulation on the left side (2s train, 8s inter-train interval) and continuous stimulation on the right for 40s. All participants were taking antidepressant medication. The study found twice as many responders in the active condition (OR =3.86) and a higher likelihood for remission (OR = 9) as compared to sham. These findings warrant further investigations for TBS stimulation as a treatment for depression. cTMS coupled with cTBS could be even more potent.

As reviewed by Hoogendam [84], there are several lines of evidence supporting the view that TMS-induced alterations in cortical excitability reflect changes in neuroplasticity: (i) effects outlast the period of stimulation, (ii) the temporal pattern of pulses is important, with low frequencies typically inducing LTD-like effects and high frequencies typically inducing LTP-like effects, (iii) changes in excitability depend on the history of activation, (iv) rTMS interacts with learning, (v) there is supporting evidence of synaptic plasticity changes in animal studies, (vi) pharmacological challenge studies have been supportive and (vii) BDNF polymorphism affects the effects of rTMS. Interestingly, Val-Met polymorphism on the BDNF gene has been reported to be a moderator of TMS antidepressant response [53]. Furthermore, Fidalgo *et al.* [55] reviewed biological markers relevant to rTMS, and based on 52 articles, including more than 1200 patients, they found that brain-derived neurotropic factor (BDNF) had the greatest support as a biomarker of depression and of treatment success.

Numerical modelling of the plasticity induced by different doses of rTMS stimulation may inform optimization of the paradigm. For example, Wilson *et al.* [90] presented a theoretical model of long-tem plasticity based on neural field theory and included a discussion of how modelling can be used to optimize parameters of rTMS. According to the authors, modelling has the advantage of exploring the effects of using parameters of stimulation that would not be within current safety guidelines without causing any harm to human subjects. Therefore, modelling can offer an elegant way to integrate findings about the behaviour of neuronal populations and brain circuitry and to determine optimal parameters of stimulation. There is also a role for preclinical studies in animals to validate these models, especially in light of new developments enabling single unit recording during TMS in awake-behaving primates [91].

Connectivity

Given the evidence for hypoactivity and hyperactivity of key cortical structures in depression (notably lateral prefrontal cortex and rostral cingulate, respectively), TMS has been targeted to those superficial cortical regions that are readily accessible from the scalp (namely, dorsolateral prefrontal cortex, DLPFC). Recent work has examined connectivity from DLPFC to other regions implicated in antidepressant response to TMS. Fox and colleagues [92] conducted a secondary data analysis of resting state functional connectivity in healthy and depressed subjects. They showed that regions of the DLPFC connected with the subgenual cingulate (sgACC) were most sensitive to the therapeutic effects of rTMS. Others have also shown stronger connectivity between sgACC and the prefrontal cortex in participants who remit from depression following a course of rTMS [93]. Hence, one of the mechanisms though which rTMS has antidepressant effects is the strengthening of the DLPFC-sgACC connection. In line with these findings, Fox *et al.* [92] proposed using connectivity analyses to establish coordinates in the left DLPFC that could be used to optimize rTMS targeting and, subsequently, to maximize treatment efficacy [92]. They also showed significant individual differences in identifying the exact area of the DLPFC that was most strongly connected to the sgACC, which strongly supported individualized, image-guided targeting of rTMS treatment for optimal engagement of this mechanism of action [49].

With regard to the networks involved, Liston *et al.* [54] examined two neuronal-networks with known abnormalities in depression and with likely response to rTMS, the CEN and the default-mode network (DMN). The CEN includes the DLPFC and lateral areas of the posterior parietal cortex (PPC) [54] and has been found to be hypoactive in depression [94, 95]. The DMN, including areas from the medial prefrontal cortex (mPFC), posterior cingulate, and medial areas of the PPC, has been implicated in maladaptive depressive behaviours such as rumination or faulty episodic memory retrieval [96, 97]. Using resting state functional connectivity fMRI analyses, the authors [54] tested 17 depressed and 35 healthy subjects before and after a 5-week course of HF-rTMS. Before treatment, abnormal connectivity was identified in depressed subjects (i.e. hyperconnectivity in the DMN and hypoconnectivity in the CEN). Post-treatment, improvements in depression were found across subjects corresponding to a large effect size ($d_{\text{pre-post}} = 1.32$). HF-rTMS treatment normalized the interconnectivity between CEN and DMN and attenuated the hyperconnectivity in the DMN (more precisely, in the sgACC). The strength of hyperconnectivity of the sgACC at baseline was a robust predictor of rTMS treatment response [54].

Neural oscillations

In addition to being spatially focal, TMS is temporally precise. This enables tuning of the stimulation to match or modulate endogenous neural oscillatory activity. Leuchter, Cook, Jin and Phillips [98] proposed that changes in thalamocortical oscillations induced by rTMS may be a more accurate description of the mechanism through which therapeutic effects for depression are achieved. Considering MDD as a connectivity problem, the authors suggested that the effectiveness of rTMS comes from strengthening connections within the networks that are affected by depression. Based on this theory, they proposed several ways to optimize rTMS in order to improve its efficacy for depression, including synchronizing the stimulation with the individual's alpha frequency and changing the waveform of the induced current in order to maximize the network effect of the stimulation [98]. Synchronized TMS (sTMS) has been evaluated in a randomized controlled trial, the results of which are currently under peer review.

Studying oscillatory phenomena during sleep may also be informative. Pellicciari *et al.* [99] showed that bilateral rTMS over the DLPFC induced significant decrease in alpha activity as measured by EEG over the left DLPFC during REM sleep. This change was strongly correlated with the decrease in depressive symptoms as measured by the HAM-D ($r = 0.74$). Therefore, alpha frequency reduction might be useful as a cortical marker of treatment response [99].

Magnetic seizure therapy (MST) for depression

The observation that ECT-induced seizures are so powerfully and rapidly effective for a broad range of severe psychiatric and neurological disorders is compelling. ECT has been reported to induce a wide variety of neuroplastic actions, including effects on gene transcription, induction of molecules relevant to plasticity and neuroplastic effects (Fig. 9.8). Which of these myriad neuroplastic effects are necessary and sufficient for antidepressant response is not known.

It has been hypothesized that the induction of plasticity underlies the superior therapeutic benefit of seizures, and that maladaptive plasticity in key brain structures subserving cognition is also responsible for the adverse cognitive side effects. Evidence suggests that there is regional specificity in the role of plasticity induction. For example, BDNF induction in the dorsal dentate was found to be not essential to antidepressant action of ECT in a rodent model, while BDNF reduction in the VTA was essential to antidepressant action [100].

The goal of MST is to target seizure induction in a focal fashion to achieve an uncoupling of the efficacy from the side effects, focusing the effects on regions and actions key to antidepressant response and sparing regions related to side effects. Specifically, avoiding unnecessary tetanic electrical stimulation of the hippocampus may avoid saturation of LTP seen with ECT, which is hypothesized to contribute to ECT-induced amnesia [101, 2].

We have published in vivo measurements and computational modelling supporting the superior focality of MST relative to ECT both in terms of E-field exposure in the brain and the degree of seizure generalization [11, 9, 13, 14, 59]. Non-human primate models provide support for the superior cognitive outcomes with MST relative to ECT [102–104]. MST has been shown to have a relatively benign cognitive side effect profile relative to ECT [105, 106].

We have also seen significant reductions in cognitive impairment in patients receiving MST in head-to-head blinded comparison with ultrabrief right unilateral ECT [7].

Evidence for antidepressant efficacy with MST has been mounting. Randomized comparison of ECT versus MST has shown similar efficacy, but with superior cognitive outcomes with MST [107]. Future research needs include methods to prevent relapse following acute response, and exploration of indications beyond depression, into other conditions where ECT shows therapeutic benefit.

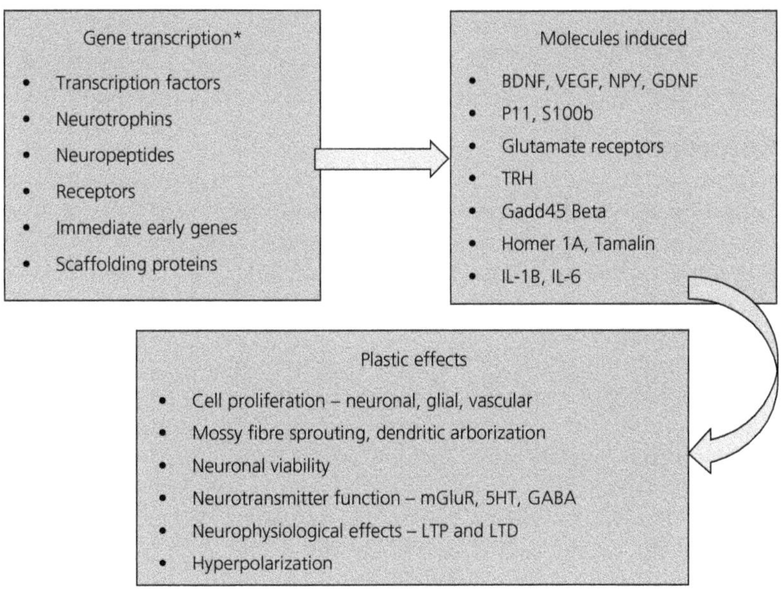

Figure 9.8 Reported neuroplastic actions of ECT. *Greater than 120 genes reported.

Conclusions

TMS induces tetanic trains of induced electrical pulses in the brain in a far more focal fashion than is possible with ECT, and TMS does so without inducing seizure. That TMS has the evidence of antidepressant efficacy tells us that indeed the repeated application of electrical pulses in the absence of a seizure can have therapeutic benefit.

MST induces a generalized seizure, but it does so without exposing deep brain structures to strong electric fields. The fact that MST has a superior neurocognitive profile to ECT suggests that the E-field exposure, rather than seizure induction, is a potential cause of ECT-induced amnesia.

Whether one uses magnetic fields to induce repetitive trains of pulses that induce plasticity, or whether one uses these pulses to trigger a seizure that itself induces plasticity, it is the induction of lasting neuroplastic changes in the brain that is thought to underlie the antidepressant efficacy of magnetic stimulation.

Future research is needed to elucidate the underlying mechanisms and to determine how best to combine TMS and MST with medications and psychotherapy to optimize acute and long-term outcomes.

References

1 Lisanby S, Maddox J, Prudic J, Devanand D, Sackeim H. The effects of electroconvulsive therapy on memory of autobiographical and public events. Archives of General Psychiatry. 2000;57(6):581–90.

2 McClintock SM, Choi J, Deng ZD, Appelbaum LG, Krystal AD, Lisanby SH. Multifactorial determinants of the neurocognitive effects of electroconvulsive therapy. The Journal of ECT. 2014;30(2):165–76.

3 O'Reardon JP, Solvason HB, Janicak PG, Sampson S, Isenberg KE, Nahas Z, *et al.* Efficacy and safety of transcranial magnetic stimulation in the acute treatment of major depression: a multisite randomized controlled trial. Biological Psychiatry. 2007;62(11):1208–16.

4 Lisanby SH, Husain MM, Rosenquist PB, Maixner D, Gutierrez R, Krystal A, *et al.* Daily left prefrontal repetitive transcranial magnetic stimulation in the acute treatment of major depression: clinical predictors of outcome in a multisite, randomized controlled clinical trial. Neuropsychopharmacology. 2009;34(2):522–34.

5 Deng ZD, Peterchev AV, Lisanby SH. Coil design considerations for deep-brain transcranial magnetic stimulation (dTMS). Conf Proc IEEE Eng Med Biol Soc 2008;2008:5675–9.

6 Lisanby S, Luber B, Finck A, Schroeder C, Sackeim H. Deliberate seizure induction with repetitive transcranial magnetic stimulation in nonhuman primates. Archives of General Psychiatry. 2001;58(2):199–200.

7 Lisanby S, Luber B, Schlaepfer T, Sackeim H. Safety and feasibility of magnetic seizure therapy (MST) in major depression: randomized within-subject comparison with electroconvulsive therapy. Neuropsychopharmacology. 2003;28(10):1852–65.

8 Lisanby S, Schlaepfer T, Fisch H, Sackeim H. Magnetic seizure therapy of major depression. Archives of General Psychiatry. 2001;58(3):303–5.

9 Deng Z-D, Lisanby SH, Peterchev AV. Electric field strength and focality in electroconvulsive therapy and magnetic seizure therapy: a finite element simulation study. Journal of Neural Engineering. 2011;8(1):016007.

10 Deng Z-D, Lisanby SH, Peterchev AV. Electric field depth-focality tradeoff in transcranial magnetic stimulation: simulation comparison of 50 coil designs. Brain Stimulation. 2013;6(1):1–13.

11 Lisanby SH, Moscrip TD, Morales O, Luber B, Schroeder C, Sackeim HA. Neurophysiological characterization of magnetic seizure therapy (MST) in non-human primates. Supplements to Clinical Neurophysiology. 2003;56:81–99.

12 Lee WH, Deng ZD, Kim TS, Laine AF, Lisanby SH, Peterchev AV. Regional electric field induced by electroconvulsive therapy in a realistic finite element head model: influence of white matter anisotropic conductivity. NeuroImage. 2012;59(3):2110–23.

13 Cycowicz YM, Luber B, Spellman T, Lisanby SH. Neurophysiological characterization of high-dose magnetic seizure therapy: comparisons with electroconvulsive shock and cognitive outcomes. The Journal of ECT. 2009;25(3): 157–64.
14 Cycowicz YM, Luber B, Spellman T, Lisanby SH. Differential neurophysiological effects of magnetic seizure therapy (MST) and electroconvulsive shock (ECS) in non-human primates. Clinical EEG and Neuroscience. 2008;39(3): 144–9.
15 Rossi S, Hallett M, Rossini PM, Pascual-Leone A. Safety, ethical considerations, and application guidelines for the use of transcranial magnetic stimulation in clinical practice and research. Clinical Neurophysiology. 2009;120(12):2008–39.
16 Gomez L, Morales L, Trapaga O, Zaldivar M, Sanchez A, Padilla E, *et al.* Seizure induced by sub-threshold 10-Hz rTMS in a patient with multiple risk factors. Clinical Neurophysiology. 2011;122(5):1057–8.
17 Barker AT, Jalinous R, Freeston IL. Non-invasive magnetic stimulation of human motor cortex. Lancet. 1985;1(8437):1106–7.
18 Gross M, Nakamura L, Pascual-Leone A, Fregni F. Has repetitive transcranial magnetic stimulation (rTMS) treatment for depression improved? A systematic review and meta-analysis comparing the recent vs. the earlier rTMS studies. Acta Psychiatrica Scandinavica. 2007;116(3):165–73.
19 Slotema CW, Blom JD, Hoek HW, Sommer IE. Should we expand the toolbox of psychiatric treatment methods to include Repetitive Transcranial Magnetic Stimulation (rTMS)? A meta-analysis of the efficacy of rTMS in psychiatric disorders. The Journal of Clinical Psychiatry. 2010;71(7):873–84.
20 George MS, Wassermann EM, Williams WA, Callahan A, Ketter TA, Basser P, *et al.* Daily repetitive transcranial magnetic stimulation (rTMS) improves mood in depression. Neuroreport. 1995; 6(14):1853–6.
21 Solvason HB, Husain M, Fitzgerald PB, Rosenquist P, McCall WV, Kimball J, *et al.* Improvement in quality of life with left prefrontal transcranial magnetic stimulation in patients with pharmacoresistant major depression: acute and six month outcomes. Brain Stimulation. 2014;7(2):219–25.
22 George MS, Lisanby SH, Avery D, McDonald WM, Durkalski V, Pavlicova M, *et al.* Daily left prefrontal transcranial magnetic stimulation therapy for major depressive disorder: a sham-controlled randomized trial. Archives of General Psychiatry. 2010;67(5):507–16.
23 McDonald WM, Durkalski V, Ball ER, Holtzheimer PE, Pavlicova M, Lisanby SH, *et al.* Improving the antidepressant efficacy of transcranial magnetic stimulation: maximizing the number of stimulations and treatment location in treatment-resistant depression. Depression and Anxiety. 2011;28(11):973–80.
24 Mantovani A, Pavlicova M, Avery D, Nahas Z, McDonald WM, Wajdik CD, *et al.* Long-term efficacy of repeated daily prefrontal transcranial magnetic stimulation (TMS) in treatment-resistant depression. Depression and Anxiety. 2012;29(10):883–90.
25 Lam RW, Chan P, Wilkins-Ho M, Yatham LN. Repetitive transcranial magnetic stimulation for treatment-resistant depression: a systematic review and metaanalysis. Canadian Journal of Psychiatry. 2008;53(9):621–31.
26 Carpenter LL, Janicak PG, Aaronson ST, Boyadjis T, Brock DG, Cook IA, *et al.* Transcranial magnetic stimulation (TMS) for major depression: a multisite, naturalistic, observational study of acute treatment outcomes in clinical practice. Depression and Anxiety. 2012;29(7): 587–96.
27 Janicak PG, Dunner DL, Aaronson ST, Carpenter LL, Boyadjis TA, Brock DG, *et al.* Transcranial magnetic stimulation (TMS) for major depression: a multisite, naturalistic, observational study of quality of life outcome measures in clinical practice. CNS Spectrums. 2013;18(6): 322–32.
28 Connolly KR, Helmer A, Cristancho MA, Cristancho P, O'Reardon JP. Effectiveness of transcranial magnetic stimulation in clinical practice post-FDA approval in the United States: results observed with the first 100 consecutive cases of depression at an academic medical center. The Journal of Clinical Psychiatry. 2012;73(4):e567–73.
29 Dell'osso B, Camuri G, Castellano F, Vecchi V, Benedetti M, Bortolussi S, *et al.* Meta-review of metaanalytic studies with repetitive transcranial magnetic stimulation (rTMS) for the

treatment of major depression. Clinical Practice and Epidemiology in Mental Health. 2011;7: 167–77.

30 Schutter DJ. Quantitative review of the efficacy of slow-frequency magnetic brain stimulation in major depressive disorder. Psychological Medicine. 2010;40(11):1789–95.

31 Berlim MT, van den Eynde F, Tovar-Perdomo S, Daskalakis ZJ. Response, remission and drop-out rates following high-frequency repetitive transcranial magnetic stimulation (rTMS) for treating major depression: a systematic review and meta-analysis of randomized, double-blind and sham-controlled trials. Psychological Medicine. 2014;44(2):225–39.

32 Ren J, Li H, Palaniyappan L, Liu H, Wang J, Li C, *et al.* Repetitive transcranial magnetic stimulation versus electroconvulsive therapy for major depression: a systematic review and meta-analysis. Progress in Neuro-Psychopharmacology & Biological Psychiatry. 2014;51:181–9.

33 Lepping P, Schonfeldt-Lecuona C, Sambhi RS, Lanka SV, Lane S, Whittington R, *et al.* A systematic review of the clinical relevance of repetitive transcranial magnetic stimulation. Acta Psychiatrica Scandinavica. 2014;130:341.

34 Berlim MT, Van den Eynde F, Daskalakis ZJ. High-frequency repetitive transcranial magnetic stimulation accelerates and enhances the clinical response to antidepressants in major depression: a meta-analysis of randomized, double-blind, and sham-controlled trials. The Journal of Clinical Psychiatry. 2013;74(2): e122–9.

35 Chen J, Zhou C, Wu B, Wang Y, Li Q, Wei Y, *et al.* Left versus right repetitive transcranial magnetic stimulation in treating major depression: a meta-analysis of randomised controlled trials. Psychiatry Research. 2013;210(3):1260–4.

36 Berlim MT, Van den Eynde F, Daskalakis ZJ. Clinically meaningful efficacy and acceptability of low-frequency repetitive transcranial magnetic stimulation (rTMS) for treating primary major depression: a meta-analysis of randomized, double-blind and sham-controlled trials. Neuropsychopharmacology. 2013;38(4):543–51.

37 George MS, Raman R, Benedek DM, Pelic CG, Grammer GG, Stokes KT, *et al.* A two-site pilot randomized 3 day trial of high dose left prefrontal repetitive transcranial magnetic stimulation (rTMS) for suicidal inpatients. Brain Stimulation. 2014;7(3):421–31.

38 Krstic J, Buzadzic I, Milanovic SD, Ilic NV, Pajic S, Ilic TV. Low-frequency repetitive transcranial magnetic stimulation in the right prefrontal cortex combined with partial sleep deprivation in treatment-resistant depression: a randomized sham-controlled trial. The Journal of ECT. 2014;30:325–31.

39 Speer AM, Wassermann EM, Benson BE, Herscovitch P, Post RM. Antidepressant efficacy of high and low frequency rTMS at 110% of motor threshold versus sham stimulation over left prefrontal cortex. Brain Stimulation. 2014; 7(1):36–41.

40 Trojak B, Meille V, Jonval L, Schuffenecker N, Haffen E, Schwan R, *et al.* Interest of targeting either cortical area Brodmann 9 or 46 in rTMS treatment for depression: a preliminary randomized study. Clinical Neurophysiology. 2014; 125:2384–9.

41 Wang H, Xue Y, Chen Y, Zhang R, Wang H, Zhang Y, *et al.* Efficacy of repetitive transcranial magnetic stimulation in the prevention of relapse of depression: study protocol for a randomized controlled trial. Trials. 2013;14:338.

42 Daskalakis ZJ, Levinson AJ, Fitzgerald PB. Repetitive transcranial magnetic stimulation for major depressive disorder: a review. Canadian Journal of Psychiatry. 2008;53(9):555–66.

43 Schutter DJ. Antidepressant efficacy of high-frequency transcranial magnetic stimulation over the left dorsolateral prefrontal cortex in double-blind sham-controlled designs: a meta-analysis. Psychological Medicine. 2009;39(1): 65–75.

44 Chen C, Bian J, Zhang W, Zhang W, Zhao C, Wei H. Unilateral versus bilateral vertebroplasty for severe osteoporotic vertebral compression fractures. Journal of Spinal Disorders & Techniques. 2014;27:E301–4.

45 Dang T, Avery DH, Russo J. Within-session mood changes from TMS in depressed patients. The Journal of Neuropsychiatry and Clinical Neurosciences. 2007;19(4):458–63.

46 Richieri R, Guedj E, Michel P, Loundou A, Auquier P, Lancon C, *et al.* Maintenance transcranial magnetic stimulation reduces depression relapse: a propensity-adjusted analysis. Journal of Affective Disorders. 2013;151(1):129–35.

47 Herwig U, Padberg F, Unger J, Spitzer M, Schonfeldt-Lecuona C. Transcranial magnetic stimulation in therapy studies: examination of the reliability of 'standard' coil positioning by neuronavigation. Biological Psychiatry. 2001; 50(1):58–61.
48 Ahdab R, Ayache SS, Brugieres P, Goujon C, Lefaucheur JP. Comparison of 'standard' and 'navigated' procedures of TMS coil positioning over motor, premotor and prefrontal targets in patients with chronic pain and depression. Clinical Neurophysiology. 2010; 40(1):27–36.
49 Fox MD, Liu H, Pascual-Leone A. Identification of reproducible individualized targets for treatment of depression with TMS based on intrinsic connectivity. NeuroImage. 2012;66C: 151–60.
50 Mitchell PB, Loo CK. Transcranial magnetic stimulation for depression. The Australian and New Zealand Journal of Psychiatry. 2006;40(5): 406–13.
51 Downar J, Geraci J, Salomons TV, Dunlop K, Wheeler S, McAndrews MP, *et al.* Anhedonia and reward-circuit connectivity distinguish nonresponders from responders to dorsomedial prefrontal repetitive transcranial magnetic stimulation in major depression. Biological Psychiatry. 2013; 76:176–85.
52 Gershon AA, Dannon PN, Grunhaus L. Transcranial magnetic stimulation in the treatment of depression. The American Journal of Psychiatry. 2003;160(5):835–45.
53 Cheeran B, Talelli P, Mori F, Koch G, Suppa A, Edwards M, *et al.* A common polymorphism in the brain-derived neurotrophic factor gene (BDNF) modulates human cortical plasticity and the response to rTMS. The Journal of Physiology. 2008;586(Pt 23):5717–25.
54 Liston C, Chen AC, Zebley BD, Drysdale AT, Gordon R, Leuchter B, *et al.* Default mode network mechanisms of transcranial magnetic stimulation in depression. Biological Psychiatry. 2014;76:517–26.
55 Fidalgo TM, Morales-Quezada JL, Muzy GS, Chiavetta NM, Mendonca ME, Santana MV, *et al.* Biological markers in noninvasive brain stimulation trials in major depressive disorder: a systematic review. The Journal of ECT. 2014; 30(1):47–61.
56 Yang XR, Kirton A, Wilkes TC, Pradhan S, Liu I, Jaworska N, *et al.* Glutamate alterations associated with transcranial magnetic stimulation in youth depression: a case series. The Journal of ECT. 2014;30:242–7.
57 Donaldson AE, Gordon MS, Melvin GA, Barton DA, Fitzgerald PB. Addressing the needs of adolescents with treatment resistant depressive disorders: a systematic review of rTMS. Brain Stimulation. 2014;7(1):7–12.
58 Figiel GS, Epstein C, McDonald WM, Amazon-Leece J, Figiel L, Saldivia A, *et al.* The use of rapid-rate transcranial magnetic stimulation (rTMS) in refractory depressed patients. The Journal of Neuropsychiatry and Clinical Neurosciences. 1998;10(1):20–5.
59 Deng ZD, Lisanby SH, Peterchev AV. Effect of anatomical variability on neural stimulation strength and focality in electroconvulsive therapy (ECT) and magnetic seizure therapy (MST). Conference proceedings: ... Annual International Conference of the IEEE Engineering in Medicine and Biology Society. 2009; 2009:682–8.
60 Nahas Z, Teneback CC, Kozel A, Speer AM, DeBrux C, Molloy M, *et al.* Brain effects of TMS delivered over prefrontal cortex in depressed adults: role of stimulation frequency and coil-cortex distance. The Journal of Neuropsychiatry and Clinical Neurosciences. 2001;13(4):459–70.
61 Levkovitz Y, Segal M. Aging affects transcranial magnetic modulation of hippocampal evoked potentials. Neurobiology of Aging. 2001;22(2): 255–63.
62 Jorge RE, Moser DJ, Acion L, Robinson RG. Treatment of vascular depression using repetitive transcranial magnetic stimulation. Archives of General Psychiatry. 2008;65(3):268–76.
63 Roth Y, Zangen A, Hallett M. A coil design for transcranial magnetic stimulation of deep brain regions. Journal of Clinical Neurophysiology. 2002;19(4):361–70.
64 Roth Y, Amir A, Levkovitz Y, Zangen A. Three-dimensional distribution of the electric field induced in the brain by transcranial magnetic stimulation using figure-8 and deep H-coils. Journal of Clinical Neurophysiology. 2007; 24(1):31–8.
65 Levkovitz Y, Harel EV, Roth Y, Braw Y, Most D, Katz LN, *et al.* Deep transcranial magnetic

stimulation over the prefrontal cortex: evaluation of antidepressant and cognitive effects in depressive patients. Brain Stimulation. 2009;2(4):188–200.

66 Deng ZD, Lisanby SH, Peterchev AV. Coil design considerations for deep transcranial magnetic stimulation. Clinical Neurophysiology. 2014;125(6):1202–12.

67 Rohan ML, Yamamoto RT, Ravichandran CT, Cayetano KR, Morales OG, Olson DP, *et al.* Rapid mood-elevating effects of low field magnetic stimulation in depression. Biological Psychiatry. 2014;76:186–93.

68 Isserles M, Rosenberg O, Dannon P, Levkovitz Y, Kotler M, Deutsch F, *et al.* Cognitive-emotional reactivation during deep transcranial magnetic stimulation over the prefrontal cortex of depressive patients affects antidepressant outcome. Journal of Affective Disorders. 2011;128(3):235–42.

69 Levkovitz Y, Sheer A, Harel EV, Katz LN, Most D, Zangen A, *et al.* Differential effects of deep TMS of the prefrontal cortex on apathy and depression. Brain Stimulation. 2011;4(4):266–74.

70 Harel EV, Rabany L, Deutsch L, Bloch Y, Zangen A, Levkovitz Y. H-coil repetitive transcranial magnetic stimulation for treatment resistant major depressive disorder: an 18-week continuation safety and feasibility study. The World Journal of Biological Psychiatry. 2014;15(4):298–306.

71 McGirr A, Van den Eynde F, Chachamovich E, Fleck MP, Berlim MT. Personality dimensions and deep repetitive transcranial magnetic stimulation (DTMS) for treatment-resistant depression: a pilot trial on five-factor prediction of antidepressant response. Neuroscience Letters. 2014;563:144–8.

72 Vanneste S, Ost J, Langguth B, De Ridder D. TMS by double-cone coil prefrontal stimulation for medication resistant chronic depression: a case report. Neurocase. 2014;20(1):61–8.

73 Bersani FS, Girardi N, Sanna L, Mazzarini L, Santucci C, Kotzalidis GD, *et al.* Deep transcranial magnetic stimulation for treatment-resistant bipolar depression: a case report of acute and maintenance efficacy. Neurocase. 2013;19(5):451–7.

74 Rapinesi C, Kotzalidis GD, Serata D, Del Casale A, Bersani FS, Solfanelli A, *et al.* Efficacy of add-on deep transcranial magnetic stimulation in comorbid alcohol dependence and dysthymic disorder: three case reports. The Primary Care Companion to CNS Disorders. 2013;15(1):pii:PCC.12m01438.

75 Harvey PO, Van den Eynde F, Zangen A, Berlim MT. Neural correlates of clinical improvement after deep transcranial magnetic stimulation (DTMS) for treatment-resistant depression: a case report using functional magnetic resonance imaging. Neurocase. 2015;21:16–22.

76 Machii K, Cohen D, Ramos-Estebanez C, Pascual-Leone A. Safety of rTMS to non-motor cortical areas in healthy participants and patients. Clinical Neurophysiology. 2006;117(2):455–71.

77 Janicak PG, O'Reardon JP, Sampson SM, Husain MM, Lisanby SH, Rado JT, *et al.* Transcranial magnetic stimulation in the treatment of major depressive disorder: a comprehensive summary of safety experience from acute exposure, extended exposure, and during reintroduction treatment. The Journal of Clinical Psychiatry. 2008;69(2):222–32.

78 Huang YZ, Rothwell JC. The effect of short-duration bursts of high-frequency, low-intensity transcranial magnetic stimulation on the human motor cortex. Clinical Neurophysiology. 2004;115(5):1069–75.

79 Sakkas P, Mihalopoulou P, Mourtzouhou P, Psarros C, Masdrakis V, Politis A, *et al.* Induction of mania by rTMS: report of two cases. European Psychiatry. 2003;18(4):196–8.

80 Pridmore S, Fernandes Filho JA, Nahas Z, Liberatos C, George MS. Motor threshold in transcranial magnetic stimulation: a comparison of a neurophysiological method and a visualization of movement method. The Journal of ECT. 1998;14(1):25–7.

81 Rossini PM, Barker AT, Berardelli A, Caramia MD, Caruso G, Cracco RQ, *et al.* Non-invasive electrical and magnetic stimulation of the brain, spinal cord and roots: basic principles and procedures for routine clinical application. Report of an IFCN committee. Electroencephalography and Clinical Neurophysiology. 1994;91(2):79–92.

82 Westin GG, Bassi BD, Lisanby SH, Luber B, New York State Psychiatric Institute NU. Determination of motor threshold using visual observation overestimates transcranial magnetic

stimulation dosage: safety implications. Clinical Neurophysiology. 2014;125(1):142–7.
83 Player MJ, Taylor JL, Weickert CS, Alonzo A, Sachdev P, Martin D, *et al.* Neuroplasticity in depressed individuals compared with healthy controls. Neuropsychopharmacology. 2013;38(11): 2101–8.
84 Hoogendam JM, Ramakers GM, Di Lazzaro V. Physiology of repetitive transcranial magnetic stimulation of the human brain. Brain Stimulation. 2010;3(2):95–118.
85 Peterchev AV, Goetz SM, Westin GG, Luber B, Lisanby SH. Pulse width dependence of motor threshold and input-output curve characterized with controllable pulse parameter transcranial magnetic stimulation. Clinical Neurophysiology. 2013;124(7):1364–72.
86 Peterchev AV, Murphy DL, Lisanby SH. Repetitive transcranial magnetic stimulator with controllable pulse parameters. Journal of Neural Engineering. 2011;8(3):036016.
87 Goetz S, Luber B, Lisanby SH, Kozyrkov CI, Grill WM, Peterchev AV. Enhancement of rTMS neuromodulatory effects with novel waveforms demonstrated via controllable pulse parameter TMS (cTMS). Neuropsychopharmacology. 2013;38:S246.
88 Huang YZ, Edwards MJ, Rounis E, Bhatia KP, Rothwell JC. Theta burst stimulation of the human motor cortex. Neuron. 2005;45(2):201–6.
89 Plewnia C, Pasqualetti P, Grosse S, Schlipf S, Wasserka B, Zwissler B, *et al.* Treatment of major depression with bilateral theta burst stimulation: a randomized controlled pilot trial. Journal of Affective Disorders. 2014;156:219–23.
90 Wilson MT, Goodwin DP, Brownjohn PW, Shemmell J, Reynolds JN. Numerical modelling of plasticity induced by transcranial magnetic stimulation. Journal of Computational Neuroscience. 2014;36(3):499–514.
91 Mueller JK, Grigsby EM, Prevosto V, Petraglia FW, Rao H, Deng Z-D, *et al.* Simultaneous transcranial magnetic stimulation and single neuron recording in alert non-human primates. Nature Neuroscience. 2014;17:1130–6.
92 Fox MD, Buckner RL, White MP, Greicius MD, Pascual-Leone A. Efficacy of transcranial magnetic stimulation targets for depression is related to intrinsic functional connectivity with the subgenual cingulate. Biological Psychiatry. 2012;72(7):595–603.
93 Baeken C, Marinazzo D, Wu GR, Van Schuerbeek P, De Mey J, Marchetti I, *et al.* Accelerated HF-rTMS in treatment-resistant unipolar depression: insights from subgenual anterior cingulate functional connectivity. The World Journal of Biological Psychiatry. 2014; 15(4):286–97.
94 Baxter LR, Jr., Schwartz JM, Phelps ME, Mazziotta JC, Guze BH, Selin CE, *et al.* Reduction of prefrontal cortex glucose metabolism common to three types of depression. Archives of General Psychiatry. 1989;46(3): 243–50.
95 Davidson RJ, Pizzagalli D, Nitschke JB, Putnam K. Depression: perspectives from affective neuroscience. Annual Review of Psychology. 2002;53:545–74.
96 Fox MD, Raichle ME. Spontaneous fluctuations in brain activity observed with functional magnetic resonance imaging. Nature Reviews Neuroscience. 2007;8(9):700–11.
97 Raichle ME, MacLeod AM, Snyder AZ, Powers WJ, Gusnard DA, Shulman GL. A default mode of brain function. Proceedings of the National Academy of Sciences of the United States of America. 2001;98(2):676–82.
98 Leuchter AF, Cook IA, Jin Y, Phillips B. The relationship between brain oscillatory activity and therapeutic effectiveness of transcranial magnetic stimulation in the treatment of major depressive disorder. Frontiers in Human Neuroscience. 2013;7:37.
99 Pellicciari MC, Cordone S, Marzano C, Bignotti S, Gazzoli A, Miniussi C, *et al.* Dorsolateral prefrontal transcranial magnetic stimulation in patients with major depression locally affects alpha power of REM sleep. Frontiers in Human Neuroscience. 2013;7:433.
100 Taliaz D, Stall N, Dar DE, Zangen A. Knockdown of brain-derived neurotrophic factor in specific brain sites precipitates behaviors associated with depression and reduces neurogenesis. Molecular Psychiatry. 2010; 15(1):80–92.
101 Stewart C, Reid I. Electroconvulsive stimulation and synaptic plasticity in the rat. Brain Research. 1993;620(1):139–41.
102 Moscrip T, Terrace H, Sackeim H, Lisanby S. Randomized controlled trial of the cognitive side-effects of magnetic seizure therapy (MST)

and electroconvulsive shock (ECS). International Journal of Neuropsychopharmacology. 2006; 9(1):1–11.

103 Spellman T, McClintock S, Terrace H, Luber B, Husain M, Lisanby S. Differential effects of high-dose magnetic seizure therapy and electroconvulsive shock on cognitive function. Biological Psychiatry. 2008;63: 1163–70.

104 McClintock SM, DeWind NK, Husain MM, Rowny SB, Spellman TJ, Terrace H, *et al.* Disruption of component processes of spatial working memory by electroconvulsive shock but not magnetic seizure therapy. International Journal of Neuropsychopharmacology. 2013; 16(1):177–87.

105 Polster JD, Kayser S, Bewernick BH, Hurlemann R, Schlaepfer TE. Effects of electroconvulsive therapy and magnetic seizure therapy on acute memory retrieval. The Journal of ECT. 2015;31:13–9.

106 Fitzgerald PB, Hoy KE, Herring SE, Clinton AM, Downey G, Daskalakis ZJ. Pilot study of the clinical and cognitive effects of high-frequency magnetic seizure therapy in major depressive disorder. Depression and Anxiety. 2013;30(2):129–36.

107 Kayser S, Bewernick BH, Grubert C, Hadrysiewicz BL, Axmacher N, Schlaepfer TE. Antidepressant effects, of magnetic seizure therapy and electroconvulsive therapy, in treatment-resistant depression. Journal of Psychiatric Research. 2011;45(5):569–76.

CHAPTER 10

Repetitive transcranial magnetic stimulation for psychiatric disorders other than depression

Daniel M. Blumberger[1], Mera S. Barr[1,2] and Zafiris J. Daskalakis[1]
[1]*Temerty Centre for Therapeutic Brain Intervention, Toronto, Canada*
[2]*University of Toronto, Toronto, Canada*

Introduction

Despite progress in behavioural treatments and pharmacotherapy in recent years, a significant percentage of persons suffering from mental disorders and addictions fail to achieve sufficient improvement from these treatments. As such, brain stimulation modalities have been investigated as potential strategies to achieve an improvement in symptoms. Repetitive transcranial magnetic stimulation (rTMS) is a safe and non-invasive form of brain stimulation and has been shown to achieve an improvement in depression in numerous clinical trials [1–4]. The ability to modulate circuits involved in other psychiatric disorders has led investigators to study the treatment in a variety of other disorders. Herein, we will review the use of rTMS to treat other neuropsychiatric disorders and addictions.

rTMS in schizophrenia

Schizophrenia is thought to be a heterogeneous syndrome rather than a single disease with a unified pathophysiology. As a result, targeting individual sub-components of the illness, such as hallucinations or negative symptoms, may yield greater success than non-specific treatments such as pharmacotherapy [5]. Hypoactivation in the dorsolateral prefrontal cortex (DLPFC) has been correlated with negative symptoms [6]. Thus, studies have employed high-frequency (HF) rTMS to the DLPFC to improve negative symptoms, as HF stimulation can increase cortical excitability [7]. In contrast, the temporoparietal cortex (TPC) has been targeted to treat auditory hallucinations (AHs) as numerous studies suggest that hyperactivity in the left TPC is associated with AHs [8, 9]. Accordingly, the majority of studies attempting to treat AH with rTMS have used low-frequency (LF; ≤1 Hz) rTMS protocols to the left TPC [10, 11]. Studies will be reviewed based on the cortical region targeted as well as the target symptoms.

rTMS applied to the DLPFC in schizophrenia

Early studies of rTMS in schizophrenia investigated the effect of LF (1 Hz) stimulation over the DLPFC, without a symptomatic focus. Improvements in non-specific symptoms such as anxiety and tension were found in two open studies, one using 30 rTMS pulses in a

Neuromodulation in Psychiatry, First Edition. Edited by Clement Hamani, Paul Holtzheimer, Andres M. Lozano and Helen Mayberg.

single session [12] and the other in 10 sessions [13]. However, a sham-controlled trial failed to find an improvement in schizophrenia-specific symptoms [14].

rTMS to the DLPFC for positive symptoms of schizophrenia

The study of rTMS for the treatment of positive symptoms in schizophrenia has focused on HF rTMS applied over the left DLPFC. This protocol was first studied in a small crossover design comparing left vs. sham stimulation (20 Hz; 80% motor threshold (MT)) for 10 sessions [15]. A significant reduction in Brief Psychiatric Rating Scale (BPRS) scores was found with active but not sham stimulation. Three subsequent studies of comparable duration and higher intensity have failed to demonstrate an improvement in positive symptoms [16–18]. In addition, meta-analytic analyses have shown that HF stimulation of the DLPFC does not lead to an improvement in positive symptoms when either the Positive subscale of the Positive and Negative Symptom Scale (PANSS-P) or the Scale for the Assessment of Positive Symptoms (SAPS) is used [19].

rTMS to the DLPFC for negative symptoms of schizophrenia

The treatment of negative symptoms utilizing HF rTMS to the DLPFC has yielded more encouraging results. While several studies found no differences between active and sham groups [16, 20–22], a number of studies have shown a significant advantage of active over sham stimulation [18, 23–26]. Higher intensities (>100% of the resting motor threshold (RMT)) and longer treatment durations may underlie the enhanced response [18, 23, 24, 27].

One positive study controlled for improved depressive symptoms using the Calgary Depression Scale for Schizophrenia as a covariate, and found that the change in depressive symptoms did not account for the an improvement in negative symptoms [18]. Other studies have compared HF left stimulation to other treatment protocols. One study compared 20 Hz stimulation to stimulation provided at the patient's individual α-frequency, based on the hypothesis that impaired oscillations at this frequency may underlie the negative symptoms [28]. Stimulation at the patient's α-frequency resulted in a significantly greater reduction in negative symptoms than in the other conditions. Another sham-controlled study compared LF (1 Hz) to HF (10 Hz) rTMS (110% MT) over the left DLPFC for 4 weeks and found that HF led to a larger reduction in the Scale for the Assessment of Negative Symptoms (SANS) [29].

While these studies of unilateral HF rTMS to the left DLPFC show promise, a recent sham-controlled study of bilateral HF (10 Hz) rTMS (110% MT; 2000 pulses) to the DLPFC for 15 days did not find any differences in negative symptoms or cognition between the active and sham groups [30]. However, this study included only participants with moderate-to-severe treatment-resistant symptoms, which may be a more difficult to treat population. A recent meta-analysis of all rTMS protocols targeting negative symptoms in schizophrenia (16 studies with 348 participants) found a treatment effect size of 0.8 compared to placebo [31]. Longer illness duration was a negative predictor of response and treatment with HF stimulation, for at least 3 weeks at 110% MT intensity targeting the left DLPFC, yielded the best results.

rTMS to the DLPFC for cognition in schizophrenia

Cognitive functioning is recognized as a primary deficit in schizophrenia [32, 33]. A study using HF stimulation to the left DLPFC led to an improvement in working memory and negative symptoms compared to sham stimulation [26]. A bilateral, HF (20 Hz), DLPFC treatment protocol has also shown some promise in improving working memory in patients with schizophrenia [34].

rTMS of the TPC for AHs

The most widely investigated application of rTMS in schizophrenia is the use of LF stimulation to the left TPC, to improve AHs. Initial studies of a relatively short duration as well as several controlled studies with larger sample sizes have demonstrated a significant reduction in AH frequency and intensity with LF stimulation compared to sham [10, 11, 34, 35]. Furthermore, one study found that the improvement was sustained in more than half of the improved subjects at 15 weeks post treatment [36]. The largest controlled study to date of AHs in patients with schizophrenia found a significant decrease in hallucination frequency but not the severity of the hallucinations. rTMS targeted both left and right Wernicke's areas at 1 Hz frequency, and an intensity of 90% MT for 15 treatments [37].

Unfortunately, other investigators have attempted to replicate and extend these findings using open, crossover and parallel randomized controlled designs with mixed results [38–51]. The variable results relate to heterogeneity in the duration and intensity of treatment. The crossover studies were of considerably shorter duration than subsequent parallel controlled trials [42–44]. Two randomized controlled trials (RCTs) found a significant reduction in frequency and intensity of AHs with less than 10 days of treatment, [38, 39] while another found no difference between active and sham stimulation after 10 days [41]. Other negative studies utilized a lower stimulation intensity of 80% MT [52] or provided stimulation for only 5 min per day, substantially less than 15–20 min used in most of the positive studies [53]. However, other RCTs of longer duration, utilizing higher intensities, and neuro-navigation or functional magnetic resonance imaging (fMRI) targeting techniques have also failed to find an effect of LF rTMS over sham [54, 55].

An initial meta-analysis of rTMS treatment of AH found an effect size of 0.76 (95% CI = 0.36–1.17) for LF rTMS applied to the left TPC [56]. Two recent meta-analyses confirm the finding of a medium-to-large effect size [19, 57, 58]. An analysis of all rTMS treatments for AH, regardless of target location, yielded a smaller effect size of 0.44 [58]. The authors describe a large degree of heterogeneity in these studies with issues including protocol duration and intensity, differing placebo controls, lack of adequate control of medications and inadequate assessment of treatment resistance [19, 57, 58].

In an attempt to optimize efficacy, investigators have explored LF (1 Hz) right and bilateral TPC stimulation. However, RCTs have failed to demonstrate an advantage of either treatment over sham [47, 49]. HF stimulation has also been investigated. One case report found a decrease in hallucination severity and frequency when HF (10 Hz) rTMS (80% MT; 2600 pulses) was delivered over the left TPC for 15 days [59]. On the basis of an earlier case report [60], one study identified the area of highest activation during a language task using individual fMRI scans, and subsequently targeted this site with HF (20 Hz) rTMS [61]. A resultant decrease in AH severity and frequency was reported within 10 days after treatment and sustained for a mean of 2 months. A significant discrepancy was found between the site of optimal stimulation established using their language task and the 10–20 EEG coordinate used in non-imaging studies. The investigators hypothesize that the use of a generic target site may account for the negative findings in previous studies, suggesting that the use of individual anatomic and functional targets within the temporal language network may improve treatment efficacy.

Multiple other studies have used imaging techniques to more specifically target neuroanatomical structures. The use of fMRI localization did not show a significant benefit when used to selectively stimulate Broca's area and the superior temporal gyrus [62], or when used to identify and target the area of greatest activation during an AH [63]. Conversely, LF rTMS applied to multiple sites activated on an fMRI scan during a hallucination in patients with intermittent hallucinations, or to a series of sites functionally coupled to Wernicke's area in patients with continual hallucinations, significantly reduced AH severity. Specifically, stimulation to the left Wernicke's area and adjacent supramarginal gyrus using fMRI localization led to a greater decrease in AH severity compared to sham or other stimulation sites [64].

Positron emission tomography (PET) activation has also been used to guide treatment. In one case study, LF (1 Hz) rTMS (90% MT) was administered based on PET activation in the left Wernicke's area for 4 weeks. A reduction in hypermetabolism was observed after treatment, but no change in AHs. The PANSS total score reflected these results with baseline scores of 36 declining to 28 at outcome, whereas the BPRS, Auditory Hallucination subscale of Psychotic Symptoms Rating Scales (PSYRATS-AH) and PANSS (hallucination subscale) showed little to no change from baseline [65]. Conversely, one open study utilizing PET imaging found a correlation between response to treatment and reduction in cortical metabolism beneath the site of stimulation [46]. Furthermore, a controlled study found a significant improvement in AH scores in the PET-guided group compared to the standard localization and sham groups [35] (Table 10.1).

These findings suggest that future imaging-targeted studies need to compare LF to HF stimulation and must continue to evaluate the relative efficacy of fMRI or PET individualized treatment compared to anatomically localized protocols. As the cost of fMRI or PET localization may prevent application to the wider population of patients with refractory AH, improved methods for targeting within the TPC using approximation are needed.

A paucity of data exists on rTMS treatment follow-up and maintenance studies. Other than some 4–12 weeks follow-up data provided in a minority of studies, there are little data on the longer-term implications of treating AH with rTMS [61, 66]. Fitzgerald *et al.* reported the successful re-treatment of two patients who relapsed following successful rTMS treatment [67]. There is a report of maintenance rTMS in a patient for 6 months with some decrease in severity but no delay in relapse [68]. One case study reported successful maintenance of reduced AH severity using LF stimulation to the TPC over an 8-month period, with a tapering protocol of once weekly for 6 weeks, once every 2 weeks for 12 weeks and once a month for 3 months [69]. Another case study reported a patient who relapsed after experiencing a 35% improvement in AH after 1 week of treatment (twice daily LF stimulation to the left TPC) who subsequently improved with the same treatment protocol, with sustained improvement over 1 year with once monthly treatment [70].

Novel approaches to AH include continuous theta burst stimulation (TBS) rTMS and stimulation at alternative sites. TBS is a novel application of rTMS involving short bursts of HF stimulation (50 Hz) repeated at the theta frequency (5 Hz) [71]. A recent study comparing 1 Hz rTMS to continuous theta burst found equivalent effects of both treatments with a significant improvement in hallucination changes scores in both groups. Nine subjects had a greater than 50% change in scores and the improvement appeared to last longer in the theta burst group [72]. Conversely, stimulation of alternate sites has not proved effective, with one group attempting vermal cerebellar stimulation leading to a 30% increase in the PSYRATS-AH subscale [73].

Conclusion

There is a pressing need to develop novel treatments for patients with schizophrenia, especially given the high rate of treatment resistance and suboptimal therapeutic response in this disorder. While the use of rTMS targeted to the

Table 10.1 Controlled rTMS studies for AHs in schizophrenia.

Articles	Number of patients	Target, coil type	Control condition	Stimulation frequency and intensity	Number of pulses/ session and number of sessions	Superior to sham
Hoffman *et al.* [11]	12	Left TPC, F8c	Tilted coil	1 Hz, 80% RMT	Pulse number increasing at each session from 240 to 1000 pulses, 4 sessions	Yes
McIntosh *et al.* [43]	16	Left TPC, F8c	Tilted coil	1 Hz, 80% RMT	240–1000 pulses, 4 sessions	No
Poulet *et al.* [44]	10	Left TPC, F8c	Sham coil	1 Hz, 90% RMT	1000 pulses, 10 sessions	Yes
Jandl *et al.* [42]	16	Left or right TPC, F8c	Tilted coil	1 Hz, 100% RMT	900 pulses, 5 sessions	Yes
Hoffman *et al.* [64]	16	fMRI-defined target, F8c	Tilted coil	1 Hz, 90% RMT	3 sessions	Yes (to the TPC region)
Loo *et al.* [49]	18	Left or right TPC, F8c	Vertex stimulation	1 Hz, 90% RMT	240–480 pulses, 3 sessions	No
Klirova *et al.* [35]	15	TPC or 18 FDG PET-defined target	Tilted coil	0.9 Hz, 100% RMT	1080 pulses, 10 sessions	Yes (PET guided better than standard and sham)
Hoffman *et al.* [36]	24 (active: 12; control: 12)	Left TPC, F8c	Tilted coil	1 Hz, 90% RMT	9 sessions	Yes
Schonfeldt-Lecuona *et al.* [62]	11 (active: 11 left STG, 8 Broca's area; control: 10)	Left STG, Broca's, fMRI defined target, F8c	Parieto-occipital junction	1 Hz, 90% RMT	960 pulses, 5 sessions	No
Chibbaro *et al.* [39]	16 (active: 8 ; control: 8)	Left TPC, F8c	Tilted coil	1 Hz, 90% RMT	4 sessions	No
Fitzgerald *et al.* [41]	33 (active: 17; control: 16)	Left TPC, F8c	Tilted coil	1 Hz, 90% RMT	960 pulses, 10 sessions	No

(continued)

Table 10.1 (Continued)

Articles	Number of patients	Target, coil type	Control condition	Stimulation frequency and intensity	Number of pulses/ session and number of sessions	Superior to sham
Hoffman *et al.* [66]	50 (active: 27; control: 23)	Left TPC, F8c	Tilted coil	1 Hz, 90% RMT	480–960 pulses, 9 sessions	Yes
Brunelin *et al.* [38]	24 (active: 14; control: 10)	Left TPC, F8c	Sham coil	1 Hz, 90% RMT	1000 pulses, 5 sessions	Yes
Rosa *et al.* [50]	11 (active: 6; control: 5)	Left TPC, F8c	Sham coil	1 Hz, 90% RMT	960 pulses, 10 sessions	No
Vercammen *et al.* [48]	36 (active: 12 unilateral, 12 bilateral; control: 12)	Left TPC or bilateral TPC, F8c	Sham coil	1 Hz, 90% RMT	1200 pulses, 6 sessions	Yes (left TPC)
de Jesus *et al.* [52]	17 (active: 8; control: 9)	Left TPC, F8c	Tilted coil	1 Hz, 90% RMT	20 sessions	No
Slotema *et al.* [55]	62 (active: 42; control: 20)	Left TPC or fMRI-defined target, F8c	Tilted coil	1 Hz, 90% RMT	1200 pulses, 15 sessions	No
Blumberger *et al.* [54]	51 (active: 17 of 1 Hz; 17 primed; control: 17)	Left TPC, F8c	Tilted coil	1 Hz, 115% RMT or 6 Hz – primed 1 Hz, 90% RMT	1200 pulses, 20 sessions	No
Hoffman *et al.* [37]	83 (active: 55; control: 28)	Wernicke's area or right homologue, F8c	Tilted coil	1 Hz, 90% RMT	960 pulses, 15 sessions	Yes

F8c, figure-of-8 coil; RMT, resting motor threshold; STG, superior temporal gyrus; TPC, temporoparietal cortex.

DLPFC in an attempt to improve global positive symptoms has yielded conflicting results, the use of HF rTMS applied to the DLPFC for treatment of negative symptoms and cognitive deficits has shown some encouraging results. It is possible that with further refinements in the protocols (i.e. MRI targeting and coil-to-cortex distance calculations), the DLPFC may become a valid target of rTMS for schizophrenia. In contrast to the studies that have targeted the DLPFC, rTMS of the left TPC to target refractory AH has yielded more encouraging results with a moderate effect size [58]. However, several of recent larger studies have failed to demonstrate improvement over sham stimulation [54, 55]. Further research is required in comparing HF to LF rTMS for AHs, the use of imaging techniques to guide stimulation and novel protocols such as TBS all of which may lead to improved treatment efficacy. In addition, future research should focus on determining the long-term implications of rTMS treatment for AHs including follow-up and maintenance studies.

rTMS in addiction

A number of brain stimulation modalities have been investigated in the treatment of substance use disorders including rTMS [74, 75]. Although rTMS is limited to the stimulation of surface cortical areas, connectivity within the cortex allows for more distant effects [76, 77]. By targeting rTMS to the DLPFC, downstream effects in the mesocorticolimbic system may affect addiction. The DLPFC has been suggested as a cortical region underlying drug- and cue-induced craving [78], and has been consistently associated with decision-making processes [79] and abnormal decision-making behaviours [80]. Taken together, there is solid rationale to target the DLFPC with rTMS in the treatment of addiction.

From a mechanistic standpoint, rTMS applied to the DLPFC may modulate prefrontal control over other regions [81], thereby muting impulsive drug use [82]. Furthermore, rTMS to the DLPFC may affect subcortical regions involved in the reward system. For example, rTMS studies have demonstrated increased dopamine release from the nucleus accumbens [83] and caudate nucleus [84] as well as a modulation of dopamine release in the orbitofrontal cortex (OFC) and subgenual anterior cingulate cortex [85]. Herein we will review the literature on the use of rTMS to treat substance use disorders including tobacco addiction, alcohol use disorders and stimulant disorders. There has not been investigation into the use of rTMS for opiate, cannabis or benzodiazepine dependence.

rTMS in tobacco dependence

The majority of research on rTMS in substance use disorders has focused on HF stimulation to the left DLPFC for tobacco dependence. An initial crossover study compared sham to HF (20 Hz) rTMS (90% RMT, 1000 pulses) over the left DLPFC on nicotine seeking in tobacco-dependent smokers following 12 h of abstinence [86]. Using a visual analogue scale (VAS) at 30 min before and 30 min following treatment, craving was significantly decreased following active compared to sham rTMS. A subsequent study administered two sessions of treatment and sham and found that active rTMS did not affect craving levels, but a decrease in smoking consumption immediately following rTMS treatment was reported [87]. Recent RCTs report similar results with significant reductions in cigarette consumption and nicotine-dependence scores in treatment groups compared to sham [88, 89].

The effects of HF rTMS to the DLPFC on cue-induced cravings have also been investigated. One study demonstrated that HF (10 Hz) rTMS (100% RMT; 1000 pulses) reduced cue-induced cigarette craving over 10 days of treatment [88]. However, these effects were not sustained over time, as no difference in cigarette consumption was present 6 months after treatment [88]. Another study also demonstrated a significant reduction in cue-induced cravings after only one session with 3000 pulses [89]. The observed effects were greater in those with higher levels of nicotine dependence, suggesting that rTMS may have more robust effects in more severe cases of nicotine dependence [89]. A within-subject study examined the effects of HF rTMS to the left DLPFC on EEG brain wave activity, specifically delta power that is known to be abnormal with nicotine use [90]. Delta power and craving ratings decreased significantly after active rTMS compared to sham, persisting up to 40 min; however, smoking cues did not modulate this effect [91].

Because of a high degree of comorbid substance use disorders among patients with neuropsychiatric illnesses, two studies investigated the effects of rTMS in smokers with a concurrent psychotic disorder. In one study, 15 patients received either HF (20 Hz) rTMS (90% RMT; 750 pulses) to the DLPFC bilaterally or sham rTMS for 20 sessions, in addition to weekly group therapy and transdermal nicotine patch (21 mg) [92]. Active rTMS significantly reduced cravings with no effect on consumption. A maximum effect was found following the first week of treatment. This is in keeping with other studies that observed early positive effects of rTMS on tobacco craving but not consumption. The second study compared HF (10 Hz) rTMS (110% RMT; 2000 pulses) over the left DLPFC to sham for 15 sessions and found the rTMS group smoked significantly fewer cigarettes [93]. Changes were seen as early as the second week of stimulation. After 3 weeks, rTMS decreased cigarette consumption by almost 13%, while the number of cigarettes smoked among those in the sham group increased. The effects on decreased consumption persisted for up to 3 weeks.

The superior frontal gyrus (SFG) has also been targeted to treat nicotine dependence. One within-subject study compared HF rTMS (10 Hz) and LF rTMS (1 Hz) delivered to the SFG to a control condition (LF rTMS (1 Hz) to the motor cortex) in modulating cravings to cigarette and neutral cues [94]. HF rTMS led to increased craving when presented with smoking cues suggesting that this treatment protocol may exacerbate tobacco addiction. However, reduced craving was reported with HF rTMS when presented with neutral cues compared to LF rTMS and control. Thus, the SFG may be involved in modulating craving and is a potential target for future investigation.

These preliminary studies show promise for rTMS to treat tobacco dependence in those with and without concurrent psychiatric disorders. Work is needed to replicate these findings, establish optimal treatment parameters and determine neuroanatomical targets. As rTMS can involve multiple daily visits, methods that enhance the effect while reducing the number of visits are required.

rTMS for cocaine dependence

The use of rTMS to treat cocaine dependence has been examined in several studies. The first study used a randomized crossover design to assess the effect of a single session of HF (10 Hz) rTMS (90% RMT; 1000 pulses) over the left or right DLPFC on cocaine craving [95]. After completion of substance withdrawal, six male cocaine-dependent inpatients were studied. Cocaine cravings were measured with a VAS 10 min before, immediately after and 4 h post rTMS treatment. HF rTMS over the right, but not the left DLPFC, was found to decrease craving levels immediately after and 4 h after treatment. Conversely, a larger study investigating the effects of 10 daily rTMS sessions over the left DLPFC found that ratings of craving gradually decreased with each session [96]. This study had a larger sample size, used a higher frequency of 15 Hz, higher intensity of 100% RMT and had a longer duration. However, the persistence of the effect was not measured and participants had not undergone detoxification.

These earliest findings suggest that HF rTMS to the right DLPFC may reduce cocaine cravings. However, larger RCTs must replicate this finding and compare rTMS of the right and left DLPFC.

rTMS for methamphetamine dependence

One study has compared LF (1 Hz) rTMS (100% RMT; 900 pulses) delivered over the left DLPFC to sham on cue-induced craving in methamphetamine users. LF rTMS was chosen as a safety measure in light of the increased incidence of seizures in methamphetamine users [97]. Ten non-treatment-seeking methamphetamine-dependent individuals and eight healthy controls (HCs) received one session of both active and sham rTMS administered 1 h apart. The active rTMS treatment significantly increased self-reported cue-induced methamphetamine cravings compared to sham, while no effect was observed in controls. These findings are in keeping with studies conducted in tobacco and cocaine users where LF rTMS leads to a reduction in inhibitory control and an enhancement of cue-induced cravings. In contrast, HF rTMS used in tobacco and alcohol studies seems to reduce cravings perhaps via increased inhibitory control [89].

rTMS in alcohol dependence

Few studies have investigated the effect of rTMS on alcohol dependence compared to tobacco. In a sham-controlled study, 45 individuals with alcohol dependence were randomized to receive 10 daily sessions of HF (10 Hz) rTMS (110% RMT; 1000 pulses) to the right DLPFC in addition to treatment with anti-craving medications (i.e. naltrexone) on an as needed basis. While active rTMS significantly reduced craving scores compared to sham rTMS, the effect was not sustained after 1 month [98]. Another study of HF rTMS to the right DLPFC found no effect on craving compared to sham [99]. However, the study consisted of only one treatment session and all participants were patients hospitalized for alcohol dependence. HF rTMS to the left DLPFC also showed no effect on reported craving after 10 treatment sessions [100].

One case study in an alcohol-dependent patient targeted the dorsal anterior cingulate cortex (dACC) with 3 weeks of daily 1 Hz rTMS to investigate the effects on alcohol craving and resting-state neural oscillations. Before rTMS, increased beta (22–23 Hz) activity in the right ACC, right insula and left prefrontal cortex (PFC), and bilateral hyperactivity in the gamma (31–35 Hz) frequency range were observed. Following 1 week of treatment, alcohol cravings decreased from 9/10 to 1/10 on a VAS. After 3 weeks, resting-state EEG revealed a decrease in beta and gamma activity in the bilateral posterior insula, anterior and retrosplenial posterior cingulate cortex (PCC).

These findings suggest that there may be therapeutic effects observed with rTMS that may be linked to an alteration in neural oscillations. Further work is needed to delineate the effect of rTMS on alcohol dependence, including optimal treatment targets and protocols.

Conclusion

The effect of rTMS on various components of addiction has been investigated to some extent. Drug craving and consumption have been the primary outcomes studied. rTMS targeted to the DLPFC may hold promise for decreasing cravings and consumption of tobacco in those with and without concurrent psychiatric disorders. HF rTMS has shown promise for treating tobacco and cocaine dependence, while LF rTMS may be more efficacious for treating methamphetamine and alcohol dependence. Possibly due to the natural history of withdrawal and addiction, investigators have not examined the effect of sequential daily rTMS treatments. In other disorders, longer treatment courses have shown the most benefit. Thus, while single sessions may provide a signal, it is likely that studies involving repeated rTMS sessions will be required.

rTMS for post-traumatic stress disorder

Post-traumatic stress disorder (PTSD) can be a debilitating disorder and available psychotherapeutic and psychopharmacological options are not effective in about one-third of patients due to non-adherence and treatment resistance [101] A limited number of trials have studied the effect of rTMS on reducing PTSD symptoms. Hyperactivity in medial prefrontal and limbic structures is thought to be part of the underlying pathophysiology of this disorder. Thus, rTMS has been used to modulate these circuits to achieve symptomatic relief.

Early investigation consisted of some promising results using open-study designs and a variety of treatment protocols. A case study using LF (1 Hz) rTMS (80% MT; 1200) delivered over the right frontal region for 3–5 weeks significantly reduced PTSD symptoms, but the effect was not sustained at 1 month [102]. Another case study showed an improvement in response to trauma-related visual stimuli when LF (1 Hz) rTMS was delivered to the right but not left frontal region [103]. LF rTMS also improved avoidance symptoms in an open-label study of 10 subjects applied over the left and right frontal regions [104]. The left DLPFC has also been targeted with some positive results including reductions in the Mississippi Scale of Combat Severity (MSCS) and the Profile of Mood States Subscales (anger–hostility, tension–anxiety and depression–dejection) [105, 106]. However, little decline in the overall MSCS score was found [106]. Overall treatment was well tolerated in all open studies with limited adverse effects including headache [104, 106] and reports of intrusive thoughts [104].

Subsequent controlled trials have also demonstrated positive effects. An RCT targeting the right DLPFC compared HF (10 Hz; 400 pulses per day), LF (1 Hz; 100 pulses per day) and sham (400 pulses per day) stimulation and found only HF rTMS significantly reduced PTSD symptoms [107]. Conversely, subsequent sham-controlled trials of LF rTMS to the right DLPFC have found an improvement in intrusion and avoidance symptoms [108], clinician and self-rated PTSD symptoms [109], re-experiencing and total PTSD symptom scores [110] as compared to sham. These more recent trials used higher intensities for similar or longer treatment duration. Another sham-controlled trial compared HF (20 Hz) rTMS (80%MT, 1600 pulses) to the right and left DLPFC over 10 sessions. Using the 'PTSD Checklist and Treatment Outcome PTSD Scale', the right DLPFC rTMS improved core PTSD symptoms while the left improved depression symptoms [111]. A recent meta-analysis of all rTMS treatments targeting PTSD symptoms supports these positive findings, reporting a mean-weighted effect size of 2.67 [112]. Similar to open-label studies, rTMS treatment was generally well tolerated; however, there were reports of dizziness, headache, neck pain, sleepiness [110, 111], an increase in anxiety and worsening of PTSD symptoms post treatment [109].

Another study delivered HF (20 Hz) deep TMS (DTMS) (120 MT; 1680 pulses; 12 sessions) during activation of memories in an attempt to cause extinction of the hyperarousal response. DTMS utilizes an H-coil that generates a magnetic field that can penetrate twice the distance of standard figure-of-eight coils [113]. Thus, DTMS can target more medial prefrontal structures and deeper within the PFC due to the coil geometry. Thirty subjects were randomized into three groups: (i) DTMS administered after script-driven imagery of the traumatic experience followed by neutral imagery, (ii) DTMS administered after script-driven imagery of a positive experience followed by neutral imagery and (iii) sham administered after script-driven imagery of a traumatic experience followed by neutral imagery. Using a clinician-rated PTSD scale, there was an improvement of over 50% (compared to baseline) in the active imagery group compared to only one responder in the other active group and no responders in the sham group [114]. DTMS was well tolerated with mild adverse effects of headache and slightly increased anxiety. One subject experienced a short, self-limiting, tonic–clonic generalized seizure during the eighth session and thus did not receive any more DTMS treatments.

Conclusion

These early findings suggest that both LF and HF rTMS may have beneficial effects on PTSD symptoms. As PTSD is associated with hyperactivity in the medial prefrontal and limbic structures, most research has focused on LF rTMS to inhibit this response. However, a recent fMRI study demonstrated a pattern of hypoactivation of the ventromedial PFC during fear extinction, suggesting that HF rTMS to this area may be effective [115]. Hyperactivity of the dACC during fear extinction is also seen on fMRI, suggesting that this area may also be a potential treatment target [115]. Right-sided stimulation appears to be more effective than left, consistent with right-sided brain laterality in fear circuitry found in animal and human studies [112]. However, much future research is required in identifying the optimal treatment targets and stimulation frequencies. In addition, much further investigation is needed to explore the effect of combined active imagery and rTMS in attenuating PTSD symptoms.

rTMS for cognitive disorders

The need for treatments for cognitive disorders is increasing with the ageing population [116]. Current treatments are only partially effective at slowing cognitive decline, and no treatments exist that improve cognition in patients with dementia [117]. As rTMS can target areas related to cognition, it has been studied as a potential method of enhancing cognition in patients with early cognitive decline.

Most studies of rTMS in cognitive disorders have focused on memory. A controlled study of adults with subjective memory complaints found that HF (5 Hz) rTMS (80% MT) delivered to the left DLPFC in one session increased associative memory compared to sham [118]. In a case study of a patient with a mild cognitive impairment (MCI), a similar improvement was seen in associative memory when HF (20 Hz) rTMS (100% MT; 2000 pulses) was delivered to the left inferior parietal lobule (IPL). However, no improvement was seen when delivered to the right or left DLPFC. The patient was subsequently given daily rTMS to the left IPL for 10 sessions. The effect on associative memory persisted, remaining significant for 24 weeks following initiation of stimulation [119].

TBS has also been investigated in patients with MCI. A study of 100 HCs and 8 patients with a MCI investigated the effects of TBS on the right and left DLPFC. Inhibitory TBS (i.e. continuous TBS) improved verbal and non-verbal memory recognition in the right but not left DLPFC. Conversely, excitatory stimulation (i.e. intermittent TBS) of the right DLPFC impaired non-verbal memory recognition whereas intermittent TBS to the left DLPFC did not affect memory recognition [120]. On the basis of these findings, a subsequent sham-controlled study including both HCs and those with an MCI examined the effects of both LF (1 Hz) rTMS (90% MT, 900 pulses) and intermittent TBS applied to the left or right DLPFC. Stimulation of the right DLPFC with LF rTMS led to an improvement in non-verbal memory and verbal recognition memory in both HCs and those with an MCI. Furthermore, intermittent TBS over the right DLPFC led to impairment in non-verbal memory in both groups. Stimulation of the left DLPFC with LF rTMS or TBS had no effect compared to sham [121].

A number of studies have also investigated rTMS in patients with Alzheimer's disease (AD) with promising effects. Two initial sham-controlled studies applied HF (20 Hz) rTMS (90% MT) to both the left and right DLPFC. The first found an improvement in action naming [122], while the second found an increase in object naming [123]. A subsequent case study also targeting the left and right DLPFC with HF (10 Hz) rTMS (100% MT, 2000 pulses) found an increase in episodic memory and speed processing after 10 sessions [124]. Targeting of the left DLPFC alone with HF (20 Hz) rTMS (100% MT, 1200 pulses) led to an increase in auditory sentence comprehension compared to sham, after 20 sessions [125]. Furthermore, both an RCT and open study targeting the left and right DLPFC, Broca's and Wernicke's areas and the left and right parietal somatosensory association cortex with HF (10 Hz) rTMS (90/110% MT, 1200/1300 pulses) found an improvement in cognition with the Alzheimer's Disease Assessment Scale cognitive function (ADAS-cog) [126, 127]. In addition, the open study also found an improvement in the MMSE and activities of daily living test scores [127].

Limited research has compared rTMS treatment protocols in AD. One study compared HF (20 Hz) to LF (1 Hz) rTMS to the DLPFC bilaterally for five sessions. HF rTMS was superior to LF rTMS in improving global cognition, depression and activities of daily living [128]. Another study compared 10 Hz (1000 pulses) vs. 15 Hz (1500 pulses) stimulation to the DLPFC bilaterally and found no difference between in effect between the treatment protocols, with both stimulation protocols demonstrating an improvement in verbal and non-verbal agility [22].

Conclusion

These findings highlight the therapeutic potential for rTMS in patients with MCI and AD. Continuous TBS and LF rTMS delivered to the right DLPFC have shown promising effects on memory in patients with MCI. While these findings suggest that rTMS may modulate brain processes involved in memory, the interpretation of these results is limited because of small sample sizes. Thus, future research is required to replicate these results in larger samples. In AD, HF rTMS delivered to both the right and left DLPFC appears to improve cognition. However, due to the variability in outcome measures, it is difficult to compare the effects of rTMS on cognition across studies. Future research should involve the selection of consistent outcome measures as well as comparison of treatment protocols with a sham condition.

rTMS for obsessive–compulsive disorder

Obsessive–compulsive disorder (OCD) is a serious and debilitating illness. Despite advances in pharmacotherapy and behavioural treatments, a significant proportion of patients with OCD struggle with refractory symptoms. rTMS has been investigated as an adjunctive treatment in patients with difficult to treat OCD. A number of HF and LF protocols targeting several cortical regions have been investigated.

Several studies investigating the effects of HF rTMS applied to the DLPFC for treatment of OCD showed early success. The first study of rTMS in OCD randomized 12 participants to receive 20 Hz rTMS (80% MT, 800 pulses) to either the left or right DLPFC or the occipital cortex as a control. In both the right and left DLPFC groups compulsive urges declined significantly from baseline, while the control site was associated with a non-significant increase in compulsions [129]. Similar findings were seen in a randomized study of 10 Hz rTMS

(100% MT) to either the left or right DLPFC. Significant improvements were reported on the obsessions, compulsions and total scores of the Yale–Brown Obsessive Compulsive Scale (YBOCS) following 2 weeks of treatment and 1 month after treatment completion. No differences were found between treatment groups [130]. Improvement on the YBOCS scale was also seen with HF rTMS targeted only to the right DLPFC when given for 30 treatment sessions [131].

Unfortunately, other studies including those with larger sample sizes have found no difference between rTMS to the DLPFC and sham. HF (10 Hz) rTMS did not lead to a significant improvement in YBOCS scores when applied over the left [132] or right [133] DLPFC. Similar non-significant results were reported with LF (1 Hz) rTMS applied to the left [134] and right DLPFC [135]. Another sham-controlled study stimulated the DLPFCs bilaterally at a frequency matching the subject's intrinsic alpha-EEG frequency for 10 sessions. While high rates of response and remission were found, active treatment did not differ from sham. However, treatment was given at a lower intensity of 80% MT [136].

The discouraging results found in stimulating the DLPFC prompted the investigation of treatment at alternate cortical regions, primarily the supplementary motor area (SMA). Initially, five OCD patients on pharmacotherapy were treated with LF (1 Hz) rTMS (100% MT; 1200 pulses) to the SMA bilaterally for 10 daily sessions. A large reduction in YBOCS scores was found following treatment, with three subjects experiencing a decrease of greater than 40% [137]. Similarly, another uncontrolled study of LF (1 Hz) rTMS (100%MT; 1000 pulses) found a decline in YBOCS scores from 26.17 to 17.17 following 15 treatment sessions [138].

Sham-controlled studies of LF (1 Hz) rTMS to the SMA have had less promising results. One RCT of 21 patients with OCD found no differences in YBOCS scores between active and sham groups when LF (1 Hz) rTMS (110% MT; 1200 pulses) was given over the right SMA for 10 sessions [139]. Another study randomized 18 medication-resistant subjects to either LF rTMS (100% MT; 1200 pulses) stimulation to the SMA bilaterally or sham for 20 sessions. Although the number of responders (≥25% decrease in YBOCS score) in the active group was greater than sham, the difference was not significant. In an open-label continuation of the study, additional participants initially randomized to active treatment demonstrated improvement in YBOCS scores, suggesting that longer treatment duration may optimize treatment effects [140]. Targeting of the pre-SMA has demonstrated more promising results with LF (1 Hz) rTMS (100% MT; 1200 pulses) delivered bilaterally leading to a significant reduction in YBOCS scores and a greater number of responders than sham stimulation [141].

Another site of stimulation that has demonstrated a potential therapeutic effect is the left OFC. In an RCT of 23 treatment-resistant OCD patients, LF (1 Hz) rTMS (80% MT) was delivered for 15 treatments. About 93.75% of subjects receiving active rTMS had a reduction in YBOCS score, with 50% experiencing a greater than 25% reduction and 25% a greater than 35% reduction. The reduction in symptoms in the active group was significantly larger than the sham group [142].

Conclusion

The results for rTMS in OCD are mixed. A recent meta-analysis evaluating all rTMS treatments in OCD using YBOCS scores found an overall effect size of 0.59, representing a significant and medium-sized difference [143]. Stimulation appears to be most effective when given at an LF and targeted at non-DLPFC regions. Some positive results have been reported with SMA and pre-SMA treatment, warranting larger scale trials of longer treatment duration. Future research is required in targeting the left OFC as a treatment for OCD. Functional neuroimaging studies show an association of hyperactivity in the OFC with OCD symptoms [142]. Thus, stimulation of the OFC may prove an OCD-specific treatment. In addition, coils that target deeper structures may be beneficial and warrant future investigation in rTMS treatment of OCD.

Summary

rTMS is an emerging therapy for the treatment of psychiatric disorders. The efficacy of rTMS in depression has led to the investigation of multiple other neuropsychiatric illnesses. To date, the most research has been conducted on rTMS in schizophrenia. Promising results have been shown with the use of HF rTMS targeting the DLPFC for the treatment of negative symptoms and cognition. In addition, much research has been conducted on the use of LF rTMS to the left TPC for the treatment of AH. While large effect sizes have been demonstrated, a number of negative trials in larger samples have failed to replicate the positive findings from smaller studies. Although meta-analyses demonstrate a moderate effect size for LF rTMS to treat AH, the efficacy of rTMS in AH has been questioned due to the negative findings from several larger trials.

Preliminary research shows that rTMS can modulate neural circuits involved in addiction, PTSD, cognitive disorders and OCD. The modulation of these circuits with rTMS may translate into therapeutic improvement that will need to be confirmed through larger confirmatory efficacy studies. In addition, identifying optimal targets and parameters of stimulation is required to enhance the efficacy of rTMS in these disorders and optimize treatment outcomes. Innovative treatment protocols such as TBS for AH and MCI and combining circuitry activation using imagery in PTSD may further improve treatment outcomes.

References

1 Berlim MT, Van den Eynde F, Daskalakis ZJ. A systematic review and meta-analysis on the efficacy and acceptability of bilateral repetitive transcranial magnetic stimulation (rTMS) for treating major depression. Psychol Med. Nov 2013;43(11):2245–2254.

2 Berlim MT, Van den Eynde F, Daskalakis ZJ. Clinically meaningful efficacy and acceptability of low-frequency repetitive transcranial magnetic stimulation (rTMS) for treating primary major depression: a meta-analysis of randomized, double-blind and sham-controlled trials. Neuropsychopharmacology. Mar 2013; 38(4):543–551.

3 George MS, Lisanby SH, Avery D, *et al.* Daily left prefrontal transcranial magnetic stimulation therapy for major depressive disorder: a sham-controlled randomized trial. Arch Gen Psychiatry. May 2010;67(5):507–516.

4 O'Reardon JP, Solvason HB, Janicak PG, *et al.* Efficacy and safety of transcranial magnetic stimulation in the acute treatment of major depression: a multisite randomized controlled trial. Biol Psychiatry. Dec 1 2007;62(11):1208–1216.

5 Citrome L. Unmet needs in the treatment of schizophrenia: new targets to help different symptom domains. J Clin Psychiatry. 2014; 75(Suppl 1):21–26.

6 Andreasen NC, O'Leary DS, Flaum M, *et al.* Hypofrontality in schizophrenia: distributed dysfunctional circuits in neuroleptic-naive patients. Lancet. 1997;349(9067):1730–1734.

7 Cohen E, Bernardo M, Masana J, *et al.* Repetitive transcranial magnetic stimulation in the treatment of chronic negative schizophrenia: a pilot study. J Neurol Neurosurg Psychiatry. 1999;67(1): 129–130.

8 Shergill SS, Brammer MJ, Williams SC, Murray RM, McGuire PK. Mapping auditory hallucinations in schizophrenia using functional magnetic resonance imaging. Arch Gen Psychiatry. Nov 2000;57(11):1033–1038.

9 Silbersweig DA, Stern E, Frith C, *et al.* A functional neuroanatomy of hallucinations in schizophrenia. Nature. 1995;378(6553):176–179.

10 Hoffman RE, Boutros NN, Berman RM, *et al.* Transcranial magnetic stimulation of left temporoparietal cortex in three patients reporting

hallucinated 'voices'. Biol Psychiatry. 1999; 46(1):130–132.
11 Hoffman RE, Boutros NN, Hu S, Berman RM, Krystal JH, Charney DS. Transcranial magnetic stimulation and auditory hallucinations in schizophrenia. Lancet. 2000;355(9209):1073–1075.
12 Geller V, Grisaru N, Abarbanel JM, Lemberg T, Belmaker RH. Slow magnetic stimulation of prefrontal cortex in depression and schizophrenia. Prog Neuropsychopharmacol Biol Psychiatry. 1997;21(1):105–110.
13 Feinsod M, Kreinin B, Chistyakov A, Klein E. Preliminary evidence for a beneficial effect of low-frequency, repetitive transcranial magnetic stimulation in patients with major depression and schizophrenia. Depress Anxiety. 1998; 7(2):65–68.
14 Klein E, Kolsky Y, Puyerovsky M, Koren D, Chistyakov A, Feinsod M. Right prefrontal slow repetitive transcranial magnetic stimulation in schizophrenia: a double-blind sham-controlled pilot study. Biol Psychiatry. 1999;46(10): 1451–1454.
15 Rollnik JD, Huber TJ, Mogk H, *et al.* High frequency repetitive transcranial magnetic stimulation (rTMS) of the dorsolateral prefrontal cortex in schizophrenic patients. Neuroreport. 2000;11(18):4013–4015.
16 Holi MM, Eronen M, Toivonen K, Toivonen P, Marttunen M, Naukkarinen H. Left prefrontal repetitive transcranial magnetic stimulation in schizophrenia. Schizophr Bull. 2004;30(2): 429–434.
17 Sachdev P, Loo C, Mitchell P, Malhi G. Transcranial magnetic stimulation for the deficit syndrome of schizophrenia: a pilot investigation. Psychiatry Clin Neurosci. Jun 2005;59(3): 354–357.
18 Hajak G, Marienhagen J, Langguth B, Werner S, Binder H, Eichhammer P. High-frequency repetitive transcranial magnetic stimulation in schizophrenia: a combined treatment and neuroimaging study. Psychol Med. Oct 2004;34(7): 1157–1163.
19 Freitas C, Fregni F, Pascual-Leone A. Meta-analysis of the effects of repetitive transcranial magnetic stimulation (rTMS) on negative and positive symptoms in schizophrenia. Schizophr Res. Mar 2009;108(1–3):11–24.
20 Mogg A, Purvis R, Eranti S, *et al.* Repetitive transcranial magnetic stimulation for negative symptoms of schizophrenia: a randomized controlled pilot study. Schizophr Res. Jul 2007; 93(1–3):221–228.
21 Novak T, Horacek J, Mohr P, *et al.* The double-blind sham-controlled study of high-frequency rTMS (20 Hz) for negative symptoms in schizophrenia: negative results. Neuro Endocrinol Lett. Feb–Apr 2006;27(1–2):209–213.
22 Barr MS, Farzan F, Tran LC, Fitzgerald PB, Daskalakis ZJ. A randomized controlled trial of sequentially bilateral prefrontal cortex repetitive transcranial magnetic stimulation in the treatment of negative symptoms in schizophrenia. Brain Stimul. 2012 Jul;5(3):337–346.
23 Prikryl R, Kasparek T, Skotakova S, Ustohal L, Kucerova H, Ceskova E. Treatment of negative symptoms of schizophrenia using repetitive transcranial magnetic stimulation in a double-blind, randomized controlled study. Schizophr Res. Sep 2007;95(1–3):151–157.
24 Jandl M, Bittner R, Sack A, *et al.* Changes in negative symptoms and EEG in schizophrenic patients after repetitive transcranial magnetic stimulation (rTMS): an open-label pilot study. J Neural Transm. Jul 2005;112(7):955–967.
25 Goyal N, Nizamie SH, Desarkar P. Efficacy of adjuvant high frequency repetitive transcranial magnetic stimulation on negative and positive symptoms of schizophrenia: preliminary results of a double-blind sham-controlled study. J Neuropsychiatry Clin Neurosci. Fall 2007;19(4): 464–467.
26 Prikryl R, Mikl M, Prikrylova Kucerova H, *et al.* Does repetitive transcranial magnetic stimulation have a positive effect on working memory and neuronal activation in treatment of negative symptoms of schizophrenia? Neuro Endocrinol Lett. 2012;33(1):90–97.
27 Prikryl R, Ustohal L, Prikrylova Kucerova H, *et al.* A detailed analysis of the effect of repetitive transcranial magnetic stimulation on negative symptoms of schizophrenia: a double-blind trial. Schizophr Res. Sep 2013;149(1–3):167–173.
28 Jin Y, Potkin SG, Kemp AS, *et al.* Therapeutic effects of individualized alpha frequency transcranial magnetic stimulation (alphaTMS) on the negative symptoms of schizophrenia. Schizophr Bull. Jul 2006;32(3):556–561.

29 Schneider AL, Schneider TL, Stark H. Repetitive transcranial magnetic stimulation (rTMS) as an augmentation treatment for the negative symptoms of schizophrenia: a 4-week randomized placebo controlled study. Brain Stimul. Apr 2008;1(2):106–111.
30 Fitzgerald PB, Herring S, Hoy K, *et al.* A study of the effectiveness of bilateral transcranial magnetic stimulation in the treatment of the negative symptoms of schizophrenia. Brain Stimul. Jan 2008;1(1):27–32.
31 Shi C, Yu X, Cheung EF, Shum DH, Chan RC. Revisiting the therapeutic effect of rTMS on negative symptoms in schizophrenia: a meta-analysis. Psychiatry Res. Mar 30 2014;215(3): 505–513.
32 Heinrichs RW. The primacy of cognition in schizophrenia. Am Psychol. Apr 2005;60(3):229–242.
33 Heinrichs RW, Zakzanis KK. Neurocognitive deficit in schizophrenia: a quantitative review of the evidence. Neuropsychology. 1998;12(3): 426–445.
34 Barr MS, Farzan F, Rajji TK, *et al.* Can repetitive magnetic stimulation improve cognition in schizophrenia? Pilot data from a randomized controlled trial. Biol Psychiatry. Mar 15 2013; 73(6):510–517.
35 Klirova M, Horacek J, Novak T, *et al.* Individualized rTMS neuronavigated according to regional brain metabolism ((18)FGD PET) has better treatment effects on auditory hallucinations than standard positioning of rTMS: a double-blind, sham-controlled study. Eur Arch Psychiatry Clin Neurosci. Sep 2013;263(6): 475–484.
36 Hoffman RE, Hawkins KA, Gueorguieva R, *et al.* Transcranial magnetic stimulation of left temporoparietal cortex and medication-resistant auditory hallucinations. Arch Gen Psychiatry. Jan 2003;60(1):49–56.
37 Hoffman RE, Wu K, Pittman B, *et al.* Transcranial magnetic stimulation of Wernicke's and Right homologous sites to curtail 'voices': a randomized trial. Biol Psychiatry. May 15 2013; 73(10):1008–1014.
38 Brunelin J, Poulet E, Bediou B, *et al.* Low frequency repetitive transcranial magnetic stimulation improves source monitoring deficit in hallucinating patients with schizophrenia. Schizophr Res. Jan 1 2006;81(1):41–45.
39 Chibbaro G, Daniele M, Alagona G, *et al.* Repetitive transcranial magnetic stimulation in schizophrenic patients reporting auditory hallucinations. Neurosci Lett. Jul 22–29 2005; 383(1–2):54–57.
40 d'Alfonso AA, Aleman A, Kessels RP, *et al.* Transcranial magnetic stimulation of left auditory cortex in patients with schizophrenia: effects on hallucinations and neurocognition. J Neuropsychiatry Clin Neurosci. Winter 2002;14(1):77–79.
41 Fitzgerald PB, Benitez J, Daskalakis ZJ, *et al.* A double-blind sham-controlled trial of repetitive transcranial magnetic stimulation in the treatment of refractory auditory hallucinations. J Clin Psychopharmacol. Aug 2005;25(4): 358–362.
42 Jandl M, Steyer J, Weber M, *et al.* Treating auditory hallucinations by transcranial magnetic stimulation: a randomized controlled cross-over trial. Neuropsychobiology. 2006; 53(2):63–69.
43 McIntosh AM, Semple D, Tasker K, *et al.* Transcranial magnetic stimulation for auditory hallucinations in schizophrenia. Psychiatry Res. Jun 30 2004;127(1–2):9–17.
44 Poulet E, Brunelin J, Bediou B, *et al.* Slow transcranial magnetic stimulation can rapidly reduce resistant auditory hallucinations in schizophrenia. Biol Psychiatry. Jan 15 2005; 57(2):188–191.
45 Saba G, Schurhoff F, Leboyer M. Therapeutic and neurophysiologic aspects of transcranial magnetic stimulation in schizophrenia. Neurophysiol Clin. May–Jun 2006;36(3):185–194.
46 Horacek J, Brunovsky M, Novak T, *et al.* Effect of low-frequency rTMS on electromagnetic tomography (LORETA) and regional brain metabolism (PET) in schizophrenia patients with auditory hallucinations. Neuropsychobiology. 2007;55(3–4):132–142.
47 Bagati D, Nizamie SH, Prakash R. Effect of augmentatory repetitive transcranial magnetic stimulation on auditory hallucinations in schizophrenia: randomized controlled study. Aust N Z J Psychiatry. Apr 2009;43(4): 386–392.
48 Vercammen A, Knegtering H, Bruggeman R, *et al.* Effects of bilateral repetitive transcranial magnetic stimulation on treatment resistant

auditory-verbal hallucinations in schizophrenia: a randomized controlled trial. Schizophr Res. Oct 2009;114(1–3):172–179.

49 Loo CK, Sainsbury K, Mitchell P, Hadzi-Pavlovic D, Sachdev PS. A sham-controlled trial of left and right temporal rTMS for the treatment of auditory hallucinations. Psychol Med. Apr 2010;40(4):541–546.

50 Rosa MO, Gattaz WF, Rosa MA, *et al.* Effects of repetitive transcranial magnetic stimulation on auditory hallucinations refractory to clozapine. J Clin Psychiatry. Oct 2007;68(10):1528–1532.

51 Subramanian P, Burhan A, Pallaveshi L, Rudnick A. The experience of patients with schizophrenia treated with repetitive transcranial magnetic stimulation for auditory hallucinations. Case Rep Psychiatry. 2013;2013:183582.

52 de Jesus DR, Gil A, Barbosa L, *et al.* A pilot double-blind sham-controlled trial of repetitive transcranial magnetic stimulation for patients with refractory schizophrenia treated with clozapine. Psychiatry Res. Jul 30 2011;188(2):203–207.

53 Saba G, Verdon CM, Kalalou K, *et al.* Transcranial magnetic stimulation in the treatment of schizophrenic symptoms: a double blind sham controlled study. J Psychiatr Res. Mar 2006; 40(2):147–152.

54 Blumberger DM, Christensen BK, Zipursky RB, *et al.* MRI-targeted repetitive transcranial magnetic stimulation of Heschl's gyrus for refractory auditory hallucinations. Brain Stimul. Oct 2012;5:577–585.

55 Slotema CW, Blom JD, de Weijer AD, *et al.* Can low-frequency repetitive transcranial magnetic stimulation really relieve medication-resistant auditory verbal hallucinations? Negative results from a large randomized controlled trial. Biol Psychiatry. Mar 1 2011;69(5):450–456.

56 Aleman A, Sommer IE, Kahn RS. Efficacy of slow repetitive transcranial magnetic stimulation in the treatment of resistant auditory hallucinations in schizophrenia: a meta-analysis. J Clin Psychiatry. Mar 2007;68(3):416–421.

57 Tranulis C, Sepehry AA, Galinowski A, Stip E. Should we treat auditory hallucinations with repetitive transcranial magnetic stimulation? A metaanalysis. Can J Psychiatry. Sep 2008; 53(9):577–586.

58 Slotema CW, Blom JD, van Lutterveld R, Hoek HW, Sommer IE. Review of the efficacy of transcranial magnetic stimulation for auditory verbal hallucinations. Biol Psychiatry. Jul 15 2014;76(2):101–110.

59 Marras A, Pallanti S. Transcranial magnetic stimulation for the treatment of pharmacoresistant nondelusional auditory verbal hallucinations in dementia. Case Rep Psychiatry. 2013; 2013:930304.

60 Dollfus S, Larmurier-Montagne A, Razafimandimby A, *et al.* Treatment of auditory hallucinations by combining high-frequency repetitive transcranial magnetic stimulation and functional magnetic resonance imaging. Schizophr Res. Jul 2008;102(1–3):348–351.

61 Montagne-Larmurier A, Etard O, Razafimandimby A, Morello R, Dollfus S. Two-day treatment of auditory hallucinations by high frequency rTMS guided by cerebral imaging: a 6 month follow-up pilot study. Schizophr Res. Aug 2009;113(1): 77–83.

62 Schonfeldt-Lecuona C, Gron G, Walter H, *et al.* Stereotaxic rTMS for the treatment of auditory hallucinations in schizophrenia. Neuroreport. Jul 19 2004;15(10):1669–1673.

63 Sommer IE, de Weijer AD, Daalman K, *et al.* Can fMRI-guidance improve the efficacy of rTMS treatment for auditory verbal hallucinations? Schizophr Res. Jul 2007;93(1–3):406–408.

64 Hoffman RE, Hampson M, Wu K, *et al.* Probing the pathophysiology of auditory/verbal hallucinations by combining functional magnetic resonance imaging and transcranial magnetic stimulation. Cereb Cortex. Feb 13 2007;17: 2733–2743.

65 Schulz T, Berger C, Krecklow B, *et al.* Repetitive transcranial magnetic stimulation (rTMS) in schizophrenia with treatment-refractory auditory hallucinations and major self-mutilation. J Neural Transm. Jan 8 2014. [Epub ahead of print]

66 Hoffman RE, Gueorguieva R, Hawkins KA, *et al.* Temporoparietal transcranial magnetic stimulation for auditory hallucinations: safety, efficacy and moderators in a fifty patient sample. Biol Psychiatry. Jul 15 2005;58(2):97–104.

67 Fitzgerald PB, Benitez J, Daskalakis ZJ, De Castella A, Kulkarni J. The treatment of recurring auditory hallucinations in schizophrenia with rTMS. World J Biol Psychiatry. 2006;7(2):119–122.

68 Poulet E, Brunelin J, Kallel L, *et al.* Is rTMS efficient as a maintenance treatment for auditory verbal hallucinations? A case report. Schizophr Res. May 2006;84(1):183–184.
69 Thirthalli J, Bharadwaj B, Kulkarni S, Gangadhar BN, Kharawala S, Andrade C. Successful use of maintenance rTMS for 8 months in a patient with antipsychotic-refractory auditory hallucinations. Schizophr Res. Mar 2008;100(1–3):351–352.
70 Poulet E, Brunelin J, Kallel L, D'Amato T, Saoud M. Maintenance treatment with transcranial magnetic stimulation in a patient with late-onset schizophrenia. Am J Psychiatry. Apr 2008;165(4):537–538.
71 Huang YZ, Edwards MJ, Rounis E, Bhatia KP, Rothwell JC. Theta burst stimulation of the human motor cortex. Neuron. Jan 20 2005; 45(2):201–206.
72 Kindler J, Homan P, Flury R, Strik W, Dierks T, Hubl D. Theta burst transcranial magnetic stimulation for the treatment of auditory verbal hallucinations: results of a randomized controlled study. Psychiatry Res. Aug 30 2013;209(1): 114–117.
73 Garg S, Goyal N, Tikka SK, Sinha VK. Exacerbation of auditory verbal hallucinations with adjunctive high-frequency cerebellar vermal repetitive transcranial magnetic stimulation in schizophrenia: a case report. J ECT. Mar 2013;29(1):65–66.
74 Barr MS, Fitzgerald PB, Farzan F, George TP, Daskalakis ZJ. Transcranial magnetic stimulation to understand the pathophysiology and treatment of substance use disorders. Curr Drug Abuse Rev. Nov 2008;1(3):328–339.
75 Wing VC, Barr MS, Wass CE, *et al.* Brain stimulation methods to treat tobacco addiction. Brain Stimul. May 2013;6(3):221–230.
76 Ziemann U. TMS induced plasticity in human cortex. Rev Neurosci. 2004;15(4):253–266.
77 Burt T, Lisanby SH, Sackeim HA. Neuropsychiatric applications of transcranial magnetic stimulation: a meta analysis. Int J Neuropsychopharmacol. Mar 2002;5(1):73–103.
78 Franklin TR, Wang Z, Wang J, *et al.* Limbic activation to cigarette smoking cues independent of nicotine withdrawal: a perfusion fMRI study. Neuropsychopharmacology. Nov 2007;32(11): 2301–2309.
79 Krain AL, Wilson AM, Arbuckle R, Castellanos FX, Milham MP. Distinct neural mechanisms of risk and ambiguity: a meta-analysis of decision-making. Neuroimage. Aug 1 2006;32(1): 477–484.
80 Bechara A, Damasio AR, Damasio H, Anderson SW. Insensitivity to future consequences following damage to human prefrontal cortex. Cognition. Apr–Jun 1994;50(1–3):7–15.
81 Hayashi MJ, Kanai R, Tanabe HC, *et al.* Interaction of numerosity and time in prefrontal and parietal cortex. J Neurosci. Jan 16 2013;33(3):883–893.
82 Goldstein RZ, Volkow ND. Dysfunction of the prefrontal cortex in addiction: neuroimaging findings and clinical implications. Nat Rev Neurosci. Nov 2011;12(11):652–669.
83 Erhardt A, Sillaber I, Welt T, Muller MB, Singewald N, Keck ME. Repetitive transcranial magnetic stimulation increases the release of dopamine in the nucleus accumbens shell of morphine-sensitized rats during abstinence. Neuropsychopharmacology. Nov 2004;29(11): 2074–2080.
84 Ko JH, Monchi O, Ptito A, Bloomfield P, Houle S, Strafella AP. Theta burst stimulation-induced inhibition of dorsolateral prefrontal cortex reveals hemispheric asymmetry in striatal dopamine release during a set-shifting task: a TMS-[(11)C]raclopride PET study. Eur J Neurosci. Nov 2008;28(10):2147–2155.
85 Cho SS, Strafella AP. rTMS of the left dorsolateral prefrontal cortex modulates dopamine release in the ipsilateral anterior cingulate cortex and orbitofrontal cortex. PLoS One. 2009;4(8):e6725.
86 Johann MWR, Kharraz A, Bobbe G, *et al.* Repetitive transcranial magnetic stimulation in nicotine dependence. Psychiatr Prax. May 2003;30(Suppl 2):129–131.
87 Eichhammer P, Johann M, Kharraz A, *et al.* High-frequency repetitive transcranial magnetic stimulation decreases cigarette smoking. J Clin Psychiatry. Aug 2003;64(8):951–953.
88 Amiaz R, Levy D, Vainiger D, Grunhaus L, Zangen A. Repeated high-frequency transcranial magnetic stimulation over the dorsolateral prefrontal cortex reduces cigarette craving and consumption. Addiction. Apr 2009;104(4): 653–660.

89 Li X, Hartwell KJ, Owens M, *et al.* Repetitive transcranial magnetic stimulation of the dorsolateral prefrontal cortex reduces nicotine cue craving. Biol Psychiatry. Apr 15 2013;73(8): 714–720.

90 Knott VJ. Electroencephalographic characterization of cigarette smoking behavior. Alcohol. Jun 2001;24(2):95–97.

91 Pripfl J, Neumann R, Kohler U, Lamm C. Effects of transcranial direct current stimulation on risky decision making are mediated by 'hot' and 'cold' decisions, personality, and hemisphere. Eur J Neurosci. Dec 2013;38(12):3778–3785.

92 Wing VC, Bacher I, Wu BS, Daskalakis ZJ, George TP. High frequency repetitive transcranial magnetic stimulation reduces tobacco craving in schizophrenia. Schizophr Res. Aug 2012;139(1–3):264–266.

93 Prikryl R, Ustohal L, Kucerova HP, *et al.* Repetitive transcranial magnetic stimulation reduces cigarette consumption in schizophrenia patients. Prog Neuropsychopharmacol Biol Psychiatry. Mar 3 2014;49:30–35.

94 Rose JE, McClernon FJ, Froeliger B, Behm FM, Preud'homme X, Krystal AD. Repetitive transcranial magnetic stimulation of the superior frontal gyrus modulates craving for cigarettes. Biol Psychiatry. Oct 15 2011;70(8):794–799.

95 Camprodon JA, Martinez-Raga J, Alonso-Alonso M, Shih MC, Pascual-Leone A. One session of high frequency repetitive transcranial magnetic stimulation (rTMS) to the right prefrontal cortex transiently reduces cocaine craving. Drug Alcohol Depend. Jan 5 2007; 86(1):91–94.

96 Politi E, Fauci E, Santoro A, Smeraldi E. Daily sessions of transcranial magnetic stimulation to the left prefrontal cortex gradually reduce cocaine craving. Am J Addict. Jul–Aug 2008; 17(4):345–346.

97 Slamberova R, Hruba L, Matejovska I, Bernaskova K, Rokyta R. Increased seizure susceptibility induced by prenatal methamphetamine exposure in adult female rats is not affected by early postnatal cross-fostering. Epilepsy Behav. Jan 2011;20(1):6–11.

98 Mishra BR, Nizamie SH, Das B, Praharaj SK. Efficacy of repetitive transcranial magnetic stimulation in alcohol dependence: a sham-controlled study. Addiction. Jan 2010;105(1):49–55.

99 Herremans SC, Baeken C, Vanderbruggen N, *et al.* No influence of one right-sided prefrontal HF-rTMS session on alcohol craving in recently detoxified alcohol-dependent patients: results of a naturalistic study. Drug Alcohol Depend. Jan 1 2012;120(1–3):209–213.

100 Hoppner J, Broese T, Wendler L, Berger C, Thome J. Repetitive transcranial magnetic stimulation (rTMS) for treatment of alcohol dependence. World J Biol Psychiatry. Sep 2011;12(Suppl 1):57–62.

101 Berger W, Mendlowicz MV, Marques-Portella C, *et al.* Pharmacologic alternatives to antidepressants in posttraumatic stress disorder: a systematic review. Prog Neuropsychopharmacol Biol Psychiatry. Mar 17 2009; 33(2):169–180.

102 McCann UD, Kimbrell TA, Morgan CM, *et al.* Repetitive transcranial magnetic stimulation for posttraumatic stress disorder. Arch Gen Psychiatry. Mar 1998;55(3):276–279.

103 Tillman GD, Kimbrell TA, Calley CS, Kraut MA, Freeman TW, Hart J, Jr. Repetitive transcranial magnetic stimulation and threat memory: selective reduction of combat threat memory p300 response after right frontal-lobe stimulation. J Neuropsychiatry Clin Neurosci. Winter 2011;23(1):40–47.

104 Grisaru N, Amir M, Cohen H, Kaplan Z. Effect of transcranial magnetic stimulation in posttraumatic stress disorder: a preliminary study. Biol Psychiatry. Jul 1 1998;44(1):52–55.

105 Nakama H, Garcia A, O'Brien K, Ellis N. Case report of a 24-year-old man with resolution of treatment-resistant major depressive disorder and comorbid PTSD using rTMS. J ECT. Mar 2014;30(1):e9–e10.

106 Rosenberg PB, Mehndiratta RB, Mehndiratta YP, Wamer A, Rosse RB, Balish M. Repetitive transcranial magnetic stimulation treatment of comorbid posttraumatic stress disorder and major depression. J Neuropsychiatry Clin Neurosci. Summer 2002;14(3):270–276.

107 Cohen H, Kaplan Z, Kotler M, Kouperman I, Moisa R, Grisaru N. Repetitive transcranial magnetic stimulation of the right dorsolateral prefrontal cortex in posttraumatic stress disorder: a double-blind, placebo-controlled study. Am J Psychiatry. Mar 2004;161(3): 515–524.

108 Osuch EA, Benson BE, Luckenbaugh DA, Geraci M, Post RM, McCann U. Repetitive TMS combined with exposure therapy for PTSD: a preliminary study. J Anxiety Disord. Jan 2009;23(1):54–59.
109 Watts BV, Landon B, Groft A, Young-Xu Y. A sham controlled study of repetitive transcranial magnetic stimulation for posttraumatic stress disorder. Brain Stimul. Jan 2012; 5(1):38–43.
110 Nam DH, Pae CU, Chae JH. Low-frequency, repetitive transcranial magnetic stimulation for the treatment of patients with posttraumatic stress disorder: a double-blind, sham-controlled study. Clin Psychopharmacol Neurosci. Aug 2013;11(2):96–102.
111 Boggio PS, Rocha M, Oliveira MO, *et al.* Noninvasive brain stimulation with high-frequency and low-intensity repetitive transcranial magnetic stimulation treatment for posttraumatic stress disorder. J Clin Psychiatry. Aug 2010;71(8):992–999.
112 Karsen EF, Watts BV, Holtzheimer PE. Review of the effectiveness of transcranial magnetic stimulation for post-traumatic stress disorder. Brain Stimul. March–April 2014;7(2):151–157.
113 Roth Y, Zangen A, Hallett M. A coil design for transcranial magnetic stimulation of deep brain regions. J Clin Neurophysiol. Aug 2002;19(4):361–370.
114 Isserles M, Shalev AY, Roth Y, *et al.* Effectiveness of deep transcranial magnetic stimulation combined with a brief exposure procedure in post-traumatic stress disorder – a pilot study. Brain Stimul. May 2013;6(3):377–383.
115 Rougemont-Bucking A, Linnman C, Zeffiro TA, *et al.* Altered processing of contextual information during fear extinction in PTSD: an fMRI study. CNS Neurosci Ther. Aug 2011;17(4):227–236.
116 Andrade C, Radhakrishnan R. The prevention and treatment of cognitive decline and dementia: an overview of recent research on experimental treatments. Indian J Psychiatry. Jan 2009;51(1):12–25.
117 Daviglus ML, Bell CC, Berrettini W, *et al.* NIH state-of-the-science conference statement: preventing Alzheimer's disease and cognitive decline. NIH Consens State Sci Statements. Apr 28 2010;27(4):1–30.
118 Sole-Padulles C, Bartres-Faz D, Junque C, *et al.* Repetitive transcranial magnetic stimulation effects on brain function and cognition among elders with memory dysfunction. A randomized sham-controlled study. Cereb Cortex. Oct 2006;16(10):1487–1493.
119 Cotelli M, Calabria M, Manenti R, *et al.* Brain stimulation improves associative memory in an individual with amnestic mild cognitive impairment. Neurocase. Jun 2012;18(3): 217–223.
120 Turriziani P, Smirni D, Oliveri M, Semenza C, Cipolotti L. The role of the prefrontal cortex in familiarity and recollection processes during verbal and non-verbal recognition memory: an rTMS study. Neuroimage. Aug 1 2010; 52(1):348–357.
121 Turriziani P, Smirni D, Zappala G, Mangano GR, Oliveri M, Cipolotti L. Enhancing memory performance with rTMS in healthy subjects and individuals with mild cognitive impairment: the role of the right dorsolateral prefrontal cortex. Front Hum Neurosci. 2012;6:62.
122 Cotelli M, Manenti R, Cappa SF, *et al.* Effect of transcranial magnetic stimulation on action naming in patients with Alzheimer disease. Arch Neurol. Nov 2006;63(11):1602–1604.
123 Cotelli M, Manenti R, Cappa SF, Zanetti O, Miniussi C. Transcranial magnetic stimulation improves naming in Alzheimer disease patients at different stages of cognitive decline. Eur J Neurol. Dec 2008;15(12):1286–1292.
124 Haffen E, Chopard G, Pretalli JB, *et al.* A case report of daily left prefrontal repetitive transcranial magnetic stimulation (rTMS) as an adjunctive treatment for Alzheimer disease. Brain Stimul. Jul 2012;5(3):264–266.
125 Cotelli M, Calabria M, Manenti R, *et al.* Improved language performance in Alzheimer disease following brain stimulation. J Neurol Neurosurg Psychiatry. Jul 2011;82(7): 794–797.
126 Rabey JM, Dobronevsky E, Aichenbaum S, Gonen O, Marton RG, Khaigrekht M. Repetitive transcranial magnetic stimulation combined with cognitive training is a safe and effective modality for the treatment of Alzheimer's disease: a randomized, double-blind study. J Neural Transm. May 2013; 120(5):813–819.

127 Bentwich J, Dobronevsky E, Aichenbaum S, *et al.* Beneficial effect of repetitive transcranial magnetic stimulation combined with cognitive training for the treatment of Alzheimer's disease: a proof of concept study. J Neural Transm. Mar 2011;118(3):463–471.
128 Ahmed MA, Darwish ES, Khedr EM, El Serogy YM, Ali AM. Effects of low versus high frequencies of repetitive transcranial magnetic stimulation on cognitive function and cortical excitability in Alzheimer's dementia. J Neurol. Jan 2012;259(1):83–92.
129 Greenberg BD, George MS, Martin JD, *et al.* Effect of prefrontal repetitive transcranial magnetic stimulation in obsessive-compulsive disorder: a preliminary study. Am J Psychiatry. Jun 1997;154(6):867–869.
130 Sachdev PS, McBride R, Loo CK, Mitchell PB, Malhi GS, Croker VM. Right versus left prefrontal transcranial magnetic stimulation for obsessive-compulsive disorder: a preliminary investigation. J Clin Psychiatry. Dec 2001; 62(12):981–984.
131 Mansur CG, Myczkowki ML, de Barros Cabral S, *et al.* Placebo effect after prefrontal magnetic stimulation in the treatment of resistant obsessive-compulsive disorder: a randomized controlled trial. Int J Neuropsychopharmacol. Nov 2011;14(10):1389–1397.
132 Sachdev PS, Loo CK, Mitchell PB, McFarquhar TF, Malhi GS. Repetitive transcranial magnetic stimulation for the treatment of obsessive compulsive disorder: a double-blind controlled investigation. Psychol Med. Nov 2007; 37(11):1645–1649.
133 Sarkhel S, Sinha VK, Praharaj SK. Adjunctive high-frequency right prefrontal repetitive transcranial magnetic stimulation (rTMS) was not effective in obsessive-compulsive disorder but improved secondary depression. J Anxiety Disord. Jun 2010;24(5):535–539.
134 Prasko J, Paskova B, Zalesky R, *et al.* The effect of repetitive transcranial magnetic stimulation (rTMS) on symptoms in obsessive compulsive disorder. A randomized, double blind, sham controlled study. Neuro Endocrinol Lett. Jun 2006;27(3):327–332.
135 Alonso P, Pujol J, Cardoner N, *et al.* Right prefrontal repetitive transcranial magnetic stimulation in obsessive-compulsive disorder: a double-blind, placebo-controlled study. Am J Psychiatry. Jul 2001;158(7):1143–1145.
136 Ma X, Huang Y, Liao L, Jin Y. A randomized double-blinded sham-controlled trial of alpha electroencephalogram-guided transcranial magnetic stimulation for obsessive-compulsive disorder. Chin Med J (Engl). 2014;127(4): 601–606.
137 Mantovani A, Lisanby SH, Pieraccini F, Ulivelli M, Castrogiovanni P, Rossi S. Repetitive transcranial magnetic stimulation (rTMS) in the treatment of obsessive-compulsive disorder (OCD) and Tourette's syndrome (TS). Int J Neuropsychopharmacol. Feb 2006;9(1):95–100.
138 Kumar N, Chadda RK. Augmentation effect of repetitive transcranial magnetic stimulation over the supplementary motor cortex in treatment refractory patients with obsessive compulsive disorder. Indian J Psychiatry. Oct 2011;53(4):340–342.
139 Kang JI, Kim CH, Namkoong K, Lee CI, Kim SJ. A randomized controlled study of sequentially applied repetitive transcranial magnetic stimulation in obsessive-compulsive disorder. J Clin Psychiatry. Dec 2009;70(12):1645–1651.
140 Mantovani A, Simpson HB, Fallon BA, Rossi S, Lisanby SH. Randomized sham-controlled trial of repetitive transcranial magnetic stimulation in treatment-resistant obsessive-compulsive disorder. Int J Neuropsychopharmacol. Mar 2010;13(2):217–227.
141 Gomes PV, Brasil-Neto JP, Allam N, Rodrigues de Souza E. A randomized, double-blind trial of repetitive transcranial magnetic stimulation in obsessive-compulsive disorder with three-month follow-up. J Neuropsychiatry Clin Neurosci. Fall 2012;24(4):437–443.
142 Ruffini C, Locatelli M, Lucca A, Benedetti F, Insacco C, Smeraldi E. Augmentation effect of repetitive transcranial magnetic stimulation over the orbitofrontal cortex in drug-resistant obsessive-compulsive disorder patients: a controlled investigation. Prim Care Companion J Clin Psychiatry. 2009;11(5):226–230.
143 Berlim MT, Neufeld NH, Van den Eynde F. Repetitive transcranial magnetic stimulation (rTMS) for obsessive-compulsive disorder (OCD): an exploratory meta-analysis of randomized and sham-controlled trials. J Psychiatr Res. Aug 2013;47(8):999–1006.

CHAPTER 11

Direct current stimulation: Introduction and technical aspects

André Russowsky Brunoni[1] and Felipe Fregni[2]

[1] *University of São Paulo, São Paulo, Brazil*

[2] *Spaulding Rehabilitation Hospital, Harvard Medical School, Boston, USA*

Introduction

'Transcranial direct current stimulation' (tDCS), once referred to as brain polarization or DC polarization, is one of the many techniques of transcranial electric stimulation (TES), which also encompasses transcranial alternating current stimulation, transcranial random noise stimulation, cranial electrical stimulation or transcranial pulse current stimulation and others (for a review, see Guleyupoglu *et al.* [1]). The modern nomenclature of 'TES' excludes other forms of brain stimulation such as electroconvulsive therapy (ECT) and repetitive transcranial magnetic stimulation (rTMS). TES techniques are characterized by delivering weak electric currents (usually between 1 and 2 mA) to the brain applied transcranially through two or more electrodes over the scalp. TES techniques are not neurostimulation methods (in comparison to rTMS and ECT) as they do not directly generate action potentials and depolarize cortical neurons; rather, these are neuromodulatory techniques that modify net cortical excitability according to the parameters of stimulation. tDCS differs from other TES techniques due to its technical aspects, being characterized by the application of a direct, usually constant current in the form of an uninterrupted, unidirectional current flow [1–3].

From a clinical and research perspective, tDCS is currently the most investigated TES technique, drawing attention from basic and clinical investigators due to some of its characteristics such as the non-invasive delivery of relatively potent neuromodulatory effects, affordability, ease of use, low rate of adverse effects and its potentially unique mechanism of action that may allow its use in combination with behavioural techniques to enhance learning [4]. In this chapter, we will review the main technological and mechanistic aspects of this technique.

Historical remarks

The use of electrical currents to stimulate the brain is not new. Reports of discharging electric currents over the brain to achieve therapeutic effects are found more than 2000 years ago – for instance, Scribonius Largus, a physician from the Roman Empire, anecdotally reported how placing a live electric ray ('torpedo fish') over the scalp to deliver a strong electric current could ameliorate a headache in his medical textbook *Compositiones Medicae* [5]. In the 11th century, the physician Ibn-Sidah suggested using a live electric

Neuromodulation in Psychiatry, First Edition. Edited by Clement Hamani, Paul Holtzheimer, Andres M. Lozano and Helen Mayberg.

catfish for the treatment of epilepsy [6]. Given the difficulties to manipulate electrical currents and also lack of reporting, no significant advances were made in this area until the 18th century.

From the late 18th century onwards, with the development of the 'voltaic' electric battery, it was possible to control the electric discharge and, therefore, more researchers started to investigate the role of electricity in biological tissues and living animals. Galvani, for instance, demonstrated muscle contractions from the leg of a frog after an electric discharge [6]. Later on, Aldini described the successful treatment of a patient with melancholia after several days of stimulation with a voltaic pile. Aldini also discharged potent electric currents over a dead body, provoking intense contractions in the corpse [6]. His experiment later inspired Mary Shelley in her famous novel, 'Frankenstein'.

From 1800 to the 1950s, there are numerous reports of using electric currents over the brain (directly or transcranially), with mixed results (for a review, see Zago *et al.* [6]). In fact, systematic research on non-invasive and invasive brain stimulation only started in the end of the first half of the 20th century, with the development of ECT by Ugo Cerletti and Lucino Bini, the neurosurgeries performed by William Penfield and the experiments of Purpura and McMurtry [7] showing neuromodulatory effects of electric stimulation in the neurons of cats, as discussed below.

In the 1950s and 1960s, several clinical experiments tested the use of direct current stimulation for the treatment of psychiatric conditions. During this period, most of the reports called this method as brain polarization. In fact, these initial studies with brain polarization gave the initial results to support the contemporary tDCS methods. At least two randomized clinical trials and four open-label trials were performed during this time period for the treatment of depression, achieving initially positive but overall mixed results (for a review, see Nitsche *et al.* [8]). In fact, brain polarization was largely forgotten as a therapeutic strategy between 1970 and 2000 for several reasons such as the stigma associated with ECT and the 'golden age' of psychopharmacotherapy in terms of clinical practice and research. The reappraisal of brain polarization with novel changes in its use gave the birth of the redesigned tDCS method after the seminal studies of Priori *et al.* [9] and Nitsche and Paulus [10] who were able to demonstrate that weak, direct electric currents delivered to the brain via two electrodes positioned over the scalp effectively induced polarity-dependent changes in cortical excitability, which is, respectively, increased and decreased by anodal and cathodal stimulation, as discussed below. In fact, contemporary use of tDCS is marked by a rigorous scientific validation and testing using, in most of the studies, neurophysiological methods to further develop this technique.

Technical aspects

The tDCS device has four main components: (i) two electrodes (anode and cathode), (ii) one ampere-meter (that measures the intensity of the electric current), (iii) a variable resistor (to maintain the electric current fixed at the desired intensity) and (iv) batteries. Figure 11.1 depicts two standard tDCS devices used in research settings.

Although most tDCS studies employ only one anode and one cathode, novel studies increasingly investigate variations of tDCS by changing electrode set-up. One of them is the 4X1 tDCS method, also called as 'high-definition' tDCS (HD-tDCS), in which one large electrode is placed in the centre and four smaller electrodes are placed at the edges [11].

The location of the electrodes is determined by the brain area involved with the behaviour that is being investigated. For instance, some studies describe the anode as the 'active' (or

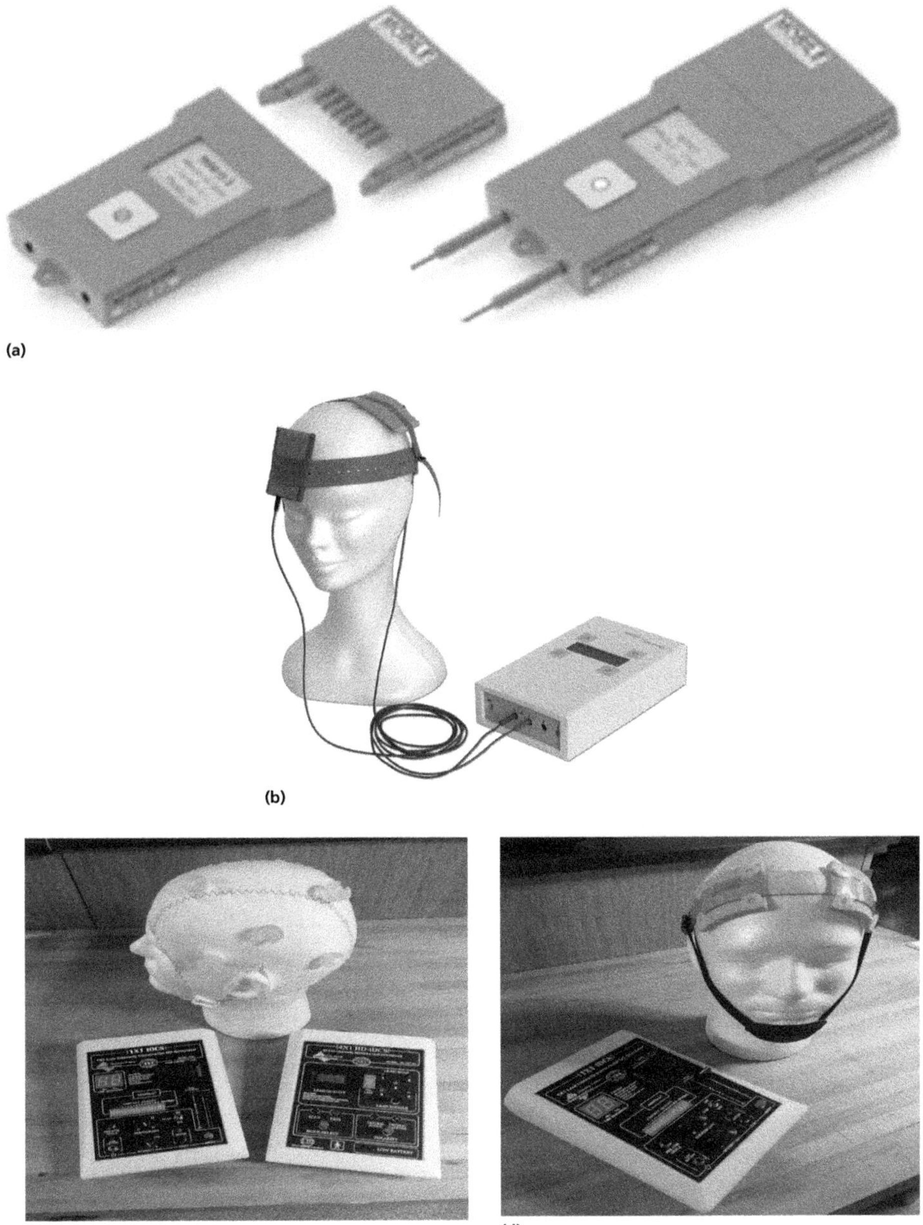

Figure 11.1 Examples of commercial tDCS devices. All devices are composed by a power generator (batteries) and electrodes that are placed over the scalp. (**a**) 'Mobile' tDCS device of Neuroconn™ DC-stimulator, presenting increased portability, due to its low size. (**b**) Neuroconn™ device, one 'standard' tDCS device used in clinical research. The electrodes and the sponges placed over the scalp are illustrated. (**c**) Soterix™ 1-1 and 4×1 (high-definition) tDCS devices, also 'standard' tDCS devices used in clinical research. (**d**) Soterix™ device with EASYstraps™ (headbands) and EASYpads™ (sponges). Source: Reproduced with permission of neuroConn and Copyright Soterix Medical. (*See insert for colour representation of the figure.*)

'stimulating') and the cathode as the 'reference' (or 'neutral') electrode. Nonetheless, such terms should not be used as both electrodes present neuromodulatory effects. In fact, researchers should only use these terms to emphasize that, in their particular montage, one electrode is used as 'active' and the other as 'reference'. Other inaccurate terms are 'unipolar' and 'bipolar' montages to describe when one or two electrodes are placed over the scalp, respectively. As the DC stimulations always generate a dipole (i.e. there are two poles) between electrodes, better terms would be, for instance, 'mono-cephalic' and 'bi-cephalic'.

Electrode positioning

The site of placement of the electrodes is determined by the brain area that the researcher wants to investigate. This rule is valid even considering that the technique of tDCS is relatively non-focal – for instance, anodal tDCS over the occipital cortex does not exert antidepressant effects [12] whereas phosphene visualization only occurs during anodal tDCS over the visual cortex [13]. Electrode placement is usually described according to the 10/20 EEG international system.

Also, tDCS is a polarity-dependent neuromodulatory technique, in which, usually, the anode increases and the cathode decreases local cortical excitability. However, such rule is not universally valid, especially when considering the neuromodulation of non-motor areas, such as the prefrontal cortex. For instance, Jacobson *et al.* [14], in a meta-analysis of motor and cognitive studies using tDCS, showed that the effects of 'anodal-excitation/cathodal-inhibition' were observed when evaluating motor cortical excitability, but were not replicated when tDCS was applied in non-motor areas, such as the prefrontal cortex, when cognitive functions were explored – specifically, cathodal stimulation rarely caused an inhibition of the function. The authors discussed that compensation processes by other brain networks could explain the lack of inhibitory cathodal effects, as cognitive functions encompass several brain networks.

Finally, the term 'mono-cephalic' is used when only one electrode (either the anode or the cathode) is positioned over the scalp (the other being positioned in an extra-cephalic position, usually over the deltoid muscle). In contrast, the term 'bi-cephalic' is used when both electrodes are placed over the scalp [3]. Choosing the position of both electrodes is important; changing either's position can fundamentally modify the stimulation effect. For instance, it has been shown that changing the reference electrode from a cephalic position to an extra-cephalic position modified significantly induced current fields and abolished clinical effects [15].

Parameters associated with tDCS effects

The 'dose' of a tDCS session is determined by the following factors: (i) the size of the electrodes, (ii) the current intensity, (iii) the duration of the sessions and (iv) the total number of sessions (and the interval between them).

- **a** Size – The electrodes usually measure 25–35 cm^2 (5 × 5 to 5 × 7 cm) in size. Larger electrodes make the stimulus less focal; conversely, smaller electrodes increase the focality of the stimulus [16, 17].
- **b** Electric current intensity – the earlier tDCS studies used low current intensities of 0.5 mA [9, 10], whereas most tDCS studies and clinical trials currently apply higher doses in the range of 1–2 mA [18]. As the electrode size varies between 25 and 35 cm^2, the current density is in the range of 0.4–0.8 A/m^2. Electric currents lower than 0.5 mA do not seem to exert neuromodulatory effects, especially when applied for a short period of time [10]; in turn, current doses between 1.5 and 2 mA are often perceived by the subject, and doses greater than 2 mA might be perceived as painful or

exceedingly uncomfortable by participants. Higher electric currents seem to be associated with higher current densities at a fixed target point in the brain, although such a relationship is nonlinear [19]. However, it is unclear whether higher doses are associated with an increased impact on neuroplasticity. Some studies have shown greater cognitive improvement with higher current doses [20, 21], whereas recent meta-analyses did not show intensity-dependent effects of tDCS in cognitive tDCS studies [14] and in clinical trials of tDCS for depression [22].

c Duration of the tDCS session – the length of a tDCS session varies between 5 and 35 min. As the applied current is constant during virtually the entire session (excluding the relatively brief fade-in and fade-out phases), it is possible to estimate the applied electric current according to the formula:

$Q = i * t$, where Q is the current charge, in coulombs (C), i is the current intensity (A) and t is the time (s)

Both maximum 'safe' time period that tDCS can be applied and the optimal time period for clinical efficacy are not yet established. For practical purposes, tDCS sessions lasting more than 30 min are undesirable in both cognitive studies (as longer stimulation periods could increase fatigue and compromise performance in cognitive tasks) and clinical trials, in which patients should return to receive tDCS for several days consecutively.

d Total number and interval between sessions – in neuropsychological studies tDCS is usually applied two or three times only (anodal, cathodal and sham sessions). Such studies are designed to address mechanistic questions and usually do not aim to evaluate the cumulative effects of tDCS. Therefore, these studies usually employ a 2- to 7-day interval between two tDCS sessions. In clinical trials, the aim is to induce tDCS cumulative effects, and therefore tDCS is applied once to twice daily for several days, excluding weekends (for a review, see [23]). For instance, in clinical studies, most studies for major depression [24–26] applied tDCS once a day for 10–15 days. On the other hand, the largest randomized clinical trial using tDCS for schizophrenia used two sessions per day, for five consecutive days [27]. Further studies are warranted to elucidate the optimal interval between tDCS sessions, as well as to explore how long the effects of tDCS endure after several tDCS sessions.

Safety and contraindications

There are few contraindications for tDCS. As the electrodes are placed over the skin, they should not be placed directly above areas of impaired skin (including areas with chronic skin diseases) to avoid skin damage and skin burn. Also, tDCS should not be applied directly over areas with implanted metallic plates, to avoid heating and shunting over this area. For patients with a history of previous neurosurgical procedures, neurologic malformations or brain neoplasias, tDCS can be modelled individually – using high-definition, computational forward models – to correctly and optimally predict the brain area that will receive most of the electrical current [28]. Likewise, the use of tDCS in special populations such as children and pregnant women should be carefully stipulated, as discussed below. Finally, there are no data that support the use of tDCS beyond the standard parameters used in research settings, that is, tDCS sessions are not usually performed in clinical settings in the following situations: (i) more than twice daily, (ii) for more than 30 min per day or (iii) using current densities above $0.125\,A/m^2$ [2, 3].

Mechanisms of action of tDCS

As described, tDCS is unique regarding other forms of non-invasive brain stimulation such as rTMS as it does not elicit neuronal firing by suprathreshold neuronal membrane depolarization but rather modulates spontaneous neuronal network activity [2, 29]. At the neuronal level, the primary mechanism of action is a polarity-dependent shift (polarization) on resting membrane potential, with anodal tDCS stimulation generally enhancing cortical activity and excitability, and cathodal tDCS stimulation having opposite effects [10]. Nonetheless, the effects of tDCS on neuronal processing are much more complex [30], and might even invert according to stimulation intensity and the nature of ongoing activity [31]. The exact mechanisms of action of tDCS are indeed still elusive;, nonetheless, it is known that tDCS produces a low-intensity electric field (<1 V/m) [32] in the brain leading to small changes (<1 mV) [33] in the membrane potential. In fact, early animal studies have shown that changes in excitability are reflected in both spontaneous firing rates [34, 35] and responsiveness to afferent synaptic inputs [36, 37].

Moreover, tDCS elicits after-effects lasting for up to 1 h [38, 39], suggesting that it not only involves electric changes in membrane potential but also modifies the synaptic microenvironment, for instance, by altering the activity of gamma-aminobutyric acid-ergic (GABAergic) neurons or enhancing the synaptic strength of *N*-methyl-D-aspartate receptor (NMDA)-dependent receptors [40–42]. tDCS also interferes with brain excitability via modulation of intracortical and corticospinal neurons [43, 44]. Moreover, although most early tDCS studies have been performed in the motor cortex, tDCS not only induce long-lasting alterations of motor-evoked potentials (MEPs) but also affects somatosensory and visual-evoked potentials. This activity is dependent on the area stimulated [45–47]. Ferrucci *et al.* [48] and Galea *et al.* [49] provided evidence that tDCS can also influence the human cerebellum. Cogiamanian *et al.* [50] and Winkler *et al.* [51] demonstrated that transcutaneous DC stimulation modulates conduction along the spinal cord and the segmental reflex pathways.

The effects of direct current stimulation promotes brain-derived neurotrophic factor (BDNF)-dependent synaptic plasticity, as shown by one recent animal study that applied anodal motor cortex stimulation and showed a lasting increase in postsynaptic excitatory potentials and also in BDNF [52]. The effects of tDCS might also be non-synaptic, perhaps involving transient changes in the density of protein channels localized below the stimulating electrode, as suggested by experiments with spinal cord [50] and peripheral nerve [44]. Finally, considering that a constant electric field displaces all polar molecules and most of the neurotransmitters and receptors in the brain have electrical properties, tDCS might also influence neuronal function by inducing neurochemical changes [53]. For instance, magnetic resonance spectroscopy showed that, after anodal, tDCS brain myoinositol significantly increased, whereas *n*-acetyl-aspartate failed to change [54].

tDCS also exerts 'indirect' effects, as observed in studies showing connectivity-driven alterations of distant cortical and subcortical areas [55, 56]. Interestingly, tDCS modulates not only single neuron activity and evoked neuronal activity but also spontaneous neuronal oscillations. Animal and modelling studies suggest that a network of tightly coupled active neurons (e.g. oscillations) may be more sensitive to applied weak current than neurons in isolation [57–59].

To conclude, although the mechanisms of action of tDCS are still elusive, it is known that these mechanisms likely involve different synaptic and non-synaptic effects on neurons and effects on non-neuronal cells and tissues within the central nervous system that are also associated with a temporal effect. By understanding these effects, it is possible to design more effective protocols of stimulation to induce the optimal behavioural modulation and also to understand further brain–behaviour relationships.

Electrophysiological studies

Nitsche and Paulus [10] demonstrated, in a seminal study, that weak, direct electric currents applied through the scalp was able to potently modulate motor cortical excitability for a short period of time beyond the period of stimulation. In several experimental studies, 10–19 healthy subjects underwent anodal or cathodal stimulation over the motor cortex using different current intensities (from 0.2 to 1 mA) and periods of stimulation (from 1 to 5 min). Although the author found that stimulations lasting less than 3 min or using less than 0.6 mA were physiologically inert in terms of changing motor cortical excitability, they observed that a single 5-min, 1 mA tDCS session exerted polarity-dependent effects in cortical excitability; that is, after anodal stimulation, motor cortical excitability increased, whereas it decreased after cathodal stimulation (Figure 11.2). To measure motor cortical excitability, the authors measured the amplitude of the MEP obtained from the resting motor threshold of the individuals. Therefore, after anodal stimulation the MEPs were larger, and after cathodal stimulation the MEPs were smaller.

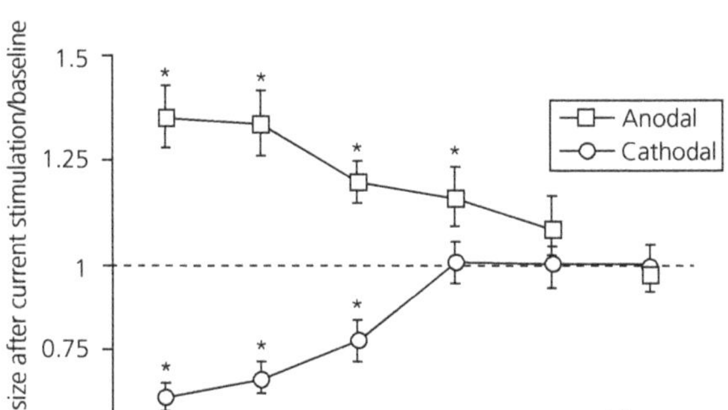

Figure 11.2 Polarity-dependent effects of tDCS. The picture illustrates an increase in cortical excitability after anodal stimulation and a decrease of cortical excitability after cathodal stimulation. Source: From Nitsche and Paulus [10]. Reproduced with permission of Wiley.

Subsequent studies by this group verified that longer stimulation periods would induce even larger neuromodulatory effects beyond the period of stimulation, such as that 13 min of cathodal stimulation would present neuromodulatory effects (also measured by MEPs) for 90 min after the end of the tDCS session [38].

More recent studies by the group of Nitsche and collaborators evaluated the impact of the time interval between two tDCS sessions on motor cortical excitability, as assessed by the changes in MEPs. Monte-Silva *et al.* [60] performed two 9-min tDCS sessions with different time intervals between them – the second session could have been performed immediately (0, 3 or 20 min) or after (3 or 24 h) the first one. The authors observed that when the second tDCS session is performed immediately after the first one, the effects are enhanced; although when it is performed after 3 or 24 h, the effects are attenuated. Possibly, in the first case, the second session occurs when the effects of the first tDCS session are still ongoing, therefore the enhancement, whereas in the latter scenario it is possible that some type of homeostatic attenuation occurs after the first tDCS session, thus decreasing the effects of the second session. Nonetheless, such attenuation was immediate, as the effects of tDCS after 30 min of the end of the session were similar regardless of the time interval between two sessions. Interestingly, in another study from other group, Alonzo *et al.* [61] investigated the effects of daily vs. second daily tDCS on motor cortical excitability finding that tDCS induced greater increases in MEP amplitude when given daily rather than second daily, an effect that reflected greater cumulative effects between sessions rather than a greater response to each individual tDCS session.

Finally, it is important to underscore that the transferability of the findings of these studies, although revealing regarding the mechanisms of action of tDCS, is limited as these studies were conducted in healthy subjects. Other factors such as the underlying neuropsychiatric disorder, the concomitant use of medications and the application of daily tDCS for several days play an important role in clinical studies. In fact, a study in Parkinson's disease has shown that tDCS impact on cortical excitability is fundamentally different than studies in healthy subjects [62].

Pharmacological studies

Several tDCS studies combined techniques of cortical excitability measurement with different pharmacological agents, such as antidepressants, anticonvulsants, antipsychotics and benzodiazepines, to investigate the mechanisms of action of tDCS, as represented in Table 11.1.

Table 11.1 Pharmacological studies with tDCS.

Drug	Effects
Citalopram	Anodal tDCS effects are increased; cathodal inhibitory effects are turned to excitatory effects [63]
Amphetamine	After-effects of anodal tDCS effects are longer [64]
l-DOPA	Cathodal tDCS effects are increased; anodal excitatory effects are turned to inhibitory effects [65]
Pergolide	After-effects of cathodal tDCS are longer [66, 67]
Lorazepam	Anodal effects are initially delayed, but later enhanced and longer [68]
Dextromethorpan	Anodal and cathodal effects are abolished [40, 41]
d-cycloserine	Anodal effects are longer [69]
Carbamazepine	Anodal effects are abolished [40, 41]
Flunarizine	Similar effects than carbamazepine

Source: From Brunoni *et al.* [3]. Reproduced with permission of Elsevier.
tDCS, transcranial direct current stimulation.

On the basis of these studies, it can be shown that the effects of anodal tDCS are complex, encompassing not only neuronal membrane depolarization but also synaptic modulation and inhibitory (GABAergic) interneurons. For instance, calcium-dependent channel blockers (carbamazepine and flunarizine) abolish the effects of anodal tDCS [41], demonstrating that such effects are partly dependent on these channels. Furthermore, glutamatergic, serotonergic and dopaminergic neurotransmitters are also implicated in the mechanisms of action of anodal tDCS. The use of an NMDA-channel blocker (dextromethorphan) and an NMDA agonist (D-cycloserine), respectively, decreases and increases tDCS effects [40, 41]. This suggests that synaptic mechanisms are involved in the effects of anodal tDCS. For the serotoninergic system, the 5-HT reuptake inhibitor citalopram enhances facilitatory plasticity and converts inhibitory plasticity into facilitation [63]. Regarding the dopaminergic system, tDCS plasticity seems to occur in a dose-dependent manner (U curve). Application of L-DOPA converts the cortical excitability enhancement effects of anodal stimulation into inhibition and prolongs the cathodal tDCS inhibitory effects [70]. Furthermore, blocking D_2 receptors seems to abolish tDCS-induced plasticity [16] and D_2 agonists, applied at high or low dosages, decrease plasticity. Moreover, plasticity is restored by medium-dosage D_2 agonists [71].

For cathodal tDCS, the use of calcium and sodium channel blockers does not seem to influence its inhibitory effects. On the other hand, NMDA blockers, similar to their effects with anodal tDCS, abolish cathodal after-effects [53]. Finally, the effects of cathodal tDCS are also related to the GABA system, according to a study using brain spectroscopy showing that GABA levels decrease after cathodal stimulation [42].

Computer-modelling studies

Computer-modelling studies are useful to predict current flow and distribution from the electrodes through the central nervous system.

Computer models are increasingly more complex, taking into consideration gyral and sulcal geometry. High-precision models are based on high-resolution (1 mm or less) anatomical brain scans to acquire precision and accuracy in aspects such as tissue dimensions, inhomogeneity and anisotropy [3].

Computer-modelling studies have suggested, for instance, that electric current can concentrate on the edge of gyri [32], which implies that the effects might not be homogeneous throughout the stimulated area. Increased appreciation of the complexity of current flow through the head (reflecting the complexity of neuro-anatomy) reinforces the utility of applying computational models to assist in tDCS dose design [72].

Computer-modelling studies do not only predict brain current flow, but also give insight into electrode design by predicting current flow patterns through the skin. Modelling studies reinforce that current does not pass uniformly through the skin but concentrates near electrode edges or skin inhomogeneities [73]. Electrode design can vary between saline-soaked cotton, sponge pads or specifically designed patches that can aid in maximizing stimulation magnitude and focality. Modelling studies also showed that decreasing the salinity of the pads reduces peak current concentration at the edges [74].

Modelling studies have also described the current density gradient starting at the electrode and up to grey matter. Wagner *et al.* [75] observed that the highest current densities are observed over the skin and in the cerebrospinal fluid, with lower current densities in the skull and grey matter. In fact, the lowest current densities are observed in the grey and white matter, with only 10–20% of the total injected current reaching the CNS. However, the current density in the CNS varies according to several factors such as electrode positioning and presence of brain lesions (e.g. stroke).

Therefore, computer modelling is expected to be increasingly used and play a critical role in the development of basic and applied tDCS research. tDCS modelling might be a more applied tool in the upcoming years with the recent development of web-based interfaces and commercial softwares, as illustrated in Figure 11.3. Although it is important to consider limitations of modelling studies and use them not in isolation but together with other useful data such as neurophysiological data.

Preclinical studies of tDCS

In a seminal study from the 1960s, Purpura and McMutry explored the polarity-dependent effect of direct current stimulation of the motor cortex of cats, observing that anodal stimulation increased the rate of action potentials in the neuronal tissue, whereas cathodal stimulation presented opposite effects, that is, a decrease in the frequency of action potentials observed in the neuronal tissue [7]. This preclinical study experimentally demonstrated the polarity-dependent effects of direct current stimulation in the neuronal tissue.

Preclinical studies from the 2000s onwards evaluated the effects of *transcranial* DC stimulation *per se*, by placing one electrode over the animal's head and the other one in an extracephalic position. In a systematic review of experimental animal studies, we [76] reviewed 12 studies evaluating the use of tDCS in animals. The reviewed studies generally demonstrated the intensity-dependent and polarity-dependent effects of tDCS, and also the tDCS after-effects (i.e. changes in cortical activity that persist beyond the period of stimulation).

In an important study, Liebetanz *et al.* [77] explored the safety limits of tDCS stimulation in rats by using increasingly larger current intensities and thereafter performing histological evaluations. The authors found that the threshold necessary to induce brain lesions in rats was two orders of magnitude higher than the charge density applied in humans. Although these results cannot be directly transferred to human studies, they corroborate

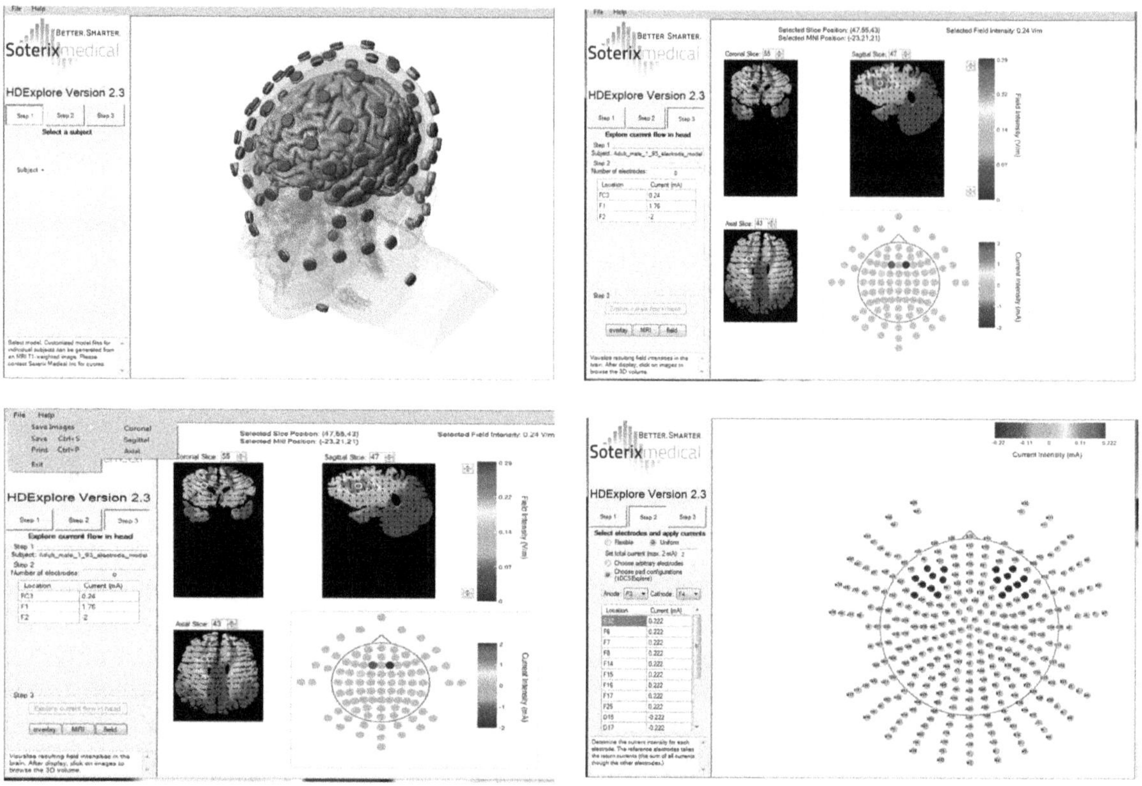

Figure 11.3 Software used for tDCS modelling studies. The dots in the phantoms' head represent possible spots for electrode placement. The software simulates current density under the anode and the cathode according to the placement of the electrodes. Source: Images provided by Soterix Medical. (*See insert for colour representation of the figure.*)

clinical studies showing that the technique is safe when used according to standardized parameters.

Clinical aspects

Adverse effects, safety and tolerability

According to the standard parameters of use, tDCS seems to be a well-tolerated technique, with few, mild side effects. In a recent literature review, we collected data from all tDCS clinical studies performed from 1998 to August 2010 [18]. Of 209 studies (172 articles, encompassing almost 4000 subjects), 56% described adverse effects and, of those, 63% reported at least one adverse effect. Only eight studies systematically addressed the frequency and intensity of adverse effects. According to the retrieved studies, we found similar rates in the active vs. sham arms of the most commonly reported adverse effects, namely headache, itching, burning, discomfort and tingling (Tables 11.2 and 11.3).

It should be underscored, though, that, in our review, we found that almost all studies failed to systematically report the frequency and intensity of adverse effects. Although this could point out that these effects might be benign and well tolerated, this also indicates that the prevalence of tDCS-related adverse effects is probably underestimated in the literature. We therefore recommend that all tDCS clinical studies provide estimates of the

Table 11.2 Adverse effects of tDCS.

Sensation	Active group	Sham group
Itching	46 (39.3%)	27 (32.9%)
Tingling	26 (22.2%)	15 (18.3%)
Headache	17 (14.8%)	13 (16.2%)
Burning	10 (8.7%)	8 (10%)
Discomfort	12 (10.4%)	11 (13.4%)
Total	117 studies	82 studies

Source: From Brunoni *et al.* [18]. Reproduced with permission of Cambridge University Press.
The rate of adverse effects observed from a systematic review performed in all clinical transcranial direct current stimulation from 1998 to August 2009 is described.

frequency and intensity of adverse effects observed.

Although in this systematic review we were not able to correlate the presence of the local adverse effects with the total amount of charge delivered, it is clinically observed that high current intensities (>2 mA) are associated with more adverse effects. Also, electrolyte solutions with lower NaCl concentrations (15 mM) seem to be more comfortable during tDCS than those solutions with higher NaCl concentrations (220 mM) – as the ionic strength of deionised water is much less than that of NaCl, there is a significantly larger voltage required to carry current through the skin compared to NaCl solutions. Dundas *et al.* [78] recommended the use of solutions with relatively low NaCl concentration, in the range of 15–140 mM, as tDCS at these concentrations is more likely to be perceived as comfortable, requires low voltage and still allows good conduction of current. It has also been proposed to apply topical anaesthetics to alleviate local adverse effects associated with tDCS [2, 3].

tDCS-induced erythema, that is, the reddening of the skin that occurs after one tDCS session, is a common adverse effect. Such erythema is caused by increased blood flow in the dermal vessels that occurs as a direct result of the current application, and also probably due to the release of multiple neuropeptides by primary afferent nerves following noxious and non-noxious stimulation, with secondary release of vasoactive substances, histamine and prostaglandins. In a study investigating this issue (data not yet published), our group observed the effects of 2 mA, 30-min anodal/cathodal tDCS on skin reddening. We observed that the erythema was more prominent over the anode than the cathode, although it was mild in both conditions. The erythema was also short-lived, lasting less than 18–24 min. The importance of tDCS-induced erythema for blinding is discussed below.

No serious adverse effects regarding tDCS have been reported in contemporary literature, including induction of seizure, stroke, cardiac arrest and other life-threatening events. Safety studies revealed that tDCS does not change heart rate variability at rest [79], does not increase the serum levels of enolase, a brain enzyme associated with neuronal death [80], and does not qualitatively alter electroencephalographic activity [81]. It should be noted, though, that most tDCS studies were performed so far in healthy subjects and not in neuropsychiatric samples. For instance, in patients with depression, several cases of tDCS-induced hypomania/mania have been reported [82–84]. Further studies assessing the safety of tDCS in patients with neuropsychiatric disorders are therefore still warranted.

Finally, the drop-out rate of patients in the active vs. sham arms of tDCS clinical trials is similar, according to the recent meta-analysis of Berlim *et al.* [22] who investigated this issue by collecting data from randomized, sham-controlled tDCS trials for depression. This suggests that continuous, daily application of tDCS for several days is an acceptable and tolerable procedure.

A final note regarding 'safety': although tDCS is considered 'safe' – and indeed the (battery-driven) tDCS device is biomedically secure as it

Table 11.3 tDCS adverse effects questionnaire.

Adverse effect	No	Yes	Severity	Relationship with stimulation
Headache	( )	( )	1 2 3 4	1 2 3 4 5
Neck pain	( )	( )	1 2 3 4	1 2 3 4 5
Local pain (anode)	( )	( )	1 2 3 4	1 2 3 4 5
Local pain (cathode)	( )	( )	1 2 3 4	1 2 3 4 5
Itching (anode)	( )	( )	1 2 3 4	1 2 3 4 5
Itching (cathode)	( )	( )	1 2 3 4	1 2 3 4 5
Scratching (anode)	( )	( )	1 2 3 4	1 2 3 4 5
Scratching (cathode)	( )	( )	1 2 3 4	1 2 3 4 5
Tingling (anode)	( )	( )	1 2 3 4	1 2 3 4 5
Tingling (cathode)	( )	( )	1 2 3 4	1 2 3 4 5
Burning (anode)	( )	( )	1 2 3 4	1 2 3 4 5
Burning (cathode)	( )	( )	1 2 3 4	1 2 3 4 5
Skin redness (anode)	( )	( )	1 2 3 4	1 2 3 4 5
Skin redness (cathode)	( )	( )	1 2 3 4	1 2 3 4 5
Somnolence	( )	( )	1 2 3 4	1 2 3 4 5
Concentration changes	( )	( )	1 2 3 4	1 2 3 4 5
Mood improvement	( )	( )	1 2 3 4	1 2 3 4 5
Mood worsening	( )	( )	1 2 3 4	1 2 3 4 5
Fatigue	( )	( )	1 2 3 4	1 2 3 4 5
Nausea	( )	( )	1 2 3 4	1 2 3 4 5
Dizziness	( )	( )	1 2 3 4	1 2 3 4 5
Other effects:				
	( )	( )	1 2 3 4	1 2 3 4 5
	( )	( )	1 2 3 4	1 2 3 4 5
	( )	( )	1 2 3 4	1 2 3 4 5

Source: Adapted from Brunoni *et al.* [18].
Proposal of questionnaire surveying for tDCS adverse effects. The patient is asked to describe whether the adverse effect was experienced. If it was experienced, the patient is asked to rate its severity (1 – none; 2 – mild; 3 – moderate; 4 – severe) and relationship with tDCS (1 – none; 2 – remote; 3 – possible; 4 – probable; 5 – definite).

delivers low-dose current with sub-threshold effects in cortical excitability and also no major or serious adverse effects for tDCS have been reported, such findings do not implicate that tDCS is 'universally safe' and therefore should be applied with caution. First, there are no data regarding tDCS use beyond the limits commonly used in experimental setting regarding current intensity, session duration and interval between sessions. Second, it is possible that tDCS enhances activity in one brain area at the expense of decreasing activity in another brain area – for instance, in our clinical trial in which tDCS presented antidepressant effects, we also found that it prevented implicit-learning acquisition during a probabilistic classification learning task, possibly by decreasing activity in brain areas responsible for implicit memory learning [85]. In this context, it is possible that 'wrong' stimulation parameters for several days would have unwanted consequences leading to maladaptive plasticity. Finally, tDCS is a relatively novel and long-term technique; follow-up studies are still warranted for fully addressing the clinical safety of tDCS.

Sham methods of tDCS

The most employed sham tDCS method was investigated by Gandiga *et al.* [86] and consists in mimicking the usually reported side effects of active tDCS stimulation, namely itching, burning and pain sensations. In order to perform this, a sham tDCS session encompasses an initial, brief period of active tDCS that lasts for less than 30–60 s, a period that is insufficient to generate any neuromodulatory effects [10]. As the tingling sensation seems to be related to the 'fade-in' and 'fade-out' periods of the tDCS sessions, the increase in current delivery should be less than 0.1–0.2 mA/s to generate no discomfort in subjects [86]. Although other methods of sham stimulation have been employed, such as the use of a very low current (0.1 mA) during the entire stimulation session [87], the method of Gandiga *et al.* is employed almost ubiquitously in tDCS clinical research and, in fact, all tDCS clinical trials for psychiatric disorders employed this sham method (for a review, see Kuo *et al.* [23]). Earlier tDCS studies employed a 'double single-blinded' approach – that is, one member of the staff was unblinded and responsible solely for switching the device off, without performing any further contact with the patient and the clinical evaluators regarding the clinical condition of the patient. Therefore, the evaluators and the patients remained blinded regarding the patient's allocation. Nonetheless, recent tDCS studies are increasingly adopting automated tDCS devices that might interrupt the electric stimulation according to a randomly generated code previously imputed for 'sham' or 'active' conditions. In this sense, such trials present a better double-blind design.

Nonetheless, recent studies claimed that, under certain conditions, the method of Gandiga *et al.* might not be adequate for proper blinding. For instance, O'Connell *et al.* [88] showed that investigators and subjects were able to correctly guess whether they received active or sham stimulation. Such correct guessing was mainly related to skin reddening in the active group, although O'Connell *et al.* also employed short fade-in/fade-out periods that might have compromised blinding. Furthermore, Palm *et al.* [89] also observed that researchers were able to distinguish between active vs. sham stimulation, also possibly due to skin reddening. Our group observed, in a recent randomized, double-blinded, sham-controlled trial enrolling 120 patients to receive active/sham tDCS or verum/placebo sertraline pill, in a factorial design, that skin reddening was indeed the only adverse effect more prevalent in the active vs. sham tDCS groups. However, in a subsequent analysis of blinding integrity of this trial, we found that [87] the sham tDCS method used was as effective as the placebo-pill method to guarantee blinding, measured by the percentage of subjects correctly guessing the type of stimulation (active/sham) and the type of pharmacological treatment (placebo-pill/sertraline) – the percentages were similar. We concluded that correct guessing was mainly related to clinical improvement (as guessing was inquired at the end of the treatment) rather than blind breaking and that the sham method employed was effective.

Truly, skin reddening is an important blinding issue, especially in clinical trials in which the patient is stimulated for several days. This increases the odds of the staff, other patients, and the patient him/herself being unblended, especially as the patient reports this adverse event. Possible approaches would be as follows: (i) using skin creams that could decrease skin reddening intensity and duration, such as a topical solution of ketoprofen 2% before the tDCS session, as recently observed by our group (unpublished data); (ii) avoiding direct visualization of the head and forehead during interviewing (e.g. through the use of hats) and/or (iii) interviewing patients before stimulation. We also recommend that if an evaluator perceives skin redness, another interviewer for the remaining of the trial must substitute him/her.

Similarities and differences of tDCS compared to other neuromodulatory techniques

It is important to underscore the main differences and similarities between tDCS and rTMS, another non-invasive brain stimulation technique used for clinical practice and research. Fundamentally, rTMS generates an electric current via electromagnetic *induction*. This induced electric current is generated over the scalp, at the coil, and is able to penetrate 20–25 mm inwards. tDCS, on the other hand, *injects* an electric current through two electrodes of different polarities that are placed over the scalp. The injected current penetrates to the central nervous system from the electrodes; therefore, the current also permeates through the skin, skull and CSF. Importantly, the induced electric current generated by rTMS is strong enough to cause neuronal depolarization and action potentials, therefore being a *suprathreshold* brain stimulation technique. Conversely, tDCS causes small changes in the neuronal potential that is not sufficient to generate action potentials *per se*; therefore, tDCS is a *subthreshold* brain stimulation technique, its effects being, as discussed, primarily in facilitating or limiting the activity (frequency of action potentials) of a neuronal network.

rTMS has greater spatial resolution than tDCS or, in other words, tDCS is much less focal than rTMS. rTMS generates an electromagnetic field in a 'conic' pattern, with the base of the cone situated in the centre of the coil. tDCS, conversely, stimulates not only the areas situated beneath the large 5 × 5 cm (or 5 × 7 cm) electrodes but also the brain regions between these electrodes. Therefore, several brain areas are more or less stimulated during a tDCS session, although generally the peak of the current flow is situated under the electrodes.

rTMS also presents greater temporal resolution than tDCS, as the stimulatory effects of a single electromagnetic pulse of TMS are immediate, whereas the neuromodulatory effects of tDCS might take some minutes to occur and depend more on the ongoing cortical activity – in fact, there seems to be no neuromodulatory effect when the tDCS session lasts for less than 1 min [10]. Furthermore, the property of inducing 'virtual brain lesions' (acute disruption of local network activity) is observed only for rTMS. Conversely, some neuromodulatory aspects are unique for tDCS such as the property of modulate two different brain areas simultaneously and the property of inducing polarity-dependent effects, with the anode and the cathode, respectively, increasing and decreasing cortical excitability beyond the period of stimulation.

Apart from these fundamental differences, tDCS and rTMS are very akin from a clinical perspective, both being non-pharmacological techniques with few adverse effects and good tolerability. Clinical treatments of both tDCS and rTMS consist in daily sessions during several weekdays, each session lasting approximately 15–30 min according to the clinical condition. In this regard, sham stimulation of tDCS is easier to achieve than that of rTMS (see discussion above). From a clinical perspective, rTMS has been more investigated and is already clinically approved for the treatment of major depression and auditory hallucinations in schizophrenia, although tDCS will probably gain more space in the future if proven to be clinically effective, as tDCS is easier to use, is easier to learn than the rTMS technique and is also more affordable.

tDCS in special populations

As the basic and clinical knowledge of tDCS advances, its use in special populations can also be considered. Recent reports have described that the use of tDCS is feasible in adolescents (5- to 12-year-olds), with the main side effects being similar as described in adults [90]. A computational modelling also explored the peak electrical field patterns of children (8- and 12-year-olds) and adults, showing that children are likely to be exposed to higher peak electrical fields than adults, although there is an overlap between children and adults with small head size [91] – therefore suggesting caution when exposing children to higher tDCS doses. In a recent review of non-invasive brain stimulation in paediatric populations, Vicario and Nitsche [92] found studies using tDCS in epilepsy, autism and schizophrenia. The authors concluded that there is therapeutic potential for using tDCS in childhood, although the studies performed hitherto present several methodological limitations that impede further conclusions. The risk of inducing maladaptive neural plasticity during this critical age of brain development should also be considered when performing tDCS studies. Finally, tDCS might not be a feasible technique in very young children, as cooperation is required to maintain the electrodes correctly positioned over the scalp.

tDCS might also be a useful strategy in pregnant women with mental and neurological disorders, as many pharmacological interventions are proscribed in this population [93]. However, no clinical or computer modelling study has prospectively explored the safety of this approach. Nonetheless, it is unlikely that that the electric currents induced by tDCS could have a direct effect in the uterus or in foetus development, as the current applied is very low. Another theoretical risk is that tDCS could modify the release of neuro-hormones associated with pregnancy. Of note, rTMS studies performed in pregnancy showed that rTMS was a safe and clinically effective intervention in the treatment of depression in this population [94, 95].

Another group of interest are the elderly. tDCS could be a useful tool to treat the many disorders associated with cognitive decline observed in this population. Furthermore, the benign profile of adverse effects, compared to medicines, makes tDCS an interesting tool, as many old patients use several medications or have clinical conditions that impede the proper use of pharmacotherapy. However, as previously observed, further studies are needed to explore the safety and effectiveness of tDCS in this group.

Ethical aspects

Because of some appealing characteristics of tDCS, namely low-cost, ease of use, tolerable adverse effects and positive results regarding enhancement and modification of normal cognitive functioning (for a review, see Utz *et al.* [96]), there is an ongoing debate to whether tDCS has also a role as a *cognitive enhancement* tool. This debate is important because tDCS is a non-expensive device to manufacture, being theoretically possible to be assembled by lay people to use at home – this means that tDCS might be more readily accessible as a 'cognitive enhancer' than, for instance, prescribed medicines used for this purpose.

In fact, one dilemma is how to craft regulatory policy regarding the use of tDCS. For instance, one company (www.foc.us) recently started to offer 'tDCS Headsets for extreme gamers' with the motto 'Overclock your head!' Such tDCS applications, outside the controlled environmental setting, put subjects at risk and might jeopardize proper research on the field [97]. Moreover, there are several *YouTube* videos fostering people in a 'do it yourself' (DIY) approach to manufacture and use their very own tDCS device. It cannot be overstated that such manufactured devices would hardly comply on any safety specifications, nor the users would necessarily follow the parameters of stimulation (duration, current, number and frequency of sessions) used in clinical research. However, crafting regulatory policy for DIY tDCS is challenging, for the reasons pointed out by Fitz and Reiner [98]: first, neither the range of applications of tDCS nor what a tDCS device 'is' is clearly defined – these issues make it difficult to enact regulation to cover for all the range of possible applications; second, users manufacture DIY tDCS for cognitive enhancement, and such topic is usually not in the scope of regulatory and medical authorities; and finally, 'regulating DIY tDCS is not a zero sum game', meaning that costly regulatory requirements may drive the DIY approach further underground. To overcome these challenges, some authorities have suggested a positive approach, favouring open communication and education to the DIY tDCS developers, to develop a culture of responsibility regarding home tDCS use, whereas critics see that such approach would not successfully mitigate the risks of using tDCS in non-experimental settings.

Even if tDCS is successfully regulated, there is still the question to whom and in which cases the use of tDCS as a cognitive enhancement tool is legit. One important discussion is the use of tDCS for educational purposes and its biological and ethical issues of, respectively, performing brain stimulation in the developing brain (when considering children and adolescents with typical and atypical development) and 'cheating' [99]. The former aspect has been discussed in the section 'tDCS in special populations'. The latter aspect is important because several studies showed cognitive enhancement in psychological functions after tDCS in healthy subjects [96]. Therefore, it should be debated whether such 'cognitive boost' would not mean cheating – that is, placing one person in unrightfully advantage over the others. However, there are many other forms of cognitive enhancements such as caffeine and private tutors, and many other cognitive tools such as computers and the Internet [100]. Furthermore, cognitive enhancement could be considered cheating if it only boosts performance temporarily (for an examination purpose, for instance), whereas its use could be considered fair when used for long-term learning, perhaps associated with standard educational methods – and, in fact, tDCS is more effective when coupled with behavioural training [99, 100]. As tDCS could be theoretically used for short- as well as long-term purposes, it would be necessary to develop regulatory protocols in order to guarantee its 'fair' use in academic and intellectual competitions.

Another lively debate is the coercive use of tDCS against one's will, potentially violating the biomedical principle of autonomy. The coercion might be implicit or explicit. For instance, 25% of university students have ever used stimulants to increase their academic performance [100] – in a theoretical scenario where tDCS use is widespread; students could find themselves 'obliged' to use tDCS in order to not stand intellectually behind their peers. Explicit coercion is using one intervention, chiefly for legal/penalty purposes, against the will of the individual. Hamilton *et al.* [101] exemplifies that tDCS could be used by the police force in the detection of deception as it interferes in the ability to lie. Other authors suggested that tDCS could be used for military purposes as this technique is able to favourably modify inhibition, impulsive behaviour, risk-taking, planning, working memory and deceptive capacities [102]. However, such findings derived from experimental settings might not be transferable into real-life situations and in fact tDCS could also be used coercively in military scenarios [103], endangering one's undeniable right to decide whether or not they want to receive an intervention.

To conclude, tDCS is being remarkably referred as 'the thinking cap' [101], not only due to its physical aspect but also because it has a true potential of improving cognition in healthy people. However, in order to verify the extent of such potential, methodological advances and bioethical discussion are warranted. Both aspects are linked, since only adequate trial methodology can be set when the consequences of the research outcome are properly discussed. The use of tDCS as a 'thinking cap' involves important bioethical questions that should be discussed by researchers, physicians and society.

Conclusion

tDCS is gaining reputation as an important non-invasive brain stimulation intervention in basic and clinical research. tDCS presents a wide range of potential applications and can be used to explore the basic aspects of neurosciences and also for the treatment of mental and neurological disorders. tDCS has some unique and appealing aspects, namely the ability to induce polarity-dependent shifts in cortical excitability, non-invasiveness, low-cost and portability, making it suitable for increasing access to novel therapies. However, such characteristics also bring challenges regarding neuroethical aspects and there is still uncertainty regarding the parameters of stimulation that should be used to achieve optimal response in clinical research. Although tDCS is still in its infancy regarding its development, in the past few years, there has been a rapid development in this technique resulting in significant more clinical data that have been guiding the initial clinical use of tDCS and also being important to optimize its clinical effects.

Appendix 11.A Positioning and montage of electrodes for tDCS

The application of tDCS can be visualized online in www.jove.com/video/2744 [104]. Here, we describe the main steps necessary to perform a tDCS session.

Materials

The necessary materials are as follows:

a One tDCS device, which should be battery-driven and deliver a constant electric current with a range of 0.5–3 mA. The batteries can be chargeable according to the device. It is not recommended to use electric outlets to power the device during the stimulation session as this could unexpectedly deliver a large discharge of electric current.

b Electrodes, generally consisted of metal or conductive-rubber electrodes enclosed by sponges that can be humidified by saline. The sponges should remain humidified during the entire stimulation session. Alternatively, conductive gels can be used instead of humidified sponges.

c It is possible to apply solutions before the stimulation sessions (such as anaesthetics or anti-inflammatory agents) to reduce adverse effects.

d Head straps should be used to place the electrodes in the desired position.

Identification of scalp areas for electrode positioning

The references used in tDCS research are mainly based according to the convention of the EEG 10/20 system. One should take into account that, according to the size of the electrodes and the distance between them, there is a possibility of shunting, that is, the electric current will not penetrate across the skin to the central nervous system, rather it will go through the skin from one electrode to the other. In this scenario, the neuromodulatory effects of tDCS would be virtually absent.

The procedure

a The first step is to identify the brain area(s) to be stimulated and prepare the corresponding skin regions to receive the electrodes. The skin should be inspected for pre-existing lesions and the electrodes should not be placed above damaged skin. The skin can be prepared by removing the hair from the site of the stimulation and gently cleaned with saline or alcohol swabs to remove lotion, dirt, sebum, hair products, etc.

b After that, the electrodes should be placed over the desired area, fixed with the head straps and then humidified with saline or other electrolyte solution. It is useful to use a syringe to add the proper amount of solution in the electrode. The electrodes should not be fully soaked and water leaking should be avoided as this increases the risk of shunting.

c Conventionally, the red cable is usually the anode (positive terminal, where the current 'enters' the body) and the blue or black cable is the cathode (negative terminal, where the current 'leaves' the body).

d The session can be started. Most modern tDCS devices present the following characteristics: (i) an automatic impedance detector that will not deliver the electric current whether the impedance is too high (>5 kΩ); (ii) pre-programmable, automatic fade-in and fade-out phases (it is recommended to avoiding increasing the current up more than 0.1 mA/s to prevent discomfort and other adverse effects); (iii) other programmable parameters such as current intensity (mA) and total session length (minutes); (iv) an automatic sham condition that turns off the device after a brief (30–60 s) period of stimulation.

e After the end of the stimulation, the device must be turned off, the electrodes removed and the skin inspected for possible lesions. According to the protocol, questionnaires evaluating adverse effects and the integrity of blinding might be applied.

References

1 Guleyupoglu B, Schestatsky P, Edwards D, Fregni F, Bikson M (2013) Classification of methods in transcranial electrical stimulation (tES) and evolving strategy from historical approaches to contemporary innovations. J Neurosci Methods 219: 297–311.

2 Nitsche MA, Cohen LG, Wassermann EM, Priori A, Lang N, *et al.* (2008) Transcranial direct current stimulation: state of the art 2008. Brain Stimul 1: 206–223.

3 Brunoni AR, Nitsche MA, Bolognini N, Bikson M, Wagner T, *et al.* (2012) Clinical research with transcranial direct current stimulation (tDCS): challenges and future directions. Brain Stimul 5: 175–195.

4 Clark VP, Parasuraman R (2014) Neuroenhancement: enhancing brain and mind in health and in disease. Neuroimage 85 Pt 3: 889–894.

5 Largus S (1529) De compositionibus medicamentorum. Wechel, Paris.

6 Zago S, Ferrucci R, Fregni F, Priori A (2008) Bartholow, Sciamanna, Alberti: pioneers in the electrical stimulation of the exposed human cerebral cortex. Neuroscientist 14: 521–528.

7 Purpura DP, McMurtry JG (1965) Intracellular activities and evoked potential changes during polarization of motor cortex. J Neurophysiol 28: 166–185.

8 Nitsche MA, Boggio PS, Fregni F, Pascual-Leone A (2009) Treatment of depression with transcranial direct current stimulation (tDCS): a review. Exp Neurol 219: 14–19.

9 Priori A, Berardelli A, Rona S, Accornero N, Manfredi M (1998) Polarization of the human motor cortex through the scalp. Neuroreport 9: 2257–2260.

10 Nitsche MA, Paulus W (2000) Excitability changes induced in the human motor cortex by weak transcranial direct current stimulation. J Physiol 527 Pt 3: 633–639.

11 Villamar MF, Volz MS, Bikson M, Datta A, Dasilva AF, *et al.* (2013) Technique and considerations in the use of 4x1 ring high-definition transcranial direct current stimulation (HD-tDCS). J Vis Exp 77: e50309.

12 Boggio PS, Rigonatti SP, Ribeiro RB, Myczkowski ML, Nitsche MA, *et al.* (2008) A randomized, double-blind clinical trial on the efficacy of cortical direct current stimulation for the treatment of major depression. Int J Neuropsychopharmacol 11: 249–254.

13 Antal A, Kincses TZ, Nitsche MA, Paulus W (2003) Manipulation of phosphene thresholds

by transcranial direct current stimulation in man. Exp Brain Res 150: 375–378.
14 Jacobson L, Koslowsky M, Lavidor M (2012) tDCS polarity effects in motor and cognitive domains: a meta-analytical review. Exp Brain Res 216: 1–10.
15 Mendonca ME, Santana MB, Baptista AF, Datta A, Bikson M, *et al.* (2011) Transcranial DC stimulation in fibromyalgia: optimized cortical target supported by high-resolution computational models. J Pain 12: 610–617.
16 Nitsche MA, Doemkes S, Karakose T, Antal A, Liebetanz D, *et al.* (2007) Shaping the effects of transcranial direct current stimulation of the human motor cortex. J Neurophysiol 97: 3109–3117.
17 Parazzini M, Fiocchi S, Rossi E, Paglialonga A, Ravazzani P (2011) Transcranial direct current stimulation: estimation of the electric field and of the current density in an anatomical human head model. IEEE Trans Biomed Eng 58: 1773–1780.
18 Brunoni AR, Amadera J, Berbel B, Volz MS, Rizzerio BG, *et al.* (2011) A systematic review on reporting and assessment of adverse effects associated with transcranial direct current stimulation. Int J Neuropsychopharmacol 14: 1133–1145.
19 Miranda PC, Faria P, Hallett M (2009) What does the ratio of injected current to electrode area tell us about current density in the brain during tDCS? Clin Neurophysiol 120: 1183–1187.
20 Boggio PS, Ferrucci R, Rigonatti SP, Covre P, Nitsche M, *et al.* (2006) Effects of transcranial direct current stimulation on working memory in patients with Parkinson's disease. J Neurol Sci 249: 31–38.
21 Iyer MB, Mattu U, Grafman J, Lomarev M, Sato S, *et al.* (2005) Safety and cognitive effect of frontal DC brain polarization in healthy individuals. Neurology 64: 872–875.
22 Berlim MT, Van den Eynde F, Daskalakis ZJ (2013) Clinical utility of transcranial direct current stimulation (tDCS) for treating major depression: a systematic review and meta-analysis of randomized, double-blind and sham-controlled trials. J Psychiatr Res 47: 1–7.
23 Kuo MF, Paulus W, Nitsche MA (2014) Therapeutic effects of non-invasive brain stimulation with direct currents (tDCS) in neuropsychiatric diseases. Neuroimage 85(part 3);948–960.
24 Brunoni AR, Valiengo L, Baccaro A, Zanao TA, Oliveira AC, *et al.* (2013) The sertraline versus electrical current therapy for treating depression clinical study: results from a factorial, randomized, controlled trial. JAMA Psychiatry 70: 383–391.
25 Loo CK, Alonzo A, Martin D, Mitchell PB, Galvez V, *et al.* (2012) Transcranial direct current stimulation for depression: 3-week, randomised, sham-controlled trial. Br J Psychiatry 200: 52–59.
26 Shiozawa P, Fregni F, Bensenor IM, Lotufo PA, Berlim MT, *et al.* (2014) Transcranial direct current stimulation for major depression: an updated systematic review and meta-analysis. Int. J Neuropsychopharmacol 17;1443–1452.
27 Brunelin J, Mondino M, Gassab L, Haesebaert F, Gaha L, *et al.* (2012) Examining transcranial direct-current stimulation (tDCS) as a treatment for hallucinations in schizophrenia. Am J Psychiatry 169: 719–724.
28 Bikson M, Rahman A, Datta A, Fregni F, Merabet L (2012) High-resolution modeling assisted design of customized and individualized transcranial direct current stimulation protocols. Neuromodulation 15: 306–315.
29 Priori A, Hallett M, Rothwell JC (2009) Repetitive transcranial magnetic stimulation or transcranial direct current stimulation? Brain Stimul 2: 241–245.
30 Rahman A, Reato D, Arlotti M, Gasca F, Datta A, *et al.* (2013) Cellular effects of acute direct current stimulation: somatic and synaptic terminal effects. J Physiol 591: 2563–2578.
31 Batsikadze G, Moliadze V, Paulus W, Kuo MF, Nitsche MA (2013) Partially non-linear stimulation intensity-dependent effects of direct current stimulation on motor cortex excitability in humans. J Physiol 591: 1987–2000.
32 Datta A, Bansal V, Diaz J, Patel J, Reato D, *et al.* (2009) Gyri-precise head model of transcranial direct current stimulation: improved spatial focality using a ring electrode versus conventional rectangular pad. Brain Stimul 2: 201–207.
33 Radman T, Ramos RL, Brumberg JC, Bikson M (2009) Role of cortical cell type and morphology in subthreshold and suprathreshold uniform electric field stimulation in vitro. Brain Stimul 2: 215–228, 228 e211–213.

34 Creutzfeld D, Fromm GH, Kapp H (1962) Influence of transcortical d-c currents on cortical neuronal activity. Exp Neurol 5: 436–452.
35 Bindman LJ, Lippold OC, Redfearn JW (1964) The action of brief polarizing currents on the cerebral cortex of the rat (1) during current flow and (2) in the production of long-lasting after-effects. J Physiol 172: 369–382.
36 Jefferys JG (1981) Influence of electric fields on the excitability of granule cells in guinea-pig hippocampal slices. J Physiol 319: 143–152.
37 Bikson M, Inoue M, Akiyama H, Deans JK, Fox JE, *et al.* (2004) Effects of uniform extracellular DC electric fields on excitability in rat hippocampal slices in vitro. J Physiol 557: 175–190.
38 Nitsche MA, Liebetanz D, Antal A, Lang N, Tergau F, *et al.* (2003) Modulation of cortical excitability by weak direct current stimulation – technical, safety and functional aspects. Suppl Clin Neurophysiol 56: 255–276.
39 Nitsche MA, Paulus W (2001) Sustained excitability elevations induced by transcranial DC motor cortex stimulation in humans. Neurology 57: 1899–1901.
40 Liebetanz D, Nitsche MA, Tergau F, Paulus W (2002) Pharmacological approach to the mechanisms of transcranial DC-stimulation-induced after-effects of human motor cortex excitability. Brain 125: 2238–2247.
41 Nitsche MA, Fricke K, Henschke U, Schlitterlau A, Liebetanz D, *et al.* (2003) Pharmacological modulation of cortical excitability shifts induced by transcranial direct current stimulation in humans. J Physiol 553: 293–301.
42 Stagg CJ, Best JG, Stephenson MC, O'Shea J, Wylezinska M, *et al.* (2009) Polarity-sensitive modulation of cortical neurotransmitters by transcranial stimulation. J Neurosci 29: 5202–5206.
43 Nitsche MA, Seeber A, Frommann K, Klein CC, Rochford C, *et al.* (2005) Modulating parameters of excitability during and after transcranial direct current stimulation of the human motor cortex. J Physiol 568: 291–303.
44 Ardolino G, Bossi B, Barbieri S, Priori A (2005) Non-synaptic mechanisms underlie the after-effects of cathodal transcutaneous direct current stimulation of the human brain. J Physiol 568: 653–663.
45 Accornero N, Li Voti P, La Riccia M, Gregori B (2007) Visual evoked potentials modulation during direct current cortical polarization. Exp Brain Res 178: 261–266.
46 Matsunaga K, Nitsche MA, Tsuji S, Rothwell JC (2004) Effect of transcranial DC sensorimotor cortex stimulation on somatosensory evoked potentials in humans. Clin Neurophysiol 115: 456–460.
47 Antal A, Nitsche MA, Kincses TZ, Kruse W, Hoffmann KP, *et al.* (2004) Facilitation of visuo-motor learning by transcranial direct current stimulation of the motor and extrastriate visual areas in humans. Eur J Neurosci 19: 2888–2892.
48 Ferrucci R, Marceglia S, Vergari M, Cogiamanian F, Mrakic-Sposta S, *et al.* (2008) Cerebellar transcranial direct current stimulation impairs the practice-dependent proficiency increase in working memory. J Cogn Neurosci 20: 1687–1697.
49 Galea JM, Jayaram G, Ajagbe L, Celnik P (2009) Modulation of cerebellar excitability by polarity-specific noninvasive direct current stimulation. J Neurosci 29: 9115–9122.
50 Cogiamanian F, Vergari M, Pulecchi F, Marceglia S, Priori A (2008) Effect of spinal transcutaneous direct current stimulation on somatosensory evoked potentials in humans. Clin Neurophysiol 119: 2636–2640.
51 Winkler T, Hering P, Straube A (2010) Spinal DC stimulation in humans modulates post-activation depression of the H-reflex depending on current polarity. Clin Neurophysiol 121: 957–961.
52 Fritsch B, Reis J, Martinowich K, Schambra HM, Ji Y, *et al.* (2010) Direct current stimulation promotes BDNF-dependent synaptic plasticity: potential implications for motor learning. Neuron 66: 198–204.
53 Stagg CJ, Nitsche MA (2011) Physiological basis of transcranial direct current stimulation. Neuroscientist 17: 37–53.
54 Rango M, Cogiamanian F, Marceglia S, Barberis B, Arighi A, *et al.* (2008) Myoinositol content in the human brain is modified by transcranial direct current stimulation in a matter of minutes: a 1H-MRS study. Magn Reson Med 60: 782–789.

55 Boros K, Poreisz C, Munchau A, Paulus W, Nitsche MA (2008) Premotor transcranial direct current stimulation (tDCS) affects primary motor excitability in humans. Eur J Neurosci 27: 1292–1300.
56 Lang N, Siebner HR, Ward NS, Lee L, Nitsche MA, *et al.* (2005) How does transcranial DC stimulation of the primary motor cortex alter regional neuronal activity in the human brain? Eur J Neurosci 22: 495–504.
57 Parra LC, Bikson M (2004) Model of the effect of extracellular fields on spike time coherence. Conf Proc IEEE Eng Med Biol Soc 6: 4584–4587.
58 Deans JK, Powell AD, Jefferys JG (2007) Sensitivity of coherent oscillations in rat hippocampus to AC electric fields. J Physiol 583: 555–565.
59 Frohlich F, McCormick DA (2010) Endogenous electric fields may guide neocortical network activity. Neuron 67: 129–143.
60 Monte-Silva KK, Kuo MF, Liebetanz D, Paulus W, Nitsche MA (2010) Shaping the optimal repetition interval for cathodal transcranial direct current stimulation (tDCS). J Neurophysiol 103: 1735–1740.
61 Alonzo A, Brassil J, Taylor JL, Martin D, Loo CK (Jul 2011) Daily transcranial direct current stimulation (tDCS) leads to greater increases in cortical excitability than second daily transcranial direct current stimulation. Brain Stimul 5(3):208–213.
62 Fregni F, Boggio PS, Santos MC, Lima M, Vieira AL, *et al.* (2006) Noninvasive cortical stimulation with transcranial direct current stimulation in Parkinson's disease. Mov Disord 10: 1693–1702.
63 Nitsche MA, Kuo MF, Karrasch R, Wachter B, Liebetanz D, *et al.* (2009) Serotonin affects transcranial direct current-induced neuroplasticity in humans. Biol Psychiatry 66: 503–508.
64 Nitsche MA, Grundey J, Liebetanz D, Lang N, Tergau F, *et al.* (2004) Catecholaminergic consolidation of motor cortical neuroplasticity in humans. Cereb Cortex 14: 1240–1245.
65 Kuo MF, Paulus W, Nitsche MA (2008) Boosting focally-induced brain plasticity by dopamine. Cereb Cortex 18: 648–651.
66 Nitsche MA, Lampe C, Antal A, Liebetanz D, Lang N, *et al.* (2006) Dopaminergic modulation of long-lasting direct current-induced cortical excitability changes in the human motor cortex. Eur J Neurosci 23: 1651–1657.
67 Terney D, Bergmann I, Poreisz C, Chaieb L, Boros K, *et al.* (2008) Pergolide increases the efficacy of cathodal direct current stimulation to reduce the amplitude of laser-evoked potentials in humans. J Pain Symptom Manage 36: 79–91.
68 Nitsche MA, Liebetanz D, Schlitterlau A, Henschke U, Fricke K, *et al.* (2004) GABAergic modulation of DC stimulation-induced motor cortex excitability shifts in humans. Eur J Neurosci 19: 2720–2726.
69 Nitsche MA, Jaussi W, Liebetanz D, Lang N, Tergau F, *et al.* (2004) Consolidation of human motor cortical neuroplasticity by d-cycloserine. Neuropsychopharmacology 29: 1573–1578.
70 Kuo MF, Unger M, Liebetanz D, Lang N, Tergau F, *et al.* (2008) Limited impact of homeostatic plasticity on motor learning in humans. Neuropsychologia 46: 2122–2128.
71 Monte-Silva K, Kuo MF, Thirugnanasambandam N, Liebetanz D, Paulus W, *et al.* (2009) Dose-dependent inverted U-shaped effect of dopamine (D2-like) receptor activation on focal and nonfocal plasticity in humans. J Neurosci 29: 6124–6131.
72 Sadleir RJ, Vannorsdall TD, Schretlen DJ, Gordon B (2010) Transcranial direct current stimulation (tDCS) in a realistic head model. Neuroimage 51: 1310–1318.
73 Miranda PC, Lomarev M, Hallett M (2006) Modeling the current distribution during transcranial direct current stimulation. Clin Neurophysiol 117: 1623–1629.
74 Minhas P, Bansal V, Patel J, Ho JS, Diaz J, *et al.* (2010) Electrodes for high-definition transcutaneous DC stimulation for applications in drug delivery and electrotherapy, including tDCS. J Neurosci Methods 190: 188–197.
75 Wagner T, Fregni F, Fecteau S, Grodzinsky A, Zahn M, *et al.* (2007) Transcranial direct current stimulation: a computer-based human model study. Neuroimage 35: 1113–1124.
76 Brunoni AR, Fregni F, Pagano RL (2011) Translational research in transcranial direct

current stimulation (tDCS): a systematic review of studies in animals. Rev Neurosci 22: 471–481.
77 Liebetanz D, Koch R, Mayenfels S, Konig F, Paulus W, *et al.* (2009) Safety limits of cathodal transcranial direct current stimulation in rats. Clin Neurophysiol 120: 1161–1167.
78 Dundas JE, Thickbroom GW, Mastaglia FL (2007) Perception of comfort during transcranial DC stimulation: effect of NaCl solution concentration applied to sponge electrodes. Clin Neurophysiol 118: 1166–1170.
79 Vandermeeren Y, Jamart J, Ossemann M (2010) Effect of tDCS with an extracephalic reference electrode on cardio-respiratory and autonomic functions. BMC Neurosci 11: 38.
80 Nitsche MA, Nitsche MS, Klein CC, Tergau F, Rothwell JC, *et al.* (2003) Level of action of cathodal DC polarisation induced inhibition of the human motor cortex. Clin Neurophysiol 114: 600–604.
81 Tadini L, El-Nazer R, Brunoni AR, Williams J, Carvas M, *et al.* (2011) Cognitive, mood, and electroencephalographic effects of noninvasive cortical stimulation with weak electrical currents. J ECT 27: 134–140.
82 Arul-Anandam AP, Loo C, Mitchell P (2010) Induction of hypomanic episode with transcranial direct current stimulation. J ECT 26: 68–69.
83 Baccaro A, Brunoni AR, Bensenor IM, Fregni F (2010) Hypomanic episode in unipolar depression during transcranial direct current stimulation. Acta Neuropsychiatr 22: 316–318.
84 Brunoni AR, Valiengo L, Zanao T, de Oliveira JF, Bensenor IM, *et al.* (2011) Manic psychosis after sertraline and transcranial direct-current stimulation. J Neuropsychiatry Clin Neurosci 23: E4–E5.
85 Brunoni AR, Zanao TA, Ferrucci R, Priori A, Valiengo L, *et al.* (2012) Bifrontal tDCS prevents implicit learning acquisition in antidepressant-free patients with major depressive disorder. Prog Neuropsychopharmacol Biol Psychiatry 43C: 146–150.
86 Gandiga PC, Hummel FC, Cohen LG (2006) Transcranial DC stimulation (tDCS): a tool for double-blind sham-controlled clinical studies in brain stimulation. Clin Neurophysiol 117: 845–850.
87 Brunoni AR, Schestatsky P, Lotufo PA, Bensenor IM, Fregni F (2013) Comparison of blinding effectiveness between sham tDCS and placebo sertraline in a 6-week major depression randomized clinical trial. Clin Neurophysiol 2;298–305.
88 O'Connell NE, Cossar J, Marston L, Wand BM, Bunce D, *et al.* (2012) Rethinking clinical trials of transcranial direct current stimulation: participant and assessor blinding is inadequate at intensities of 2 mA. PLoS One 7: e47514.
89 Palm U, Reisinger E, Keeser D, Kuo MF, Pogarell O, *et al.* (2013) Evaluation of sham transcranial direct current stimulation for randomized, placebo-controlled clinical trials. Brain Stimul 6: 690–695.
90 Andrade AC, Magnavita GM, Allegro JV, Neto CE, Lucena RD, *et al.* (2013) Feasibility of transcranial direct current stimulation use in children aged 5 to 12 years. J Child Neurol 10:1360–5.
91 Kessler SK, Minhas P, Woods AJ, Rosen A, Gorman C, *et al.* (2013) Dosage considerations for transcranial direct current stimulation in children: a computational modeling study. PLoS One 8: e76112.
92 Vicario CM, Nitsche MA (2013) Non-invasive brain stimulation for the treatment of brain diseases in childhood and adolescence: state of the art, current limits and future challenges. Front Systems Neurosci 7: 94.
93 Valiengo LC, Bensenor IM, Lotufo PA, Fraguas R, Jr., Brunoni AR (2013) Transcranial direct current stimulation and repetitive transcranial magnetic stimulation in consultation-liaison psychiatry. Braz J Med Biol Res 46: 815–908.
94 Hizli Sayar G, Ozten E, Tufan E, Cerit C, Kagan G, *et al.* (2013) Transcranial magnetic stimulation during pregnancy. Arch Womens Ment Health 4: 311–5.
95 Kim DR, Sockol L, Barber JP, Moseley M, Lamprou L, *et al.* (2011) A survey of patient acceptability of repetitive transcranial magnetic stimulation (TMS) during pregnancy. J Affect Disord 129: 385–390.
96 Utz KS, Dimova V, Oppenlander K, Kerkhoff G (2010) Electrified minds: transcranial direct current stimulation (tDCS) and Galvanic Vestibular Stimulation (GVS) as methods of non-invasive brain stimulation in neuropsychology: a review of current data and future implications. Neuropsychologia 48: 2789–2810.

97 Bikson M, Bestmann S, Edwards D (2013) Neuroscience: transcranial devices are not playthings. Nature 501: 167.
98 Fitz NS, Reiner PB (2015) The challenge of crafting policy for do-it-yourself brain stimulation. J Med Ethics (5):410–2.
99 Cohen Kadosh R, Levy N, O'Shea J, Shea N, Savulescu J (2012) The neuroethics of non-invasive brain stimulation. Curr Biol 22: R108–R111.
100 Greely H, Sahakian B, Harris J, Kessler RC, Gazzaniga M, *et al.* (2008) Towards responsible use of cognitive-enhancing drugs by the healthy. Nature 456: 702–705.
101 Hamilton R, Messing S, Chatterjee A (2011) Rethinking the thinking cap: ethics of neural enhancement using noninvasive brain stimulation. Neurology 76: 187–193.
102 Levasseur-Moreau J, Brunelin J, Fecteau S (2013) Non-invasive brain stimulation can induce paradoxical facilitation. Are these neuroenhancements transferable and meaningful to security services? Front Hum Neurosci 7: 449.
103 Sehm B, Ragert P (2013) Why non-invasive brain stimulation should not be used in military and security services. Front Hum Neurosci 7: 553.
104 DaSilva AF, Volz MS, Bikson M, Fregni F (2011) Electrode positioning and montage in transcranial direct current stimulation. J Vis Exp 51: pii: 2744.

CHAPTER 12

Transcranial direct current stimulation

Colleen Loo[1,2,3,4] and Donel Martin[1,5]
[1]University of New South Wales, Sydney, Australia
[2]St George Hospital, Sydney, Australia
[3]Black Dog Institute, Sydney, Australia
[4]Wesley Hospital, Sydney, Australia
[5]Advanced Neuropsychological Treatment Services, Sydney, Australia

Introduction and technical aspects

History of transcranial direct current stimulation (tDCS)

The approach of using weak electric fields (e.g. <1 milliampere (mA) current intensity) for therapeutic purposes in medicine has a history over centuries. In previous decades, this technique, applied to the brain, was known as 'brain polarization'. Early scientists understood from animal models that passing a weak, sustained direct current across neuronal tissue resulted in polarization of the neuronal membrane [1].

Since around 2000, there has been a resurgence of interest in the therapeutic potential of this stimulation technique, which has been rebranded as 'transcranial Direct Current Stimulation' (tDCS). Studies before 2000 used relatively low stimulus intensities (0.02–0.5 mA) with considerable variability in stimulation technique. As a result, outcomes were highly variable [2]. From then, the development of commercial equipment enabling the reliable delivery of currents in the 1–3 mA range has facilitated a steep increase in research studies in tDCS.

Technical aspects

A typical tDCS machine is a small, battery driven device, which measures the impedance (resistance) of the head, and delivers a constant current of set amplitude, passed between two electrodes (anode and cathode) that are placed on the scalp. Modern tDCS machines deliver up to about 3 mA. The term 'direct' refers to the current being unidirectional, that is, flowing in one direction, from the anode to the cathode, in contrast to a bidirectional current (e.g. alternating current) in which alternate pulses are in the opposite direction (see Figure 12.1). Thus, neuronal effects are often different under the anode and the cathode and the electrodes are not interchangeable (in contrast to, say, electrodes used in electroconvulsive therapy (ECT)). tDCS may involve a single anode and a single cathode, or multiple anodes and/or cathodes.

Given the unidirectional nature of the current, rubber electrodes are often used to minimize electrochemical interactions at the electrode–skin interface. Furthermore, a sponge soaked in an electrolyte solution is often placed between the rubber electrode and the skin (see below for a safe stimulation technique).

Neuromodulation in Psychiatry, First Edition. Edited by Clement Hamani, Paul Holtzheimer, Andres M. Lozano and Helen Mayberg.

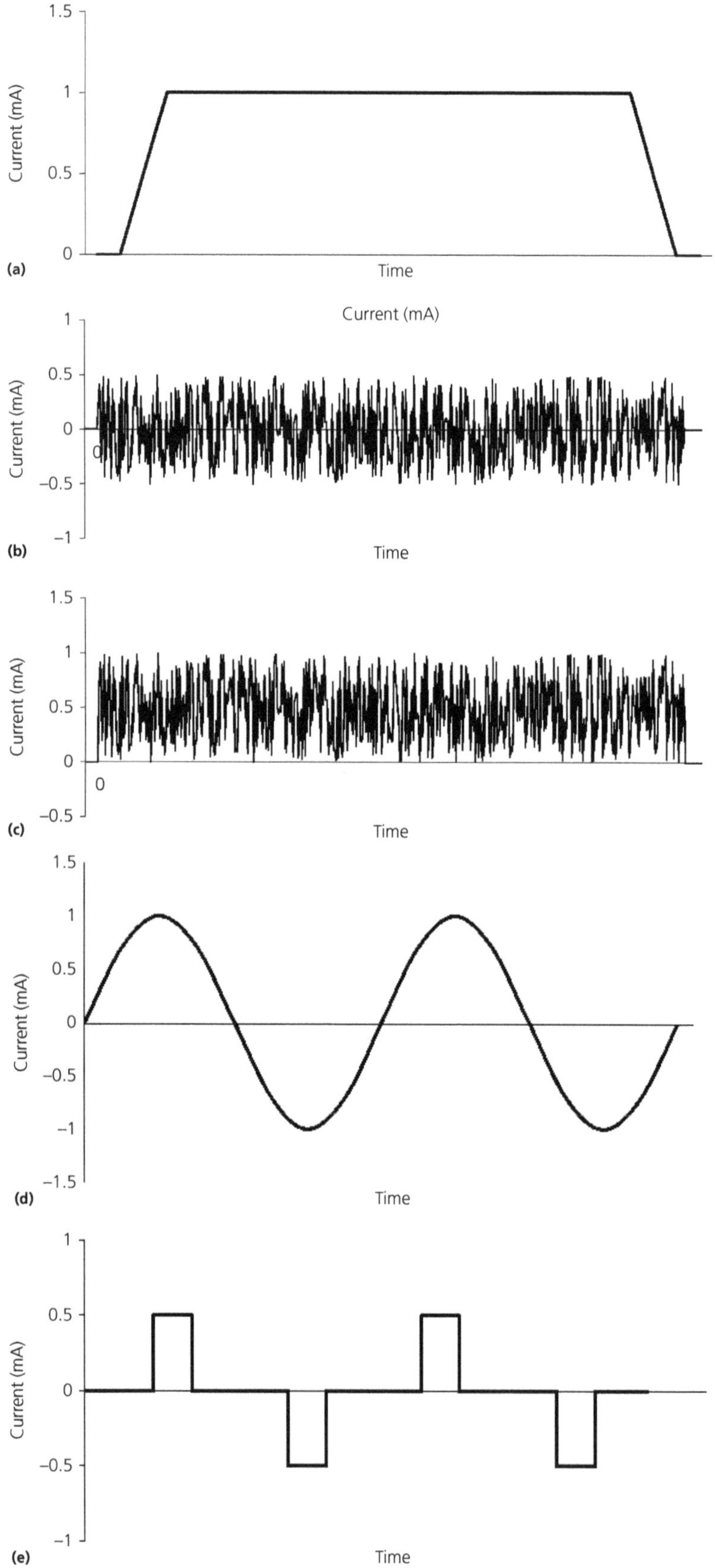

Figure 12.1 Schematic showing different waveforms used in transcranial electrical stimulation: **(a)** direct current stimulation (1 mA); **(b)** random noise stimulation (1 mA, 0 offset); **(c)** random noise stimulation (1 mA, 0.5 mA offset); **(d)** alternating current stimulation (2 mA); **(e)** pulsed, square wave, alternating current.

Adequate distance between electrodes is important, as close spacing of the electrodes will result in most of the current being shunted over the scalp, rather than penetrating the skull to stimulate neuronal tissue. Unlike transcranial magnetic stimulation (TMS), tDCS is a relatively diffuse stimulation [3]. Nevertheless, computer modelling studies suggest that the placement of the electrodes in different montage arrangements may result in significant differences in cerebral stimulation patterns [4]. Recently, the technique of 'High definition' tDCS was developed to deliver more focal stimulation [5]. In this approach, the main target electrode is surrounded by multiple return electrodes, such that the stimulatory effect is focused under the target electrode.

Recent research has shown that the electric field density induced in the cortex by tDCS is influenced by the anatomy of the gyri and sulci [6]. Neuronal effects are also dependent on the anatomy and orientation of the neuron relative to the tDCS electric field [7]. Overall, the effects of tDCS stimulation depend on the combination of electrode shape, size and number, electrode montage and inter-electrode distance, and stimulus parameters (amplitude, duration and spacing of stimulation sessions) [8–10].

Mechanisms of action

tDCS shifts the resting membrane potential, with anodal stimulation depolarizing the soma of pyramidal cells whereas cathodal stimulation results in hyperpolarization [1]. tDCS can change neuronal excitability, as demonstrated in neuroimaging and physiological studies [2, 11]. These studies show that (i) anodal and cathodal stimulation have specific and different effects; (ii) electrode montage (where the anode and cathode are positioned) determines the resultant neuronal effects; (iii) lasting changes of up to 90 min occur after a single stimulation session, the magnitude and duration of effects depending on the duration of the stimulus [12]; and (iv) sustained effects occur after repeated stimulation sessions [13, 14]. In clinical trials, tDCS sessions are often repeated every weekday, over a period of several weeks, to induce cumulative and lasting neuroplastic effects.

tDCS is a very mild form of brain stimulation and does not, in itself, depolarize neurons sufficiently to initiate action potentials. Rather, by changing the resting membrane potential, tDCS alters the threshold for neuronal depolarization. tDCS changes the background spontaneous neuronal firing rate. A preclinical study showed that background neuronal firing is essential for lasting effects of tDCS [15]. Apart from direct, immediate effects on membrane potential, tDCS also acts through synaptic mechanisms. This has been demonstrated by pharmacological challenge studies, in which specific receptor antagonists are given before tDCS, altering the effects of stimulation. These studies have shown that the NMDA, dopamine and other receptors mediate the effects of tDCS. Other mechanisms have also been proposed for the effects of tDCS (see [2, 16]).

Safety considerations

tDCS as practised in its modern form is relatively safe and well tolerated. It is estimated that current density induced in neuronal tissue is well within safety limits [17, 18]. The side effects most commonly observed with tDCS include mild tingling, itching or burning sensation felt underneath the electrodes during stimulation, and skin redness immediately following stimulation [19, 20]. Other less common side effects include fatigue and mild headache. More serious adverse side effects, however, have also been reported, including several cases of skin burns and lesions [21], and mood switch in bipolar depressed patients [22–24].

The risk for skin burns and lesions is increased with the use of increased stimulation parameters (e.g. higher current strength and longer exposure), repeated treatment sessions, poor tDCS technique and inadequate patient monitoring. Current studies have safely administered up to 2.5 mA current for 35 min [25]. A protocol for safe administration of tDCS has been published [26].

For patients receiving tDCS, it is important to check for existing skin disease, irritation, or lesion, or use of any skin treatment at or around the electrode sites before commencing each tDCS treatment. All of these factors can affect the likelihood of skin damage from tDCS and may exclude the patient from being able to safely receive tDCS. For example, it is recommended that tDCS should not be given over areas where the skin is broken (cut and abrasion) [19]. Before treatment, light cleaning of the skin underneath the electrode sites with an alcohol swab is also recommended to remove residual dirt and oils that can affect impedance levels. Single-use sponges soaked in an electrolyte solution are placed between the rubber electrode and skin. A low concentration saline solution ('normal saline', <140 nM) is recommended. Good contact with the skin over the whole electrode surface is important, to avoid concentration of current in focal areas. Before commencing treatment and at regular intervals during treatment, impedance levels should be monitored as an indicator of electrode contact. During treatment, it may be necessary to add small amounts of additional electrolyte to the sponges at regular intervals to prevent the sponges drying out, which will also increase impedance. Note that the use of too much electrolyte (e.g. so that it drips down the skin) will affect the direction of the current path through the skin. During treatment patients should also be carefully monitored and told to immediately report if the stimulation feels painful. Following stimulation, the electrode sites should then be checked for damage or skin irritation and the patients questioned in regard to the occurrence of other possible side effects (e.g. headache).

Mood switching has been reported to occur in depressed bipolar patients receiving tDCS. Careful patient screening is therefore important to determine whether a patient is bipolar before commencing treatment. Risk can be then further potentially minimized by ensuring that bipolar patients are taking mood stabilizer medication at an adequate therapeutic dose for the duration of the treatment course. Regular clinical monitoring for changes in mood and symptoms of mania is further recommended. Preliminary evidence additionally suggests that risk for induction of mania may be modulated by the choice of electrode montage, with a higher risk from montages that stimulate deeper regions [23].

Clinical results

Studies of tDCS to treat depression

The major focus of clinical trials in psychiatry has been the treatment of depression. Positive reports of antidepressant effects of tDCS span several decades [2, 16]. From 2000, facilitated by the commercial availability of modern tDCS machines, several randomized controlled trials have been conducted, using higher stimulus parameters than trials of previous decades. Stimulation has mainly been premised on excitatory, anodal stimulation of the left dorsolateral prefrontal cortex (left DLPFC, corresponding to F3 on the 10/20 EEG system), that is, a similar premise to the use of TMS in treating depression. The cathode has been placed at a distance on the contralateral frontal lobe, the exact position varying from F4, F8, to supraorbital. The optimal montage for antidepressant efficacy is yet to be clarified (see future directions). Most trials have given tDCS every weekday, for 1 or more weeks. Overall, from 2006 to the present, the stimulation parameters used in treatment trials (current intensity, stimulation duration and number of treatment sessions) have been gradually increased. See Table 12.1 for

Table 12.1 Controlled clinical trials investigating transcranial direct current stimulation (tDCS) for the treatment of depression.

Study	Participants and treatment groups (*N*)	Treatment resistance (mean number of antidepressant trials failed)	tDCS montage (anode, cathode)	tDCS parameters (e.g. 2 mA, 20 min)	Treatment sessions (number, frequency)	Mean % change in depression scores at end acute course	Response rate at end treatment (1 month follow-up)	Remission rate at end treatment (1 month follow-up)
Fregni *et al.* [27]	*N*=10, MDD Active tDCS [5] Sham tDCS [5]	NR	F3, RSO	1 mA, 20 min	Five sessions, alternate days	HAM-D:* **Active:** 60% **Sham**: 13% $p<0.05$ BDI-II **Active:** 70% **Sham**: 30% $p<0.05$	**Active**: 4/5 **Sham**: 0/5	NR
Boggio *et al.* [28]	*N*=40, MDD DLPFC tDCS [21] Occipital tDCS [9] Sham tDCS [10]	**DLPFC**: 1.6 **Occipital:** 1.7 **Sham**: 1.5	F3, RSO for DLPFC; anodal tDCS over occipital cortex for Occipital	2 mA, 20 min	Ten sessions	HDRS* **DLPFC:** 45.5% **Occipital**: 22.7% **Sham:** 13.6% DLPFC vs. sham: $p=0.0018$; DLPFC vs. occipital: $p=0.009$; Occipital vs. sham: $p=0.6$ BDI-II* **DLPFC:** 41% **Occipital**: 20% **Sham:** 11%	**DLPFC:** 8/21 **Occipital**: 0/9 **Sham:** 2/10 $p=0.019$	**DLPFC:** 5/21 **Occipital**: 0/9 **Sham:** 0/10 $p=0.02$

(*continued*)

Table 12.1 (Continued)

Study	Participants and treatment groups (*N*)	Treatment resistance (mean number of antidepressant trials failed)	tDCS montage (anode, cathode)	tDCS parameters (e.g. 2 mA, 20 min)	Treatment sessions (number, frequency)	Mean % change in depression scores at end acute course	Response rate at end treatment (1 month follow-up)	Remission rate at end treatment (1 month follow-up)
Loo *et al.* [29]	$N=40$, MDD Active tDCS [20] Sham tDCS [20]	**Active**: 1.0 **Sham**: 1.7	F3, RSO	1 mA, 20 min	Five sessions, three times per week (then open label)	MADRS* **Active**: 31.5% **Sham**: 29.6% NS	N/A for comparison period	N/A for comparison period
Loo *et al.* [19]	$N=64$, MDD Active tDCS [30] Sham tDCS [31]	**Active:** 1.7 **Sham:** 1.8	F3, RSO	2 mA, 20 min	Fifteen sessions, consecutive weekdays	MADRS: **Active:** 31.1% **Sham**: 16.2% Time × Treatment: $p=0.04$ IDS **Active:** 29.2% **Sham**: 18.1% NS QIDS-C **Active:** 28.7% **Sham**: 15.3% NS QIDS-SR: **Active:** 26.4% **Sham**: 22.8% Treatment: $p<0.05$ CGI **Active:** 14.9% **Sham**: 9.4% NS	**Active**: 4/33 **Sham**: 4/31	**Active**: 0/33 **Sham**: 0/31

Palm *et al.* [32]	N=22 (20 MDD, 2 BPAD) Active tDCS (then sham) [11] Sham tDCS (then active) [11]	**Active first**: 2.9 **Sham first**: 2.91	F3, RSO	1 mA (first 10 patients) or 2 mA (next 12 patients), 20 min	Ten sessions before crossover, consecutive weekdays	HAM-D: **Active first, active condition:** 16% **Sham first, sham condition**: 12% **Active first, sham condition:** 8% **Sham first, active condition**: 14% No effects of stimulation intensity on HAM-D (p=0.38)	N/A	N/A
Blumberger *et al.* [33]	N=24, MDD without psychotic features Active tDCS [13] Sham tDCS [11]	**Active:** 4.3 **Sham:** 4.1	F3, F4	2 mA, 20 min	Fifteen daily sessions, consecutive weekdays	HDRS-17: **Active:** 24.5% **Sham**: 24.9% NS, p=0.80 *Completers only*: NS, p=0.59 MADRS **Active:** 19.4% **Sham**: 13.4% NS, p=0.55 BDI-II **Active:** 35.0% **Sham**: 27.5% NS, p=0.38	HDRS-17 **Active:** 1/13 **Sham**: 1/11 MADRS **Active:** 1/13 **Sham**: 0/11 BDI-II **Active:** 3/13 **Sham**: 1/11	HDRS-17 **Active:** 0/13 **Sham**: 0/11 MADRS **Active:** 1/13 **Sham**: 0/11 BDI-II **Active:** 2/13 **Sham**: 1/11

(*continued*)

Table 12.1 (Continued)

Study	Participants and treatment groups (*N*)	Treatment resistance (mean number of antidepressant trials failed)	tDCS montage (anode, cathode)	tDCS parameters (e.g. 2 mA, 20 min)	Treatment sessions (number, frequency)	Mean % change in depression scores at end acute course	Response rate at end treatment (1 month follow-up)	Remission rate at end treatment (1 month follow-up)
Brunoni *et al*. [30]	*N* = 120, MDD	1.7	F3 and F4	2 mA, 30 min	Ten daily sessions, over 2 weeks.	MADRS	**Combined:** 16/30 [19/30]	**Combined:** 6/30 [14/30]
	Four groups: Combined (tDCS + sertraline) [34] tDCS (tDCS + placebo) [34] Sertraline (sertraline + sham tDCS) [34] Placebo (sham tDCS + placebo) [34]		*Note*: Sertraline fixed dose of 50 mg/day		Two sessions, given once a fortnight, following this.	**Combined:** 48.5% **Sertraline**: 28.9% **tDCS**: 34.0% **Placebo**: 30.2% Combined group vs. placebo ($p = 0.02$) vs. sertraline ($p = 0.01$) vs. tDCS ($p = 0.05$) Other comparisons NS	**Sertraline**: 10/30 [10/30] **tDCS**: 9/30 [13/30] **Placebo**: 11/30 [5/30]	**Sertraline**: 5/30 [9/30] **tDCS**: 4/30 [12/30] **Placebo**: 6/30 [4/30]

BDI-II, Beck Depression Inventory; BPAD, bipolar affective disorder; CGI, Clinical Global Impression Scale; DLPFC, dorsolateral prefrontal cortex; HAM-D, Hamilton Depression Scale; HDRS-17, 17 item Hamilton Depression Rating Scale; IDS, Inventory of Depressive Symptomatology; mA, milliamps; MADRS, Montgomery Asberg Depression Rating Scale; MDD, major depressive disorder; NR, not reported; NS, not significant; QIDS-C, Quick Inventory of Depression Symptomatology, Clinician; QIDS-SR, Quick Inventory of Depressive Symptomatology, Self-Rated; RSO, right supraorbital area.

* Approximate figures based on published graph.

placebo-controlled trials of tDCS to date, summarizing the treatment approach used and results obtained. Patients enrolled in these trials ranged from non-treatment resistant to highly treatment resistant. The majority of these trials reported significant efficacy for tDCS compared with sham stimulation, although trials with more treatment-resistant patients did not find tDCS effective [32, 33].

Two meta-analyses of placebo-controlled trials based on mean changes in depression scores found that tDCS had significant antidepressant efficacy compared to placebo 'sham' stimulation [34, 35]. Blumberger *et al.* [33] A meta-analysis based on response rates found no difference between active and sham tDCS [31]. Overall, the results of double-blind, placebo-controlled trials to date suggest that tDCS has antidepressant efficacy, although apart from the early trial of Fregni *et al.* [27] and the large trial of Brunoni *et al.* [30], response and remission rates have been relatively low (see Table 12.1). Research into optimizing tDCS treatment approach to improve outcomes is in its infancy.

The role of tDCS relative to antidepressant medications and other treatments is as yet unclear. Trials that included moderate pharmacotherapy-resistant patients (failed one to two antidepressants in current episode) mostly reported positive results. Trials with high treatment-resistant patients (failure of three to four antidepressant medications in current episode) did not find tDCS superior to sham stimulation (see Table 12.1). Other clinical predictors of response (e.g. depression subtype and patient demographics such as age) are as yet unclear. tDCS has only been specifically tested in bipolar depression in one small, open-label trial [36]. The response in bipolar depressed patients during the treatment week was comparable to that of unipolar depressed patients. Of interest, bipolar patients seemed to have better maintenance of response over the 1-month follow-up period. It is unclear whether this is a feature of the response of bipolar disorder to tDCS, or whether it may be explained by the fact that bipolar patients were treated with concurrent mood stabilizer medications during the trial and follow-up period.

Evidence from pharmacological challenge studies in healthy volunteers, testing which agents may block or modify the effects of tDCS [37–40], and from treatment studies in depressed patients, suggests that the effects of tDCS may be moderated by some medications. The trial in depressed patients by Brunoni *et al.* [30] found that the combination of prefrontal tDCS and sertraline, commenced together, was more effective than either treatment alone. This is consistent with an earlier proof of concept study in the motor cortex of healthy volunteers, which found sertraline may enhance changes in neuronal excitability induced by tDCS [41]. Conversely, analysing results from a naturalistic study, Brunoni and colleagues [36] suggested that concurrent treatment with benzodiazepines may reduce the antidepressant efficacy of tDCS. This is consistent with earlier findings from a motor cortex study in healthy volunteers that lorazepam altered the effects of anodal tDCS [42]. Studies in the motor cortex of healthy volunteers also suggest that anticonvulsant medications that block sodium channels (e.g. carbamazepine) may block the effects of anodal tDCS (though interestingly, not cathodal tDCS) [38], but the impact of this in clinical treatment studies (e.g. in depression) is as yet unclear.

tDCS in the treatment of schizophrenia

Interest has been growing in the potential of tDCS to treat symptoms of schizophrenia, in particular auditory hallucinations and cognitive deficits (see section below). Typically, cathodal (inhibitory) tDCS has been given over the temporoparietal cortex to treat auditory hallucinations, whereas anodal tDCS to the left prefrontal cortex has been used to enhance cognition. There have been several case reports of beneficial effects of tDCS on hallucinations and catatonia (for a review of studies of tDCS in schizophrenia, see Ref. 43). A particular advantage of tDCS is the potential for its ongoing use on a domiciliary basis in patients with chronic schizophrenia, given the portability and relatively low expense of the equipment [44]. There has been one RCT of tDCS in the treatment of schizophrenia. This double-blind, placebo-controlled trial by Brunelin and colleagues [45] gave tDCS twice per day for 5 days to 30 patients with schizophrenia and treatment refractory auditory hallucinations, using the electrode configuration described above. Results were promising, with significant reduction in hallucination scores (effects lasting up to 3 months), as well as significant reduction in negative symptom scores.

Maintenance of treatment effects

With pharmacotherapies, continuation or maintenance treatment is generally recommended to assist with prevention of relapse of depression. However, unlike those methods of treatment, therapeutic brain stimulation techniques, including tDCS and ECT, have a more distinct continuation and maintenance phase due in part to logistical and methodological considerations, including safety. Several different treatment options are therefore available for the prevention of relapse following response to the acute treatment phase, including changing the frequency of treatments, re-administration of an acute treatment phase when relapse occurs or introduction of a new treatment (e.g. psychological treatment).

Until now, a combination of the first two options has been investigated with moderate success. This approach was first used in a patient with schizophrenia in the 1960s, where after relapse an additional acute course was given followed by continuation treatment at a frequency of one or two tDCS sessions a week [46]. A recent report detailed ongoing successful treatment of a patient with severe schizophrenia, with tDCS sessions continued once to twice daily on a domiciliary basis (given the portability of the tDCS device) over a period of 3 years, maintaining excellent clinical response to treatment [44].

Two recent open-label studies have explored different treatment frequency schedules for up to 6 months following clinical response in depressed patients. One study investigated the efficacy of tDCS given on a weekly basis for the first 3 months, then fortnightly for the second 3 months. The majority or patients (84%) survived without relapse after the first 3 months of weekly treatment, although this dropped to 51% at the 6 month time point [47]. In the other study, tDCS was instead given fortnightly for the first 3 months, then monthly for the second 3 months, with results showing that 60 and 47% of patients survived without relapse, respectively [48]. These preliminary reports suggest that ongoing continuation/maintenance treatment may have a role, although this has yet to be tested in a placebo-controlled trial, and the optimal treatment frequency or protocol for continuation treatment remains to be determined. Notwithstanding, these early results suggest that a treatment frequency of at least one session a week may be effective at least in the short term. The level of treatment resistance may be an important consideration in determining the treatment frequency [47, 48]. Therefore, the optimal frequency and duration of continuation treatment may need to be determined on an individual level.

Cognitive enhancing effects of tDCS

The cognitive enhancing effects of tDCS have gained increasing attention. The majority of research has been conducted in healthy participants, where studies have focused on primarily, but not limited to, tDCS effects on attention, learning and memory, and executive functioning (e.g. working memory, problem solving, response inhibition and generativity). There is now strong evidence to suggest that tDCS can modulate and enhance these and potentially other cognitive processes [49]. A further line of investigation has involved using tDCS to enhance the effects of cognitive training, based on the principle that anodal tDCS lowers the threshold for neuronal activation, and thus stimulation before, or during cognitive training, may facilitate the activation and reinforcement of the specific neural circuits involved [50–52]. These findings have direct relevance for clinical populations including psychiatric conditions, where cognitive dysfunction is a common symptom or phenotype. Cognitive dysfunction is directly associated with day-to-day functional abilities of patients, so the potential for cognitive enhancement using tDCS offers promising therapeutic potential.

A growing number of studies have investigated the effects of tDCS on cognition in psychiatric conditions. The majority of this research has been conducted in depressed patients where RCTs investigating antidepressant effects have evaluated both acute (i.e. during and immediately after treatment) and cumulative effects following repeated treatments. Interestingly, reports of acute cognitive effects of tDCS in depressed patients date back to the 1960s. For example, in an early double-blind trial, it was reported that bifrontal anodal stimulation transiently increased both alertness and talkativeness in some patients, whilst cathodal stimulation, in contrast, had a subduing effect during stimulation [53]. Similar acute cognitive enhancing effects have been reported in trials conducted since 2000 which have primarily focused on anodal tDCS stimulation given to the left DLPFC. In a large double-blind trial, an acute cognitive enhancing effect was found on a test of processing speed and attention which was administered immediately before and after the first treatment session [19]. Acute performance-enhancing effects on working memory [54] and emotional bias [55–57] have similarly been reported. The latter effects are of particular interest, as they may represent a potential mechanism for antidepressant effects. In contrast, bifrontal tDCS was found to decrease implicit learning in another study, which potentially may be attributed to cathodal stimulatory effects on the right DLPFC [58].

Findings in relation to cumulative cognitive enhancing effects following repeated treatments, however, have been less clear. A small trial reported significant improvements in working memory performance, assessed using the Digit Span test, following five treatment sessions [27]. Other larger trials though have failed to find any cumulative cognitive effects following up to 15 treatment sessions using this same measure, or using other cognitive measures that have also evaluated effects on learning and memory and executive functions [19, 30, 59]. It is possible that the failure to detect cumulative effects may be due to confounding of antidepressant effects. Assessment of these effects earlier in the treatment course may therefore help to delineate this issue. Indeed, in a study that analysed a large dataset comprising several clinical trials of TMS for depression, significant improvement on a visual memory test was found midway during the treatment course, which in turn significantly predicted final antidepressant response [60]. In addition, it is possible that cumulative cognitive enhancing effects may be best obtained when tDCS treatment is combined with performance on a cognitive task. In a recent pilot study, for example, significant improvement on an affective working memory task was found at follow-up with tDCS combined with cognitive control training [61, 62].

Compared to in depression, the cognitive enhancing effects of tDCS in other psychiatric conditions have been minimally studied. Preliminary work has investigated acute cognitive effects in patients with schizophrenia and substance use disorders. Patients with schizophrenia show significant cognitive deficits across multiple domains, including attention, learning and memory, executive function and social cognition. The modulation and enhancement of cognitive functioning with tDCS therefore may be useful for the development of new therapeutic treatments for cognition. Two studies so far have investigated acute effects with promising results. Vercammen and colleagues [63] investigated the effect of anodal left DLPFC stimulation on performance on a difficult probabilistic decision-making task. Whilst no overall effect on performance was found across the entire sample, in a subset of patients who demonstrated the ability to learn on the task at baseline, performance was significantly improved. In a second study, right but not left anodal posterior parietal cortex stimulation modulated and partially corrected the absence of a left attentional bias observed in patients, an approach that may be useful for remediating right hemispheric dysfunction associated with the disorder [64].

There is also growing interest in the cognitive effects of tDCS in substance use disorders. Both left anodal/right cathodal DLPFC and right anodal/left cathodal DLPFC stimulation were shown to increase risky decision making in chronic cannabis users [65]. In contrast, acute improvement in executive functioning was found following anodal left DLPFC stimulation in alcohol-dependent patients, but only in the type characterized by poorer baseline cognitive functioning [66]. Cumulative effects have also been examined in alcoholic patients, with a trend improvement in change in executive functioning found following repeated tDCS sessions given once a week [67]. These results therefore provide preliminary evidence for acute modulation of executive functioning with prefrontal tDCS in these disorders. These effects may assist with the development of new treatment approaches that focus on improving impulse control and/or regulating mood. Increased response inhibition, for example, has been demonstrated with tDCS combined with training in healthy adults [68]. Such a new treatment may have potential therapeutic applications in other impulse control disorders, including attention-deficit hyperactivity disorder, obsessive–compulsive disorder and eating disorders.

Future directions

There is much scope for the further optimization of tDCS treatment technique to maximize therapeutic effects. Recent clinical trials have used incrementally higher stimulus amplitudes and stimulus durations. However, these parameter increases are limited by tolerability (higher stimulus amplitudes are uncomfortable or painful) and the risk of skin damage. Several studies have investigated the use of two or more stimulus sessions separated by intervals of minutes to hours, showing that the interaction between sessions can be critical to enhancing, negating or even reversing anodal or cathodal effects [9, 15, 69, 70]. This is based on the principle of metaplasticity, that is, the first stimulation session 'primes' the brain, influencing the response to subsequent stimulation sessions when the latter are given within a certain critical period of after effects.

Fine-tuning the electrode montage may also be an important factor in optimizing tDCS for the treatment of specific psychiatric disorders, with electrodes placed such as to maximize stimulation to key brain regions. For example, a small pilot trial suggested that antidepressant effects may be enhanced by targeting deep brain regions [71].

As discussed in the review of experimental data above, there may be benefits from combining tDCS with pharmacological agents or cognitive-based interventions, such that neuroplastic and/or therapeutic effects are additive or synergistic.

Finally, other forms of transcranial electrical stimulation in the low-amplitude range are also being explored. These include random noise stimulation (in which the amplitude and frequency of the current change continuously and randomly), transcranial alternating current (in which the current is bidirectional, unlike in tDCS) and other manipulations of current waveform (for a review, see Ref. 72). There is preliminary evidence that these may also have useful therapeutic effects [73–75].

In conclusion, tDCS and related forms of low-amplitude transcranial electrical stimulation show promising potential in the treatment of neuropsychiatric disorders. It has large potential for translation into the clinical sphere as the equipment is relatively inexpensive and portable, and early reports suggest that selected patients could be trained to continue with maintenance treatment sessions at home. Research has already begun to explore methods of optimizing stimulation efficacy, such that more potent forms of therapeutic tDCS are tested in future clinical trials.

References

1 Bindman LJ, Lippold OC, Redfearn JW. The action of brief polarizing currents on the cerebral cortex of the rat (1) during current flow and (2) in the production of long-lasting after-effects. The Journal of Physiology. 1964 Aug;172:369–82. PubMed PMID: 14199369. Pubmed Central PMCID: 1368854.

2 Arul-Anandam AP, Loo C. Transcranial direct current stimulation: a new tool for the treatment of depression? Journal of Affective Disorders. 2009 Feb 6;117:137–45. PubMed PMID: 19201483. Epub 2009/02/10. Eng.

3 Sadleir RJ, Vannorsdall TD, Schretlen DJ, Gordon B. Transcranial direct current stimulation (tDCS) in a realistic head model. NeuroImage. 2010 Jul 15;51(4):1310–8. PubMed PMID: 20350607.

4 Bai S, Dokos S, Ho KA, Loo C. A computational modelling study of transcranial direct current stimulation montages used in depression. NeuroImage. 2014 Feb 15;87:332–44. PubMed PMID: 24246487.

5 Datta A, Bansal V, Diaz J, Patel J, Reato D, Bikson M. Gyri-precise head model of transcranial direct current stimulation: improved spatial focality using a ring electrode versus conventional rectangular pad. Brain Stimulation. 2009 Oct;2(4):201–7, 7 e1. PubMed PMID: 20648973. Pubmed Central PMCID: 2790295.

6 Miranda PC, Mekonnen A, Salvador R, Ruffini G. The electric field in the cortex during transcranial current stimulation. NeuroImage. 2013 Apr 15;70:48–58. PubMed PMID: 23274187.

7 Radman T, Ramos RL, Brumberg JC, Bikson M. Role of cortical cell type and morphology in subthreshold and suprathreshold uniform electric field stimulation in vitro. Brain Stimulation. 2009 Oct;2(4):215–28, 28 e1–3. PubMed PMID: 20161507. Pubmed Central PMCID: 2797131.

8 Nitsche MA, Seeber A, Frommann K, Klein CC, Rochford C, Nitsche MS, *et al.* Modulating parameters of excitability during and after transcranial direct current stimulation of the human motor cortex. The Journal of Physiology. 2005 Oct 1;568(Pt 1):291–303. PubMed PMID: 16002441. Pubmed Central PMCID: 1474757.

9 Monte-Silva K, Kuo MF, Liebetanz D, Paulus W, Nitsche MA. Shaping the optimal repetition interval for cathodal transcranial direct current stimulation (tDCS). Journal of Neurophysiology. 2010 Apr;103(4):1735–40. PubMed PMID: 20107115.

10 Moliadze V, Antal A, Paulus W. Electrode-distance dependent after-effects of transcranial direct and random noise stimulation with extracephalic reference electrodes. Clinical Neurophysiology. 2010 Dec;121(12):2165–71. PubMed PMID: 20554472.

11 Nitsche MA, Cohen LG, Wassermann EM, Priori A, Lang N, Antal A, *et al.* Transcranial direct current stimulation: state of the art 2008. Brain Stimulation. 2008 Jul;1(3):206–23. PubMed PMID: 20633386.

12 Nitsche MA, Paulus W. Sustained excitability elevations induced by transcranial DC motor cortex stimulation in humans. Neurology. 2001 Nov 27;57(10):1899–901. PubMed PMID: 11723286.

13 Alonzo A, Brassil J, Taylor JL, Martin D, Loo CK. Daily transcranial direct current stimulation (tDCS) leads to greater increases in cortical

excitability than second daily transcranial direct current stimulation. Brain Stimulation. 2012 Jul;5(3):208–13. PubMed PMID: 22037139.

14 Galvez V, Alonzo A, Martin D, Loo CK. Transcranial direct current stimulation treatment protocols: should stimulus intensity be constant or incremental over multiple sessions? The International Journal of Neuropsychopharmacology. 2013 Feb;16(1):13–21. PubMed PMID: 22310245.

15 Fricke K, Seeber AA, Thirugnanasambandam N, Paulus W, Nitsche MA, Rothwell JC. Time course of the induction of homeostatic plasticity generated by repeated transcranial direct current stimulation of the human motor cortex. Journal of Neurophysiology. 2011 Mar;105(3):1141–9. PubMed PMID: 21177994.

16 Nitsche MA, Boggio PS, Fregni F, Pascual-Leone A. Treatment of depression with transcranial direct current stimulation (tDCS): a review. Experimental Neurology. 2009 Sep;219(1):14–9. PubMed PMID: 19348793.

17 Nitsche MA, Liebetanz D, Lang N, Antal A, Tergau F, Paulus W. Safety criteria for transcranial direct current stimulation (tDCS) in humans. Clinical Neurophysiology. 2003 Nov;114(11):2220–2; author reply 2–3. PubMed PMID: 14580622.

18 Bikson M, Datta A, Elwassif M. Establishing safety limits for transcranial direct current stimulation. Clinical Neurophysiology. 2009 Jun; 120(6):1033–4. PubMed PMID: 19394269. Pubmed Central PMCID: 2754807.

19 Loo CK, Alonzo A, Martin D, Mitchell PB, Galvez V, Sachdev P. Transcranial direct current stimulation for depression: 3-week, randomised, sham-controlled trial. The British Journal of Psychiatry. 2012 Jan;200(1):52–9. PubMed PMID: 22215866.

20 Brunoni AR, Amadera J, Berbel B, Volz MS, Rizzerio BG, Fregni F. A systematic review on reporting and assessment of adverse effects associated with transcranial direct current stimulation. The International Journal of Neuropsychopharmacology. 2011 Sep;14(8): 1133–45. PubMed PMID: 21320389.

21 Palm U, Keeser D, Schiller C, Fintescu Z, Nitsche M, Reisinger E, *et al.* Skin lesions after treatment with transcranial direct current stimulation (tDCS). Brain Stimulation. 2008 Oct;1(4):386–7. PubMed PMID: 20633396.

22 Arul-Anandam AP, Loo C, Mitchell P. Induction of hypomanic episode with transcranial direct current stimulation. The Journal of ECT. 2010 Mar;26(1):68–9. PubMed PMID: 19483641.

23 Galvez V, Alonzo A, Martin D, Mitchell PB, Sachdev P, Loo CK. Hypomania induction in a patient with bipolar II disorder by transcranial direct current stimulation (tDCS). The Journal of ECT. 2011 Sep;27(3):256–8. PubMed PMID: 21206371.

24 Brunoni AR, Valiengo L, Zanao T, de Oliveira JF, Bensenor IM, Fregni F. Manic psychosis after sertraline and transcranial direct-current stimulation. The Journal of Neuropsychiatry and Clinical Neurosciences. 2011 Summer;23(3): E4–5. PubMed PMID: 21948925.

25 Koenigs M, Ukueberuwa D, Campion P, Grafman J, Wassermann E. Bilateral frontal transcranial direct current stimulation: failure to replicate classic findings in healthy subjects. Clinical Neurophysiology. 2009 Jan;120(1):80–4. PubMed PMID: 19027357. Pubmed Central PMCID: 2650218.

26 Loo CK, Martin DM, Alonzo A, Gandevia S, Mitchell PB, Sachdev P. Avoiding skin burns with transcranial direct current stimulation: preliminary considerations. The International Journal of Neuropsychopharmacology. 2011 Apr;14(3):425–6. PubMed PMID: 20923600.

27 Fregni F, Boggio PS, Nitsche MA, Marcolin MA, Rigonatti SP, Pascual-Leone A. Treatment of major depression with transcranial direct current stimulation. Bipolar Disorders. 2006 Apr;8(2):203–4. PubMed PMID: 16542193.

28 Boggio PS, Rigonatti SP, Ribeiro RB, Myczkowski ML, Nitsche MA, Pascual-Leone A, *et al.* A randomized, double-blind clinical trial on the efficacy of cortical direct current stimulation for the treatment of major depression. The International Journal of Neuropsychopharmacology. 2008 Mar;11(2):249–54. PubMed PMID: 17559710. Pubmed Central PMCID: 3372849.

29 Loo CK, Sachdev P, Martin D, Pigot M, Alonzo A, Malhi GS, *et al.* A double-blind, sham-controlled trial of transcranial direct current stimulation for the treatment of depression. International Journal of Neuropsychopharmacology. 2010 Feb; 13(1): 61-69. PubMed PMID: 19671217

30 Brunoni AR, Valiengo L, Baccaro A, Zanao T, de Oliveira JF, Goulart AC, *et al.* The sertraline vs

electrical current therapy for treating depression clinical study: results from a factorial, randomised, controlled trial. JAMA Psychiatry. 2013;70(4):383–91.
31 Berlim MT, Van den Eynde F, Daskalakis ZJ. Clinical utility of transcranial direct current stimulation (tDCS) for treating major depression: a systematic review and meta-analysis of randomized, double-blind and sham-controlled trials. Journal of Psychiatric Research. 2013 Jan;47(1):1–7. PubMed PMID: 23084964.
32 Palm U, Schiller C, Fintescu Z, Obermeier M, Keeser D, Reisinger E, *et al*. Transcranial direct current stimulation in treatment resistant depression: a randomized double-blind, placebo-controlled study. Brain Stimulation. 2012 Jul;5(3):242–51. PubMed PMID: 21962978.
33 Blumberger DM, Tran LC, Fitzgerald PB, Hoy KE, Daskalakis ZJ. A randomized double-blind sham-controlled study of transcranial direct current stimulation for treatment-resistant major depression. Frontiers in Psychiatry. 2012;3:74. PubMed PMID: 22912618. Pubmed Central PMCID: 3421236.
34 Shiozawa P, Fregni F, Bensenor IM, Lotufo PA, Berlim MT, Daskalakis JZ, *et al*. Transcranial direct current stimulation for major depression: an updated systematic review and meta-analysis. The International Journal of Neuropsychopharmacology. 2014 Sep;17(9):1443–52. PubMed PMID: 24713139.
35 Kalu UG, Sexton CE, Loo CK, Ebmeier KP. Transcranial direct current stimulation in the treatment of major depression: a meta-analysis. Psychological Medicine. 2012 Sep;42(9):1791–800. PubMed PMID: 22236735.
36 Brunoni AR, Ferrucci R, Bortolomasi M, Vergari M, Tadini L, Boggio PS, *et al*. Transcranial direct current stimulation (tDCS) in unipolar vs. bipolar depressive disorder. Progress in Neuro-Psychopharmacology & Biological Psychiatry. 2011 Jan 15;35(1):96–101. PubMed PMID: 20854868.
37 Liebetanz D, Nitsche MA, Tergau F, Paulus W. Pharmacological approach to the mechanisms of transcranial DC-stimulation-induced after-effects of human motor cortex excitability. Brain. 2002 Oct;125(Pt 10):2238–47. PubMed PMID: 12244081.
38 Nitsche MA, Fricke K, Henschke U, Schlitterlau A, Liebetanz D, Lang N, *et al*. Pharmacological modulation of cortical excitability shifts induced by transcranial direct current stimulation in humans. The Journal of Physiology. 2003 Nov 15;553(Pt 1):293–301. PubMed PMID: 12949224. Pubmed Central PMCID: 2343495.
39 Nitsche MA, Liebetanz D, Schlitterlau A, Henschke U, Fricke K, Frommann K, *et al*. GABAergic modulation of DC stimulation-induced motor cortex excitability shifts in humans. The European Journal of Neuroscience. 2004 May;19(10):2720–6. PubMed PMID: 15147306.
40 Kuo MF, Paulus W, Nitsche MA. Boosting focally-induced brain plasticity by dopamine. Cerebral Cortex. 2008 Mar;18(3):648–51. PubMed PMID: 17591596.
41 Nitsche MA, Kuo MF, Karrasch R, Wachter B, Liebetanz D, Paulus W. Serotonin affects transcranial direct current-induced neuroplasticity in humans. Biological Psychiatry. 2009 Sep 1;66(5):503–8. PubMed PMID: 19427633.
42 Nitsche MA, Niehaus L, Hoffmann KT, Hengst S, Liebetanz D, Paulus W, *et al*. MRI study of human brain exposed to weak direct current stimulation of the frontal cortex. Clinical Neurophysiology. 2004 Oct;115(10):2419–23. PubMed PMID: 15351385.
43 Agarwal SM, Shivakumar V, Bose A, Subramaniam A, Nawani H, Chhabra H, *et al*. Transcranial direct current stimulation in schizophrenia. Clinical Psychopharmacology and Neuroscience. 2013 Dec;11(3):118–25. PubMed PMID: 24465247. Pubmed Central PMCID: 3897759.
44 Andrade C. Once- to twice-daily, 3-year domiciliary maintenance transcranial direct current stimulation for severe, disabling, clozapine-refractory continuous auditory hallucinations in schizophrenia. The Journal of ECT. 2013 Sep;29(3):239–42. PubMed PMID: 23377748.
45 Brunelin J, Mondino M, Gassab L, Haesebaert F, Gaha L, Suaud-Chagny MF, *et al*. Examining transcranial direct-current stimulation (tDCS) as a treatment for hallucinations in schizophrenia. American Journal of Psychiatry. 2012 Jul;169(7): 719-24. PubMed PMID: k
46 Herjanic M, Moss-Herjanic B. Clinical report on a new therapeutic technique: polarization.

Canadian Psychiatric Association Journal. 1967 Aug;12(4):423–4. PubMed PMID: 6064676.
47 Martin DM, Alonzo A, Ho KA, Player M, Mitchell PB, Sachdev P, *et al.* Continuation transcranial direct current stimulation for the prevention of relapse in major depression. Journal of Affective Disorders. 2013 Jan 25;144(3):274–8. PubMed PMID: 23146197.
48 Valiengo L, Bensenor IM, Goulart AC, de Oliveira JF, Zanao TA, Boggio PS, *et al.* The sertraline versus electrical current therapy for treating depression clinical study (select-TDCS): results of the crossover and follow-up phases. Depression and Anxiety. 2013 Jul;30(7):646–53. PubMed PMID: 23625554.
49 Coffman BA, Clark VP, Parasuraman R. Battery powered thought: enhancement of attention, learning, and memory in healthy adults using transcranial direct current stimulation. NeuroImage. 2014 Jan 15;85(Pt 3):895–908. PubMed PMID: 23933040.
50 Martin DM, Liu R, Alonzo A, Green M, Player MJ, Sachdev P, *et al.* Can transcranial direct current stimulation enhance outcomes from cognitive training? A randomized controlled trial in healthy participants. The International Journal of Neuropsychopharmacology. 2013 Oct;16(9):1927–36. PubMed PMID: 23719048.
51 Park SH. Long-term effects of transcranial direct current stimulation combined with computer-assisted cognitive training in healthy older adults. Neuroreport. 2014;25(2):122–6.
52 Martin DM, Liu R, Alonzo A, Green M, Loo CK. Use of transcranial direct current stimulation (tDCS) to enhance cognitive training: effect of timing of stimulation. Experimental Brain Research. 2014 Oct;232:3345–51. PubMed PMID: 24992897.
53 Lippold OC, Redfearn JW. Mental changes resulting from the passage of small direct currents through the human brain. The British Journal of Psychiatry 1964 Nov;110:768–72. PubMed PMID: 14211693.
54 Oliveira JF, Zanao TA, Valiengo L, Lotufo PA, Bensenor IM, Fregni F, *et al.* Acute working memory improvement after tDCS in antidepressant-free patients with major depressive disorder. Neuroscience Letters. 2013 Mar 14;537:60–4. PubMed PMID: 23370288.
55 Brunoni AR, Zanao TA, Vanderhasselt MA, Valiengo L, de Oliveira JF, Boggio PS, *et al.* Enhancement of affective processing induced by bifrontal transcranial direct current stimulation in patients with major depression. Neuromodulation. 2014 Feb;17(2):138–42. PubMed PMID: 23710817.
56 Boggio PS, Rocha RR, da Silva MT, Fregni F. Differential modulatory effects of transcranial direct current stimulation on a facial expression go-no-go task in males and females. Neuroscience Letters. 2008 Dec 12;447(2–3):101–5. PubMed PMID: 18926878.
57 Wolkenstein L, Plewnia C. Amelioration of cognitive control in depression by transcranial direct current stimulation. Biological Psychiatry. 2013 Apr 1;73(7):646–51. PubMed PMID: 23219367.
58 Brunoni AR, Zanao TA, Ferrucci R, Priori A, Valiengo L, de Oliveira JF, *et al.* Bifrontal tDCS prevents implicit learning acquisition in antidepressant-free patients with major depressive disorder. Progress in NeuroPsychopharmacology & Biological Psychiatry 2013 Jun 3;43:146–50. PubMed PMID: 23274503.
59 Loo CK, Sachdev P, Martin D, Pigot M, Alonzo A, Malhi GS, *et al.* A double-blind, sham-controlled trial of transcranial direct current stimulation for the treatment of depression. The International Journal of Neuropsychopharmacology. 2010 Feb;13(1):61–9. PubMed PMID: 19671217.
60 Hoy KE, Segrave RA, Daskalakis ZJ, Fitzgerald PB. Investigating the relationship between cognitive change and antidepressant retrospective study. Brain Stimulation. 2012;5(4):539–46.
61 Segrave RA, Arnold S, Hoy K, Fitzgerald PB. Concurrent cognitive control training augments the antidepressant efficacy of tDCS: a pilot study. Brain Stimulation. 2014 Mar–Apr; 7(2):325–31. PubMed PMID: 24486425.
62 Brunoni AR, Boggio PS, De Raedt R, Bensenor IM, Lotufo PA, Namur V, *et al.* Cognitive control therapy and transcranial direct current stimulation for depression: a randomized, double-blinded, controlled trial. Journal of Affective Disorders. 2014 Jun;162:43–9. PubMed PMID: 24767004.
63 Vercammen A, Rushby JA, Loo C, Short B, Weickert CS, Weickert TW. Transcranial direct

current stimulation influences probabilistic association learning in schizophrenia. Schizophrenia Research. 2011 Sep;131(1–3):198–205. PubMed PMID: 21745726.
64 Ribolsi M, Lisi G, Di Lorenzo G, Koch G, Oliveri M, Magni V, *et al.* Perceptual pseudoneglect in schizophrenia: candidate endophenotype and the role of the right parietal cortex. Schizophrenia Bulletin. 2013 May;39(3):601–7. PubMed PMID: 22419195. Pubmed Central PMCID: 3627750.
65 Boggio PS, Zaghi S, Villani AB, Fecteau S, Pascual-Leone A, Fregni F. Modulation of risk-taking in marijuana users by transcranial direct current stimulation (tDCS) of the dorsolateral prefrontal cortex (DLPFC). Drug and Alcohol Dependence. 2010 Dec 1;112(3):220–5. PubMed PMID: 20729009.
66 Nakamura-Palacios EM, de Almeida Benevides MC, da Penha Zago-Gomes M, de Oliveira RW, de Vasconcellos VF, de Castro LN, *et al.* Auditory event-related potentials (P3) and cognitive changes induced by frontal direct current stimulation in alcoholics according to Lesch alcoholism typology. The International Journal of Neuropsychopharmacology. 2012 Jun;15(5):601–16. PubMed PMID: 21781352.
67 da Silva MC, Conti CL, Klauss J, Alves LG, do Nascimento Cavalcante HM, Fregni F, *et al.* Behavioral effects of transcranial direct current stimulation (tDCS) induced dorsolateral prefrontal cortex plasticity in alcohol dependence. Journal of Physiology, Paris 2013 Dec; 107(6):493–502. PubMed PMID: 23891741.
68 Ditye T, Jacobson L, Walsh V, Lavidor M. Modulating behavioral inhibition by tDCS combined with cognitive training. Experimental Brain Research. 2012 Jun;219(3):363–8. PubMed PMID: 22532165.
69 Monte-Silva K, Kuo MF, Hessenthaler S, Fresnoza S, Liebetanz D, Paulus W, *et al.* Induction of late LTP-like plasticity in the human motor cortex by repeated non-invasive brain stimulation. Brain Stimulation. 2013 May;6(3):424–32. PubMed PMID: 22695026.
70 Bastani A, Jaberzadeh S. Within-session repeated a-tDCS: the effects of repetition rate and inter-stimulus interval on corticospinal excitability and motor performance. Clinical Neurophysiology. 2014 Sep;125:1809–18. PubMed PMID: 24582469.
71 Martin DM, Alonzo A, Mitchell PB, Sachdev P, Galvez V, Loo CK. Fronto-extracephalic transcranial direct current stimulation as a treatment for major depression: an open-label pilot study. Journal of Affective Disorders. 2011 Nov;134(1–3):459–63. PubMed PMID: 21641047.
72 Guleyupoglu B, Schestatsky P, Edwards D, Fregni F, Bikson M. Classification of methods in transcranial electrical stimulation (tES) and evolving strategy from historical approaches to contemporary innovations. Journal of Neuroscience Methods. 2013 Oct 15;219(2):297–311. PubMed PMID: 23954780. Pubmed Central PMCID: 3833074.
73 Chan HN, Alonzo A, Martin DM, Player M, Mitchell PB, Sachdev P, *et al.* Treatment of major depressive disorder by transcranial random noise stimulation: case report of a novel treatment. Biological Psychiatry. 2012 Aug 15;72(4):e9–10. PubMed PMID: 22425412.
74 Vanneste S, Fregni F, De Ridder D. Head-to-head comparison of transcranial random noise stimulation, transcranial AC stimulation, and transcranial DC stimulation for tinnitus. Frontiers in Psychiatry. 2013;4:158. PubMed PMID: 24391599. Pubmed Central PMCID: 3866637.
75 Palm U, Hasan A, Keeser D, Falkai P, Padberg F. Transcranial random noise stimulation for the treatment of negative symptoms in schizophrenia. Schizophrenia Research. 2013 May; 146(1–3):372–3. PubMed PMID: 23517664.

CHAPTER 13

Deep brain stimulation: Introduction and technical aspects

Willard S. Kasoff[1] and Robert E. Gross[2]
[1] University of Arizona College of Medicine, Tucson, USA
[2] Emory University School of Medicine, Atlanta, USA

Introduction

History of stereotaxy and deep brain stimulation

Although neuromodulation for psychiatric disorders has attracted increasing attention in recent years, the historical connections between stereotactic neurosurgery and modern psychiatry date to the earliest foundations of both fields. Indeed, interest in psychiatric disease was the major driving force in the development of early stereotactic lesioning procedures in the 1940s and 1950s as well as that of deep brain stimulation (DBS) in the 1970s and 1980s. In their pioneering 1947 description of a human stereotactic apparatus (which was adapted from the Horsley–Clarke animal apparatus developed in 1908), Spiegel and Wycis noted that 'this apparatus is being used for psychosurgery. In a series of patients … lesions have been placed in the region of the medial nucleus of the thalamus (medial thalamotomy) in order to reduce the emotional reactivity by a procedure much less drastic than frontal lobotomy' [1]. As reported by Gildenberg, who had worked as a medical student with Spiegel and Wycis, the desire to avoid the 'often devastating' effects of prefrontal lobotomy motivated the development of an apparatus to allow discrete lesions in the dorsomedial thalamus, which 'reverberated' with the prefrontal area [2]. The stereotactic apparatuses developed by Spiegel and Wycis, and shortly thereafter by Leksell and others, found widespread applications in non-psychiatric disorders, including movement disorders, pain and epilepsy, while surgery for psychiatric disorders fell out of favour in the 1970s due to ethical and public-opinion concerns [2–7]. Leksell's frame, in particular, the target-centred arc of which was perfectly suited for early efforts in radiosurgery (and which continues to be used for this purpose), was used for gamma capsulotomies for severe anxiety and obsessive–compulsive disorder (OCD); however, Leksell noted in 1983 that 'psychosurgery meets much opposition from ideologists in Sweden and elsewhere in the world' [8]. Whether for psychiatric disorders (e.g. dorsal thalamotomy and capsulotomy) or other functional disorders, the primary use of the stereotactic frame was to provide access to deep structures for ablative lesions, including radiosurgery (Figure 13.1).

The use of the stereotactic frame to deliver electrodes for electrical stimulation of deep structures of the brain followed surprisingly quickly, and again found early application in psychiatric disorders. An early pioneer of neuromodulation, Lawrence Pool, at the Neurological Institute at

Neuromodulation in Psychiatry, First Edition. Edited by Clement Hamani, Paul Holtzheimer, Andres M. Lozano and Helen Mayberg.

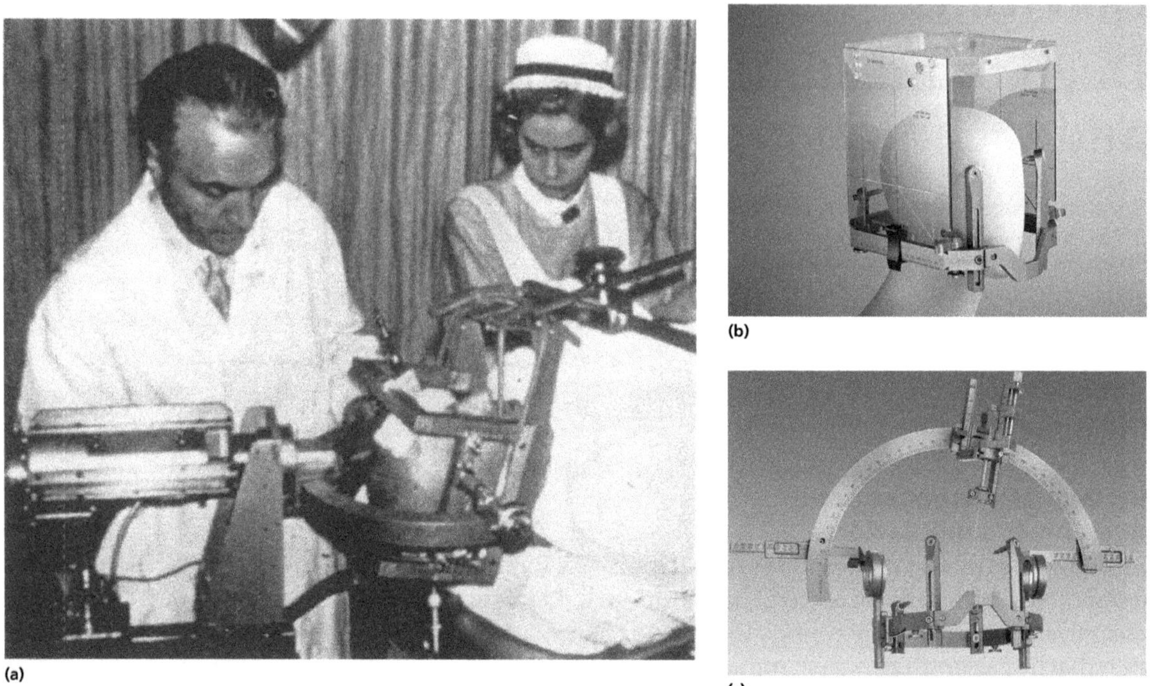

(a)

(b)

(c)

Figure 13.1 Leksell arc-centred stereotactic frame. Lars Leksell was an influential early pioneer in stereotactic and functional neurosurgery, here (**a**) performing a radiosurgical anterior capsulotomy, which he pioneered. He designed the Leksell stereotactic frame, a version of which remains in popular usage today, for functional stereotactic procedures including psychiatric surgery. Source: From Leksell [8]. Reproduced with permission from BMJ Publishing Group Ltd. The present-day Leksell G frame (**b** and **c**) shown with the fiducial localizer box (**b**) for imaging and with the stereotactic arc with instrument holder (**c**). This is a classic arc-centred device: with the frame set for the target coordinates, all angles of approach will direct an instrument to the target. (Source: b and c reproduced with permission of Elekta).

Columbia University, reasoned that electrical stimulation might provide a non-destructive, reversible alternative to ablative procedures such as subfrontal leucotomy, which were performed all too commonly at that time. Having implanted an earlier patient with an induction coil for stimulating the femoral nerve for paraparesis [9], in 1948 Pool placed a silver electrode in the caudate nucleus of a patient with Parkinson's disease afflicted with intractable depression, coupled to a permanent mini induction coil placed in the skull, and reported that the patient had some benefits from daily stimulation for 8 weeks; a wire broke and the therapy was discontinued [10]. Pool also implanted a psychotic patient in 1948 with a cingulate gyrus stimulator [11]. In 1954, Heath at Tulane reported pain relief in schizophrenic patients following electrical stimulation of the septal nuclei via a stereotactic approach (first performed in 1950 [12]), and similar results were reported by Pool using Heath's technique in a patient treated exclusively for pain (with an externalized electrode wire) [10]. Heath reported stimulation of the amygdala in schizophrenia in 1955 [13]. In these and other reports of brain stimulation, only acute stimulation through externalized wires was used. However, Glenn pioneered the use of his radiofrequency-coupled device – first introduced for cardiac pacing in 1959 [14, 15] – for nervous system stimulation, which was then applied to stimulation of the peripheral nervous system, the dorsal spinal columns and ultimately intracranial stimulation.

Early observations of the beneficial effects of high-frequency stimulation (HFS) of the thalamus on tremor [16–18] provided the basis for chronic thalamic stimulation for tremor [19, 20], and DBS dominated the therapeutic literature thenceforth. The ensuing technical availability of stimulation equipment, combined with the published results of stereotactic ablation of various intracranial targets (e.g. ventral capsule and subgenual cingulate), as well as increased understanding of networks underlying neuropsychiatric disorders resulting from new investigative tools (e.g. positron emission tomography (PET) and functional magnetic resonance imaging (fMRI)) propelled the renewed interest in DBS for various psychiatric disorders [21].

Mechanism of action

The homologous clinical effects of ablation and HFS in the motor thalamus, globus pallidus and even subthalamic nucleus suggested the notion that DBS conferred some sort of electrical (e.g. depolarization) blockade of local cellular activity. Thus, the inductive leap to DBS from lesioning procedures such as gamma or radiofrequency capsulotomy was small, following the leap from thalamotomy to thalamic DBS, and pallidotomy to pallidal DBS, for movement disorders. However, subsequent research has shown this simple understanding of the mechanism of action of DBS to be at best incomplete. In fact, current understanding is that, at the cellular level at least, DBS activates axons, including neuronal afferents and efferents – the latter predominating. For example, experiments have shown that electrical stimulation of motor thalamus (ventral intermediate nucleus) during human mapping studies suppresses action potentials recorded extracellularly from cell bodies [22, 23]. At the same time, however, a significant body of work supports that the same parameters will activate axons – be they cell body afferents (which may indeed underlie cell body suppression via activation of inhibitory afferents) or, more importantly, efferents – the latter rendering cell body suppression moot [24–26]. Efferent axonal fibres affected may include those originating from local cell bodies as well as axons *en passage* within the stimulation field [27].

High-frequency DBS activates subpopulations of local neurons based on complex interactions between stimulation parameters, cell characteristics and local anatomy. Both orthodromic and antidromic activation may occur [28], as well as resonance effects within stimulated circuits [29]. DBS may also disrupt pathological or disordered rhythms in involved circuits, overriding pathological activity or allowing normal rhythms to re-emerge [30, 31]. Regional, network and, ultimately, clinical effects will depend on the connectivity of the activated neurons, and immediate network effects may continue to evolve over weeks to months via neuromodulatory and adaptive effects. While each stage of the interaction between DBS and neural tissue is highly complex and incompletely understood, known networks have demonstrated measurable and consistent functional imaging changes in response to high-frequency DBS [32–35], and both the electrical properties and clinical effects of chronically implanted DBS systems have proven relatively stable in the movement-disorder population.

The clinical effects of DBS on neural networks thus need to be interpreted or reinterpreted within the context of the present understanding of mechanism(s) of action – and, conversely, clinical observations need to continue to propel further experiments to elucidate mechanism(s) of action. Ultimately, clinical observations should be taken at face value (when adequately established) and explanations of those effects sought, to further inform and drive advances in therapies. Finally, mechanism(s) of action no doubt vary from system to system depending on the composition of neural elements (e.g. fibre diameter and orientation) and the precise anatomical arrangement of grey matter/white matter pathways and their proximity and orientation with respect to the electrode. Moreover, stimulation effects vary based on several stimulation parameters: amplitude, frequency, pulse width, pulse waveform, train pattern, as well as constant current vs. voltage stimulation [27, 36, 37]. The volume of tissue affected will vary with the selected electrode configuration and with local variations in tissue impedance, such as those between white and grey matter.

Advantages of DBS vs. ablation

Some advantages of DBS are obvious: adjustability and reversibility, with associated clinical, ethical and practical benefits. While adjustability typically is thought to refer to the ability to alter the field of stimulation with voltage/current adjustments, the ability to alter frequency and pulse width – and with more advanced systems, possibility additional parameters such as pattern and waveform – conceivably allows the actual mechanism to be altered. In the face of incomplete understanding of the mechanism, and the experimental nature of surgery for psychiatric disorders, this is arguably the most important advantage. For clinical and translational research, moreover, the relative ease of double-blinding allows well-controlled evaluation of DBS therapy, including the ability to use patients as their own controls with crossover designs. Thus, DBS permits a level of investigational rigour that is, theoretically, difficult to achieve with ablation.

Procedural and technical aspects of DBS

DBS equipment

In the United States, Medtronic is the only DBS manufacturer that is currently approved by FDA for any indication; it has full market approval for DBS for Parkinson's disease and tremor, while DBS for dystonia is at present only available under a humanitarian device exemption (HDE). DBS is approved under a HDE for OCD as well, but for no other psychiatric indications. Medtronic is also approved in Canada and all settled continents for movement disorders. Other DBS equipment manufacturers – St. Jude Medical Corp. (SJMC, Plano, TX) and Boston Scientific Corp. (BSCI, Marlborough, MA), while at present in clinical trials in the United States, are approved in Europe for Parkinson's disease and dystonia.

The essential components of the DBS systems are similar across manufacturers, consisting of three components. The first part is the DBS lead, whose active tip consists of individual cylindrical platinum contacts, typically 1.5 long and approximately 1.25 mm in diameter. Medtronic and SJM offer four-contact (tetrapolar) leads, whereas BSCI offers an eight-contact lead (neither SJM nor BSCI electrodes are approved by FDA at the time of this writing). Designs are available with contact spacing of 0.5 or 1.5 mm; these can be chosen based on the anatomical region being targeted (Figure 13.2a). A lead specific for anterior capsule DBS for OCD is available, with larger contacts and intercontact distances (3 mm) for spanning a greater distance (21 mm). The DBS lead attaches under the scalp to an extension cable, which is passed subcutaneously behind the ear, down the neck and over the clavicle to attach to the implantable pulse generator (IPG) implanted subcutaneously in the anterior chest (or, alternatively, in the abdomen for special circumstances) (Figure 13.2). IPGs are also available in various configurations (Figure 13.2). The three main variables are as follows: (i) single vs. dual channel: bilateral implantations can be performed either using the dual channel IPG or using two single channel IPGs, based on both patient and physician preference; (ii) primary cell vs. rechargeable, the former needing to be replaced every 2–5 years typically, depending on DBS site and stimulation parameters,

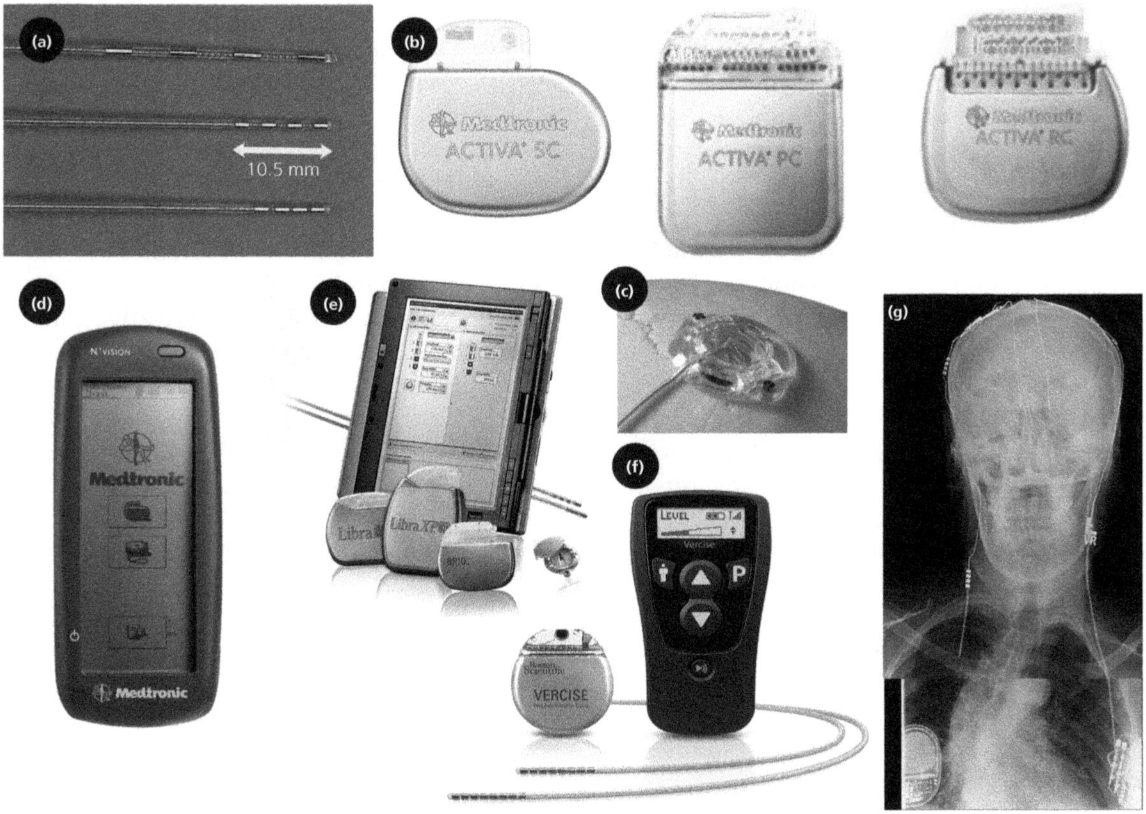

Figure 13.2 Deep brain stimulation equipment. (**a**) DBS leads of different configurations. The contacts of the bottom two leads are 1.5 mm long cylinders, separated by 1.5 mm (middle lead) or 0.5 mm (bottom lead). The upper electrode array has larger contacts (3.0 mm) and wider spacing (3.0 mm) adapted for use in the anterior internal capsule (e.g. for OCD; in the United States, this is the only use for which this lead is approved by the FDA, under a HDE). (**b**) Internal pulse generators (IPGs) are primary cell (left and middle) or rechargeable (right), and either single channel (left) or dual-channel (middle, right). (**c**) StimLoc ring for anchoring the DBS lead to the bone and covering the burr hole. (**d**) IPGs are programmed telemetrically. Source: a–d reproduced with permission of Medtronic. (**e**) St. Jude Medical also offers single (left) and dual-channel (centre, right) IPGs, as well as a dual-channel rechargeable IPG (right); depicted also are the DBS electrodes, and the burr-hole anchoring device. Source: Reproduced with permission of St Jude Medical. (**f**) Boston Scientific offers a dual-channel rechargeable IPG, and DBS leads with eight closely spaced contacts. Source: Reproduced with permission of Roshini Jain. (**g**) X-ray showing bilateral DBS leads, extension cables connected in the head (left side of figure) and neck (right side of figure), and IPGs. In fact, the latter is a poor location for the DBS-to-extension connection to be located, which predisposes to breakage, which occurred with a previous right extension cable where the connection was in the neck (left side of figure). (*See insert for colour representation of the figure.*)

whereas the latter lasts significantly longer between replacements, but requires daily to weekly recharging; the rechargeable IPG is also thinner than primary cell models; (iii) constant voltage vs. constant current: the latter essentially automatically compensates for variations in tissue impedance (the alternating current (AC) variable reflecting resistance), whereas constant voltage leads to variable current in the face of varying impedance.

Whether there is a difference in effectiveness or side effects has yet to be demonstrated.

Implantation of the DBS equipment occurs in two stages: the implantation of the DBS lead(s) in one stage, and the extension cable and IPG in the second stage. The latter can be performed immediately following the DBS leads, following induction of general anaesthesia. Alternatively, the second stage can be performed days to weeks subsequently, for patient-related and/or reimbursement-related reasons. Another way that procedures can be staged is by performing the procedure unilaterally with the contralateral side months (typically) later; this is advantageous for minimizing adverse cognitive effects, most relevant for older patients and those with Parkinson's disease.

Patient selection: general considerations

As with all surgery, careful, evidence-based patient selection is the most important determinant of successful outcome. Screening and selection criteria for specific diseases will be discussed in other chapters; however, several general principles of presurgical evaluation will be outlined here. Of critical importance is a multidisciplinary, team-based approach to patient evaluation and selection, including evaluations by, at a minimum, a psychiatrist, neuropsychologist and neurosurgeon. Formal protocols for patient selection should be employed wherever possible, following approval by an institutional review board for all experimental procedures. Several consensus publications have been produced to guide responsible practices in patient selection and follow-up [38–41].

Medical fitness and pre-operative evaluation

Candidates for psychiatric neuromodulation tend to present for surgery at younger ages than their movement-disorder counterparts and consequently tend to have fewer medical comorbidities [42]. Potential contraindications to surgery include severe cardiopulmonary disease, coagulopathy and platelet dysfunction. Although age is a consideration, DBS and lesioning have been performed in properly selected movement disorder patients up to the eighth and even ninth decade with a high degree of surgical and anaesthetic safety. The presence of cognitive deficits as detected on neuropsychological testing is a relative contraindication, particularly when bilateral surgery is to be performed. However, mild loss of memory or executive function in an elderly patient, or in chronically ill psychiatric patients, perhaps contributed to by electroconvulsive therapy, is not a barrier to surgery. Morbidly obese patients or those with a history of snoring or obstructive sleep apnoea may present airway or ventilation challenges while under sedation; these can usually be managed by an experienced anaesthesiology team but are best identified before surgery. As always, decisions regarding medical fitness for surgery are best made on an individual basis, in close consultation with the patient's primary-care provider and the anaesthesiology team.

All patients should undergo non-contrast brain MRI before surgical evaluation to rule out the presence of an underlying lesion or structural abnormality, which may both complicate the diagnosis and increase the risk of surgery. MRI findings of excessive brain atrophy may indicate undiagnosed degenerative disease and may increase the risk of haemorrhage or misplacement due to brain shift [43].

Medical comorbidities, particularly hypertension and hyperglycaemia, should be well controlled in order to limit the risk of haemorrhage and infection, respectively. Nutrition should be optimized to promote wound healing. Routine pre-operative blood work should be performed and anaesthesia consultation obtained. Potential polypharmacy issues in the psychiatric population include the use of agents with anti-platelet effects (e.g. valproic acid) or anaesthetic interactions (e.g. monoamine oxidase inhibitors). Aspirin, non-steroidal anti-inflammatory drugs, anti-coagulants and dietary supplements that interfere with haemostasis (e.g. garlic, ginger and vitamin E) are discontinued at least 1 week before surgery and may generally be restarted 1–2 weeks after surgery in uncomplicated cases. Patients with significant cardiac or pulmonary comorbidities, clotting disorders, immune compromise or other medical issues should be evaluated and cleared for surgery by their appropriate medical specialist.

Many patients will be apprehensive, especially given the elective nature of psychiatric surgery, fears associated with awake surgery and the potential, however small, for permanent neurological morbidity. Ample opportunity should be given for questions to be answered, over more than one clinic visit if necessary. The patient should be familiarized with the expected workflow on the day of surgery, as well as reasonable expectations for inpatient and outpatient recovery. Preparatory videos are available from DBS manufacturers and on the websites of many major DBS centres and may be integrated into the surgical consultation. Many patients benefit from peer-to-peer discussion, and patients who have already undergone DBS placement at the same institution can be an invaluable resource for the surgical team. Finally, patients should be counselled that future electroconvulsive therapy will be contraindicated after DBS placement.

DBS: procedural considerations

A wide variety of tools and techniques are available to the stereotactic surgeon, and practice patterns will differ between – and even within – specialized centres, based on surgeon experience, preference and local capability [44–46]. Although detailed comparisons are beyond the scope of this chapter, we will attempt to provide an overview of common options and their relative merits. An individual team's experience with a given strategy is likely the most important predictor of successful and safe DBS placement.

Coordinate systems and atlases

Stereotactic planning and analysis take place in a three-dimensional coordinate space aligned with the commissural plane, a horizontal plane containing the anterior commissure (AC) and posterior commissure (PC) (Figure 13.3). The midcommissural point (MCP) is generally used as the origin of the coordinate system. By convention, the X dimension is horizontal, expressed in millimetres to the right (positive) or left (negative) of the midsagittal plane. The Y dimension is anterior (positive) or posterior (negative) to the MCP. The Z dimension is vertical and is expressed in millimetres superior (positive) or inferior (negative) to the commissural plane.

The Talairach brain atlas, first published in 1967, established the AC–PC coordinate system and defined the Talairach grid, which predicts the size and location of intracranial structures in constant proportion to the AC–PC distance. The updated Talairach–Tourneau [47] and Schaltenbrand–Wahren [48] atlases are the two references most commonly used in clinical settings (Figure 13.3). Both contain high-resolution photomicrographs of sections in all three planes, with successive sections separated by 1–1.5 mm. Large-format reproductions of parasagittal sections are still used by many centres for manual plotting of microelectrode data (see below); however, the reliance of these two classic atlases on a small number of cadaveric specimens somewhat limits their universal application, and the use of a different specimen in each plane yields measurable internal inconsistencies as well [49–52]. Thus, electronic versions of the atlases are increasingly being integrated into commercial planning workstations with the ability to deform the Talairach grid in three dimensions to fit an individual patient's anatomy (Figure 13.3f). Several DBS centres

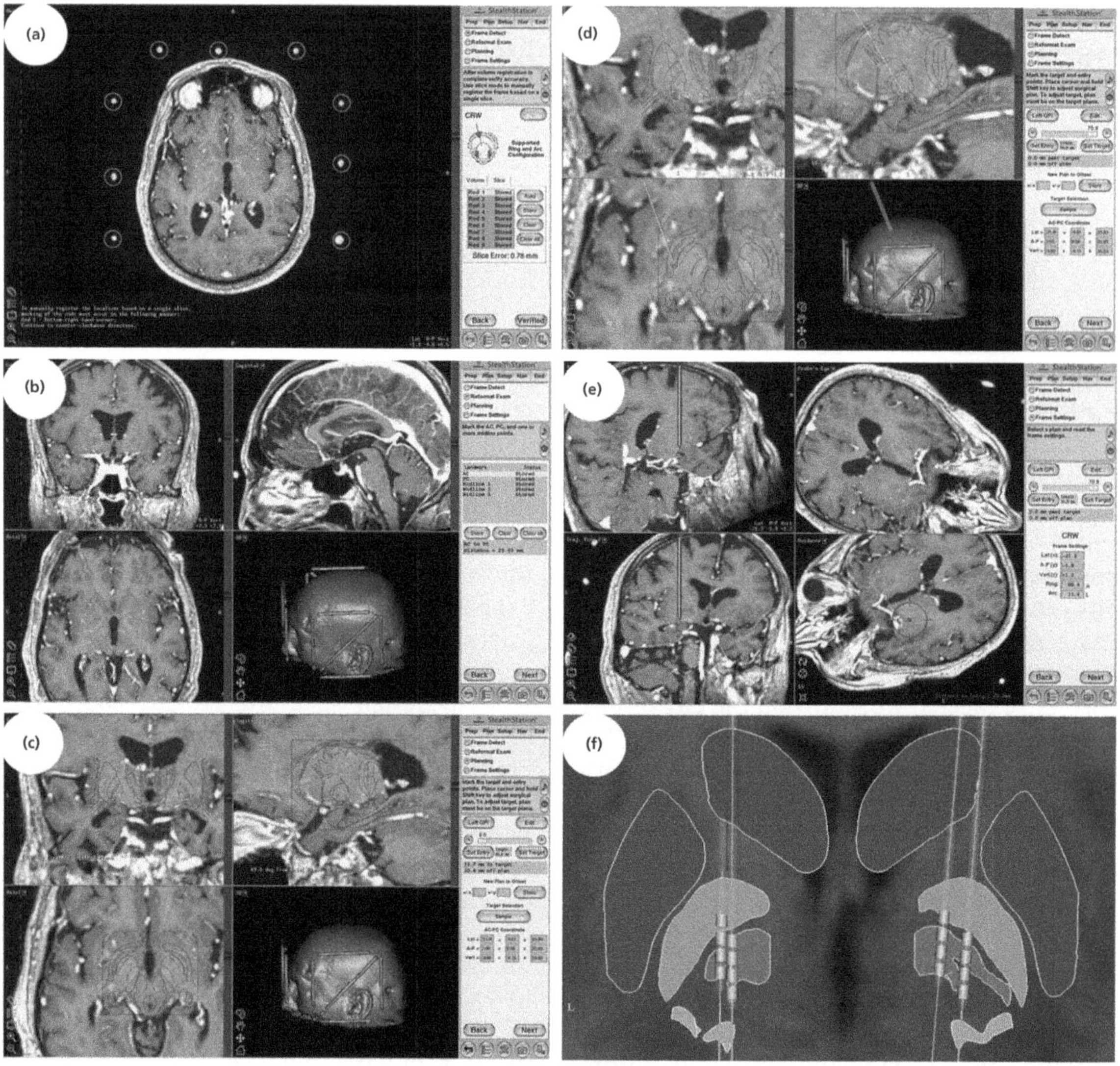

Figure 13.3 Stereotactic planning of DBS electrodes. Images from the Stealth Framelink software (Medtronic), showing the stages of planning a DBS electrode insertion. (**a**) The contrast-enhanced MRI is performed after affixing the stereotactic frame base ring (in this case a CRW Stereotactic System, Integra). The locations of the fiducial bars (9 circled points) is noted by the software, to register the brain MRI space to the physical space of the frame allowing transformations of brain targets to the instrument holder. (**b**) The locations of the anterior commissure (AC) and posterior commissure (PC), and the line connecting them, provide a consistent internal reference for a 3D space in which common functional stereotactic targets such as the basal ganglia can be targeted. Here AC and PC are noted in the software for targeting with respect to the AC–PC line (synonymous with a so-called Talairach space). The 3D reconstruction of the fiducial localizer box is seen in the bottom right corner. (**c**) Most software programs allow a digital version of the classic Schaltenbrand and Wahren (or other) atlas to be co-registered to the patient's MRI scan via AC/PC coordinates, to aid in so-called indirect targeting. Here the target in the globus pallidus (red dot) has been selected based on its relationship to the AC–PC line and the atlas. (**d**) The entry point is chosen to provide a rational trajectory for the DBS lead (i.e. here proceeding rostrally through the globus

use locally developed software for detailed, probabilistic modelling of the basal ganglia and other subcortical targets [53, 54], potentially enabling more accurate target localization and post-operative analysis. An example from our own centre is shown in Figure 13.3f; however, this technology is not currently available for routine clinical use.

Stereotactic frames and 'frameless' aiming devices

There are various apparatuses available for stereotactic implantation of DBS electrodes, from classic frames in which imaging fiducials (points assumed as a fixed basis for comparison, i.e. to register brain space to physical space) are contained within the instrument-holder platform (Figures 13.1b and 13.4a), to so-called frameless systems, which are really reduced instrument holders separated from the imaging fiducials (Figure 13.4b–d). In all systems, fiducials serve to link ('co-register') the imaging space, in which the individual patient's anatomy is visualized, to the physical space containing the instruments at the time of surgery. This relationship is established by physical contiguity (using a classic headframe), or by virtual connection of the fiducials to the instrument holder using an optical camera/computer that 'sees' both (e.g. frameless neuronavigation systems), or a tactile system that 'touches' both (e.g. stereotactic robot).

Frames can be generally be characterized as having translational, arc-centred, burr-hole-mounted or interlocking-arc designs [55]. The frames most commonly used in North America are the Cosman–Roberts–Wells (CRW) frame (Figure 13.4a) (Integra Life Sciences, Plainsboro, NJ; www.integralife.com) and the Leksell Series G frame (Figure 13.1b and c) (Elekta AB, Stockholm, Sweden; www.elekta.com). Both are arc-centred designs: once the frame is adjusted to the coordinates (X, Y, Z) of the desired target, the working channel of the frame may be moved freely along two perpendicular interlocking arcs that form a quadrant around the target, enabling the surgeon to easily adjust the entry point and trajectory (to avoid surface vessels, for example) while remaining aimed precisely at the target (Figures 13.1c and 13.4). The CRW frame features an external 'phantom' base, whose pointer can be set to the desired target coordinates and used to check frame accuracy before use. Systems popular in Europe, in addition to the Leksell, are the Riechert–Mundinger frame and the Zamorano–Duchovny (ZD) frame (inomed, Emmendingen, Germany, www.inomed.com), which are also arc-centred. With these classic stereotactic frames, the fiducials are contained on a localizer that affixes to the frame base for imaging (CT, MRI and positive-contrast venticulography) (Figure 13.1b). The relationship of the frame fiducials to defined anatomical points (e.g. AC and PC) is calculated and this provides the measurements by which to adjust the X, Y and Z of the frame; this is most often accomplished using a neuronavigation workstation with integrated software (Figure 13.3).

So-called 'frameless' stereotactic frames are essentially variants of the burr-hole frame.

Figure 13.3 (Continued) pallidus) and to avoid critical neurovascular structures. This image shows the trajectory on coronal (upper left), sagittal (upper right) and axial (bottom left) images; in each plane the oblique trajectory is out-of-plane. (**e**) The path is in 'trajectory' views that depict the whole trajectory in one plane allowing easy visualization of veins and arteries and the ventricle that may lay in the path. (**f**) Planning can include a depiction of the location of the DBS lead(s) with respect to brain structures. In this case, we have used our proprietary software (OneTrack) to depict a coronal trajectory view of the basal ganglia in a patient-specific fashion, allowing us to see the location of the DBS leads with respect to the globus pallidus in this patient who underwent bilateral anteromedial and posterolateral globus pallidus DBSs for Tourette Syndrome. Source: Courtesy of K. Mewes, Emory University. (*See insert for colour representation of the figure.*)

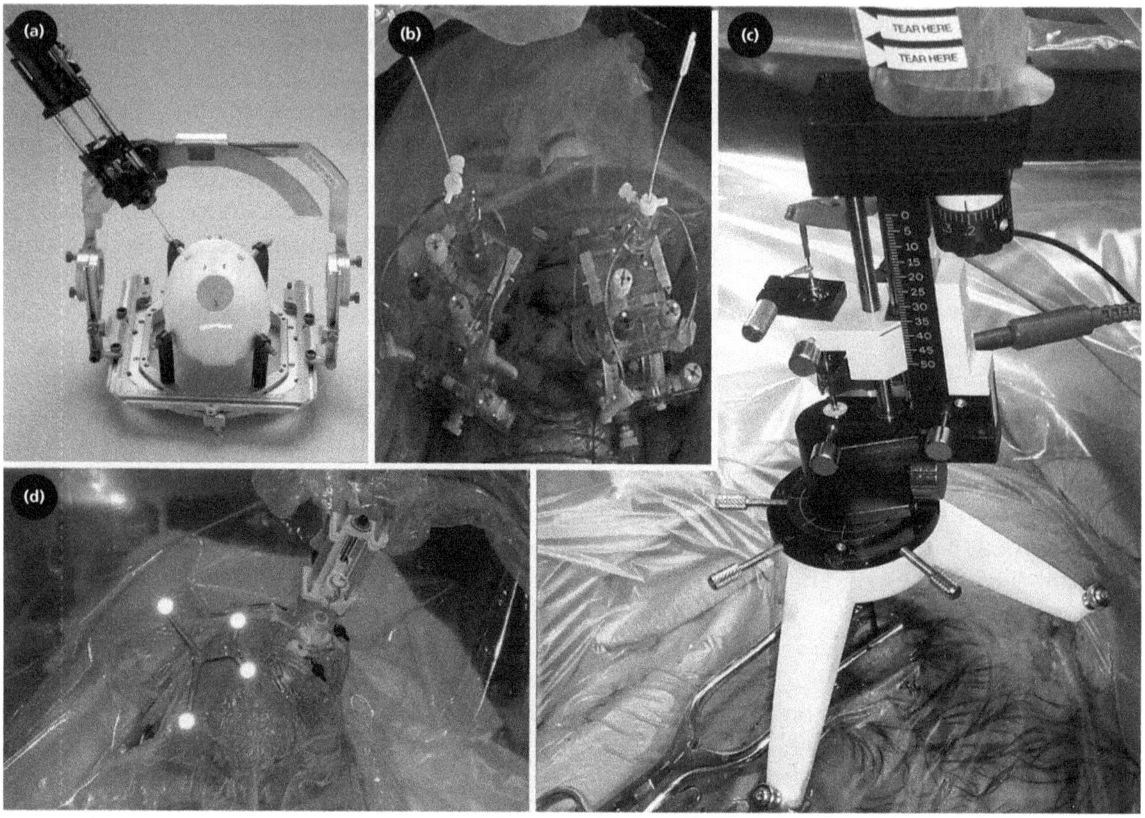

Figure 13.4 Classic and modern stereotactic devices. Classic frames, such as the CRW (**a**, Integra), incorporate the fiducials into the stereotactic device using an attached localizer (see Figure 13.1b) during imaging to relate and transform the brain imaging (MRI, CT) space to the physical frame space. The relationship, yielding frame coordinates for adjusting the instrument holder (stereotactic arc, as shown), is calculated using software or by direct measurement on X-ray, CT and/or MRI. Newer stereotactic devices use different approaches. The microTargeting platform (**c**, Fred Haer Corp.) physically separates the imaging fiducials from the frame. The fiducials are physically attached to the patient's head before CT and MRI imaging and the trajectory is planned on proprietary software. An acrylic stereotactic platform is custom-manufactured (white tripod in **c**) that attaches to the fiducials, instantiating in physical space the imaging-planned trajectory (the picture shows the microelectrode drive attached to the platform). The NexFrame (**d**, Medtronic) also separates the fiducials from the frame. A CT is performed with fiducials attached and co-registered to an MRI for trajectory planning. In the operating room, the relationship of the imaging fiducials to the NexFrame, a plastic stereotactic device affixed atop the burr hole, is calculated by software after detection of their location in physical space using a camera to visualize reflective balls (seen in picture attached to the stereotactic device). The Clearpoint Smartframe (**b**, MRI Interventions) utilizes a fiducial cannula prefilled with gadolinium. The stereotactic device is affixed to the patient in the MRI scanner, and the relationship of the cannula (physical space) to the brain space is determined with an MRI. The software calculates the necessary adjustments to align the attached tower containing the fiducial cannula to the planned trajectory, which are made using four coloured knobs. The DBS is inserted through the fiducial cannula, as shown. (*See insert for colour representation of the figure.*)

Present-day versions are plastic or acrylic, and are affixed over the burr hole, e.g. NexFrame (Figure 13.4d; Medtronic, Minneapolis, MN). Fiducials, rather than being integrated with the frame, as above, are directly affixed to the bone before imaging. Not having a fixed relationship to the miniframe, in contrast to classic frames, this relationship needs to be determined and adjusted. In the operating room, the NexFrame (Figure 13.4d) is affixed to the bone after opening. Its position with respect to the fiducials is determined by an optical imaging camera system that detects fiducials attached to the NexFrame, and fiducials at the end of a wand that is used to touch each of the bone fiducials in turn. This serves to register the physical space of the NexFrame to the brain MRI space via the fiducials, which are visible in both spaces. The NexFrame movement is tracked by the camera as it is adjusted to point to the chosen target.

Another frameless system, the microTargeting platform (Figure 13.4c; Fred Haer Corp, FHC, Bowdoin, ME, www.fh-co.com), solves the relationship of the miniframe to the fiducials by custom synthesizing a frame using rapid prototype technology, based on the CT and MRI performed with bone fiducials. Using proprietary software, the fiducials are detected on the images, and the target chosen by the user, and the program prescribes the platform dimensions, which is then manufactured. The platform affixes to the bone fiducials and the mandrel inserted into the aperture of the platform directs instruments to the target. The Clearpoint system (Figures 13.4b, 13.6e and f; MRI Interventions, Irvine, CA, www.mriinterventions.com) is a MRI-targeting platform that, like the NexFrame, affixes at the burr hole. There is a contrast-lined cannula and MRI-visible fiducials within the miniframe. The proprietary software is used to calculate adjustments to the frame to direct a cannula to the target.

Frameless systems offer less restriction on patient head movement during surgery and allow a more streamlined workflow on the day of surgery. The frameless systems may reduce institutional start-up costs by eliminating the need to purchase a traditional frame, but significantly increase per-case costs.

Accuracy

Potential sources of inaccuracy and error exist at each stage of DBS placement, including imaging (e.g. limits of MRI or CT resolution, MRI distortion effects, slice thickness and 3D reconstruction inaccuracies), frame placement (e.g. over-tightening, mechanical loading and other sources of distortion), target selection (e.g. measurement inaccuracies and frame registration error) and DBS lead placement (e.g. inherent frame inaccuracy, probe deflection, cerebrospinal fluid (CSF) loss and brain shift [56, 57], and post-placement lead migration. Although sources of error can be addressed and mitigated (e.g. via CT–MRI fusion to overcome distortion effects, intraoperative fluoroscopy to detect deflection or migration, or advanced intraoperative imaging to detect and correct for lead deflection and brain shift), systematic studies using frame-based approaches generally show mean three-dimensional vector errors between 1 and 1.5 mm, although the clinical significance of these dimensions varies by target and study [58–67]. The accuracy and clinical outcomes achieved using frameless systems are comparable to those of traditional frames [59, 64, 68–78]. Accuracy assessments of the ClearPoint system appear to compare favourably with both frame-based and frameless systems [79], but clinical data have not yet been published.

Frame placement

The patient typically arrives at the hospital the morning of surgery. A peripheral IV is placed in the pre-operative holding area. The head frame is affixed, using two anterior and two posterior skull pins, under conscious sedation (e.g. midazolam and fentanyl) and local anaesthesia (e.g. 1% lidocaine/0.5%

bupivacaine/1:10 bicarbonate). Care is taken to place the frame symmetrically, with the base ring below, and parallel to, the orbitomeatal line, in order to align the frame with the commissural plane and reduce potential error in three-dimensional image reconstruction (Figure 13.1b).

Imaging

Various approaches are used for imaging and target identification (Figure 13.3). Volumetric MRI is the gold standard for targeting, using magnetization-prepared rapid gradient-echo sequence (MPRAGE) or Spoiled Gradient Recalled Acquisition (SPGR) sequences, with 1–1.5 mm slice thickness, acquired in axial, coronal or sagittal planes covering the entire head. Ideally, 3T imaging is obtained for better signal-to-noise ratio. Contrast enhancement with gadolinium allows identification of cerebral vasculature. Other MRI sequences may maximize visualization of particular structures, such as inversion recovery for grey/white differentiation and susceptibility weighted imaging for visualization of structures with higher iron content.

Volumetric imaging can be obtained before frame application, or with the frame on. The former allows the procedures to be separated in time, which is advantageous when targeting takes some time. For depression cases, for example, we obtain a 3T MRI ahead of time, including diffusion tensor imaging (DTI), which is used for careful target planning of the subgenual cingulate white matter (Figure 13.5l). In this situation, stereotactic imaging with contrast, either another MRI or a stereotactic CT scan, is obtained after frame placement on the day of surgery; the two studies are then easily co-registered in the navigation software. With frameless approaches, imaging must be performed with the bone fiducials in place. For the microTargeting platform (FHC), both MRI and CT are obtained 5 days or more ahead of surgery, with bone fiducials in place, and no further imaging is needed on the day of surgery, since the custom manufactured frame attaches to the fiducials and instantiates the target planning. Finally, it is even possible to use an intraoperative CT scan on the day of surgery to image the fiducials for planning [80].

Operating room set-up and surgical planning

Following imaging, the patient is brought to the operating room and placed on the operating room (OR) bed in a recumbent position, with the head and back slightly elevated for comfort. The frame is attached to the bed with the patient's neck in a comfortable, neutral position (Figure 13.5a). It is important to not tend too much towards a semi-sitting position that produces a pressure differential between the head and the lungs leading to excessive air entry due to negative pressure; air then becomes trapped under the frontal bone producing pneumocephalus, brain shift and increasing the risk for seizures. Pressure points are carefully padded, and the patient is kept warm using blankets or a forced-air heating blanket. After positioning, the patient is sedated with a short-acting IV agent such as propofol, and oxygen is delivered via nasal cannula or facemask. Alternatively, for psychiatric surgery, since the stereotactic target is often determined anatomically rather than with physiologic recording and stimulation, surgery may be performed under general anaesthesia (endotracheally or intravenously delivered). In that event, the anaesthesia may begin in the OR following imaging, or before frame application for greater patient comfort. A Foley catheter is placed, and prophylactic antibiotics (usually a first-generation cephalosporin, nafcillin or vancomycin in cases of allergy) are administered.

Various approaches to hair clipping may be used, dependent to some degree on the stereotactic method. Either a wide frontal shave can be used, or the incision can be estimated on the 3D scalp rendering on the navigation station. For frame cases, we use a wide coronal incision for bilateral cases, which affords some leeway and thus allows a minimal strip shave. The incision is kept behind the hairline, although this may not always be possible in patients whose hairlines are receding. The scalp is sterilely prepped and draped, with the raised plastic drape held away from the patient's face by an ether bar or the arm of the fluoroscope. The surgeon, scrub tech and instruments are thus behind the patient's line of sight, leaving the patient's view relatively unobstructed and allowing the anaesthesia, psychiatry and nursing teams easy access to the patient without contaminating the sterile field (Figure 13.5b).

Anaesthetic considerations

Standard non-invasive monitoring (pulse oximetry, blood pressure cuff and electrocorticography (ECG)) is used. Short-acting IV agents such as propofol, remifentanyl and/or dexmetetomidine are used for sedation, enabling rapid emergence for the awake portion of the procedure, if needed. Local anaesthetic is used for the incision, and additional doses of local anaesthetic may be injected into the pin sites or incision line as needed during the case. Intermittent doses of fentanyl may be given with little effect on microelectrode data. Neither anticonvulsants nor corticosteroids are needed. Alternatively, as noted above, the entire procedure may be performed under general anaesthesia. If general anaesthesia is used, microelectrode recording (MER) remains possible, using propofol, dexmetetomidine and/or sevoflurane [81–83].

Blood pressure is carefully controlled below 150 mmHg systolic to minimize the risk of intracranial haemorrhage. Particular attention must be paid to preventing hypertension during emergence from sedation at the start of MER, and an IV drip (e.g. nicardipine) may be needed in patients with a history of hypertension. An arterial line is rarely needed.

Patients with obstructive sleep apnoea or obese body habitus may have intermittent airway obstruction when sedated; if this cannot be managed with a jaw thrust or nasal trumpet, a laryngeal mask airway can be placed. While endotracheal intubation can be performed with the stereotactic frame in place, in airway emergencies the procedure should be aborted and the frame rapidly removed.

Opening

Once the target and trajectory have been selected, the stereotactic arc is set to the desired settings. The Leksell frame can be set to the final coordinates only after the arc is attached through the drapes to the base ring, since the attachment bars are used for the Y settings. The CRW frame can be fully adjusted either before or after attachment to the base ring. We prefer to set coordinates before attachment in order to verify accuracy using the phantom base. Moreover, by assembling the whole system (including X–Y stage and microelectrode drive) on the phantom, the composite system can be checked for any stereotactic inaccuracies, which can occur with error or damage to any of the components. The Leksell frame does not have an adjustable phantom base but does have a non-sterile targeting model that may be used in between surgeries to check calibration.

After the arc system is set to the desired trajectory, the approximate location of the burr hole can be marked on the scalp to direct planning of a small linear or curvilinear incision (Figure 13.5c). The incision should be made at least 1 cm from the burr hole and away from the planned path of the DBS lead [84]. We prefer a coronally oriented incision to stay behind the hairline and to minimize interruption of scalp blood supply. For bilateral procedures, a single incision spanning the two entry sites is most efficient and gives an excellent cosmetic result. The scalp is incised and held open with a small self-retaining retractor.

The skull entry point is marked using the stereotactic frame, and a 14-mm burr hole placed using a standard perforating drill bit. Since trajectories are invariably oblique to the skull, the

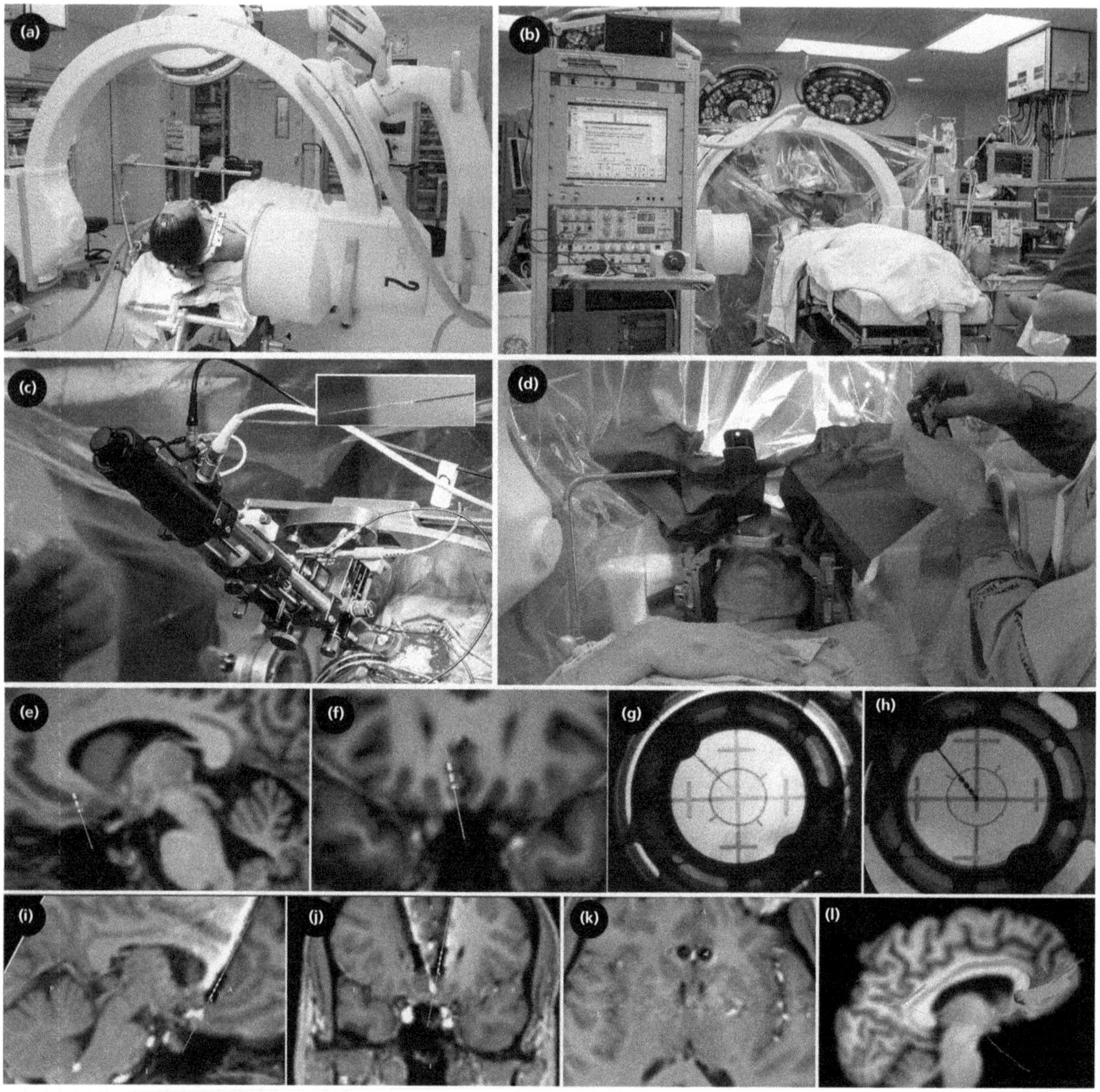

Figure 13.5 DBS insertion in the operating room, using microelectrode and/or stimulation mapping. In procedures performed in the OR, the patient is positioned comfortably supine (**a**), in this case with a CRW frame affixed to the table (in NexFrame and microTargeting platform cases, the head is held in a cervical collar rather than affixed to the table). For radiological control, a C-arm is positioned for lateral fluoroscopy (**a** and **b**): by alignment through the middle of the frame it provides stereotactic accuracy feedback in the sagittal plane (anterior/posterior and superior/inferior) but does not indicate medial/lateral accuracy (**g** and **h**). In contrast, 3D imaging with CT or MRI provides radiological control in all three planes (see Figure 13.6). The surgeon remains behind a sterile clear drape (**b**) to maintain sterility while still being able to monitor the patient, who may remain awake during some or all of the procedure. The MER equipment is seen to the left in (**b**). The microelectrode is driven in by an electric microdrive (**c**, Axon Instruments) controlled by the operator; the high-impedance microelectrode is inset in (**c**). Thus, a physiological map of the target area is developed and overlain upon the MRI scan (**e**, sagittal; **f**, coronal; in this case using our proprietary OneTrack software). Radiological accuracy is checked by lateral fluoroscopy (**g**). Following microelectrode mapping (if used), the DBS is inserted through the same cannula and

burr hole should be angled somewhat rather than being made strictly perpendicular to the skull, and additional bone removal from the inner table of the skull is advantageous to avoid deflection; this is accomplished with a small cutting burr or bone punch. Care should be taken to seal the edges of the burr hole with bone wax to prevent air embolism, as any veins within the bone are non-collapsible; if the head is significantly above the heart, these veins will not be apparent due to the negative intravenous pressure.

The dura is opened in a cruciate manner and the edges coagulated to allow maximal unobstructed access to the cortical surface. The arachnoid and pia are gently coagulated with bipolar cautery and opened as far as the dural opening will allow, again in order to provide unobstructed access for microelectrode penetration. Great care should be taken to obtain meticulous haemostasis; any subdural blood will accumulate lateral/inferior to the burr hole and may escape notice until critical. Nevertheless, it is important to avoid coagulation of any surface veins that may lead to venous stasis or infarction; gelfoam is sufficient to obtain haemostasis of venous bleeders, whereas arterial dural bleeding requires cauterization.

If a commercial burr-hole cap and lead-fixation system (e.g. StimLoc, Figure 13.2c; Medtronic, Minneapolis, MN) is being used, the ring is attached at this point. This may be recessed into the skull in patients with thin skin or for cosmetic reasons. The frame coordinates are rechecked, and the MER apparatus is assembled (Figure 13.5c). The burr hole is sealed with fibrin glue or other sealant in order to minimize CSF loss and resulting brain shift during MER.

Target selection

Target and trajectory determination is almost invariably performed using one of the available stereotactic targeting software platforms that are commercially available (Figure 13.3). Details of the method(s) to determine particular targets, e.g. for OCD or depression, are covered in detail in the chapters devoted to these topics. In some instances, co-registration of multiple data sets – e.g. MRI (contrast-enhanced to identify vasculature), stereotactic CT, DTI track maps [85] and functional imaging studies – is advantageous. The AC, PC and midline points may be used as internal references for indirect atlas-based or probabilistic targeting (Figure 13.3).

Entrance points are chosen to avoid cerebral veins, sulci and, in most circumstances, ventricular penetration. The trajectory must also consider the three-dimensional relationship of the electrode contacts to the target structure and its surrounding structures, since programming will be confined to adjustments along the linear array. Entry points are at, or anterior to, the coronal suture, in order to be well away from eloquent cortex. As needed, trajectories can come near to the midline (Figure 13.5j), but it is important to consider that the edge of the burr hole will be 7 mm from the planned entry and, especially if there is any migration of the entry, may encounter

Figure 13.5 (Continued) the accuracy checked (**h**). Stimulation mapping to check for clinical benefits and/or side effects is performed in the awake patient (**d**). After affixing the lead to the skull, post-operative imaging (MRI and/or CT) is performed, and the image can be overlain upon the intraoperative map depicted in the OneTrack software (**i**, sagittal; **j**, coronal; **k**, axial) to check for accurate implantation and to guide post-operative programming decisions with respect to contact(s) utilized for stimulation. (**l**) DTI of white matter pathways, in this case of the subgenual cingulate region, can aid in targeting as well, and may one day – in combination with 3D radiological control (see Figure 13.6) – obviate the need for microelectrode mapping. (OneTrack images – courtesy of K. Mewes, Emory University; DTI image – courtesy of K. Choi and H. Mayberg, Emory University). (*See insert for colour representation of the figure.*)

the sagittal sinus or draining veins. While the lateral ventricles may be safely traversed, they are generally avoided if possible in order to minimize CSF loss, brain shift and the possibility of probe deflection on the ependymal surface.

Physiological mapping and lead placement

The optimally effective location for a DBS lead is inherently linked to both anatomical and physiologic data. In the pre-MRI and early MRI eras, physiologic mapping and clinical feedback using MER and test stimulation in awake patients were essential to refine standardized atlas-based targeting for an individual patient. However, with the increasing anatomic resolution of clinically available MRI and the increasing ability to map function non-invasively (e.g. with DTI-based tractography, Figure 13.5l, and fMRI), MER and other direct mapping techniques will likely become less and less necessary in the coming years. Moreover, in treating psychiatric disease, as opposed to movement disorders, immediate intraoperative feedback may be less robustly predictive of clinical outcome and may again become less critical to the surgical process. Most DBS centres continue to incorporate physiologic mapping in order to directly measure the 'therapeutic window' between beneficial and adverse stimulation effects, as well as for ongoing clinical research. However, the ubiquitous role of physiologic mapping will likely undergo significant evolution in the modern era.

A variety of techniques are available for mapping and recording neuronal physiolo gic activity. High-impedance microelectrodes record extracellular action potentials from either individual cell bodies ('single units') or multiple cells ('multiunit hash') [86]. Lower-impedance semi-microelectrodes or macroelectrodes record background neuronal activity (e.g. power and root-mean-square noise) and/or local field potentials from mass dendritic activity. These categories of activity depend on the types of electrodes employed and the filtering of the activity by the data acquisition unit. All can be of localizing value depending on the target and clinical context. While, in surgery for movement disorders, the kinaesthetic or sensory-responsive properties and somatotopic arrangement of the cells encountered is used to identify relevant nuclei, these clues may not be available in MER for psychiatric disorders, and mapping may be limited to defining grey–white boundaries. Unit responses have, however, been observed in limbic regions [87–90].

Microelectrode mapping is performed using tungsten or platinum–iridium microelectrodes with impedance between 0.5 and 1 MΩ (Figure 13.5). The delicate microelectrode tip is protected by a thin guide cannula, whose uninsulated tip can also serve as an electrode for macrostimulation. The guide cannula is advanced along the trajectory by a microdrive (electric, hydraulic or manual), which permits precise depth control in 0.01 mm increments and smooth passage through the target tissue (Figure 13.5b and c). The electrode trajectory can be offset in the anterior–posterior and medial–lateral directions in millimetre increments with the use of an adjustable X–Y stage (Figure 13.5c), a mandrel with multiple channels that can be offset in various ways, or by adjustment of the stereotactic frame [86]. At the end of each microelectrode track, radiological imaging with lateral fluoroscopy (Figure 13.5g) or intraoperative CT scanning (Figure 13.6a–d; see below) is very useful to check frame accuracy as well as for visual confirmation of position adjustments made during mapping.

Macrostimulation may be delivered via a dedicated macroelectrode (such as a lesioning electrode), the DBS electrode, or via the exposed tip of the microelectrode guide cannula. Stimulation typically uses high-frequency (≥100 Hz) square-wave pulses and amplitudes typically of 0.5–10 V. The goal is both to determine the threshold for eliciting adverse effects from neighbouring regions and to assess for

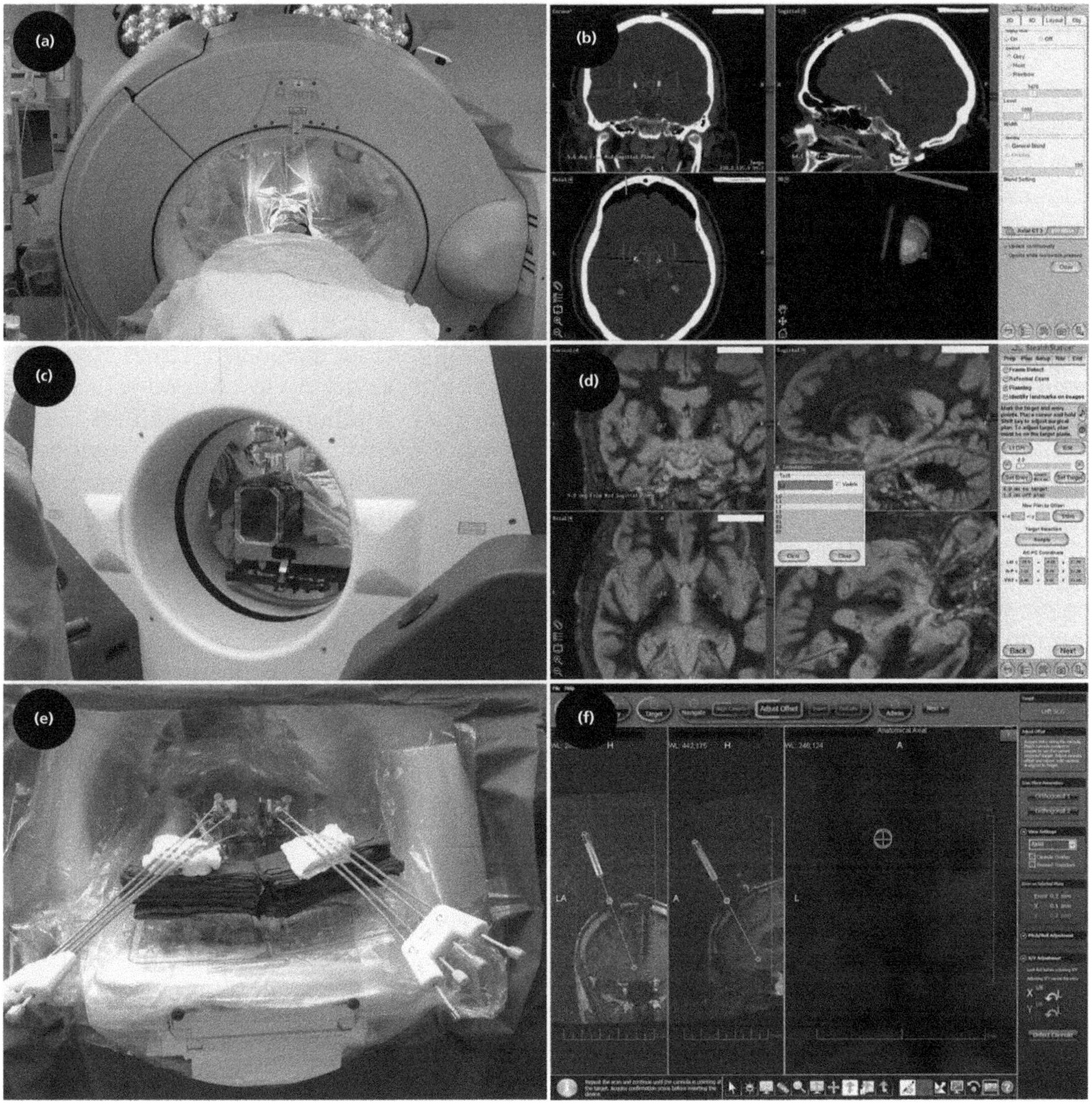

Figure 13.6 Three-dimensional (3D) radiological control. 3D radiological control is the gold standard for ascertaining final DBS implantation accuracy and is the *best* when it occurs intraoperatively when adjustments can more easily be made than post-operatively (**a**). Several options are available at present. The O-arm (Medtronic) is a flat-panel cone-beam CT scanner that provides both intraoperative lateral and anterior/posterior fluorography as well as 3D CT scanning (**b**) (albeit with somewhat less resolution that traditional fan-beam CT). It can be used for determining intraoperative accuracy by co-registration to the pre-operative MRI using the Stealth neuronavigational workstation. Source: a and b are courtesy of K. Holloway, Medical College of Virginia. True fan-beam intraoperative CT scanning is available using the Bodytom (**c**) or the smaller Ceretom (Samsung Neurologica). The intraoperative CT scans can similarly be co-registered to the pre-operative MRI using neuronavigational software (e.g. Stealth, **d**). Source: c and d are courtesy of F. Ponce, Barrow Neurological Institute. Surgery can be performed in the MRI suite (**e**), or in the operating room using an intraoperative MR unit. In this case, DBS insertion is performed after aligning the stereotactic device (e.g. Clearpoint as shown in **e** and **f**, MRI Interventions) and checking insertion accuracy with a ceramic stylet inserted through a peel-away sheath. Any inaccuracies are immediately seen on the MRI scan and can be adjusted before closure. (*See insert for colour representation of the figure.*)

clinical responses mimicking the effects of DBS current (Figure 13.5d). Again, while in movement disorders an immediate therapeutic response is often seen (e.g. tremor), test stimulation in psychiatric cases may not yield immediately obvious results. Nevertheless, clinical responses have been noted from intraoperative stimulation for depression [85, 91–93] and OCD [94–97]. The predictive value of such acute effects on chronic responses is under investigation.

Either following MER and/or macrostimulation, or in lieu of it, the DBS lead itself is inserted. Additional stimulation is then performed through the DBS lead in both monopolar and bipolar configurations, again in order to test for effectiveness and assess the threshold for stimulation-induced side effects. Testing through the DBS lead is a closer approximation of eventual therapeutic stimulation than guide cannula macrostimulation, although stimulation effects can sometime be obscured by the microlesional effect of DBS lead insertion.

Intraoperative radiological control

Radiological control is critical to insure stereotactic accuracy of the implanted lead, using lateral fluoroscopy (Figure 13.5h) or intraoperative CT (Figure 13.6a–d) or MR scan (Figure 13.6e and f) [56, 58, 63, 64, 80]. Historically, stereotactic ORs were set up with X-ray tubes positioned several metres laterally and anteriorly from a fixed anchor in the room for the stereotactic frame, to eliminate parallax and allow direct measurements to be made from the fluorography. This led to the cumbersome arrangement that the OR table would be in the corner of the room to accommodate the lateral X-ray, and the anterior X-ray tube would be in the floor above the OR. At present, portable fluoroscopy is widely available, but almost invariably limited to lateral views, thus only revealing accuracy in the dorsoventral and anteroposterior, not mediolateral, dimensions, and direct measurements are difficult due to parallax (Figure 13.5g and h). In contrast, intraoperative CT (e.g. O-arm, Medtronic; Ceretom, NeuroLogica, Danvers, MA, www.neurologica.com) or MRI (IMRIS, Winnipeg, Manitoba, www.imris.com) gives immediate three-dimensional information (Figure 13.6). Both fluoroscopy and CT can detect stereotactic error, that is, deflection of the DBS from the stereotactic target. However, neither is sufficient to determine accuracy with respect to brain tissue, and thus cannot detect the situation where the lead is stereotactically accurate with respect to the frame, but anatomically inaccurate due to brain shift [56, 57, 61, 63, 98]. (Intraoperative post-implantation CT scans can be co-registered to the pre-operative MRI (Figure 13.6b and d) but do so only by overlay of bone-derived signals, thus do not detect brain shift.) In contrast, intraoperative MRI, when available, detects both stereotactic and anatomical accuracy. Radiologic control during the stages of lead fixation and wound closure is also useful to detect inadvertent lead dislodgement while it can be easily corrected.

Closure and recovery

After lead position is finalized, the patient is sedated for closure. The proximal lead is secured in place with either a commercial burr-hole cap system (e.g. StimLoc, Medtronic) (Figure 13.2c) or a small titanium miniplate and hydroxyapatite bone cement. In the latter case, care should be taken while bending the miniplate to avoid excess pressure on the lead insulation and covering the anchor point with silastic. The exposed proximal end of the lead is protected by a temporary silastic cap and tunnelled posterolaterally beneath the galea for later connection to the internal pulse generator. In bilateral cases, the leads may be separately tunnelled on each side and connected to separate IPGs, or both leads may be tunnelled on the same side and connected to a dual-channel IPG. The wound is irrigated, haemostasis obtained and the scalp closed in layers. Some centres instil concentrated antibacterial solutions into the wound before closure [99]. The use of absorbable skin suture material may decrease the need for post-operative care in uncomplicated cases.

After skin closure, the frame is removed and the patient allowed to emerge from sedation. After recovery in the post-anaesthesia care unit, the patient is transported to a regular ward for observation overnight. Most centres obtain confirmatory imaging with CT and/or MRI during the first 24 h after surgery to assess electrode position and rule out significant haemorrhage or pneumocephalus. The majority of patients are ambulatory by the evening of surgery and are discharged on the first post-operative day, although some patients may require longer recovery time.

The time required for DBS surgery varies based on the techniques used, surgeon and hospital experience, the use of intraoperative testing or intraoperative research protocols, the target chosen and the difficulty of target localization in an individual case. MER-guided unilateral placement generally takes 3–5 h; bilateral placement, 6–8 h. OR time may be significantly shortened by reducing the use of MER guidance in favour of macrostimula tion alone or intraoperative CT/MRI; these methods have comparable success rates in uncontrolled series but have not been directly compared with MER-guided surgery.

Intraoperative emergencies

All members of the surgical team should be aware of the signs and symptoms of rare but serious intraoperative complications, and close communication and teamwork are essential for complication avoidance and management. Venous air embolism (VAE) typically presents with coughing, tachypnoea and hypoxaemia in an awake patient, and is managed by lowering the head, irrigating the surgical field, waxing exposed bone edges and addressing any dural bleeding. VAE is rare, and precordial Doppler monitoring is not routinely used. Pneumocephalus may present with seizures or decreasing level of consciousness, and is treated post-operatively with 100% inspired oxygen via a non-rebreather mask. Cortical or subcortical haemorrhage may present with seizures, decreased level of consciousness and/or progressive motor deficit. Deep intracranial haemorrhage may present with a sudden loss of microelectrode tracings, focal neurologic signs, or progressive obtundation. Regardless of cause, seizures should be treated with benzodiazepines and anticonvulsants. Concern for intracranial haemorrhage should be addressed immediately with an emergent CT scan.

Pulse generator placement

IPGs placement may be performed immediately following DBS lead placement or may be delayed and performed as an outpatient procedure 1–2 weeks later. This decision is based partially on physician and patient convenience and partially on reimbursement considerations, with staged surgery producing a more favourable revenue margin for the hospital. Either method is well tolerated, and staged surgery does not delay the initiation of therapy, which is generally scheduled for 3–4 weeks after surgery in order to allow implantation-related tissue changes to stabilize.

IPG placement is performed under general anaesthesia with standard monitoring. The patient is positioned with the head turned away from the side of lead placement. The end of the lead is palpated under the scalp in the retroauricular region and a small linear scalp incision made to expose the lead tail. A second incision is made in the infraclavicular region, parallel to and approximately two fingerbreadths inferior to the clavicle, and a subcutaneous pocket fashioned above the pectoralis fascia. A 40-cm lead extension is tunnelled to the infraclavicular area and connected to both the lead and the IPG, which is placed in the pocket and secured with permanent suture. The entire system is interrogated by a remote programming device before wound closure in order to confirm device integrity and appropriate connection between all four electrode contacts and the IPG. Both incisions are closed in a cosmetically appropriate manner using absorbable suture. Single-channel IPGs are approximately the size and shape of cardiac pacemakers; dual-channel IPGs are somewhat bulkier, approximately the size of a deck of cards; rechargeable IPGs are smaller than non-rechargeable devices.

Post-operative care

Post-operative incisional care is routine, and most patients return to their normal activities within 4 weeks of surgery. Once the skin has healed, there are no restrictions placed on daily activities by the presence of DBS hardware. Passage through airport security is routine. Brain MRIs can be safely performed using a transmit/receive head coil, although some older IPG models may need to be turned off temporarily and the voltage temporarily set to zero. Receive-only head coils and body coils are contraindicated, as are electroconvulsive therapy (ECT) and transcranial magnetic stimulation.

Internal pulse generator programming

Initial programming of the IPG using telemetry (Figure 13.2d–f) usually takes place 2–4 weeks after lead placement in order to allow any oedema to resolve and tissue impedances to return to baseline (although the latter may be obviated by constant-current IPGs). Stimulation is tested systematically at all four contacts in monopolar configuration, with the DBS contact serving as the cathode (the 'active' or 'negative' contact) and the IPG casing serving as the anode (the 'positive' contact). Adjacent pairs of contacts are then tested in bipolar configuration, which produces volumes of tissue activated (VTA) oriented towards the anode when the anode is in close proximity to the cathode. More complex configurations using three or more contacts may be used to adjust the shape and location of the VTA. For a given electrode configuration, initial frequency and pulse width settings are chosen and the voltage is gradually increased from 0.5 while observing for therapeutic and adverse effects. Charge density is kept below $30\,\mu C/cm^2$ to prevent tissue damage, but short of that, higher voltages may be needed given the VTA necessary for some psychiatric targets. Settings are tested in a systematic, empirical fashion, since DBS lead position and local anatomy will vary significantly from patient to patient. Several sessions in the first months after surgery may be required until an optimal configuration is reached. Stimulation parameters may be adjusted throughout the life of the device in response to changes in efficacy or side effects [100], possibly related to chronic changes in impedance [101–103].

IPG replacement

IPG replacement is an outpatient procedure under local anaesthesia and takes approximately 30 min to perform. In movement disorder patients, IPG lifespan is typically 5–7 years; however, our initial experience with subcallosal cingulate DBS in treatment-resistant depression patients has shown higher power consumption, with IPG replacement required every 1.5–2 years. Given the potential for severe morbidity and even mortality with symptom relapse in severe psychiatric disease, battery life should be closely monitored and IPGs replaced before they become exhausted. Batteries that are near their end of service may provide unreliable stimulation, and IPG interrogation should be performed for any changes in clinical efficacy [104, 105].

Complications

DBS is a routine procedure with low complication rates in experienced centres. However, as with any intracranial surgery and any use of chronically implanted devices, complications can and do occur, and both patients and physicians should be familiar with the range of complications and strategies for prevention and management. DBS complications can be broadly divided into surgical, stimulation-related and hardware-related adverse effects. Prospective series with standardized recording instruments have also shown a significant rate of adverse medical events in the immediate perioperative period, but these rarely have a significant effect on hospital stay or quality of life [106].

Surgical complications

For DBS in general, the vast majority of which are for patients with movement disorders, reported intracranial haemorrhage rates vary between 1.5 and 5%, of which the large majority are small, asymptomatic and do not require treatment or prolongation of hospital stay [107–115]. Reported symptomatic haemorrhage rates are between 0.2 and 2% [107–110, 113, 116].

The majority of patients with symptomatic haemorrhage or insertional oedema recover with conservative management. Risk factors for haemorrhage include perioperative hypertension, the use of MER and the number of microelectrode passes, and transventricular trajectories [107, 108]. Rates may vary in unique patient populations, such as those with psychiatric disease, due to differences in age and other comorbidities. Nevertheless, in our 30 cases, we have had one subcortical haematoma (3%) mirroring the experience with movement disorders.

In movement disorder series, the rate of lead misplacement requiring repositioning ranges from 1.2 to 7.8% [109, 114, 117], although this rate has not been well established in psychiatric series.

Stimulation-related adverse effects

Stimulation-related effects, such as paresthesias or dysarthria, are reversible if stimulation is discontinued, but can often be managed with adjustments in programming [36]. These adverse effects are target specific (see chapters on specific targets and indications).

Hardware-related complications

Reported infection rates after DBS placement are between 1.7 and 8.5%, with significant variation among centres in both reporting criteria and management strategies [99, 107, 109, 111, 118–124]. Not all cases of infection ultimately require lead removal. Cellulitis can often be successfully managed with a 2-week course of IV and/or oral antibiotics without therapy interruption (Figure 13.7c). Purulent infection of the IPG pocket usually requires removal of the IPG and extension cable, but the DBS lead itself can sometimes be preserved and connected to a new IPG system after the infection has been eradicated. Extension of a purulent collection to the scalp usually requires removal of the entire DBS system. Intracranial infection is fortunately extremely rare, with only a handful of cases reported [125–127].

Because timely treatment of low-grade infection or minor wound breakdown may be the difference between hardware salvage and hardware removal, careful surveillance by all members of the psychiatry and neurosurgery teams is essential. This is especially true during long-term follow-up, when the patient will not have regular visits with the neurosurgery team, and after IPG replacement, which usually does not require a formal post-operative visit but which may carry more infection risk than initial placement [120, 128].

Non-infectious hardware complications, such as skin erosion (Figure 13.7b and e), lead migration and lead fracture, have fortunately become less frequent with the introduction of low-profile connector systems and smaller batteries, and as surgical awareness of these issues has improved. Although early series reported hardware-related complications in up to 25% of patients, with an incidence rate of 8.4% per electrode-year [123, 128], more recent series report incidence rates under 1% per electrode-year [107]. Overall rates of hardware-related complications are between

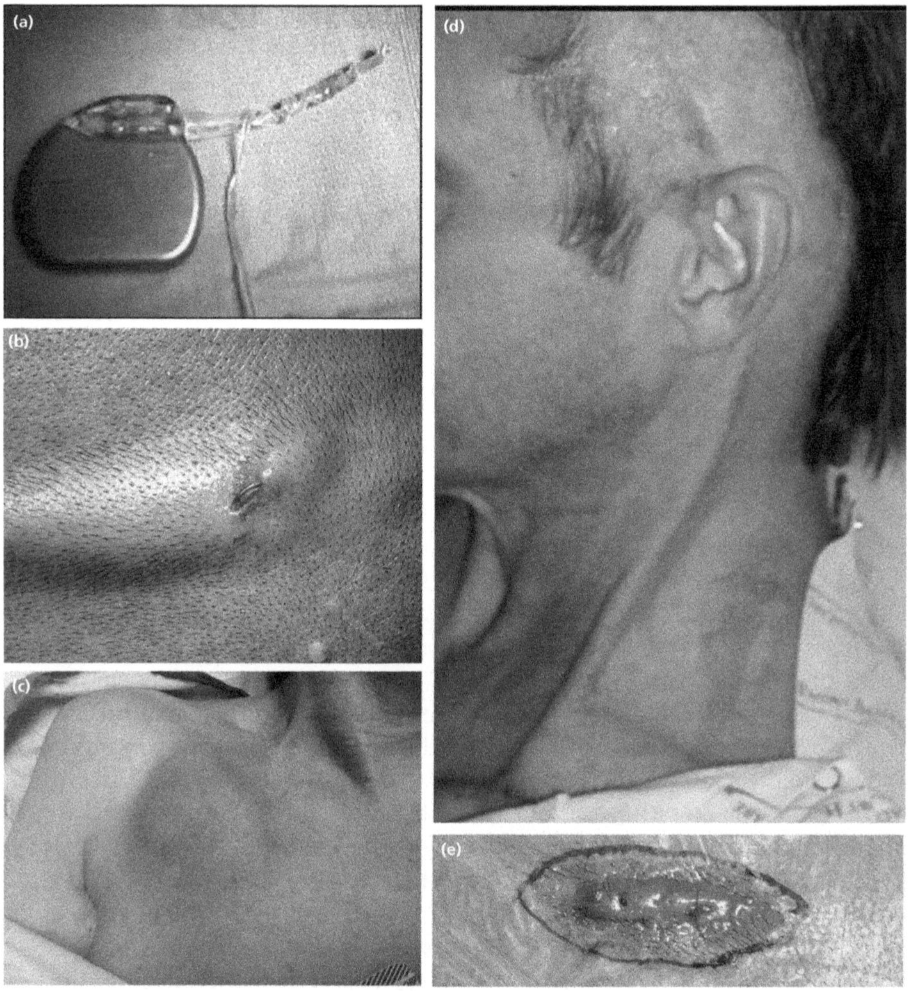

Figure 13.7 Some complications of DBS. (**a**) A case of 'twiddling': the patient rotated the IPG over and over until the tension on the wires caused them to break. This presented in a manner typical for lead or extension wire fracture, with loss of benefit and high impedance of the system detected during programming, prompting intraoperative investigation. (**b**) Erosions of the hardware through the skin can be infected, or sterile as in this case of erosion due to a loop of the DBS lead. The skin in fact has healed below the wire so that it comes out and goes back into the skin. This was repaired surgically without requiring removal. Infected systems often present with cellulitis (**c**); in many cases this can be treated with antibiotics alone, if no fluid collection has developed that envelopes and permeates the hardware. In the latter circumstance, all exposed hardware almost invariably needs to be removed and replaced at a later date. Less clear is the circumstance shown in E, a chronic erosion. We perform complete debridement of the affected region, which usually cultures positively, and rotate a scalp advancement with the assistance of plastic surgery colleagues; this is effective approximately 50% of the time for chronic erosions. Bowstringing is another hardware-related complication (**e**), due to a hypertrophic scar capsule forming around the extension wires. This tethers the DBS-to-extension wire connection to the IPG, although the extension wire within the capsule is freely mobile. Removing the extension wire is not sufficient: the picture shows the appearance in this patient *after* the wire had been removed. In these extreme cases, severing the scar capsule at four or five places releases the tension band and mitigates the tethering. (*See insert for colour representation of the figure.*)

3 and 15% [107, 109, 112, 113, 118, 122, 129], with lead migration rates between 0.5 and 3.1% [107, 130, 131], lead fracture rates between 1 and 5% [84, 107, 109, 114, 130–133] and extension cable revision rates between 0.4 and 1.5% [107, 109].

Lead migration, fracture (Figure 13.7a), short circuit or other hardware issues may present as loss of clinical benefit, or as localized electrical sensations if the lead or extension insulation is breached. Any of these circumstances should prompt interrogation of the DBS system to rule out abnormal electrode impedances. Very high impedances indicate the possibility of lead or extension break or disconnection. Although plain X-rays may be used to further investigate the physical integrity of the system, breaks are often not radiologically apparent. Low impedance raises the possibility of a short circuit between wires, which can also present with impedances that are identical (and low) on two adjacent contacts. These situations may only be resolved by open exploration and impedance testing of each component.

Long-term complications may include cases of sterile skin erosion (Figure 13.7b) with preserved DBS function. In these rare cases, hardware can frequently be preserved with debridement and closure [134–137]. Bowstringing (Figure 13.7d) is relatively uncommon but may require surgical incisions to release the scar cord, and can predispose to lead or extension fracture [138].

Future directions

After a decade or more of relative technological stability, several major advances in DBS targeting, placement, hardware and stimulation paradigms are poised to move from bench to bedside in the coming years. As detailed elsewhere in this volume, visualization of target nuclei is being greatly enhanced by high-field MRI, and white matter pathways can increasingly be seen in precise anatomic and functional detail through the use of MR tractography. The ability to relate treatment effects to specific white matter pathways and to target those pathways in individual patients despite anatomic variation is one of the most exciting prospects for the future in both psychiatric and movement-disorder stereotactic surgeries.

Surgical options for DBS lead placement have proliferated in recent years, and major DBS centres are increasingly pursuing asleep, image-guided lead placement techniques. Portable CT scanning provides accurate three-dimensional lead localization immediately after placement, which may shorten procedures and decrease the need for physiologic confirmation in many cases [63]. A more significant paradigm shift has accompanied the introduction of purely image-guided lead placement using interventional MRI, either in an MRI-equipped operating room or an interventional radiology suite. Interventional MRI technology allows real-time target selection, adjustment for brain shift, three-dimensional evaluation with resolution of individual nuclear structures and immediate assessment of any complications. Initial experience with this technique has shown fewer brain penetrations and later lead adjustments than using conventional MER guidance [139, 140]. Greater use of these two technologies may yield a less intimidating experience for patients than the use of traditional MER-based mapping and help make DBS accessible to patients with significant claustrophobia or anxiety.

Advanced DBS hardware designs are now in clinical trials. This includes leads with finer-grained contacts and leads capable of generating shaped and steerable current, which in turn allows more focused activation of target tissue, avoidance of unwanted stimulation effects and better compensation for imperfect lead placement [141]. An IPG capable of simultaneous electrical recording and stimulation has recently received FDA approval (Active PC+S, Medtronic, Minneapolis, MN), opening the door to long-term physiologic data collection and the possibility of closed-loop responsive stimulation if pathologic electrical activity can be reliably identified [142, 143]. Leads that can instantaneously and continuously sample local neurotransmitter concentrations have been tested intraoperatively in humans and may someday allow stimulation to be responsive to the extracellular chemical, as well as electrical, environment [144]. Finally, paradigms using asymmetric waveforms or non-continuous stimulation may provide additional opportunities for tissue selection and decreased power usage, enabling longer intervals between IPG changes [145, 146].

Taken together, these advances in imaging and DBS technology offer the promise of more effective, safer, longer-lasting and less expensive DBS treatment for established indications as well as the rapidly expanding list of emerging indications discussed elsewhere in this text.

References

1 Spiegel EA, Wycis HT, Marks M, Lee AJ. Stereotaxic apparatus for operations on the human brain. Science 1947 Oct 10; 106 (2754): 349–50.

2 Gildenberg PL. Spiegel and Wycis – the early years. Stereotact Funct Neurosurg. 2001 Jan; 77 (1–4):11–6.

3 Talairach J, Hecaen M, David M, Monnier M, Ajuriaguerra J. Recherches sur la coagulation therapeutique des structures sous-corticales chez l'homme. Rev Neurol. 1949;81:4–24.

4 Bailey P, Stein S. A Stereotaxic Apparatus for Use on the Human Brain. AMA Scientific Exhibit. Atlantic City; 1951.

5 Riechert T, Wolff M. Uber ein neues Zielgeraet zur intrakraniellen elektrischen Abteilung und Ausschaltung. Arch Psychiatr Z Neurol. 1951; 186:225–30.

6 Brown RA, Roberts TS, Osborn AG. Stereotaxic frame and computer software for CT-directed neurosurgical localization. Invest Radiol. 1980; 15(4):308–12.

7 Leksell L. A stereotaxic apparatus for intracerebral surgery. Acta Chir Scand. 1949;99:229–33.

8 Leksell L. Stereotactic radiosurgery. J Neurol Neurosurg Psychiatry. 1983 Sep; 46(9): 797–803.

9 Pool JL. Nerve stimulation in paraplegic patients by means of buried induction coil; preliminary report. J Neurosurg. 1946 May;3:264–7.

10 Pool JL. Psychosurgery in older people. J Am Geriatr Soc. 1954 Jul;2(7):456–66.

11 Pool L, Ransohoff J. Autonomic effects on stimulating rostral portion of cingulate gyri in man. J Neurophysiol. 1949 Nov;12(6):385–92.

12 Heath R. Studies in Schizophrenia: A Multidisciplinary Approach to Mind-Brain Relationships. Cambridge, MA: Harvard University Press; 1954.

13 Heath RG, Monroe RR, Mickle WA. Stimulation of the amygdaloid nucleus in a schizophrenic patient. Am J Psychiatry. 1955 May 1;111(11): 862–3.

14 Glenn WW, Mauro A, Longo E, Lavietes PH, Mackay FJ. Remote stimulation of the heart by radiofrequency transmission. Clinical application to a patient with Stokes-Adams syndrome. N Engl J Med. 1959 Nov 5;261:948–51.

15 Glenn WW, Furman S, Gordon AJ, Escher DJ, Van Heeckeren DW. Radiofrequency-controlled catheter pacemaker. Clinical application. N Engl J Med. 1966 Jul 21;275(3):137–40.

16 Hassler R. The influence of stimulations and coagulations in the human thalamus on the tremor at rest and its physiopathologic mechanism. Excerpta Medica Found. 1955;2:637–42.

17 Tasker RR, Organ LW, Hawrylyshyn P. Investigation of the surgical target for alleviation of involuntary movement disorders. Appl Neurophysiol. 1982 Jan;45(3):261–74.

18 Guiot G, Albe-Fessard D, Arfel G, Hertzog E, Vourc'h G, Hardy J, et al. Interpretation of the effects of thalamus stimulation in man by isolated shocks. C R Hebd Seances Acad Sci. 1962 May 14; 254:3581–3.

19 Benabid AL, Pollak P, Louveau A, Henry S, de Rougemont J. Combined (thalamotomy and stimulation) stereotactic surgery of the VIM thalamic nucleus for bilateral Parkinson disease. Appl Neurophysiol. 1987 Jan;50(1–6): 344–6.

20 Brice J, McLellan L. Suppression of intention tremor by contingent deep-brain stimulation. Lancet. 1980 Jun 7;1(8180):1221–2.
21 Rosenow J, Das K, Rovit RL, Couldwell WT, Irving S. Cooper and his role in intracranial stimulation for movement disorders and epilepsy. Stereotact Funct Neurosurg. 2002; 78:95–112.
22 Wu YR, Levy R, Ashby P, Tasker RR, Dostrovsky JO. Does stimulation of the GPi control dyskinesia by activating inhibitory axons? Mov Disord. 2001 Mar;16(2):208–16.
23 Dostrovsky JO, Levy R, Wu JP, Hutchison WD, Tasker RR, Lozano AM. Microstimulation-induced inhibition of neuronal firing in human globus pallidus. J Neurophysiol. 2000 Jul;84(1):570–4.
24 Histed MH, Bonin V, Reid RC. Direct activation of sparse, distributed populations of cortical neurons by electrical microstimulation. Neuron. 2009 Aug 27;63(4):508–22.
25 Miocinovic S, Parent M, Butson CR, Hahn PJ, Russo GS, Vitek JL, et al. Computational analysis of subthalamic nucleus and lenticular fasciculus activation during therapeutic deep brain stimulation. J Neurophysiol. 2006;96:1569–80.
26 Lafreniere-Roula M, Kim E, Hutchison WD, Lozano AM, Hodaie M, Dostrovsky JO. High-frequency microstimulation in human globus pallidus and substantia nigra. Exp brain Res. 2010 Aug;205(2):251–61.
27 Lujan JL, Chaturvedi A, McIntyre CC. Tracking the mechanisms of deep brain stimulation for neuropsychiatric disorders. Front Biosci. 2008 Jan;13:5892–904.
28 Walker HC, Huang H, Gonzalez CL, Bryant JE, Killen J, Cutter GR, et al. Short latency activation of cortex during clinically effective subthalamic deep brain stimulation for Parkinson's disease. Mov Disord. 2012 Jun;27(7):864–73.
29 Hammond C, Ammari R, Bioulac B, Garcia L. Latest view on the mechanism of action of deep brain stimulation. Mov Disord. 2008 Nov 15;23(15):2111–21.
30 Birdno MJ, Grill WM. Mechanisms of deep brain stimulation in movement disorders as revealed by changes in stimulus frequency. Neurotherapeutics. 2008 Jan;5(1):14–25.
31 McIntyre CC, Savasta M, Kerkerian-Le Goff L, Vitek JL. Uncovering the mechanism(s) of action of deep brain stimulation: activation, inhibition, or both. Clin Neurophysiol. 2004 Jun;115(6):1239–48.
32 Ballanger B, Jahanshahi M, Broussolle E, Thobois S. PET functional imaging of deep brain stimulation in movement disorders and psychiatry. J Cereb Blood Flow Metab. 2009 Nov;29(11):1743–54.
33 Boertien T, Zrinzo L, Kahan J, Jahanshahi M, Hariz M, Mancini L, et al. Functional imaging of subthalamic nucleus deep brain stimulation in Parkinson's disease. Mov Disord. 2011 Aug 15;26(10):1835–43.
34 Baker KB, Kopell BH, Malone D, Horenstein C, Lowe M, Phillips MD, et al. Deep brain stimulation for obsessive-compulsive disorder: using functional magnetic resonance imaging and electrophysiological techniques: technical case report. Neurosurgery. 2007 Nov;61(5 Suppl 2):E367–8.
35 Rauch SL, Dougherty DD, Malone D, Rezai A, Friehs G, Fischman AJ, et al. A functional neuroimaging investigation of deep brain stimulation in patients with obsessive-compulsive disorder. J Neurosurg. 2006 Apr;104(4):558–65.
36 Montgomery EB. Deep Brain Stimulation Programming: Principles and Practice. 1st ed. New York, NY: Oxford University Press; 2010.
37 Rolston JD, Desai SA, Laxpati NG, Gross RE. Electrical stimulation for epilepsy: experimental approaches. Neurosurg Clin N Am. 2011;22(4):425–42.
38 Nuttin B, Wu H, Mayberg H, Hariz M, Gabriels L, Galert T, et al. Consensus on guidelines for stereotactic neurosurgery for psychiatric disorders. J Neurol Neurosurg Psychiatry. 2014 Jan 20;85(9):1003–1008.
39 Greenberg BD, Price LH, Rauch SL, Friehs G, Noren G, Malone D, et al. Neurosurgery for intractable obsessive-compulsive disorder and depression: critical issues. Neurosurg Clin N Am. 2003 Apr;14(2):199–212.
40 Nuttin B, Gybels J, Cosyns P, Gabriels L, Meyerson B, Andreewitch S, et al. Deep brain stimulation for psychiatric disorders. Neurosurgery. 2002 Aug;51(2):519.
41 Garnaat SL, Greenberg BD, Sibrava NJ, Goodman WK, Mancebo MC, Eisen JL, et al. Who Qualifies for Deep Brain Stimulation for OCD? Data From a Naturalistic Clinical Sample.

J Neuropsychiatry Clin Neurosci. 2014 Jan 1;26(1):81–6.
42 Rughani AI, Hodaie M, Lozano AM. Acute complications of movement disorders surgery: effects of age and comorbidities. Mov Disord. 2013 Oct;28(12):1661–7.
43 Azmi H, Machado A, Deogaonkar M, Rezai A. Intracranial air correlates with preoperative cerebral atrophy and stereotactic error during bilateral STN DBS surgery for Parkinson's disease. Stereotact Funct Neurosurg. 2011 Jan;89(4):246–52.
44 Rezai AR, Kopell BH, Gross RE, Vitek JL, Sharan AD, Limousin P, et al. Deep brain stimulation for Parkinson's disease: surgical issues. Mov Disord. 2006 Jun;21 (Suppl 1):S197–218.
45 Ondo WG, Bronte-Stewart H. The North American survey of placement and adjustment strategies for deep brain stimulation. Stereotact Funct Neurosurg. 2005 Jan;83(4):142–7.
46 Abosch A, Timmermann L, Bartley S, Rietkerk HG, Whiting D, Connolly PJ, et al. An international survey of deep brain stimulation procedural steps. Stereotact Funct Neurosurg. 2013 Jan;91(1):1–11.
47 Talairach J, Tournoux P. Co-Planar Stereotaxis Atlas of the Human Brain. Direct. Thieme Medical Publishers, New York, 1988.
48 Schaltenbrand G, Wahren W. Atlas for Stereotaxy of the Human Bran. 2nd ed. Stuttgart: Thieme Medical Publishers, Inc; 1998.
49 Niemann K, van Nieuwenhofen I. One atlas – three anatomies: relationships of the Schaltenbrand and Wahren microscopic data. Acta Neurochir (Wien). 1999 Jan;141(10): 1025–38.
50 Nowinski WL. Towards construction of an ideal stereotactic brain atlas. Acta Neurochir (Wien). 2008 Jan; 150(1):1–13.
51 Nowinski WL. Atlases for deep brain stimulation. J Neurosurg. 2010 Mar;112(3):696–8.
52 Nowinski WL, Liu J, Thirunavuukarasuu A. Quantification and visualization of three-dimensional inconsistency of the ventrointermediate nucleus of the thalamus in the Schaltenbrand-Wahren brain atlas. Acta Neurochir (Wien). 2008 Jul;150(7):647–53
53 Sudhyadhom A, Okun MS, Foote KD, Rahman M, Bova FJ. A Three-dimensional Deformable Brain Atlas for DBS Targeting. I. Methodology for atlas creation and artifact reduction. Open Neuroimag J. 2012 Jan;6:92–8.
54 Gibson V, Peifer J, Gandy M, Robertson S, Mewes K. 3D visualization methods to guide surgery for Parkinson's disease. Stud Health Technol Inform. 2003 Jan;94:86–92.
55 Gildenberg P, Krauss JK. History of Stereotactic Surgery. In: Lozano AM, Gildenberg PL, Tasker RR, editors. Textbook of Stereotactic and Functional Neurosurgery. 1st ed. Berlin/ Heidelberg: Springer-Verlag; 2009. p. 3–33.
56 Hunsche S, Sauner D, Maarouf M, Poggenborg J, Lackner K, Sturm V, et al. Intraoperative X-ray detection and MRI-based quantification of brain shift effects subsequent to implantation of the first electrode in bilateral implantation of deep brain stimulation electrodes. Stereotact Funct Neurosurg. 2009 Jan;87(5):322–9.
57 Khan MF, Mewes K, Gross RE, Skrinjar O. Assessment of brain shift related to deep brain stimulation surgery. Stereotact Funct Neurosurg. 2008 Jan;86(1):44–53.
58 Maciunas RJ, Galloway RL, Latimer JW. The application accuracy of stereotactic frames. Neurosurgery. 1994 Oct;35(4):682–94.
59 Bjartmarz H, Rehncrona S. Comparison of accuracy and precision between frame-based and frameless stereotactic navigation for deep brain stimulation electrode implantation. Stereotact Funct Neurosurg. 2007 Jan;85(5):235–42.
60 Fiegele T, Feuchtner G, Sohm F, Bauer R, Anton JV, Gotwald T, et al. Accuracy of stereotactic electrode placement in deep brain stimulation by intraoperative computed tomography. Parkinsonism Relat Disord. 2008 Dec;14(8): 595–9.
61 Daniluk S, Davies KG, Novak P, Vu T, Nazzaro JM, Ellias SA. Isolation of the brain-related factor of the error between intended and achieved position of deep brain stimulation electrodes implanted into the subthalamic nucleus for the treatment of Parkinson's disease. Neurosurgery. 2009 May;64(5 Suppl 2):374–82.
62 Thani NB, Bala A, Lind CRP. Accuracy of magnetic resonance imaging-directed frame-based stereotaxis. Neurosurgery. 2012 Mar;70(1 Suppl Operative):114–23.

63 Burchiel KJ, McCartney S, Lee A, Raslan AM. Accuracy of deep brain stimulation electrode placement using intraoperative computed tomography without microelectrode recording. J Neurosurg. 2013 Aug;119(2):301–6.

64 Kelman C, Ramakrishnan V, Davies A, Holloway K. Analysis of stereotactic accuracy of the cosman-robert-wells frame and nexframe frameless systems in deep brain stimulation surgery. Stereotact Funct Neurosurg. 2010 Jan;88(5):288–95.

65 Pezeshkian P, DeSalles AAF, Gorgulho A, Behnke E, McArthur D, Bari A. Accuracy of frame-based stereotactic magnetic resonance imaging vs frame-based stereotactic head computed tomography fused with recent magnetic resonance imaging for postimplantation deep brain stimulator lead localization. Neurosurgery. 2011 Dec;69(6):1299–306.

66 Smith JS, Quiñones-Hinojosa A, Barbaro NM, McDermott MW. Frame-based stereotactic biopsy remains an important diagnostic tool with distinct advantages over frameless stereotactic biopsy. J Neurooncol. 2005;73: 173–9.

67 Winkler D, Hammer N, Oehlwein C, Schwarz J, Strecker K, Fritzsch D, et al. Implementing conventional Zamorano Dujovny frames versus individually manufactured microTargeting platforms–a comparative study on deep brain stimulation in Parkinson patients. Stereotact Funct Neurosurg. 2013 Jan;91(6): 392–8.

68 Balachandran R, Mitchell JE, Dawant BM, Fitzpatrick JM. Accuracy evaluation of microTargeting Platforms for deep-brain stimulation using virtual targets. IEEE Trans Biomed Eng. 2009 Jan 23;56(1):37–44.

69 Brontë-Stewart H, Louie S, Batya S, Henderson JM. Clinical motor outcome of bilateral subthalamic nucleus deep-brain stimulation for Parkinson's disease using image-guided frameless stereotaxy. Neurosurgery. 2010 Oct;67(4): 1088–93.

70 Cheng C-Y, Hsing M-T, Chen Y-H, Wu S-L, Sy HN, Chen C-M, et al. Deep brain stimulation for Parkinson's disease using frameless technology. Br J Neurosurg. 2014 Jun;28(3):383–6.

71 D'Haese P-F, Pallavaram S, Konrad PE, Neimat J, Fitzpatrick JM, Dawant BM. Clinical accuracy of a customized stereotactic platform for deep brain stimulation after accounting for brain shift. Stereotact Funct Neurosurg. 2010 Jan;88(2):81–7.

72 Fukaya C, Sumi K, Otaka T, Obuchi T, Kano T, Kobayashi K, et al. Nexframe frameless stereotaxy with multitract microrecording: accuracy evaluated by frame-based stereotactic X-ray. Stereotact Funct Neurosurg. 2010 Jan;88(3): 163–8.

73 Henderson JM. Frameless localization for functional neurosurgical procedures: a preliminary accuracy study. Stereotact Funct Neurosurg. 2004;82:135–41.

74 Henderson JM, Holloway KL. Achieving optimal accuracy in frameless functional neurosurgical procedures. Stereotact Funct Neurosurg. 2008 Jan;86(5):332–3.

75 Henderson JM, Holloway KL, Gaede SE, Rosenow JM. The application accuracy of a skull-mounted trajectory guide system for image-guided functional neurosurgery. Comput Aided Surg. 2004 Jan;9(4):155–60.

76 Holloway KL, Gaede SE, Starr PA, Rosenow JM, Ramakrishnan V, Henderson JM. Frameless stereotaxy using bone fiducial markers for deep brain stimulation. Journal of neurosurgery. 2005:103(3):404–13.

77 Konrad PE, Neimat JS, Yu H, Kao CC, Remple MS, D'Haese P-F, et al. Customized, miniature rapid-prototype stereotactic frames for use in deep brain stimulator surgery: initial clinical methodology and experience from 263 patients from 2002 to 2008. Stereotact Funct Neurosurg. 2011 Jan;89(1):34–41.

78 Smith AP, Bakay RAE. Frameless deep brain stimulation using intraoperative O-arm technology. Clinical article. J Neurosurg. 2011 Aug;115(2):301–9.

79 Larson PS, Starr PA, Bates G, Tansey L, Richardson RM, Martin AJ. An optimized system for interventional magnetic resonance imaging-guided stereotactic surgery: preliminary evaluation of targeting accuracy. Neurosurgery. 2012 Mar;70(1 Suppl Operative):95–103.

80 Holloway K, Docef A. A quantitative assessment of the accuracy and reliability of O-arm images for deep brain stimulation surgery. Neurosurgery. 2013 Mar;72(1 Suppl Operative):47–57.

81 Gross RE, Mewes K, Ghani GA. Anesthesia for movement disorders surgery. In: Bakay RAE, editor. Movement Disorder Surgery: The Essentials. 1st ed. New York, NY: Thieme Medical Publishers, Inc; 2009. p. 70–82.
82 Sebeo J, Deiner SG, Alterman RL, Osborn IP. Anesthesia for pediatric deep brain stimulation. Anesthesiol Res Pract. 2010 Jan;2010:1–4.
83 Venkatraghavan L, Luciano M, Manninen P. Review article: anesthetic management of patients undergoing deep brain stimulator insertion. Anesth Analg. 2010 Apr 1;110(4): 1138–45.
84 Constantoyannis C, Berk C, Honey CR, Mendez I, Brownstone RM. Reducing hardware-related complications of deep brain stimulation. Can J Neurol Sci. 2005 May;32(2):194–200.
85 Riva-Posse P, Choi KS, Holtzheimer PE, McIntyre CC, Gross RE, Chaturvedi A, et al. Defining critical white matter pathways mediating successful subcallosal cingulate deep brain stimulation for treatment-resistant depression. Biol Psychiatry. 2014 Apr 13.
86 Gross RE, Krack P, Rodriguez-Oroz MC, Rezai AR, Benabid A-L. Electrophysiological mapping for the implantation of deep brain stimulators for Parkinson's disease and tremor. Mov Disord. 2006 Jun; 21 Suppl 1:S259–83.
87 Laxton AW, Neimat JS, Davis KD, Womelsdorf T, Hutchison WD, Dostrovsky JO, et al. Neuronal coding of implicit emotion categories in the subcallosal cortex in patients with depression. Biol Psychiatry. 2013 Nov 15;74(10):714–9.
88 Sheth SA, Mian MK, Patel SR, Asaad WF, Williams ZM, Dougherty DD, et al. Human dorsal anterior cingulate cortex neurons mediate ongoing behavioural adaptation. Nature. 2012 Aug 9;488(7410):218–21.
89 Richter EO, Davis KD, Hamani C, Hutchison WD, Dostrovsky JO, Lozano AM. Cingulotomy for psychiatric disease: microelectrode guidance, a callosal reference system for documenting lesion location, and clinical results. Neurosurgery. 2008 Jun;62(6 Suppl 3):957–65.
90 Gale JT, Martinez-Rubio C, Sheth SA, Eskandar EN. Intra-operative behavioral tasks in awake humans undergoing deep brain stimulation surgery. J Vis Exp. 2011 Jan;6(47).
91 Holtzheimer PE, Kelley ME, Gross RE, Filkowski MM, Garlow SJ, Barrocas A, et al. Subcallosal cingulate deep brain stimulation for treatment-resistant unipolar and bipolar depression. Arch Gen Psychiatry. 2012 Feb; 69(2):150–8.
92 Mayberg HS, Lozano AM, Voon V, McNeely HE, Seminowicz D, Hamani C, et al. Deep brain stimulation for treatment-resistant depression. Neuron. 2005 Mar 3;45(5): 651–60.
93 Schlaepfer TE, Bewernick BH, Kayser S, Mädler B, Coenen VA. Rapid effects of deep brain stimulation for treatment-resistant major depression. Biol Psychiatry. 2013 Jun 15;73(12): 1204–12.
94 Gentil AF, Eskandar EN, Marci CD, Evans KC, Dougherty DD. Physiological responses to brain stimulation during limbic surgery: further evidence of anterior cingulate modulation of autonomic arousal. Biol Psychiatry. 2009 Oct 1;66(7):695–701.
95 Goodman WK, Foote KD, Greenberg BD, Ricciuti N, Bauer R, Ward H, et al. Deep brain stimulation for intractable obsessive compulsive disorder: pilot study using a blinded, staggered-onset design. Biol Psychiatry. 2010 Mar 15;67(6):535–42.
96 Okun MS, Mann G, Foote KD, Shapira NA, Bowers D, Springer U, et al. Deep brain stimulation in the internal capsule and nucleus accumbens region: responses observed during active and sham programming. J Neurol Neurosurg Psychiatry. 2007 Mar;78(3): 310–4.
97 Tsai H-C, Chang C-H, Pan J-I, Hsieh H-J, Tsai S-T, Hung H-Y, et al. Acute stimulation effect of the ventral capsule/ventral striatum in patients with refractory obsessive-compulsive disorder – a double-blinded trial. Neuropsychiatr Dis Treat. 2014 Jan;10:63–9.
98 Sillay KA, Kumbier LM, Ross C, Brady M, Alexander A, Gupta A, et al. Perioperative brain shift and deep brain stimulating electrode deformation analysis: implications for rigid and non-rigid devices. Ann Biomed Eng. 2013 Mar;41(2):293–304.
99 Miller JP, Acar F, Burchiel KJ. Significant reduction in stereotactic and functional neurosurgical hardware infection after local neomycin/polymyxin application. J Neurosurg. 2009 Feb;110(2):247–50.

100 Montgomery EB. Deep Brain Stimulation Programming. In: Bakay RAE, editor. Movement Disorder Surgery: The Essentials. 1st ed. New York, NY: Thieme Medical Publishers, Inc; 2009. p. 187–213.
101 Wei XF, Grill WM. Impedance characteristics of deep brain stimulation electrodes in vitro and in vivo. J Neural Eng. 2009 Aug;6(4):046008.
102 McConnell GC, Butera RJ, Bellamkonda RV. Bioimpedance modeling to monitor astrocytic response to chronically implanted electrodes. J Neural Eng. 2009 Oct;6(5):055005.
103 McConnell GC, Rees HD, Levey AI, Gutekunst C-A, Gross RE, Bellamkonda RV. Implanted neural electrodes cause chronic, local inflammation that is correlated with local neurodegeneration. J Neural Eng. 2009 Oct;6(5): 056003.
104 Vora AK, Ward H, Foote KD, Goodman WK, Okun MS. Rebound symptoms following battery depletion in the NIH OCD DBS cohort: clinical and reimbursement issues. Brain Stimul. 2012 Oct;5(4):599–604.
105 Fakhar K, Hastings E, Butson CR, Foote KD, Zeilman P, Okun MS. Management of deep brain stimulator battery failure: battery estimators, charge density, and importance of clinical symptoms. PLoS One. 2013 Jan;8(3): e58665.
106 Burdick AP, Fernandez HH, Okun MS, Chi Y-Y, Jacobson C, Foote KD. Relationship between higher rates of adverse events in deep brain stimulation using standardized prospective recording and patient outcomes. Neurosurg Focus. 2010 Aug;29(2):E4.
107 Fenoy AJ, Simpson RK. Risks of common complications in deep brain stimulation surgery: management and avoidance. J Neurosurg. 2014 Jan;120(1):132–9.
108 Zrinzo L, Foltynie T, Limousin P, Hariz MI. Reducing hemorrhagic complications in functional neurosurgery: a large case series and systematic literature review. J Neurosurg. 2012 Jan;116(1):84–94.
109 Falowski S, Ooi YC, Smith A, Verhargen Metman L, Bakay RA. An evaluation of hardware and surgical complications with deep brain stimulation based on diagnosis and lead location. Stereotact Funct Neurosurg. 2012;90(3):173–80.
110 Park JH, Chung SJ, Lee CS, Jeon SR. Analysis of hemorrhagic risk factors during deep brain stimulation surgery for movement disorders: comparison of the circumferential paired and multiple electrode insertion methods. Acta Neurochir (Wien). 2011 Aug;153(8):1573–8.
111 Boviatsis EJ, Stavrinou LC, Themistocleous M, Kouyialis AT, Sakas DE. Surgical and hardware complications of deep brain stimulation. A seven-year experience and review of the literature. Acta Neurochir (Wien). 2010 Dec; 152(12):2053–62.
112 Vergani F, Landi A, Pirillo D, Cilia R, Antonini A, Sganzerla EP. Surgical, medical, and hardware adverse events in a series of 141 patients undergoing subthalamic deep brain stimulation for Parkinson disease. World Neurosurg. 2010 Apr;73(4):338–44.
113 Bhatia S, Oh M, Whiting T, Quigley M, Whiting D. Surgical complications of deep brain stimulation. A longitudinal single surgeon, single institution study. Stereotact Funct Neurosurg. 2008;86(6):367–72.
114 Tir M, Devos D, Blond S, Touzet G, Reyns N, Duhamel A, et al. Exhaustive, one-year follow-up of subthalamic nucleus deep brain stimulation in a large, single-center cohort of Parkinsonian patients. Neurosurgery. 2007 Aug;61(2):297–304.
115 Fisher R, Salanova V, Witt T, Worth R, Henry T, Gross R, et al. Electrical stimulation of the anterior nucleus of thalamus for treatment of refractory epilepsy. Epilepsia. 2010 May;51(5): 899–908.
116 Umemura A, Oka Y, Yamamoto K, Okita K, Matsukawa N, Yamada K. Complications of subthalamic nucleus stimulation in Parkinson's disease. Neurol Med Chir (Tokyo). 2011 Jan;51(11):749–55.
117 Hu X, Jiang X, Zhou X, Liang J, Wang L, Cao Y, et al. Avoidance and management of surgical and hardware-related complications of deep brain stimulation. Stereotact Funct Neurosurg. 2010;88(5):296–303.
118 Baizabal Carvallo JF, Mostile G, Almaguer M, Davidson A, Simpson R, Jankovic J. Deep brain stimulation hardware complications in patients with movement disorders: risk factors and clinical correlations. Stereotact Funct Neurosurg. 2012 Jan;90(5):300–6.

119 Sillay KA, Larson PS, Starr PA. Deep brain stimulator hardware-related infections: incidence and management in a large series. Neurosurgery. 2008;62(2):360–6.
120 Pepper J, Zrinzo L, Mirza B, Foltynie T, Limousin P, Hariz M. The risk of hardware infection in deep brain stimulation surgery is greater at impulse generator replacement than at the primary procedure. Stereotact Funct Neurosurg. 2013 Jan;91(1):56–65.
121 Piacentino M, Pilleri M, Bartolomei L. Hardware-related infections after deep brain stimulation surgery: review of incidence, severity and management in 212 single-center procedures in the first year after implantation. Acta Neurochir (Wien). 2011 Dec;153(12): 2337–41.
122 Voges J, Waerzeggers Y, Maarouf M, Lehrke R, Koulousakis A, Lenartz D, et al. Deep-brain stimulation: long-term analysis of complications caused by hardware and surgery–experiences from a single centre. J Neurol Neurosurg Psychiatry. 2006 Jul;77(7):868–72.
123 Lyons KE, Wilkinson SB, Overman J, Pahwa R. Surgical and hardware complications of subthalamic stimulation: a series of 160 procedures. Neurology. 2004 Aug 24;63(4):612–6.
124 Temel Y, Ackermans L, Celik H, Spincemaille GH, van der Linden C, Walenkamp GH, et al. Management of hardware infections following deep brain stimulation. Acta Neurochir (Wien). 2004;146(4):355–61.
125 Brandão E, Rosas MJ, Abreu P, Linhares P, Vaz R. Intracerebral abscess: a rare complication of deep brain stimulation. Neurocirugia (Astur). 2013 Jan;24(1):33–6.
126 Blomstedt P, Bjartmarz H. Intracerebral infections as a complication of deep brain stimulation. Stereotact Funct Neurosurg. 2012 Jan; 90(2):92–6.
127 Vanderhorst VG, Papavassiliou E, Tarsy D, Shih L. Early brain abscess: a rare complication of deep brain stimulation. Mov Disord. 2009 Jul 15;24(9):1395–7.
128 Oh MY, Abosch A, Kim SH, Lang AE, Lozano AM. Long-term hardware-related complications of deep brain stimulation. Neurosurgery. 2002;50(6):1268–74.
129 Doshi PK. Long-term surgical and hardware-related complications of deep brain stimulation. Stereotact Funct Neurosurg. 2011 Apr; 89(2):89–95.
130 Baizabal Carvallo JF, Simpson R, Jankovic J. Diagnosis and treatment of complications related to deep brain stimulation hardware. Mov Disord. 2011 Jul;26(8):1398–406.
131 Kenney C, Simpson R, Hunter C, Ondo W, Almaguer M, Davidson A, et al. Short-term and long-term safety of deep brain stimulation in the treatment of movement disorders. J Neurosurg. 2007 Apr;106(4):621–5.
132 Hamani C, Lozano AM. Hardware-related complications of deep brain stimulation: a review of the published literature. Stereotact Funct Neurosurg. 2006 Jan;84(5–6):248–51.
133 Fernandez FS, Alvarez Vega MA, Antuna Ramos A, Fernandez Gonzalez F, Lozano Aragoneses B. Lead fractures in deep brain stimulation during long-term follow-up. Parkinsons Dis. 2010;2010:409356.
134 Fenoy AJ, Simpson RK. Management of device-related wound complications in deep brain stimulation surgery. J Neurosurg. 2012 Jun 7;116(6):1324–32.
135 Lanotte M, Verna G, Panciani PP, Taveggia A, Zibetti M, Lopiano L, et al. Management of skin erosion following deep brain stimulation. Neurosurg Rev. 2009;32(1):111–4.
136 Spiotta AM, Bain MD, Deogaonkar M, Hammert W, Lucas AR, Boulis NM, et al. Methods of scalp revision for deep brain stimulator hardware: case report. Neurosurgery. 2008;62(March (ONS Suppl 1)):E249–E250.
137 Gómez R, Hontanilla B. The reconstructive management of hardware-related scalp erosion in deep brain stimulation for Parkinson disease. Ann Plast Surg. 2014 Sep;73(3):291–4.
138 Miller PM, Gross RE. Wire tethering or ‘bowstringing’ as a long-term hardware-related complication of deep brain stimulation. Stereotact Funct Neurosurg. 2009 Jan;87(6): 353–9.
139 Vega RA, Holloway KL, Larson PS. Image-guided deep brain stimulation. Neurosurg Clin N Am. 2014 Jan;25(1):159–72.
140 Starr PA, Martin AJ, Ostrem JL, Talke P, Levesque N, Larson PS. Subthalamic nucleus deep brain stimulator placement using high-field interventional magnetic resonance imaging and a skull-mounted aiming device:

technique and application accuracy. J Neurosurg. 2010 Mar;112(3):479–90.
141 Martens HCF, Toader E, Decré MMJ, Anderson DJ, Vetter R, Kipke DR, et al. Spatial steering of deep brain stimulation volumes using a novel lead design. Clin Neurophysiol. 2011 Mar;122(3):558–66.
142 Tass PA, Klosterkötter J, Schneider F, Lenartz D, Koulousakis A, Sturm V. Obsessive-compulsive disorder: development of demand-controlled deep brain stimulation with methods from stochastic phase resetting. Neuropsychopharmacology. 2003 Jul;28(Suppl 1):S27–34.
143 Little S, Pogosyan A, Neal S, Zavala B, Zrinzo L, Hariz M, et al. Adaptive deep brain stimulation in advanced Parkinson disease. Ann Neurol. 2013 Sep;74(3):449–57.
144 Chang S-Y, Kimble CJ, Kim I, Paek SB, Kressin KR, Boesche JB, et al. Development of the mayo investigational neuromodulation control system: toward a closed-loop electrochemical feedback system for deep brain stimulation. J Neurosurg. 2013 Dec 1;119(6):1556–65.
145 Okun MS, Foote KD, Wu SS, Ward HE, Bowers D, Rodriguez RL, et al. A trial of scheduled deep brain stimulation for Tourette syndrome: moving away from continuous deep brain stimulation paradigms. JAMA Neurol. 2013 Jan;70(1):85–94.
146 Brocker DT, Swan BD, Turner DA, Gross RE, Tatter SB, Koop MM, et al. Improved efficacy of temporally non-regular deep brain stimulation in Parkinson's disease. Exp Neurol. 2013 Jan;239:60–7.

CHAPTER 14

Deep brain stimulation: Clinical results in treatment-resistant depression

Shane J. McInerney[1,2,3], Peter Giacobbe[1,3], Anna Cyriac[3] and Sidney H. Kennedy[1,2,3]

[1] *University of Toronto, Toronto, Canada*
[2] *St Michael's Hospital, Toronto, Canada*
[3] *University Health Network, Toronto, Canada*

Introduction and rationale for deep brain stimulation (DBS) for depression

Introduction – overview of the field

Worldwide, depression is a seriously disabling public health problem with a very high prevalence rate [1]. Despite the expansion of options for pharmacologic treatment in the past 20 years, two-thirds of depressed patients do not achieve remission with the first antidepressant prescribed [2] and one-third have not achieved remission after four sequential trials of treatment [3]. The minimum criteria for treatment-resistant depression (TRD) require failure to respond to at least two adequate trials of antidepressant medications [4]. These patients tend to have poorer functioning and a more prolonged course of illness [5] and more complex treatment regimens are required with increasing treatment resistance. A greater level of resistance is generally required for more invasive neurostimulation therapies to be considered.

Neurostimulation therapies

Neurostimulation treatments include repetitive transcranial magnetic therapy (rTMS), magnetic seizure therapy (MST), vagus nerve stimulation, electroconvulsive therapy (ECT) and deep brain stimulation (DBS). The most established brain stimulation treatment for severe depression and TRD is ECT, yet stigma and cognitive adverse effects limit its wider use [6]. With the introduction of MRI-guided techniques, rTMS has become a more targeted intervention but with little uniformity between studies (variable sample sizes, inclusion of bipolar depressed patients and low treatment resistance), its efficacy in TRD has yet to be firmly established [7]. MST uses rTMS to deliver a rapidly alternating magnetic field under anaesthesia in order to induce a seizure. MST is an investigational form of neurostimulation that has demonstrated promise as a potential alternative to ECT [8].

Indication for use of DBS in depression

The development of DBS for depression follows a course through treatments for movement disorders (Figure 14.1) [9]. It is generally accepted that the biological basis of depression cannot be attributed to abnormalities in any one neurotransmitter system, or in any discrete brain region. Heterogeneity of

Neuromodulation in Psychiatry, First Edition. Edited by Clement Hamani, Paul Holtzheimer, Andres M. Lozano and Helen Mayberg.

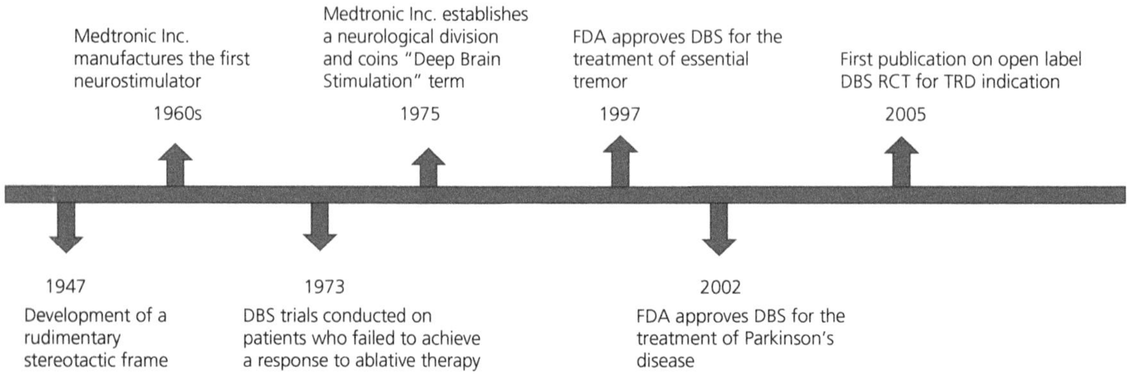

Figure 14.1 Progression in the development of DBS.

clinical symptoms can best be explained on the basis of dysfunction in neural networks involving limbic-cortical pathways [10]. Advances in the understanding of the neural circuitry of depression provide a rationale for DBS of discrete brain areas including the subcallosal cingulate gyrus (SCG) [10], the nucleus accumbens (NAcc) [11], the ventral capsule/ventral striatum (VC/VS) [12], the inferior thalamic peduncle (ITP) [13], the lateral habenula (LHb) [14] and medial forebrain bundle (MFB) [15].

DBS involves the bilateral stereotactic implantation of electrodes into specific brain structures where continuous stimulation of variable parameters is applied via neurostimulator devices placed subcutaneously in the infra-clavicular region [16, 17]. The programming of these devices is carried out by an external transmitter, and systematic adjustment of stimulation parameters (e.g. active contacts, amplitude or voltage, pulse width and frequency) is usually required, especially during the initial months after implantation [18].

Clinical targets and anatomical sites for DBS in depression

The areas that have been targeted for intervention will be outlined and the rationale for each area reviewed. The evidence to support DBS for TRD comes from open trials, often with a follow-up of 1 year or more (Table 14.1).

Subcallosal cingulate gyrus

Evidence in Parkinson's disease (PD) has demonstrated that chronic, high-frequency DBS in pathologically overactive motor circuits produces profound clinical benefit. It was hypothesized that focal stimulation of the SCG could also normalize aberrant activity throughout the depression circuit [16] and a proof-of-principle trial of the efficacy of SCG DBS in TRD began in 2003 in Toronto. Of the six patients who underwent SCG DBS for TRD, two met response criteria on the HDRS-17 (Hamilton Depression Rating Scale – 17 Item) at 1 month post-DBS activation and four achieved an antidepressant response by 6 months, with three of these subjects achieving remission [19]. In an expansion of this original cohort, the 1-year outcome of the first 20 patients who received SCG DBS for TRD identified 11 (55%) as responders and seven (35%) achieved or were within one point of remission (score of 8 or less on HDRS-17) at the end of a 12-month study period. The majority of the patients (8 of 11) who achieved an antidepressant response at 6 months continued to meet these criteria at 12 months [16]. The response to treatment was accompanied by reduction in metabolic activity in limbic and cortical areas based on ^{18}F-fluorodeoxyglucose (^{18}F-FDG) positron emission tomography (PET) [16].

Table 14.1 Neuro-anatomical targets across DBS studies.

Target	Authors	Sample size	Follow-up period	Results
Subcallosal cingulate white matter	Mayberg *et al.* [19]	6	6 months	Response: 66% Remission: 50%
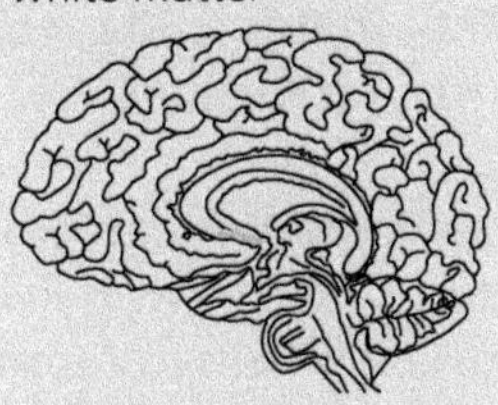	Lozano *et al.* [16]	20 (includes previous 6)	12 months	Response: 55% Remission: 33%
	Kennedy *et al.* [20]	20 long-term follow-up	Last follow-up (up to 6 years)	Response: 55% Remission: 35%
	Guinjoan *et al.* [21]	1	1 year	Remission
	Puigdemont *et al.* (2011)	8	1 year	Response: 62.5% Remission: 50%
	Holtzheimer *et al.* [22]	10 MDD,7 BD II	24 weeks	Response: 41% Remission: 18%
			1 year ($n=14$)	Response: 36% Remission: 36%
			2 years ($n=12$)	Response: 92% Remission: 58%
	Lozano *et al.* [23]	21	6 months 1 year	Response: 48% Response: 29% (62% with >40% reduction)
	Merkl *et al.* [24]	6	24–36 weeks	Response: 33% Remission: 33%
Ventral capsule/ventral striatum	Malone *et al.* [12]	15	6 months	Response: 40% Remission: 20%
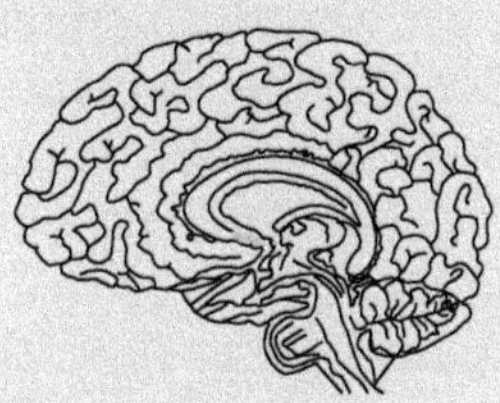			Last follow-up (23.5 + 14.9 months)	Response:53.3% Remission: 40%
	Dougherty et al. [34]	30	12 months	response 20% remission 13%
			18 months	response 26.7%
			24 months	response 23.3% remission 20%
Nucleus accumbens	Schlaepfer *et al.* [25]	3	1 week	Improvement with Stimulator 'ON'
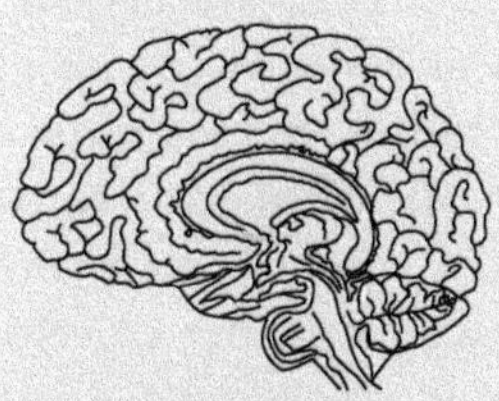	Bewernick *et al.* [11]	10 (includes previous 3)	12 months	Response: 50% Remission: 30%
	Bewernick *et al.* [26]	11 (includes previous 10)	2 years (up to 4 years; $n=5$)	Response: 45.5% Remission: 9% (1 patient)
Inferior thalamic peduncle	Jiménez *et al.* 13	1	24 months	Remission
Lateral habenula	Sartorius *et al.* [14]	1	12 months	Remission
Medial forebrain bundle	Schlaepfer *et al.* [15]	7	12–33 weeks	Response: 85% Remission: 57%

Source: Modified from Riva-Posse *et al.* [27]. Reproduced with permission of Elsevier.

Multi-site *Single site.*

The areas of reduced activity such as the orbital and medial frontal cortex are consistent with known connectivity to SCG [16].

After the initial 12-month study of DBS, patients from this cohort were assessed annually. Using intention to treat analysis (as four of the patients were lost to follow-up), response rates were 45% (9/20) at year 2, 60% (12/20) at year 3 and 55% (11/20) at the last follow-up visit of 3–6 years post-surgery. Approximately one- third of the patients were in remission at the time of their last follow-up assessment [20].

A subsequent open-label multi-centre Canadian trial of SCG DBS for TRD ($n = 21$) included 10 patients at the Toronto site who received FDG PET and 11 additional patients from either the Vancouver or Montreal sites. This study found that 57% of patients were deemed responders at 1 month, 48% at 6 months and 29% at 12 months [23]. The apparent drop in efficacy when measured in 'response rates' from 6 to 12 months occurred as 4 out of 10 patients had a reduction in their HDRS scores in the 40–50% range at the 12-month time point. Had the response rate been calculated on this 40% improvement basis, the response would be 62% [23]. A European group also reported on eight TRD patients who received SCG DBS under open-label conditions [28]. Following 1 month of active stimulation, three patients met criteria for remission while four were in remission at 1 year. The clinical and demographic characteristics of this group of patients are similar to other SCG DBS cohorts but this study used bipolar rather than monopolar stimulation. The authors found a preference for responders having electrodes located in BA24, corpus callosum and head of caudate [28].

In a further open-label trial of SCG DBS, the effect in a mixed group of 10 patients with TRD and 7 patients with bipolar II depression (BD) was examined [22]. Patients received single-blind sham stimulation for 4 weeks followed by long-term active stimulation from DBS electrodes implanted bilaterally in the white matter target in the SCG. A significant decrease in the severity of depressive symptoms was noted; three patients achieved remission at 6 months, 5 patients at 1 year and 12 patients were in remission after 2 years of active stimulation. The antidepressant effects of SCG DBS were consistent in this study, with no relapses being reported in patients who achieved remission [22].

A case report of a 55-year-old woman with major depressive disorder (MDD), who had previously undergone successful cingulotomy for MDD but relapsed after 6 months, had DBS to the SCG and remained in remission for the 30 months of the study [29]. Guinjoan *et al.* [21] found that right unilateral stimulation was more effective than bilateral stimulation but that left unilateral stimulation caused a sudden deterioration in mood in a case study of a patient with MDD who underwent SCG DBS [21]. Ramasubbu *et al.* [30] evaluated SCG DBS on four TRD patients and had a 50% response rate after 6 months of optimal stimulation [30]. Merkl *et al.* [24] conducted SCG DBS on six TRD patient and at last observation at 24–36 weeks, two patients were remitters (HDRS-24 < 10) and four were non-responders. Stimulation of the SCG for 24 h had only modest antidepressant effect while chronic stimulation of SCG had long-lasting antidepressant effects for two out of the six patients [24].

There is preliminary evidence that the integrity of white matter projections from the SCG to the amygdala should be intact to produce an antidepressant response to SCG DBS [31]. McNab *et al.* [31] described a report of a patient with TRD following a right thalamic stroke who failed to respond to SCG DBS. Both *in vivo* diffusion tensor imaging (DTI) and post-mortem neuropathology revealed a reduced number of white matter fibres projecting from the SCG to the amygdala only in the right hemisphere that was damaged by the stroke. Similarly, a superior effect of right unilateral compared to bilateral SCG stimulation has been associated with greater cross-hemispheric white matter projections seen with DTI from the right compared to left SCG [31]. Given that using gross neuroanatomical landmarks of DBS electrode placement may not be sufficient to predict long-term antidepressant outcomes with stimulation in the SCG, future studies could examine the potential role of individual differences in neuronal projections both to and from the SCG as a mediator of response.

An examination of 1-year outcomes with SCG DBS for TRD appears to be comparable across centres, with progressively better results being seen with long-term follow-up beyond 1 year [20, 22]. The reason for the elevated rates of response observed over time is unclear. Although DBS exerts its electrophysiological effects within milliseconds, positive clinical outcomes may only be evident weeks to months later. Understanding the short- and long-term neurophysiological and psychological adaptations that occur with chronic SCG DBS may help to elucidate the mechanisms of this putative treatment and improve patient selection.

Ventral capsule/ventral striatum

The VC/VS brain areas affect the cortico-striato-thalamocortical (CSTC) system including the orbitofrontal cortex, basal ganglia and anterior cingulate [32]. The rationale for targeting this network in TRD comes from findings that DBS to the VC/VS in patients with OCD resulted in improvements in depressive as well as obsessive–compulsive symptomatology [13, 33]. Malone *et al.* [12] conducted the first VC/VS DBS open-label, multi-centre trial in which 15 patients with TRD received bilateral DBS in the VC/VS areas over a period of 45 months. Responder rates on the HDRS at 3 months, 6 months and last follow-up were 46.7, 40 and 53.3%, respectively. The same group later reported on an expanded cohort of VC/VS DBS patients (the original 15 patients cited above plus two additional patients) with a 53% response rate observed at 3 months, 47% at 6 months and 71% at the last follow-up [12]. Dougherty *et al.* conducted a 16-week sham-controlled trial of VC/VS DBS in TRD patients. Response rates in the controlled phase did not differ significantly between active (20%) and control (14.3%) patients. Patients in the subsequent open-label follow-up phase achieved response rates of 20%, 26.7% and 23.3% at 12, 18, and 24 months, respectively [34].

Nucleus accumbens

Evidence from preclinical studies and human neuroimaging data implicates a prominent role for the NAcc in reward and pleasure processing. Given dense reciprocal connections of the NAcc to limbic and prefrontal regions, the NAcc is well situated to mediate reward-seeking motivational behaviour via dopaminergic circuitry [35, 36]. An increase in NAcc neuronal activity has been observed during expectations and experience of rewards. Although the pathophysiological mechanisms implicating NAcc dysfunction in MDD are not fully understood, there is evidence to link the NAcc to depressive symptoms of anhedonia and impaired motivation [36]. There is also evidence that MDD patients have significantly attenuated responsiveness to pleasurable stimuli, particularly the ability to integrate reward reinforcement history over time [37] and they exhibit less responsiveness to positive stimuli than healthy controls [38]. Furthermore, the severity of anhedonia is negatively correlated with activity in the NAcc [39].

Considering the role of the NAcc in hedonic response and depression pathophysiology, Schlaepfer *et al.* [25] observed that DBS to this site could alleviate anhedonia in TRD patients. In all three patients studied, significant improvements on the HDRS occurred when the stimulator was turned on but not when the stimulator was turned off. FDG-PET findings after 1 week of stimulation compared with pre-implantation showed bilateral increased metabolism in the VS (including the NAcc), the cingulate cortex, the amygdala and dorsolateral/dorsomedial prefrontal cortices. Decreased metabolism was observed in the caudate, thalamus and ventromedial/ventrolateral prefrontal cortices [25].

A subsequent study by the same group examined DBS to NAcc in 10 TRD patients over 1-year of continuous treatment. Relative to pre-treatment, five of the patients were classified as 'responders'. FDG-PET findings (6 months post-treatment vs. pre-treatment) in this sample revealed decreases in metabolism localized to the SCG, orbital prefrontal cortex, posterior cingulate cortex, thalamus and caudate nucleus [11]. In a subsequent report, the same authors reported on the long-term effects up to 4 years of NAcc DBS for TRD in a sample ($n=11$) that included subjects from the authors' earlier report. The five responders at 1 year to NAcc DBS sustained their therapeutic response through the last follow-up at 4 years [26].

Medial forebrain bundle

The MFB white matter tract carries both ascending and descending fibres between the ventral tegmental area and the NAcc, conferring a functional anatomy similar to the VC/VS and NAcc DBS target sites for TRD. Increased levels of dopamine after stimulation of the MFB in an animal model suggest a reward/hedonic role for the MFB similar to that associated with the NAcc. DTI is required to visualize the fibre tracts of the intended superolateral branch target of the MFB in surgical planning [32, 35]. The Schlaepfer group assessed the safety and efficacy of DBS to the superolateral branch of the MFB in six TRD patients and one patient with bipolar disorder in a sustained and severe depressive episode. At last follow-up 12–33 weeks later, six were responders and four of the six were in remission (which included the bipolar-depressed patient), which provides encouragement for further investigation of the MFB in TRD [15].

Other experimental targets – ITP and lateral habenula (LHb)

Stimulation of the ITP and the LHb have been the subject of individual case reports on DBS to their sites, but further reports are required before the potential benefits of DBS to either site can be evaluated.

The ITP courses along the ventromedial side of the thalamus to the posterior limb of the internal capsule and encompasses the VS and NAcc. The thalamo-orbitofrontal (Th-OF) system and its main fibre, ITP area, are involved in wakefulness, selective attention and motor-sensory behaviours [40]. Dysregulation of 5HT and NE induce overactivity of the orbitofrontal cortex, which then affects ITP activity. Overactivity in the Th-OF and midline thalamic nuclei has been found in patients with MDD [33]. Jiménez *et al.* [13] published a case report of DBS to the ITP in a woman who achieved remission in the ON phase of the double-blind period, while symptoms progressively recurred after 10 months OFF stimulation [13]. The sustained therapy in the absence of active stimulation could be explained by DBS of the ITP affording an induction of neurotransmitter regulatory processes but the possibility of a placebo effect in this case study of ITP DBS cannot be excluded [35].

The habenular complex, located in the medial to posterior thalamic regions, receives strong serotonergic, noradrenergic and dopaminergic innervations [41]. There is evidence of LHb overactivity in depressed states [42, 43], and strong covariation between the LHb and dorsal raphe, suggesting a convergent pathway controlling the release of 5HT [44]. The LHb has also been found to play a role in reward control via the ventral tegmentum [45, 46]. To date, there is one published case study of DBS to the LHb in a woman with TRD that resulted in a sustained full remission of depressive symptoms after 4 months of stimulation [14]. The apparent therapeutic effect conferred by DBS of the LHb awaits replication and extension to larger samples.

Current registered randomized controlled trials for TRD trials

Table 14.2 shows the current registered DBS randomized controlled trials (RCTs). The BROADEN (BROdmann Area 25 DEep brain

Table 14.2 Active DBS for TRD trials.

Study title	DBS of nucleus accumbens for chronic and resistant major depressive disorder (PRESTHYM)	DBS of the slMFB for the treatment of refractory major depression (FORESEEII)	A pilot study of DBS to the lateral habenula in TRD	DBS for TRD	A clinical evaluation of subcallosal cingulate gyrus DBS for TRD
Institution	Rennes Hospital, France	University Hospital, Germany	Mount Sinai Hospital, USA	Emory University, USA	University Health Network Toronto, Canada
Status	Active but not recruiting	Recruiting	Recruiting	Recruiting	Recruiting
Enrolment	10	12	6	20	40
Age range	30–60	20–75	21–70	18–70	21–70
Design	Open-label trial	RCT	RCT	Open-label trial	RCT
Primary outcome measure	Response after 4 months of DBS months based on HDRS score	Change in Montgomery Asberg Depression Scale (MADRS) at 6 and 12 months	Change in HDRS-17 score from baseline to 6 months	Response after 6 months based on HDRS-24	Change in HDRS-17 at 3 and 6 months

Neuromodulation) study, a US multi-site RCT that evaluated DBS to SCG under sham-controlled double-blind conditions, failed a futility analysis and was terminated prematurely. The current (FORESEE II: FOREbrain Stimulation dEprEssion) is a sham comparator study with stimulation for 8 weeks following implantation of an internal pulse generator (IPG) with DBS to the superolateral branch of the main MFB (slMFB). Emory University, Dartmouth-Hitchcock Medical Center and University Health Network, Toronto, are continuing trials examining SCG DBS. The European DBS SCG is a multi-site study that is active but no longer recruiting as an adjunctive treatment for TRD. The Calgary group (CRIO-DBS) hypothesizes that long pulse-width DBS applied to the SCC region will lead to improvements in TRD patients and that specific neuroimaging biomarkers will correlate with response to DBS; the functional recovery will be enhanced with concurrent cognitive behavioural therapy. PRESTHYM is a French preliminary study evaluating DBS of NAcc in patients with chronic and resistant MDD. The University of Texas Health Science Center, Houston, proposes a clinical study of MFB DBS as a treatment in 10 patients with TRD. The Mount Sinai Group in New York proposes an investigation of the safety, tolerability and benefit of DBS to the lateral habenula for patients with TRD. The completed multi-centre Reclaim trial to evaluate the safety and efficacy of bilateral DBS of the VC/VS reported on findings from 30 subjects of the planned cohort of 208 (see Table 14.1) [34]. While deemed a failed trial, a range of 20–27% of patients did achieve response at some time during an open label continuation phase out to 24 weeks. (All trial information can be viewed at www.clinicaltrials.gov)

Adverse effects of DBS

Table 14.3 outlines the most common complications that have been reported in the DBS for TRD literature.

Surgery

The DBS surgical procedure, not unlike other neurosurgical procedures, can have adverse events (AEs). In the first publication on DBS for TRD patients, Mayberg *et al.* [10] reported that two patients developed local infections related to the connector cable at the chest or scalp. Both were treated with intravenous antibiotics but the devices were explanted after approximately 6 months because of persistent infection in the absence of clinical benefit (with subsequent resolution of their infections). No worsening of depressive symptoms was observed in either subject following explantation. Another patient in that study developed skin erosion over the hardware and also received antibiotics. Subsequently in the expanded sample of 20 patients, four patients had wound infections (including two of the original Mayberg patients). In three cases, this occurred early in the series when electrodes were externalized for several days before the IPG was inserted. These three patients had their hardware removed. In one patient, the hardware was reimplanted after a 6-month delay with recapture of the clinical benefit. In the two others who did not receive significant benefit, the explanted hardware was not replaced [16]. All patients from patient six on (that is after the Mayberg 2005 report) had electrodes and pulse generator inserted in a single surgery. One patient had superficial scalp cellulitis 2 weeks after surgery that responded to antibiotics, and another experienced a generalized seizure the evening of surgery, which was successfully treated with phenytoin for 3 months with no further seizures. Four patients reported headache or pain at the site of the pulse generator implant in the immediate post-operative period [16]. AEs in the Schlaepfer study [26] on the NAcc were directly related to the surgical procedure (e.g. pain at sites of implantation) and no other adverse effects were observed.

Table 14.3 Common DBS for TRD adverse events.

Surgery-related effects:
Infection at the surgery sites (5%)
Pain or discomfort (5%)
Allergic or rejection response to implanted materials (<1%)
Stimulation-related effects:
Headache (5%)
Tingling sensation during stimulation (<5%)
Short- or long-term pain experienced at the impulse generator sites (<5%)
Short-term and reversible symptoms with changes in stimulator settings for example sweating, dizziness, blurred vision and strabismus (<5%)
Slowed thinking, anxiety and deterioration in mood (<5%)
Short term dizziness or nausea (<1%)
Effects not related to stimulation include:
Changes in the electrode position, loose electrical connections and/or lead failure (<5%)
Lead repositioning; lead fractures (<5%)
Skin erosion (<1%)
Component malfunction (<5%)

Malone *et al.* [12] had a total of 25 SAEs reported by six patients, four of which were identified as related to the DBS neurostimulator device, both of which required revision [12]. Adverse effects in the Bewernick *et al.* [11] were limited to those limited to the surgical procedure (such as dysphagia and pain), during the course of parameter change (erythema and sweating) or unrelated to the DBS treatment [11]. In the report by Puigdemont *et al.* (2012), both the surgical procedure and post-operative period were generally well tolerated by all eight patients. Two patients reported cephalalgia, and three reported pain in the neck at the site of the sub-dermal leads. There were no other AEs reported by previous studies, such as wound infection, scalp cellulitis or seizures. One explanation for the lack of infections, as already suggested, was that all patients had the electrodes and the pulse generator inserted in a single surgical intervention [28]. Holtzheimer *et al.* [22] reported 22 AEs in 11 patients (65%), 12 serious AEs (SAEs) occurred in 4 patients (24%) with 9 of the 12 SAEs (75%) occurring in 1 patient with bipolar disorder. No AE or SAE was related to active stimulation. No intraoperative haemorrhages occurred. Eight device- or surgery-related events included two SAEs (DBS system infections requiring explantation, both in the same patient) and six AEs [22].

In Schlaepfer's later [47] study on DBS of the superolateral branch target of the MFB, blurred vision and strabismus occurred in all patients when specific electrode contacts were activated at higher amplitudes. Other AEs related to stimulation were dizziness and increased sweating. During implantation of the first electrode (left), one patient had an intracranial bleeding with transient hemiparesis and dysarthria [47].

Post-operative

Lozano *et al.* [16] reported nausea and vomiting in 7 of 20 patients. It was unclear whether this represented a side effect of stimulating this region, a consequence of the interaction between stimulation and medications, or was due to completely unrelated causes. In other patients, there was a lead extension malfunction immediately after surgery requiring extension replacement and a case of superficial skin erosion at the burr-hole site 7 weeks after device activation, which was treated successfully with antibiotics [23]. Three additional SAEs included two syncopal episodes in one patient and an occurrence of deterioration of mood, disinhibition and impulsivity in a bipolar patient. All were addressed with changes in medication and stimulation parameters. The remaining 18 of the 25 SAEs were unrelated to DBS therapy. Increased depression was noted on several occasions to be associated with cessation of stimulation due to neurostimulator battery depletion (four patients) or accidental deactivation (three patients) [16].

In the Malone study, there were two incidents of hypomania in a bipolar patient and an incident of worsening depression during stimulation, which resolved with stimulation parameter and medication alterations [12]. Several patients reported instances of worsening depression that was caused by battery depletion (four patients) or inadvertent deactivation of the neurostimulator (three patients).

Hypomania

In Malone *et al.* [12], there were two incidents of hypomania in a bipolar patient; both resolved after modification of stimulation parameters and medications [12]. To our knowledge, no other studies reported hypomanic events following DBS.

Cognitive

There have been a number of studies examining the effect of DBS on cognition and none have found any deleterious effects. In the first examination of cognition following SCG DBS, a 12-month neuropsychological follow-up did not reveal any deterioration in cognition and in fact the majority of patients exhibited improvements in their neuropsychological functioning from the 'below average' to 'average' range [48]. The cognitive effects of NAcc DBS were also examined over a 12-month period by Grubert *et al.* [49] and revealed significantly improved cognitive performance in attention, learning and memory, executive function and visual perception and also that these effects were independent of the antidepressant effects or changes in NAcc-DBS parameters [50]. Neuropsychological follow-up of the same group over 24–36 months confirmed no deterioration in cognition along with a significantly improved score on nonverbal fluency [26]. Malone *et al.*'s [12] DBS of the VC/VS revealed no adverse effects on any cognitive domain [12]. In the 8-month period of ON stimulation for ITP DBS on a single patient with resistant MDD, neuropsychological performance progressively improved to normal levels with an improvement in the verbal, nonverbal memory and abstraction tests by the 8 month follow-up period [13]. Holtzheimer *et al.* [22] found that neuropsychological function had either improved or remained stable over a 24-week assessment period in patients who received chronic SCG DBS stimulation [22]. None of the six patients in the Merkl *et al.* [24] study who received SCG DBS had any cognitive deficits at either 6- or 12-month follow-up [24]. A 42-month follow up of four patients who had SCG DBS indicated that there was stability in cognitive functioning over this period, relative to baseline assessment [51].

Long-term outcomes

The long-term outcomes of the cohort of 20 patients who received SCG DBS for TRD at the University of Toronto centre were examined with patients reporting functional gains in their quality of life and work status post-DBS and these effects continued beyond the 1 year to last follow-up time points [20]. After 1 year of DBS, half of the patients were able to maintain employment [16] and, at the last follow-up, 65% engaged in work-related activities [20].

Existing data in patients with TRD suggest a positive correlation between long-term improvements in depressive and anxiety symptoms [16, 28], although longer times were required to reach maximal improvements in anxiety symptoms as compared to the core mood symptoms of depression [16]. However, short-term exacerbations in anxiety have been described in a minority of patients with SCG DBS [22, 23].

DBS and suicidal ideation

The most serious AEs reported in patients who have received SCG DBS are self-harm and suicide. Although it is recognized that increased all-cause mortality, including completed suicides, is an inherent feature of TRD, and has been estimated in two studies to be 13% over 4–8 years [52] and 32% over 7 years [50] in this clinical population, the emergence of suicidal ideation in patients with SCG DBS is a psychiatric emergency [53]. In the combined published case series of SCG DBS, less than 5% (3/64) of patients with TRD who have received this procedure have completed suicide [20, 22, 23, 28]. In these reports, the timing of the suicidal behaviour, including both attempts and completed suicide, has ranged from 1 week post-DBS activation [22] to over 6 years post-surgery [20]. In the Bewernick *et al.* [11] study, one patient attempted and another patient completed suicide during the follow-up period. These serious AEs were judged unrelated to the DBS treatment, as the suicide attempt was related to non-compliance of the patient (both to medication and study visits to adjust stimulation parameters), and this patient is now classified as a responder with stable stimulation parameters. Both patients also had attempted suicide previous to entering the study [11]. Kennedy *et al.* [20] reported two patients in whom suicide was considered a probable cause of death. These two patients accounted for four of the six psychiatric admissions during the 3- to 6-year follow-up period. One of the patients who died by suicide had a family history of completed suicide in four first- or second-degree relatives. There was no evidence that either death was due to DBS device failure or changes in stimulation parameters [20].

The relationship between DBS and suicide in this population is complex and multi-factorial. Inquiry as to the presence of suicidality should be a kernel part of each post-DBS implantation follow-up visit and an expression of suicidal thoughts by any patient should prompt an evaluation of the functionality of the DBS device [54]. As has been reported in TRD and in other patients with severe mental illness, suicidal behaviours may occur even in those patients who have had a marked improvement in their underlying condition [22, 55, 56]. The depletion of the DBS battery or its deactivation may herald a rapid re-emergence of depressive symptoms. Holtzheimer *et al.* [22] reported that three patients experienced an acute relapse of their depressive symptoms with suicidal ideation within 2 weeks of undergoing a single-blind discontinuation of active DBS in their protocol. There were two suicide attempts; each was temporally associated with a significant psychosocial stressor. One suicide attempt in a patient with MDD occurred after 1 week of active stimulation, but the suicidal ideation resolved without stimulation parameter or medication change; this patient was a responder at the 24-week time point and a remitter at the 1- and 2-year time points. The other suicide attempt in a patient with bipolar disorder occurred 54 weeks into the observational follow-up phase and was not associated with any treatment change, although this patient was a responder at the 2-year time point [22]. It took several months after the re-activation of stimulation for the depressive symptoms to remit. In contrast, a woman receiving SCG DBS for TRD had a rapid relapse with re-emergence of suicidality on two occasions following the cessation of active stimulation, which rapidly stabilized with the re-introduction of stimulation [57]. The role of poor psychological re-adaptation to one's interpersonal and employment situation has been suggested as a potential contributor to suicide following DBS for PD [58]. This merits further investigation in the TRD population especially given the younger age at which this group receives DBS compared to those with PD. One patient in the Spanish sample reported by Puigdemont *et al.* [28] displayed an initial clinical improvement, attempted suicide 4 months after starting DBS, was hospitalized and did not respond at 6- or 12-month follow-up periods. However, two of the five final responders had a recurrence of their depression during the first 3–4 months after starting DBS [28].

Future direction in DBS

Technical advances in DBS hardware with enhanced stimulation capabilities are now emerging. Rechargable batteries that can increase the lifetime of a battery from 3–5 to 9 years are now available [54]. Other modifications in the pipeline include nano-sized electrodes designed according to individual brain structure [59], miniaturized leads that may enhance placement and decrease AEs [60], bidirectional DBS system that is capable of capturing neural activity in real time and concurrent electrical stimulation [61]. A further development could include the combination of DBS and optogenetics, whereby wavelengths of light could affect specific cells in the brain [62].

Bioethics of DBS

The premise that neuromodulation techniques such as DBS facilitate neural malleability raises both hopes and fears as is the case in emerging neurotechnologies such as DBS [63]. Following the successful application of DBS in PD and preliminary success in TRD, the National Institutes of Health and Dana Foundation sponsored a multi-disciplinary conference to discuss the scientific and ethical implications of DBS specifically for mood and behavioural disorders. The purpose of this conference was to discuss two primary ethical issues – to establish a consensus on clinical trial design for DBS and to develop standards to ensure the protection of trial participants [64]. The conference proceedings advised that DBS be investigated within the realm of carefully designed trials [64].

The nature of DBS allows researchers to design RCTs, whereby a patient may be allocated to sham treatment for a limited time and receive no stimulation during the double-blind phase. This clinical research design is exposed to several biases. For instance, patients are subjected to tests post-surgery to ensure the functionality of the device. Post-surgery and/or randomization patients may report sensations of 'knowing' if the device has been turned on [65]. In contrast to other neurostimulation therapies, DBS presents unique situations such as the capacity to have the entire system explanted or turned off. This also presents the interesting query of how the treatment should be dispensed. Currently, patients, in some studies, are given the capability to adjust their stimulating settings within a defined window raising the question of whether the patient or the treating physician should govern the stimulator settings [65].

The most noted ethical concern that emerges from the use of DBS treatment is patient safety [64]. Recruiting an already vulnerable population increases the likelihood of patients not considering the relevant benefits and risks involved in the process of DBS [66]. DBS candidates are selected based on stringent eligibility criteria such as demonstrated chronicity and severity of MDD as well as the failure of conventional antidepressant trials [66]. These criteria highlight the susceptibility of this population as candidates may feel compelled to provide consent [67]. This is exacerbated by several factors, which include the nature of participants being recruited, the competency of patients with psychiatric disorders and, lastly, the management of patient expectations that tend to be significantly higher due to the relative invasiveness of DBS compared to other treatments [66].

In addition, the association of cognitive impairment with MDD significantly increases concern about patients being able to comprehend the procedures involved and the capacity to provide informed consent. To evaluate the issue of decisional capacity, Fisher and colleagues [68] administered the MacArthur Competence Assessment Tool for Clinical Research (MacCAT-CR) in 31 DBS participants. Their findings indicated that researchers may be underestimating the decisional capacity of MDD patients, who demonstrated decisional capacity albeit with a few therapeutic misconceptions such as overrating the likelihood of personal benefit and the degree of individual care in the study [68]. In another study using the same clinical tool to examine the thematic enrolment decisions of participants, perceived lack of other treatment options, desire to take initiative, beliefs about DBS as a novel treatment and altruism were some of the themes that emerged. None of the themes suggested that any participant had a compromised decision-making capacity [69]. Dunn *et al.*'s review paper echoed this sentiment and suggested that TRD patients are no more impaired as to their capacity but due to the invasive nature of the treatment, additional safeguards should be employed to ensure that the participant has made an autonomous decision [70].

At present, there is a drought of information on DBS and its effects on individual are experiences of his or her personal identity following DBS treatment [71, 72]. Neural interventions have the capacity to alter experiences so profoundly that they may impact the experience of personhood [73] while providing the rebuttal that treatments such as DBS do not affect the personhood or the identity of individuals any more than psychopharmacological or behavioural and cognitive therapies [67]. The ethical implications of DBS continue to be questioned and the optimal delivery methods for DBS remain to be established. Since this is the case, ethical thinking must catch up in order to incorporate these rapidly evolving developments [74].

Conclusion

With a choice of target site and the range of stimulation parameters available, preliminary evidence suggests that DBS for MDD has a substantial role to play in the treatment of this very disabling illness. A significant treatment response has been reported within 1 week in some cases [14, 35], although the most convincing response data have been derived from periods of stimulation of 6–12 months and longer. While the peri- and post-operative DBS periods must be carefully considered, DBS-related side effects have for the most part been transient and have resolved with the adjustment of stimulation parameters.

In this chapter of DBS for depression, we have discussed DBS to SCG, VC/VS and NAcc targets in particular because they have included larger sample sizes and a longer course of treatment. Importantly, results for each of these three targets yield comparable positive response rates. This rate of growth of our knowledge and experience with this procedure for TRD will continue to progress in the future with the exploration of the antidepressant effects of SCG DBS under methodologically rigorous blinded, sham-controlled conditions [35].

The optimal methods of combining the established biological and psychological treatments for depression with DBS remain unknown. Synergistic or additive effects of concurrent changes in the treatments provided to these patients in long-term follow-up are possible contributory factors to the improved response rates observed with chronic SCG DBS [20, 22]. Although offering promise for those with TRD, positive results from large-scale, multi-centre, placebo-controlled trials are vital to justify the continuous use of DBS for TRD.

Acknowledgement

The authors thank Ms. Madelin Donovan for her assistance with referencing and preparation of the chapter.

References

1 Kessler RC, Berglund P, Demler O, Jin R, Koretz D, Merikangas KR, *et al.* The epidemiology of major depressive disorder: results from the National Comorbidity Survey Replication (NCS-R). JAMA. 2003 Jun 18;289(23):3095–105.

2 Little A. Treatment-resistant depression. American Family Physician. 2009 Jul 15;80(2):167–72.

3 Warden D, Rush A, Trivedi M, Fava M, Wisniewki S. The STAR*D Project Results: a comprehensive review of findings. Current Psychiatry Reports. 2007;9(6):449–59.

4 Souery D, Amsterdam J, De Montigny C, Lecrubier Y, Montgomery S, Lipp O, *et al.* Treatment resistant depression: methodological overview and operational criteria. European Neuropsychopharmacology. 1999;9:83–91.

5 Petersen T, Papakostas GI, Mahal Y, Guyker WM, Beaumont EC, Alpert JE, *et al.* Psychosocial functioning in patients with treatment resistant depression. European Psychiatry. 2004 Jun; 19(4):196–201.

6 Blumberger DM, Mulsant BH, Daskalakis ZJ. What is the role of brain stimulation therapies in the treatment of depression? Current Psychiatry Reports. 2013;15:368.

7 Cusin C, Dougherty DD. Somatic therapies for treatment-resistant depression: ECT, TMS, VNS, DBS. Biology of Mood & Anxiety Disorders. 2012 Jan;2(1):14.

8 Lisanby SH, Luber B, Schlaepfer TE, Sackeim HA. Safety and feasibility of magnetic seizure therapy (MST) in major depression: randomized within-subject comparison with electroconvulsive therapy. Neuropsychopharmacology. 2003 Oct; 28(10):1852–65.

9 Benabid AL. What the future holds for deep brain stimulation. Expert Review of Medical Devices. 2007 Nov;4(6):895–903.

10 Mayberg HS, Lozano AM, Voon V, McNeely HE, Seminowicz D, Hamani C, *et al.* Deep brain stimulation for treatment-resistant depression. Neuron. 2005;45:651–60.

11 Bewernick BH, Hurlemann R, Matusch A, Kayser S, Grubert C, Hadrysiewicz B, *et al.* Nucleus accumbens deep brain stimulation decreases ratings of depression and anxiety in treatment-resistant depression. Biological Psychiatry. 2010 Jan 15;67(2):110–6.

12 Malone DA, Dougherty DD, Rezai AR, Carpenter LL, Friehs GM, Eskandar EN, *et al.* Deep brain stimulation of the ventral capsule/ ventral striatum for treatment-resistant depression. Biological Psychiatry. 2009;65(4): 267–75.

13 Jiménez F, Velasco F, Salin-Pascual R, Hernández JA, Velasco M, Criales JL, *et al.* A patient with a resistant major depression disorder treated with

deep brain stimulation in the inferior thalamic peduncle. Neurosurgery. 2005 Sep;57(3):585–93; discussion 585–93.

14 Sartorius A, Kiening KL, Kirsch P, von Gall CC, Haberkorn U, Unterberg AW, *et al.* Remission of major depression under deep brain stimulation of the lateral habenula in a therapy-refractory patient. Biological Psychiatry. 2010 Jan 15; 67(2):e9–11.

15 Schlaepfer TE, Bewernick BH, Kayser S, Mädler B, Coenen VA. Rapid effects of deep brain stimulation for treatment-resistant major depression. Biological Psychiatry. 2013 Jun 15;73(12):1204–12.

16 Lozano AM, Mayberg HS, Giacobbe P, Hamani C, Craddock RC, Kennedy SH. Subcallosal cingulate gyrus deep brain stimulation for treatment-resistant depression. Biological Psychiatry. 2008 Sep 15;64(6):461–7.

17 Blomstedt P, Sjöberg RL, Hansson M, Bodlund O, Hariz MI. Deep brain stimulation in the treatment of depression. Acta Psychiatrica Scandinavica. 2011 Jan;123(1):4–11.

18 Ward HE, Hwynn N, Okun MS. Update on deep brain stimulation for neuropsychiatric disorders. Neurobiology of Disease. 2010 Jun; 38(3):346–53.

19 Mayberg HS, Lozano AM, Voon V, McNeely HE, Seminowicz D, Hamani C, *et al.* Deep brain stimulation for treatment-resistant depression. Neuron. 2005 Mar 3;45(5):651–60.

20 Kennedy SH, Giacobbe P, Rizvi SJ, Placenza FM, Nishikawa Y, Mayberg HS, *et al.* Deep brain stimulation for treatment-resistant depression: follow-up after 3 to 6 years. American Journal of Psychiatry. 2011;168:502–10.

21 Guinjoan SM, Mayberg HS, Costanzo EY, Fahrer RD, Tenca E, Antico J, *et al.* Asymmetrical contribution of brain structures to treatment-resistant depression as illustrated by effects of right subgenual cingulum stimulation. The Journal of Neuropsychiatry and Clinical Neurosciences. 2010 Jan;22(3):265–77.

22 Holtzheimer PE, Kelley ME, Gross RE, Filkowski MM, Garlow SJ, Barrocas A, *et al.* Subcallosal cingulate deep brain stimulation for treatment-resistant unipolar and bipolar depression. Archives of General Psychiatry. 2012 Feb; 69(2):150–8.

23 Lozano AM, Giacobbe P, Hamani C, Rizvi SJ, Kennedy SH, Kolivakis TT, *et al.* A multicenter pilot study of subcallosal cingulate area deep brain stimulation for treatment-resistant depression. Journal of Neurosurgery. 2012 Feb; 116(2):315–22.

24 Merkl A, Schneider G-H, Schönecker T, Aust S, Kühl K-P, Kupsch A, *et al.* Antidepressant effects after short-term and chronic stimulation of the subgenual cingulate gyrus in treatment-resistant depression. Experimental Neurology. 2013 Nov;249:160–8.

25 Schlaepfer TE, Cohen MX, Frick C, Kosel M, Brodesser D, Axmacher N, *et al.* Deep brain stimulation to reward circuitry alleviates anhedonia in refractory major depression. Neuropsychopharmacology. 2008;33:368–77.

26 Bewernick BH, Sturm V, Kayser S, Schlaepfer TE. Long-term effects of nucleus accumbens deep brain stimulation in treatment-resistant depression: evidence for sustained efficacy. Neuropsychopharmacology. 2012;37:1975–85.

27 Riva-Posse P, Holtzheimer PE, Garlow SJ, Mayberg HS. Practical considerations in the development and refinement of subcallosal cingulate white matter deep brain stimulation for treatment-resistant depression. World Neurosurgery. 2013;80(3):S27.e25–34.

28 Puigdemont D, Pérez-Egea R, Portella MJ, Molet J, de Diego-Adeliño J, Gironell A, *et al.* Deep brain stimulation of the subcallosal cingulate gyrus: further evidence in treatment-resistant major depression. The International Journal of Neuropsychopharmacology. 2012 Jul 22;15:121–33.

29 Neimat JS, Hamani C, Giacobbe P, Merskey H, Kennedy SH, Mayberg HS, *et al.* Patients with prior ablative cingulotomy. American Journal of Psychiatry. 2008;165(6):687–93.

30 Ramasubbu R, Anderson S, Haffenden A, Chavda S, Kiss ZHT. Double-blind optimization of subcallosal cingulate deep brain stimulation for treatment-resistant depression: a pilot study. Journal of Psychiatry & Neuroscience. 2013 Sep;38(5):325–32.

31 McNab JA, Voets NL, Jenkinson N, Squier W, Miller KL, Goodwin GM, *et al.* Reduced limbic connections may contraindicate subgenual cingulate deep brain stimulation for intractable

depression. Journal of Neurosurgery. 2009 Oct;111(4):780–4.

32 Hernandez G, Hamdani S, Rajabi H, Conover K, Stewart J, Arvanitogiannis A, *et al.* Prolonged rewarding stimulation of the rat medial forebrain bundle: neurochemical and behavioral consequences. Behavioral Neuroscience. 2006 Aug;120(4):888–904.

33 Velasco M, Velasco F, Jiménez F, Carrillo-Ruiz JD, Velasco AL, Salín-Pascual R. Electrocortical and behavioral responses elicited by acute electrical stimulation of inferior thalamic peduncle and nucleus reticularis thalami in a patient with major depression disorder. Clinical Neurophysiology. 2006 Feb;117(2):320–7.

34 Dougherty DD, Rezai AR, Carpenter LL, Howland RH, Bhati MT, O'Reardon JP, *et al.* A randomized sham-controlled trial of deep brain stimulation of the ventral capsule/ventral striatum for chronic treatment-resistant depression. Biological Psychiatry. 2015;78:240–8.

35 Kaur N, Chou T, Corse AK, Arulpragasam AR, Deckerbach T, Evans K. Deep brain stimulation for treatment-resistant depression. Psychiatric Annals. 2013;43(8):358–65.

36 George MS, Ketter TA, Parekh PI, Horwitz B, Herscovitch P, Post RM. Brain activity during transient sadness and happiness in healthy women. The American Journal of Psychiatry. 1995;152:341–51.

37 Pizzagalli DA, Iosifescu D, Hallett LA, Ratner KG, Fava M. Reduced hedonic capacity in major depressive disorder: evidence from a probabilistic reward task. Journal of Psychiatric Research. 2008;43:76–87.

38 Epstein J, Pan H, Kocsis JH, Yang Y, Butler T, Chusid J, *et al.* Lack of ventral striatal response to positive stimuli in depressed versus normal subjects. The American Journal of Psychiatry. 2006;163:1784–90.

39 Hasler G, Fromm S, Carlson PJ, Luckenbaugh DA, Waldeck T, Geraci M, *et al.* Neural response to catecholamine depletion in unmedicated subjects with major depressive disorder in remission and healthy subjects. Archives of General Psychiatry. 2008;65:521–31.

40 Velasco F, Velasco M, Jiménez F, Velasco AL, Salin-Pascual R. Neurobiological background for performing surgical intervention in the inferior thalamic peduncle for treatment of major depression disorders. Neurosurgery. 2005 Sep;57(3):439–48; discussion 439–48.

41 Geisler S, Trimble M. The lateral habenula: no longer neglected. CNS Spectrums. 2008 Jun;13(6):484–9.

42 Ranft K, Dobrowolny H, Krell D, Bielau H, Bogerts B, Bernstein H-G. Evidence for structural abnormalities of the human habenular complex in affective disorders but not in schizophrenia. Psychological Medicine. 2010; 40:557–67.

43 Shumake J, Gonzalez-Lima F. Brain systems underlying susceptibility to helplessness and depression. Behavioral and Cognitive Neuroscience Reviews. 2003;2:198–221.

44 Morris JS, Smith KA, Cowen PJ, Friston KJ, Dolan RJ. Covariation of activity in habenula and dorsal raphé nuclei following tryptophan depletion. NeuroImage. 1999;10:163–72.

45 Li B, Piriz J, Mirrione M, Chung C, Proulx CD, Schulz D, *et al.* Synaptic potentiation onto habenula neurons in the learned helplessness model of depression. Nature. 2011;470:535–9.

46 Matsumoto M, Hikosaka O. Lateral habenula as a source of negative reward signals in dopamine neurons. Nature. 2007;447:1111–5.

47 Schlaepfer TE, Bewernick BH, Kayser S, Mädler B, Coenen VA. Rapid effects of deep brain stimulation for treatment-resistant major depression. Biological Psychiatry. 2013;73(12): 1204–12.

48 McNeely HE, Mayberg HS, Lozano AM, Kennedy SH. Neuropsychological impact of Cg25 deep brain stimulation for treatment-resistant depression: preliminary results over 12 months. The Journal of Nervous and Mental Disease. 2008 May;196(5):405–10.

49 Grubert C, Hurlemann R, Bewernick BH, Kayser S, Hadrysiewicz B, Axmacher N, *et al.* Neuropsychological safety of nucleus accumbens deep brain stimulation for major depression: Effects of 12-month stimulation. World Journal of Biological Psychiatry. 2011 Oct; 12(7):516–27.

50 O'Leary DA, Lee AS. Seven year prognosis in depression. Mortality and readmission risk in the Nottingham ECT cohort. The British Journal of Psychiatry. 1996 Oct;169(4):423–9.

51 Bogod NM, Sinden M, Woo C, Defreitas VG, J TI, Howard AK, *et al.* Neuropsychological safety of subgenual cingulate gyrus deep brain resistant depression. The Journal of Neuropsychiatry and Clinical Neurosciences. 2014; 26:126–33.
52 Shergill SS, Robertson MM, Stein G, Bernadt M, Katona CL. Outcome in refractory depression. Journal of Affective Disorders. 1999 Aug;54(3):287–94.
53 Giacobbe P, Kennedy S. Textbook of Stereotactic and Functional Neurosurgery. Lozano AM, Gildenberg PL, Tasker RR, editors. Berlin/ Heidelberg: Springer; 2009, pp. 2925–41.
54 Timmermann L, Schupbach M, Hertel F, Wolf E, Eleopra R, Franzini A, *et al.* A new rechargeable device for deep brain stimulation: a prospective patient satisfaction survey. European Neurology. 2013;69(4):193–9.
55 Abelson JL, Curtis GC, Sagher O, Albucher RC, Harrigan M, Taylor SF, *et al.* Deep brain stimulation for refractory obsessive-compulsive disorder. Biological Psychiatry. 2005 Mar 1;57(5):510–6.
56 Albanese A, Piacentini S, Romito LMA, Leone M, Franzini A, Broggi G, *et al.* Suicide after successful deep brain stimulation for movement disorders. Neurology. 2005 Aug 9;65(3): 499–500; author reply 499–500.
57 Howard A, Honey CR, Hurwitz TA, Ilcewicz-Klimek M, Woo C, Lam RW, *et al.* Deep brain stimulation interruption and suicidality. Journal of Neurosurgery. 2012 Feb;116(2):467–8.
58 Houeto J-L, Mallet L, Mesnage V, Tezenas du Montcel S, Béhar C, Gargiulo M, *et al.* Subthalamic stimulation in Parkinson disease: behavior and social adaptation. Archives of Neurology. 2006 Aug;63(8):1090–5.
59 Suyatin D., Wallman J, Thelin J, Prinz C., Jörntell H, Samuelson L, *et al.* Nanowire-based electrode for acute in vivo neural recordings in the brain. PLoS One. 2013;8(2):e56673.
60 Mohammed M, Etimadi L, Ekstrand J, Al E. Matrix Embedded Ultra Thin Electrodes for Multisite Deep Brain Stimulation and Recording. Berlin, Germany: INS Conference; 2013.
61 Medtronic Inc. First U.S. Implants of New Medtronic Deep Brain Stimulation System Advance Ground-Breaking Research Into Brain Activity While Therapy Is Delivered. 2013. Available at http://newsroom.medtronic.com/phoenix.zhtml?c=251324&p=irol-newsArticle&id=1882373 (accessed 20 Jun 2015).
62 Gradinaru V, Mogri M, Thompson K, Henderson J., Deisseroth K. Optical deconstruction of Parkinsonian neural circuitry. Science. 2009;324(5925):354–9.
63 Fins J., Shapiro ZE. Deep brain stimulation, brain maps and personalized medicine: lessons from the human genome project. Brain Topography. 2014;27:55–62.
64 Rabins P, Appleby B, Brandt J, Mahlon R, DeLong M, Dunn L, *et al.* Scientific and ethical issues related to deep brain stimulation for disorders of mood, behaviour and thought. Archives of General Psychiatry. 2009; 66(9):931–7.
65 Grant R., Halpern C., Baltuch G., O'Reardon J., Caplan A. Ethical considerations in deep brain stimulation for psychiatric illness. Journal of Clinical Neuroscience. 2014;21:1–5.
66 Lipsman N, Giacobbe P, Bernstein M, Lozano A. Informed consent for clinical trials of deep brain stimulation in psychiatric disease: challenges and implications for trial design. Journal of Medical Ethics. 2012;38:107–11.
67 Cabrera L., Evans E., Hamilton R. Ethics of the electrified mind: defining issues and perspectives on the principled use of brain stimulation in medical research and clinical care. Brain Topography. 2014;27:33–45.
68 Fisher CE, Dunn L, Christopher P, Holtzheimer PE, Leykin Y, Mayberg HS, *et al.* The ethics of research on deep brain stimulation for depression: decisional capacity and therapeutic misconception. Annals of the New York Academy of Sciences. 2012;1265:69–79.
69 Christopher PP, Leykin Y, Appelbaum PS, Holtzheimer PE, Mayberg HS, Dunn LB. Enrolling in deep brain stimulation research for depression: influences on potential subjects' decision making. Depression and Anxiety. 2012 Feb;29(2):139–46.
70 Dunn L, Holtzheimer PE, Hoop J, Mayberg HS, Roberts L, Appelbaum P. Ethical issues in deep brain stimulation research for treatment resistant

depression: focus on risk and consent. AJOB Neuroscience. 2011;2(1):29–36.

71 Witt K, Kuhn J, Timmermann L, Zurowski M, Woopen C. Deep brain stimulation and the search for identity. Neuroethics. 2013;6:499–511.

72 Kraemer F. Me, myself and my brain implant: deep brain stimulation raises questions of personal authenticity and alientation. Neuroethics. 2013;6:483–97.

73 Farah M, Wolpe P. Monitoring and manipulating brain function: new neuroscience technologies and their ethical implications. Hastings Center Report. 2004;34(3):35–45.

74 Johansson V, Garwicz M, Kanje M, Halldenius L, Shouenborg J. Thinking ahead on deep brain stimulation: an analysis of the ethical implications of a developing technology. AJOB Neuroscience. 2014;5(1):24–33.

CHAPTER 15

Deep brain stimulation for the treatment of obsessive–compulsive disorder

Michael Giffin[1], Martijn Figee[1] and Damiaan Denys[1,2]

[1] *University of Amsterdam, Amsterdam, The Netherlands*

[2] *The Netherlands Institute for Neuroscience, an Institute of the Royal Netherlands Academy of Arts and Sciences, Amsterdam, The Netherlands*

Introduction

Obsessive–compulsive disorder (OCD) is a chronic psychiatric condition characterized by invasive thoughts, repetitive compulsions, ritualistic behaviours and intense anxiety (Table 15.1). With 10% of all OCD patients being unresponsive to pharmacological regiments and behavioural therapy [1], there is an urgent need for alternative treatment strategies. Evidence from neuroimaging studies indicates that OCD is neurobiologically characterized by abnormal functioning within the orbitofronto-striato-thalamo-cortical (CSTC) network. Specifically, patients with OCD have significantly higher connectivity between ventral–striatal and orbitofrontal regions, and connectivity strength strongly correlates with OCD symptom severity [2–6]. Because of this well-evidenced link to discrete neural circuitry, OCD may be a prime candidate for deep brain stimulation (DBS). However, it was not until 1999 that a first case-series of DBS for OCD was published [7]. DBS targets for OCD were originally adopted from experience with stereotactic ablation, which was until then an accepted last-resort strategy for refractory OCD. Based on the efficacy of anterior capsulotomy for OCD [8], high-frequency DBS of the same target was expected to improve OCD by producing a functional and reversible lesion. Subsequently, with growing functional data regarding the neuroanatomical correlates of OCD, other targets within the CSTC network were explored. Following the first positive results of DBS in the original anterior capsule target (anterior limb of the internal capsule (ALIC)), targeting shifted more towards the ventral capsule/ventral striatum (VC/VS) and nucleus accumbens (NAcc). The subthalamic nucleus (STN) was tried after positive results on obsessive–compulsive symptoms from STN DBS in patients with Parkinson's disease and comorbid OCD. Finally, case studies report on DBS in other nodes of the CSTC network, that is, the inferior thalamic peduncle (ITP) or globus pallidus interna (GPi).

Efficacy

Over the past 10 years, the efficacy of DBS has been reported in six double-blind controlled studies and 15 open-label or case studies (Table 15.1) [9]. About 150 patients with OCD have been treated with DBS in the internal capsule or its connected network structures.

Neuromodulation in Psychiatry, First Edition. Edited by Clement Hamani, Paul Holtzheimer, Andres M. Lozano and Helen Mayberg.

Table 15.1 Studies of deep brain stimulation in the treatment of obsessive–compulsive disorder.

Target	Study (year)	*N*	Parameters	Follow-up	Mean Y-BOCS decrease, *points* (%)	Responders[1], n (%)	Y-BOCS on vs off, *points*
ALIC	Nuttin *et al.* [7]	4	100 Hz, 210 μs 4.7–5.0 V	NM	NA	3 (75)[2]	NA
ALIC	Nuttin *et al.* [10]	6	100 Hz 210/450 μs 4.0–10.5 V	3–31 months; crossover phase: 3 months on 5–10 weeks off	NM	3 (50)	19.8 vs 32.3
ALIC	Anderson and Ahmed *et al.* [11]	1	100 Hz, 210 μs 2.0 V	10 months	27 (79)	1 (100)	NA
ALIC	Abelson *et al.* [12]	4	130/150 Hz, 60/210 μs 5.0–10.5 V	4–2 months; crossover phase: four blinded on–off periods	9.8 (30)	2 (50)	26.5 vs 29.3
VC/VS	Greenberg *et al.* [16]	10	100–130 Hz, 90–210 μs, 8–17 V	36 months	12.3 (55)	4 (40)	NA
VC/VS	Goodman *et al.* [13]	6	135 Hz, 90–210 μs, 3.3–8.5 V	12 months; staggered onset: 30 or 60 days stimulation following surgery	15.7 (47)	4 (67)	NM Reduction: 5.33 vs 0.67
ALIC – VC/VS	Greenberg *et al.* [17][3]	26	100–130 Hz, 90–450 μs, 2–10.5 V	3–36 months	13.1 (38)	16 (62)	NA
VC/VS	Roh *et al.* [18]	4	90–130 Hz, 90–270 μs 2–5 V	24 months	22.2(60)	4 (100)	NA
VC/VS	Tsai *et al.* [19]	4	130 Hz, 210 μs, 2–8 V	15 months	12 (33)	2 (50)	NA
Right NAcc	Sturm *et al.* [22]	4	130 Hz, 90 μs, 2–6.5 V	24–30 months	NA	3 (75)[2]	NA
NAcc – VC/VS	Aouizerate *et al.* [53]	1	130 Hz, 120 μs, 4 V	27 months	13 (52)	1 (100)	NA
NAcc	Denys *et al.* [24]	16	130 Hz, 90 μs, 3.5–5.0 V	21 months; crossover phase: 2 weeks on, 2 weeks off	17.5 (52)	9 (56)	NM difference: 8.3
NAcc	Franzini *et al.* [54]	2	130 Hz, 90 μs, 5/5.5 V	24–27 months	13(38)	1 (50)	NA

Right NAcc	Huff *et al.* [23]	10	145 Hz, 90–140 μs, 3.5–6.5 V	12 months; crossover phase: 3 months on, 3 months off	6.8 (21)	1(10)	27.9 vs 31.1
STN	Mallet *et al.* [26]	2	185 + 130 Hz, 60 + 90 μs, 3.1 + 3.2 V	6 months	20 (81)	2 (100)	NA
STN	Fontaine *et al.* [25]	1	185 Hz, 60 μs, right = 3.5 V; left = 1.3 V	12 months	31 (97)	1 (100)	NA
STN	Mallet *et al.* [27]	16	130 Hz 3 60 μs, 2.0 ± 0.9 V	No follow-up; crossover: 3 months on, 3 months off	13.3 (41)	NA	19 vs 28
Left STN – left NAcc	Barcia *et al.* [29]	2	130 Hz, 90 μs, 3.5–4.0 V	15–36 months	12.5(38)	2 (100)	NA
STN	Chabardes *et al.* [28]	4	130 Hz, 60 μs, 1.2–4.0 V	6 months	21.2(65)	3 (75)	NA
ITP	Jimenez *et al.* [55]	6	130 Hz, 450 μs, 5.0 V	12–36 months	20.3 (57)	6 (100)[4]	NA
GPi	Nair *et al.* [31]	4	120–160 Hz, 90 μs, 2.3–4.4 mA	3–26 months	NA	4 (100)[5]	NA

Source: Bais *et al.* [9]. Reproduced with permission of Elsevier.

ALIC, anterior limb of the internal capsule; GPi, globus pallidus internus; ITP, inferior thalamic peduncle; N, number of patients; NA, not applicable; NAcc, nucleus accumbens; NM, not mentioned; STN, subthalamic nucleus; VC/VS, ventral capsule/ventral striatum; Y-BOCS, Yale–Brown Obsessive Compulsive Scale.

[1] Responders defined as greater than or equal to 35% reduction on the Y-BOCS.

[2] No scale: mentioned that effect was found.

[3] Combined study, including Nuttin [10], Greenberg [16] and Goodman [13].

[4] Six patients were responders after 12 months; 3 patients were lost to follow-up after 36 months.

[5] Obsessive Compulsive Inventory scale greater than 85% reduction in 4 patients.

In the meantime, DBS for OCD has received approval in Europe and a Humanitarian Device Exemption approval in the United States. In the following sections, efficacy studies of DBS in OCD will be discussed separately per target. When evaluating the studies mentioned below, it is important to note that patient samples and DBS targets from different studies often overlap. Inclusion and response criteria in DBS studies have been rather stringent and uniform: patients are all fully refractory to regular pharmacotherapy and behavioural therapy, have an illness duration of at least 5 years and have Yale–Brown Obsessive Compulsive Scale (Y-BOCS) scores of at least 25. Response was defined as an improvement of 35% or more on the Y-BOCS unless mentioned otherwise. Depressive symptoms, global functioning and anxiety symptoms were usually included as secondary outcome measures.

Anterior limb of internal capsule

The ALIC is part of the internal capsule in front of the genu, between the head of the caudate nucleus and the lenticular nucleus. It contains fibres connecting the prefrontal cortex and the subcortical nuclei, including the dorsomedial thalamus. DBS of the ALIC in patients suffering from refractory OCD was initiated in 1998 at the Karolinska Institute in Stockholm, where two patients received bilateral implantation, but these results were never published (S. Andreewitch pers. comm.). In 1999, the Leuven group published the first results of bilateral ALIC DBS in four OCD patients [7]. Although outcome was not quantified by change in Y-BOCS scores, three of the four patients exhibited positive responses, with one patient reporting a 90% reduction in compulsive and ritualistic behaviour. These four patients and two others were followed up for a period of 21 months, at which time three patients were responders with a greater than or equal to 35% decrease in symptom severity [10]. Moreover, the actual DBS effects seemed to outweigh placebo effects, as an average symptom change of 12.5 points (40%) was observed between double-blinded on and off stimulation. A subsequent case report of ALIC DBS in one patient described a 79% Y-BOCS reduction at 3 months and complete remission at 10 months follow-up [11]. Interestingly, the setting was on a much lower voltage (2 V) than Nuttin used in his study (4–10.5 V). However, these initial positive effects of ALIC DBS could not be fully replicated in a double-blind controlled study performed by the Michigan Group [12]. Of the four patients included in their study, only one patient had a decrease of more than 35% in the double-blind phase. Nevertheless, this patient further improved with 73% at 8 months follow-up, and another patient improved with 44% when intensive behavioural therapy was added. In these two responding patients, decreased orbitofrontal cortex (OFC) activity was found on positron emission tomography scans, suggesting that ALIC DBS can improve OCD when it is able to restore the inhibitory function of the ventral CSTC pathway.

Based on these first studies in small-sized OCD samples, ALIC DBS seemed to have only modestly positive effects, which warranted exploration of other targets. As high voltages were often needed to achieve positive effects with ALIC DBS, and because the most distal parts of the ALIC electrodes were located in the VS and NAcc, these ventral targets were subsequently explored for the treatment of OCD.

Ventral capsule/ventral striatum

The VS contains the ventral caudate nucleus and NAcc and is thought to be associated with reward and motivation. Combined with the ventral part of the internal capsule (VC), it is referred to as the VC/VS region. The VC/VS target was based on positive experiences of

Gamma Knife lesions and DBS at the ALIC when more ventral regions were targeted [13, 14], that is, more posterior, towards the junction of the anterior capsule, anterior commissure and bed nucleus of the stria terminalis. Moreover, a case report suggested positive results of ventral striatal (caudate nucleus) DBS in a patient with combined OCD and depression [15]. Greenberg *et al.* [16] were the first to target this region. In their study, 10 patients received 3 years of bilateral VC/VS DBS in an open-label fashion, which resulted in a mean decline in Y-BOCS of 12.3 points (38%) and four of eight responders. These first positive results with VC/VS DBS were replicated in a randomized double-blind controlled study by Goodman *et al.* in 2010 [13]. Six OCD patients were implanted with bilateral VC/VS electrodes, after which three patients received active stimulation, whereas the other three patients received 1 month of sham stimulation and 1 month of true stimulation. Although Y-BOCS reductions did not significantly differ after 1 month of sham versus active stimulation, an improvement was observed in either group only when the device was activated. At 1-year follow-up, there was an average Y-BOCS decrease of 15.6 points (46%) and four of the six patients responded to DBS. In all six patients, 1 year DBS significantly improved comorbid depressive symptoms. In the same year, Greenberg *et al.* [17] combined data of four centres, including patients implanted in the ALIC [10] and VC/VS [16] with the most distal contacts often being placed in the NAcc. In a total of 26 patients, a mean Y-BOCS decrease of 12.5 points (36.8%) was shown after 3–36 months of DBS. The percentage of patients meeting the full response criterion was 61.5% (16 of 26) at 23–36 months follow-up. Of note, patients who received implants later in the study generally experienced better results, which were accounted for by a shift of target site from ALIC to VC/VS. Finally, two open studies reported the efficacy of VC/VS DBS for OCD, with a mean Y-BOCS decrease of 22.2 points (60%) after 24 months in four patients [18] and a decrease of 12.2 points (33%) after 15 months in another four patients [19]. Again, in both patient groups, a significant decrease in depressive symptoms was also observed.

Overall, beneficial effects on OCD and depressive symptoms were observed in uncontrolled DBS studies when stimulating the VC/VS, but patient samples have been small and the only controlled study did not show significant benefits of active over sham stimulation at 2 months post-surgery. Although the efficacy of ALIC and VC/VS DBS appears to be comparable, lower voltages are generally needed to achieve efficacy when stimulating VC/VS, suggesting that the VS is decisive for the efficacy of DBS in OCD.

Nucleus accumbens

The NAcc is part of the VS. It is located where the head of the caudate and the anterior portion of the putamen meet, just beneath the ALIC, and is involved in functions ranging from reward processing to motivation and addiction. The NAcc is considered a promising target for DBS because there is evidence of dysfunction of the reward system in OCD. For instance, in a study by Figee *et al.* [20] using a monetary incentive delay task and functional MRI, OCD patients showed attenuated reward anticipation activity in the NAcc compared with healthy controls. Moreover, the NAcc has a central role in mediating neural activity between the amygdaloid complex, basal ganglia, mediodorsal thalamus and prefrontal cortex, all crucially involved in the pathophysiology of OCD [21, 22]. In 2003, Sturm *et al.* [22] implanted electrodes in a way that the anterior and ventral capsule and the shell of the NAcc could be stimulated selectively. The rationale behind this targeting was based on the aforementioned studies that used internal capsule electrodes ending in the NAcc. In the study of Sturm *et al.* [22], four patients were implanted with electrodes. The first patient improved with bipolar stimulation over the two distal electrode leads and not with stimulation of the internal capsule, which suggests that effective stimulation occurred in the NAcc itself. As bilateral stimulation did not improve the effects of right-sided unilateral stimulation, the other three patients were implanted only unilaterally in the right NAcc. In a 24- to 30-week follow-up period, nearly total recovery from both anxiety and OCD symptoms in three of four patients was reported; however, no scale was used to register the improvement. The only patient without response appeared to have the electrode placed outside the NAcc. The same group failed to replicate the efficacy of unilateral right NAcc DBS using a double-blind controlled design in 10 OCD patients [23]. After 12 months of DBS, the mean Y-BOCS reduction was 6.8 points (21%), and only 1 of 10 patients had a Y-BOCS reduction of more than 35%. The blinded phase did not show a significant difference in Y-BOCS between on and off stimulation. A second double-blind controlled study performed by Denys *et al.* [24] used the NAcc core instead of the shell as a target and stimulation was performed bilaterally instead of unilaterally. In 16 OCD patients, a significant Y-BOCS difference of 8.3 points (25%) was shown comparing active and sham DBS. In the open phase, there was a mean decline of 15.7 (46%) on the Y-BOCS score, in which 9 of 16 patients were responders with a remarkable symptom reduction of 72%. In addition, a significant reduction in anxiety and depressive symptoms was found. Different from previous studies, cognitive behavioural therapy (CBT) was systematically added to the treatment after the first Y-BOCS reduction of 6 points. While anxiety and depression improved mainly during the initial phase of DBS treatment, obsessive–compulsive symptoms continued to improve during subsequent CBT, which seemed to be particularly effective in decreasing compulsive behaviours and avoidance. Of importance, an improvement in this study was observed only when using the dorsal electrode in the area of the NAcc core around the border of the internal capsule, rather than in the NAcc shell that was targeted by Sturm *et al.* [22]. Thus, stimulation of both the NAcc and the VC seems essential for efficacy in OCD. Potentially, stimulation of this crossroad enables modulation of the NAcc as well as adjacent limbic and prefrontal regions involved in OCD pathophysiology. In agreement, a recent study showed that DBS of this region in 16 OCD patients modulated fMRI reward responses in the NAcc and found that OCD symptom improvement correlated with normalized functional connectivity between the NAcc and prefrontal cortex [2].

Subthalamic nucleus

The STN is a small nucleus within the CSTC pathway. The STN is a long-known DBS target for Parkinson's disease and became an interesting option for OCD when positive effects of STN DBS were reported in Parkinson's patients with comorbid OCD [25, 26]. The efficacy of STN DBS was confirmed in a double-blind controlled multicentre study in 17 OCD patients [27]. Compared to the target for Parkinson's disease, the more anterior and medial aspects of the STN were targeted, that is, the limbic STN. Obsessive–compulsive symptoms were significantly lower after active stimulation of the STN compared to sham stimulation, with a Y-BOCS difference of 9 points (32%). Active stimulation resulted in a mean Y-BOCS decrease of 8.9 points (31%). After the first 3 months of open DBS treatment, 75% of the patients were responders, although response was defined as at least 25% Y-BOCS decrease instead of the usual 35%. Contrary to studies using internal capsule and VS targets, no significant effects on depression and anxiety symptoms were found with STN DBS. This was replicated in a subsequent case series that included two patients of the previous study and two additional ones [28]. In these four OCD patients, 6 months of STN DBS resulted in a mean Y-BOCS decline of 21 points (65%), without effects on depressive or anxiety symptoms.

In conclusion, a case series and one controlled study demonstrate the efficacy of bilateral STN DBS for OCD; however, unlike DBS at the VC and VS, STN stimulation does not affect anxiety or mood. Of interest, a recent study implanted two OCD patients with electrodes in both the STN and the NAcc [29]. Combined stimulation improved both obsessive–compulsive and affective symptoms, and double-blind testing of all possible combinations surprisingly revealed that unilateral stimulation of the left NAcc combined with the left STN was most beneficial (Figure 15.1).

Inferior thalamic peduncle

The ITP consists of white matter fibres connecting the thalamus and OFC, and may thus be another target for modulation of aberrant activity in the CSTC circuit. One open study investigated DBS at the ITP in six OCD patients [30]. One year of bilateral bipolar ITP stimulation resulted in a mean Y-BOCS decrease of 18.3 points (51%) with five of five responders. ITP DBS did not affect comorbid drug abuse that was present in three patients.

Anteromedial globus pallidus internus

The anteromedial globus pallidus internus (GPi) is a structure in the basal ganglia that extends connecting fibres between the VS and the thalamus. The GPi is a common target for DBS in the treatment of Gilles de la Tourette and movement disorders such as dystonia and Parkinson's disease. However, its position within the indirect corticostriatal network

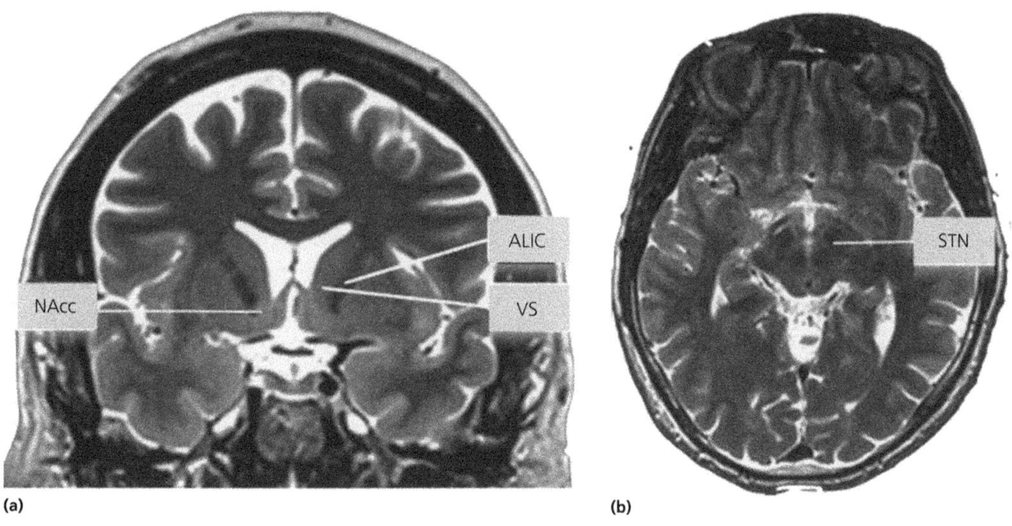

Figure 15.1 DBS target locations for OCD. Reconstructed targets onto coronal **(a)** and axial **(b)** sections. ALIC, anterior limb of the internal capsule; NAcc, nucleus accumbens; STN, subthalamic nucleus; VS, ventral striatum.

would make the GPi also an interesting DBS target for OCD. Nair *et al.* [31] recently reported an impressive improvement of obsessive–compulsive symptoms with GPi DBS in four patients with Gilles de la Tourette and prominent OCD symptoms. Here, 3–26 months of GPi DBS resulted in complete OCD resolution in two patients with the other two experiencing a greater than 85% reduction in scores on the obsessive–compulsive inventory scale.

Complications and side effects of DBS

DBS is invasive and has to be applied chronically. Therefore, appropriate attention should be paid to complications and side effects. Surgery-related intracerebral haemorrhage or infection rates of 1–2% are generally reported in DBS studies for movement disorders [32]. Although the average age of implanted OCD patients is much lower compared to patients with movement disorders, relatively high numbers of surgery-related haemorrhage were noted in DBS studies for OCD, that is, 1 of 17 OCD patients receiving STN DBS [27] and 2 of 26 patients receiving VC/VS DBS [17]. Similarly, surgical wound infection was mentioned in 1 of 16 patients with NAcc DBS [24], 1 of 26 patients with VC/VS DBS [17] and 2 of 17 patients with STN DBS [27]. With regard to device-related problems, electrode breakage was reported in 1 of 4 patients [12] and in 1 of 26 patients [17] and various studies noted that some patients disturbingly felt the material within their body [24, 33]. Acute mood changes during the first few days of stimulation of the ALIC and NAcc have been reported, specifically transient sadness, anxiety [34] and euphoria, sometimes to the extent of hypomanic and manic symptoms [35]. Transient hypomania is the side effect most commonly observed immediately after stimulation and seems to occur more often in the VC/VS–NAcc region, that is, between 50 and 67%, as contrasted with only 4–8% in STN DBS patients [36]. However, all hypomanic and manic episodes associated with DBS resolved after the field density was readjusted by changing the voltage and/or the active contact. Other transient side effects consist of olfactory or gustatory symptoms, nausea, fear, panic and impulsivity, often related to higher voltages and to more ventral electrode positions [35, 37]. All these effects reversed after DBS parameter changes or cessation. Increased libido was reported by 7 of 16 patients with NAcc DBS but this was not experienced as uncomfortable [30]. Mild and transient concentration problems, forgetfulness, word finding problems and confusion are also sometimes reported [24, 30]. Based on the available studies that investigated long-term cognitive functioning after DBS, no substantial cognitive decline was found in a total of 56 implanted OCD patients. On the contrary, most studies reported cognitive improvement following DBS [38].

Response prediction

No consistent clinical response predictor could be defined from the currently published DBS studies in OCD. In the study by Denys *et al.* [24], three of the four DBS non-responders (versus 1 in 12 of the responders) had ego-syntonic obsessive–compulsive symptoms consisting of perfectionism, hoarding or need for symmetry. No other study has specifically investigated ego-syntonic characteristics as a potential DBS response predictor. However, OCD symptoms that are more often ego-syntonic, such as hoarding and symmetry/ordering symptoms, have been found to predict poor response to capsulotomy or cingulotomy [39, 40]. Acute mood changes after implantation often precede and likely help facilitate positive response to DBS treatment [24]. One American group even reported laughter during ALIC-NAcc DBS implantation as a predictor of response, with strength of laughter during intraoperative setting refinement positively correlating with Y-BOCS score reduction at 2 years [6, 41].

Response predictors of DBS may be related to target location. All targets discussed thus far are part of the CTST network, however, with comparable efficacy, that is, on average between 46 and 65% long-term improvement. Thus, more research is still needed to determine which target can provide the greatest benefit for each patient. In a study by van den Munckhof *et al.* [42], 16 OCD patients who had received bilateral NAcc DBS were examined with MRI in order to determine whether the exact anatomical position of the active electrode predicts the reduction of OCD symptoms. Although each patient had DBS targeted at the NAcc, electrode contacts varied from patient to patient, which can be explained by individual differences in brain convulsion patterns [43]. Most patients had active contacts near the border between the NAcc and the ventral ALIC (vALIC), while some patients had active contacts in the anterior portion of the external global pallidus, medially in the caudate nucleus or on the border between these two regions. Importantly, this variability of contact placement correlated with clinical outcome. Patients who had both electrode contacts terminating in the vALIC responded to DBS with a mean Y-BOCS score reduction of 73%, while patients with contacts terminating in other nearby structures responded with a mean Y-BOCS score reduction of 43%. In agreement, Abelson *et al.* [12] found that the best responder in four implanted patients with DBS in the ALIC had one electrode terminating in the vALIC. Furthermore, it is likely that the best responders in studies by Goodman *et al.* [13] and Greenberg *et al.* [17] received stimulation of the vALIC due to the methods of target selection and large electrodes used by those researchers. Indeed, the location of the vALIC within the CSTC pathway marks it as a particularly viable candidate for modulation of the hyperactive pathways involved in OCD, as it contains fibres extending ventrally to the OFC and ventromedial prefrontal cortex (vmPFC). Abelson *et al.* [12] demonstrated that OCD responders who had contacts in the ALIC had reduced activity in the OFC, while non-responders did not exhibit any modulated effects within this structure, suggesting that stimulation of vALIC-OFC fibres is required for good response.

In general, DBS likely restores pathological networks to normalcy primarily by direct electrical stimulation of myelinated axon fibres [44, 45]. Therefore, response prediction studies should involve white matter imaging techniques such as diffusion tensor imaging (DTI). A DTI study of patients with major depression revealed that the precise anatomical location of the electrode did not predict clinical response; however, white matter tracks connecting to the contact site did predict outcome [46]. In OCD, several DTI studies have found differences in brain connectivity between OCD patients and healthy controls [47–51], yet Li *et al.* [47] note that due to the relatively narrow types of analyses employed in these studies, the clinical impact has been extremely low. However, when applying a sophisticated analytical technique known as multi-voxel pattern analysis, they were able to identify OCD patients with 84% accuracy based on white matter abnormalities in specific CSTC pathways, as well as occipital and temporal white matter areas. Using pre-surgical DTI scans, these white matter characteristics could be investigated in association with the electrode position in order to define the optimal stimulation contacts. Finally, a study that combined resting-state fMRI with DBS revealed that DBS reduced excessive frontostriatal functional connectivity, which correlated with obsessive–compulsive symptom improvement [2]. Future resting-state fMRI studies should investigate whether frontostriatal hyperconnectivity can be used as a prediction marker.

Conclusion DBS in OCD

DBS enables long-term efficacy with relatively few side effects. In open studies and case series, DBS of various targets improves obsessive–compulsive symptoms, sometimes up to complete remission, and on average 60% responders, with significant benefits of active over sham stimulation for DBS at the anterior and ventral capsule, VS or STN. All effective DBS targets for OCD are part of the CSTC circuit and efficacy for these various targets is rather comparable, although recent evidence suggests that stimulation of the vALIC may be a particularly efficacious target, and stimulation centred around the vALIC and VS additionally improves depression and anxiety, whereas this does not occur with STN DBS. Efficacy depends on bilateral stimulation, although combined unilateral stimulation of the NAcc and STN was recently shown to be a promising option as well. DBS may be more effective when patients are followed up with behavioural therapy to overcome remaining compulsive and avoidant behaviours. Finally, DBS is a relatively safe intervention, as surgery-related haemorrhage and infections are relatively rare and most side effects are transient. From all these studies together, it is hard to distinguish clinical predictors of DBS response, although acute mood changes usually precede further response to DBS at the ventral striatal targets, and egosyntonic symptoms may be negative predictors of DBS response. In addition, DTI techniques may be used in order to gain a more thorough understanding of white matter pathways that need to be stimulated for optimal outcomes. Normalized frontostriatal connectivity, as measured with resting-state fMRI, correlates with obsessive–compulsive symptom improvement in response to NAcc DBS [2]. As functional connectivity is a relatively simple and reliable measure and excessive frontostriatal connectivity is a robust finding in OCD [2–4, 52], this may be a promising prediction marker. Functional connectivity might even be used for the future development of 'closed loop' DBS systems that are able to recognize pathological network activity for automatic adjustment of stimulation parameters.

References

1 Denys D. Pharmacotherapy of obsessive-compulsive disorder and obsessive-compulsive spectrum disorders. Psychiatr Clin North Am. 2006;29(2):553–84.

2 Figee M, Luigjes J, Smolders R, Valencia-Alfonso C-E, van Wingen G, de Kwaasteniet B, *et al.* Deep brain stimulation restores frontostriatal network activity in obsessive-compulsive disorder. Nat Neurosci. 2013;16(4):386–7.

3 Harrison BJ, Pujol J, Cardoner N, Deus J, Alonso P, López-Solà M, *et al.* Brain corticostriatal systems and the major clinical symptom dimensions of obsessive-compulsive disorder. Biol Psychiatry. 2013;73(4):321–8.

4 Harrison BJ, Soriano-Mas C, Pujol J, Ortiz H, López-Solà M, Hernández-Ribas R, *et al.* Altered corticostriatal functional connectivity in obsessive-compulsive disorder. Arch Gen Psychiatry. 2009;66(11):1189–200.

5 Hou J, Wu W, Lin Y, Wang J, Zhou D, Guo J, *et al.* Localization of cerebral functional deficits in patients with obsessive-compulsive disorder: a resting-state fMRI study. J Affect Disord. 2012; 138(3):313–21.

6 Whiteside S, Port J, Abramowitz J. A meta-analysis of functional neuroimaging in obsessive compulsive disorder. Psychiatry Res Neuroimaging. 2004; 132(1):69–79.

7 Nuttin B, Cosyns P, Demeulemeester H, Gybels J, Meyerson B. Electrical stimulation in anterior limbs of internal capsules in patients with obsessive-compulsive disorder. Lancet. 1999; 354(9189):1526.

8 Mindus P, Rasmussen SA, Lindquist C. Neurosurgical treatment for refractory obsessive-compulsive disorder: implications for understanding frontal lobe function. J Neuropsychiatry Clin Neurosci. 1994;6(4):467–77.

9 Bais M, Figee M, Denys D. Neuromodulation in Obsessive-Compulsive Disorder. In: Psychiatric Clinics of North America. (Ed. Goodman W). Elsevier, Ltd, Oxford. 2014, Forthcoming.

10 Nuttin BJ, Gabriëls LA, Cosyns PR, Meyerson BA, Andréewitch S, Sunaert SG, *et al.* Long-term electrical capsular stimulation in patients with obsessive-compulsive disorder. Neurosurgery. 2003;52(6):1263–74.
11 Anderson A, Ahmed A. Treatment of patients with intractable obsessive-compulsive disorder with anterior capsular stimulation: *Case report.* J Neurosurg. 2003;98(5):1104–8.
12 Abelson JL, Curtis GC, Sagher O, Albucher RC, Harrigan M, Taylor SF, *et al.* Deep brain stimulation for refractory obsessive-compulsive disorder. Biol Psychiatry. 2005;57(5):510–6.
13 Goodman WK, Foote KD, Greenberg BD, Ricciuti N, Bauer R, Ward H, *et al.* Deep brain stimulation for intractable obsessive compulsive disorder: pilot study using a blinded, staggered-onset design. Biol Psychiatry. 2010;67: 535–42.
14 Greenberg B, Price L, Rauch S, Friehs G, Noren G, Malone D, *et al.* Neurosurgery for intractable obsessive-compulsive disorder and depression: critical issues. Neurosurg Clin N Am. 2003; 14(2):199–212.
15 Aouizerate B, Martin-Guehl C. Deep brain stimulation for OCD and major depression. Am J Psychiatry. 2005;162(11):2192.
16 Greenberg BD, Malone DA, Friehs GM, Rezai AR, Kubu CS, Malloy PF, *et al.* Three-year outcomes in deep brain stimulation for highly resistant obsessive-compulsive disorder. Neuropsychopharmacology. 2006;31(11): 2384–93.
17 Greenberg BD, Gabriels LA, Malone DA, Rezai AR, Friehs GM, Okun MS, *et al.* Deep brain stimulation of the ventral internal capsule/ventral striatum for obsessive-compulsive disorder: worldwide experience. Mol Psychiatry. 2010;15(1):64–79.
18 Roh D, Chang WS, Chang JW, Kim C-H. Long-term follow-up of deep brain stimulation for refractory obsessive-compulsive disorder. Psychiatry Res. 2012;200(2–3):1067–70.
19 Tsai H-C, Chang C-H, Pan J-I, Hsieh H-J, Tsai S-T, Hung H-Y, *et al.* Pilot study of deep brain stimulation in refractory obsessive-compulsive disorder ethnic Chinese patients. Psychiatry Clin Neurosci. 2012;66:303–12.
20 Figee M, Vink M, de Geus F, Vulink N, Veltman DJ, Westenberg H, *et al.* Dysfunctional reward circuitry in obsessive-compulsive disorder. Biol Psychiatry. 2011;69(9):867–74.
21 Saxena S, Rauch SL. Functional neuroimaging and the neuroanatomy of obsessive compulsive disorder. Psychiatr Clin North Am. 2000;23(3): 563–86.
22 Sturm V, Lenartz D, Koulousakis A, Treuer H, Herholz K, Klein JC, *et al.* The nucleus accumbens: a target for deep brain stimulation in obsessive–compulsive- and anxiety-disorders. J Chem Neuroanat. 2003;26(4):293–9.
23 Huff W, Lenartz D, Schormann M, Lee S-H, Kuhn J, Koulousakis A, *et al.* Unilateral deep brain stimulation of the nucleus accumbens in patients with treatment-resistant obsessive-compulsive disorder: outcomes after one year. Clin Neurol Neurosurg. 2010;112(2):137–43.
24 Denys D, Mantione M, Figee M, van den Munckhof P, Koerselman F, Westenberg H, *et al.* Deep brain stimulation of the nucleus accumbens for treatment-refractory obsessive-compulsive disorder. Arch Gen Psychiatry. 2010;67(10):1061–8.
25 Fontaine D, Mattei V, Borg M, von Langsdorff D, Magnie MN, Chanalet S, *et al.* Effect of subthalamic nucleus stimulation on obsessive-compulsive disorder in a patient with Parkinson disease. Case report. J Neurosurg. 2004;100: 1084–6.
26 Mallet L, Mesnage V, Houeto JL, Pelissolo A, Yelnik J, Behar C, *et al.* Compulsions, Parkinson's disease, and stimulation. Lancet. 2002;360(9342): 1302–4.
27 Mallet L, Polosan M, Jaafari N, Baup N, Welter ML, Fontaine D, *et al.* Subthalamic nucleus stimulation in severe obsessive-compulsive disorder. N Engl J Med. 2008;359(20): 2121–34.
28 Chabardès S, Polosan M, Krack P, Bastin J, Krainik A, David O, *et al.* Deep brain stimulation for obsessive-compulsive disorder: subthalamic nucleus target. World Neurosurg. 2013; 80(3–4):S31.e1–8.
29 Barcia JA, Reyes L, Arza R, Saceda J, Avecillas J, Yáñez R, *et al.* Deep brain stimulation for obsessive-compulsive disorder: is the side relevant? Stereotact Funct Neurosurg. 2014;92(1): 31–6.
30 Jiménez F, Nicolini H, Lozano AM, Piedimonte F, Salín R, Velasco F. Electrical stimulation of

the inferior thalamic peduncle in the treatment of major depression and obsessive compulsive disorders. World Neurosurg. 2012;80(3–4): S30.e17–25.

31 Nair G, Evans A, Bear RE, Velakoulis D, Bittar RG. The anteromedial GPi as a new target for deep brain stimulation in obsessive compulsive disorder. J Clin Neurosci. 2014;21(5):815–21.

32 Fenoy AJ, Simpson RK. Risks of common complications in deep brain stimulation surgery: management and avoidance. J Neurosurg. 2014;120:132–9.

33 Nuttin B, Gybels J, Cosyns P, Gabriels L, Meyerson B, Andréewitch S, *et al.* Deep brain stimulation for psychiatric disorders. Neurosurgery. 2002;51(2):519.

34 Shapira NA, Okun MS, Wint D, Foote KD, Byars JA, Bowers D, *et al.* Panic and fear induced by deep brain stimulation. J Neurol Neurosurg Psychiatry. 2006;77(3):410–2.

35 Okun MS, Mann G, Foote KD, Shapira NA, Bowers D, Springer U, *et al.* Deep brain stimulation in the internal capsule and nucleus accumbens region: responses observed during active and sham programming. J Neurol Neurosurg Psychiatry. 2007;78(3):310–4.

36 Haq IU, Foote KD, Goodman WK, Ricciuti N, Ward H, Sudhyadhom A, *et al.* A case of mania following deep brain stimulation for obsessive compulsive disorder. Stereotact Funct Neurosurg. 2010;88(5):322–8.

37 Luigjes J, Mantione M, van den Brink W, Schuurman PR, van den Munckhof P, Denys D. Deep brain stimulation increases impulsivity in two patients with obsessive-compulsive disorder. Int Clin Psychopharmacol. 2011;26(6): 338–40.

38 Bergfeld IO, Mantione M, Hoogendoorn MLC, Denys D. Cognitive functioning in psychiatric disorders following deep brain stimulation. Brain Stimul. 2013;6(4):532–7.

39 Gentil AF, Lopes AC, Dougherty DD, Rück C, Mataix-Cols D, Lukacs TL, *et al.* Hoarding symptoms and prediction of poor response to limbic system surgery for treatment-refractory obsessive-compulsive disorder. J Neurosurg. 2014; 121(1):1–8.

40 Rück C, Larsson KJ, Mataix-Cols D. Predictors of medium and long-term outcome following capsulotomy for obsessive-compulsive disorder: one site may not fit all. Eur Neuropsychopharmacol. 2012;22(6):406–14.

41 McIntyre CC, Hahn PJ. Network perspectives on the mechanisms of deep brain stimulation. Neurobiol Dis. 2010;38(3):329–37.

42 van den Munckhof P, Bosch DA, Mantione MH, Figee M, Denys DA, Schuurman PR. Active stimulation site of nucleus accumbens deep brain stimulation in obsessive–compulsive disorder is localized in the ventral internal capsule. Acta Neurochir Suppl 2013;1117:53–9.

43 van den Munckhof P, Contarino MF, Bour LJ, Speelman JD, de Bie RM, Schuurman PR. Postoperative curving and upward displacement of deep brain stimulation electrodes caused by brain shift. Neurosurgery. 2010;67(1): 49–53.

44 Kringelbach ML, Green AL, Owen SLF, Schweder PM, Aziz TZ. Sing the mind electric – principles of deep brain stimulation. Eur J Neurosci. 2010;32(7):1070–9.

45 Nowak LG, Bullier J. Axons, but not cell bodies, are activated by electrical stimulation in cortical gray matter. Exp Brain Res. 1998;118(4): 477–88.

46 Riva-Posse P, Choi KS, Holtzheimer PE, McIntyre CC, Gross RE, Chaturvedi A, *et al.* Defining critical white matter pathways mediating successful subcallosal cingulate deep brain stimulation for treatment-resistant depression. Biol Psychiatry. 2014;76(12):1–7.

47 Li F, Huang X, Tang W, Yang Y, Li B, Kemp GJ, *et al.* Multivariate pattern analysis of DTI reveals differential white matter in individuals with obsessive-compulsive disorder. Hum Brain Mapp. 2014;35(6):2643–51.

48 Li F, Huang X, Yang Y, Li B, Wu Q, Zhang T, *et al.* Microstructural brain abnormalities in patients with obsessive-compulsive disorder: diffusion tensor MR imaging. Radiology. 2011;260(1): 216–23.

49 Menzies L, Williams GB, Chamberlain SR, Ooi C, Fineberg N, Suckling J, *et al.* White matter abnormalities in patients with obsessive-compulsive disorder and their first-degree relatives. Am J Psychiatry. 2008;165(10):1308–15.

50 Yoo SY, Jang JH, Shin Y-W, Kim DJ, Park H-J, Moon W-J, *et al.* White matter abnormalities in

drug-naïve patients with obsessive-compulsive disorder: a diffusion tensor study before and after citalopram treatment. Acta Psychiatr Scand. 2007;116(3):211–9.
51 Szeszko PR, Ardekani BA, Ashtari M, Malhotra AK, Robinson DG, Bilder RM, *et al.* White matter abnormalities in obsessive-compulsive disorder: a diffusion tensor imaging study. Arch Gen Psychiatry. 2005;62(7):782–90.
52 Sakai Y, Narumoto J, Nishida S, Nakamae T, Yamada K, Nishimura T, *et al.* Corticostriatal functional connectivity in non-medicated patients with obsessive-compulsive disorder. Eur Psychiatry. 2011;26(7):463–9.
53 Aouizerate B, Cuny E, Martin-Guehl C, Guehl D, Amieva H, Benazzouz A, *et al.* Deep brain stimulation of the ventral caudate nucleus in the treatment of obsessive-compulsive disorder and major depression. Case report. J Neurosurg. 2004; 101(4):682–6.
54 Franzini A, Messina G, Gambini O, Muffatti R, Scarone S, Cordella R, *et al.* Deep-brain stimulation of the nucleus accumbens in obsessive compulsive disorder: clinical, surgical and electrophysiological considerations in two consecutive patients. Neurol Sci. 2010;31(3):353–9.
55 Jiménez F, Nicolini H, Lozano AM, Piedimonte F, Salín R, Velasco F. Electrical stimulation of the inferior thalamic peduncle in the treatment of major depression and obsessive compulsive disorders. World Neurosurg. 2013; 80(3–4): S30.e17–25.

CHAPTER 16

Deep brain stimulation: Emerging indications

Yasin Temel[1,2], Sarah Hescham[1,2], Maartje Melse[1,2] and Veerle Visser-Vandewalle[2]

[1] *Maastricht University Medical Center, Maastricht, The Netherlands*

[2] *University of Cologne, Cologne, Germany*

Introduction

The neurosurgical treatment of refractory psychiatric disorders is undergoing a revival with the application of deep brain stimulation (DBS). For a long time, neurobiological mechanisms underlying psychiatric disorders have been considered to depend on solitary systems such as neurotransmitters and specific cortical areas. Although these models might still explain individual symptoms, recent findings from both clinical and experimental studies [1] suggest a dysfunction of interrelated networks involving cortical and subcortical structures and various neuroactive substances [2, 3]. For instance, symptoms of Tourette syndrome (TS) and obsessive–compulsive disorder (OCD) have been linked to non-motor elements of the basal ganglia-thalamocortical pathways, including the nucleus accumbens (NAc), ventral pallidum and medial parts of the thalamus, along with a dysfunctional mesolimbic dopaminergic system [3–5]. This 'dysfunctional network hypothesis' has been one of the bases for exploring DBS in psychiatric disorders.

In this chapter, we describe emerging indications for DBS. Preclinical and clinical studies are ongoing. For each indication, we will briefly discuss the rationale for DBS, supporting data from preclinical studies and clinical data. As studies are all experimental, clinical data mainly include the description of individual or small series of cases. It is not the aim of this chapter to provide a complete overview of the literature, but rather a balanced selection of relevant articles, which are also summarized in Table 16.1.

Addiction

Addiction can either be classified as substance dependence (e.g. alcohol, nicotine and drugs) or compulsive behaviour (e.g. gambling, exercise and food). Hallmarks include impaired control over substance or behaviour, resulting in a withdrawal syndrome when the use is discontinued. Chronic consumption of alcohol is amongst the most common addictions and represents one of the greatest health and socioeconomic problems worldwide. The lifetime prevalence of becoming alcohol dependent is approximately 12% in the United States [6] and 4.1% in Europe [7]. The treatment of alcohol dependency relies on pharmacological and psychological interventions. However, the efficacy of these therapies is undermined by the high relapse rates of 40–70% [8].

Human neuroimaging studies have identified brain reward circuits involved in drug effects and addiction [9]. DBS has been proposed as a potential tool to alleviate addictive

Neuromodulation in Psychiatry, First Edition. Edited by Clement Hamani, Paul Holtzheimer, Andres M. Lozano and Helen Mayberg.

Table 16.1 Summary of relevant articles described in this chapter.

Disease	DBS target	Number of patients	Overall DBS results
Addiction	NAc	16	Three of three alcohol-dependent patients significantly reduced alcohol consumption. Three of three heroin-dependent patients became heroin abstinent. Three of 10 nicotine-dependent patients quit smoking.
AD	Nucleus basalis of Meynert	1	No clear clinical effect, but glucose metabolic activity was preserved in the ipsilateral temporal and parietal cortex, while it decreased on the contralateral side.
	Fornix	7	Four out of seven mild AD patients showed improvements/stabilizations of ADAS-cog and MMSE scores 12 months post-op.
Disorders of consciousness: *PVS*	Mesencephalic reticular formation and/or non-specific thalamic nuclei	8	Three out of eight patients emerged from the PVS and were able to communicate at the end of the trial, but remained bedridden.
	Centromedian–parafascicular complex	44	In 21 cases, an improvement in consciousness was attained, but all remained bedridden.
MCS	Central thalamus	1	The patient showed advances in responsiveness to commands, functional object use, intelligible vocalization and oral feeding.
	Centromedian–parafascicular complex	5	All patients emerged from MCS and could return home and live with their families. All but one remained bedridden and one required a wheelchair.
Schizophrenia	NAc	1	Improvement of psychosocial functioning.
Aggressiveness	Posterior hypothalamus	3	All patients significantly reduced aggressive behaviour.
	Projections from the frontobasal cortex to the hypothalamus	1	High-frequency stimulation induced defensive rage, whereas low-frequency settings achieved attenuation of the intermittent explosive symptomatology.
	Posteromedial hypothalamus	11	DBS showed marked and sustained improvement of aggressive behaviour in majority of patients, in some cases leading to a complete disappearance of violent outbursts.
Anorexia nervosa	Subgenual cingulate	1	Weight gain and recovery from eating disorder.
	Ventral capsule/ventral striatum	1	
	NAc	4	
	Subcallosal cingulate	6	After 9 months, half of the patients increased their BMI to 16–21 kg/m^2, while the remaining patients did not change from their historical baseline BMI.

Table is organized by indication and describes DBS target, number of patients and the overall clinical outcome.

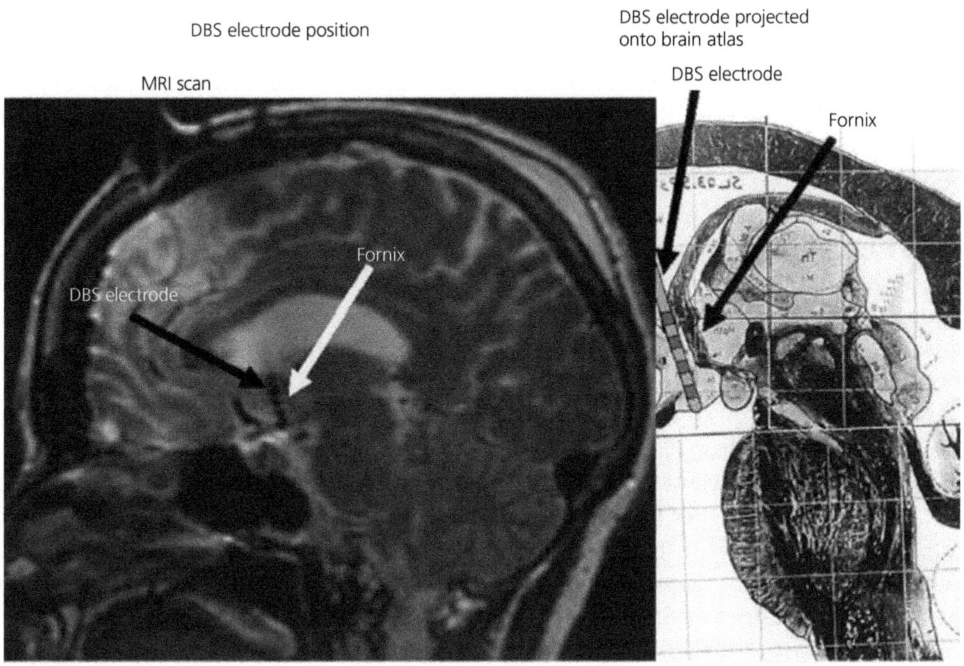

Figure 16.1 Graphic and anatomical presentations of electrode trajectories towards the NAc (cross) in different plains on a pre-operative magnetic resonance image (MRI). In addition, the figure shows main structures and pathways of the mesolimbic circuit, which are chemically dependent. Source: Kuhn *et al.* [10]. Reproduced with permission of Wolters Kluwer Health.

behaviours by modulating the reward circuits (Figure 16.1). One of the first observations was in a 54-year-old male patient suffering from severe agoraphobia and comorbid alcohol dependency. The patient received bilateral DBS of the NAc at 130 Hz, 90 µs pulse width and 3–4.5 V for a period of 12 months to treat his anxiety disorder. Although DBS had almost no effect on the phobia, the patient showed remarkable improvements in his alcohol dependency. Without a specific motivation, he rapidly and drastically reduced his alcohol consumption [11]. This unintended alleviation of alcohol dependency led to the hypothesis that DBS of the NAc could have an impact on addictive behaviours. Along this line, the same group investigated in a retrospective study whether DBS had effects on comorbid nicotine dependence in 10 patients suffering from TS, anxiety disorder or OCD. Although stimulation parameters were set to treat the primary psychiatric condition, 3 of 10 patients were able to quit smoking after DBS [10]. Recently, a prospective case study with three severely alcohol-dependent patients was conducted. The patients were treated with bilateral DBS of the NAc at 130 Hz, 90 µs and 3.5–4.5 V. Two patients were abstinent after 12 months and the third had markedly reduced his alcohol consumption [12].

Regarding chronic opioid abuse, the effect of bilateral DBS of the NAc was described in a patient suffering from heroin dependency [13]. The patient remained heroin abstinent during the 6-year follow-up period. Interestingly, the patient also reduced smoking and the stimulator was turned off after 2.5 years, while the beneficial effects of surgery persisted. Similar findings were obtained in another case study with a 2-year follow-up, in which two heroin-dependent patients were treated with DBS in the NAc [14].

Another potential target for DBS to alleviate addictive behaviour is the subthalamic nucleus (STN). This basal ganglia structure is widely targeted for DBS in patients with Parkinson's disease (PD). Besides playing a pivotal role in motor behaviour, the STN has strong limbic properties [4]. Interestingly, in PD patients, DBS of the STN can alleviate symptoms of dopamine dysregulation syndrome, which is characterized by severe dopamine drug addiction and behavioural disorders such as manic psychosis, hypersexuality, pathological gambling and mood swings [15–18]. Nevertheless, contradictory effects have been found as well. In one case report, a PD patient who had no history of addiction before his bilateral STN DBS treatment became a pathologic gambler within a few weeks with stimulation [19]. Other studies also found varying effects of STN DBS. Some patients improved their addictive behaviour, while others persisted or even worsened their addiction [20].

Preclinical studies found that the STN, ventral tegmental area and the NAc constitute essential structures within the reward circuitry [21–24]. Rats with lesions or high-frequency stimulation of the STN experience reduced motivation for cocaine seeking while increasing it to attain food rewards [21, 22]. Similar to human findings, DBS of the NAc core or shell also resulted in a significant reduction in drug-related behaviour [25–28]. However, the exact mechanisms of actions are still being investigated.

Alzheimer's disease

Alzheimer' disease (AD) is the most prevalent form of dementia. It is characterized by various pathological processes including brain atrophy, amyloid deposition, neurofibrillary tangles and synaptic dysfunction leading to chronic cognitive decline, often accompanied by psychiatric symptomatology, deterioration of functional ability, personality changes and a general decline of quality of life [29]. The inability to acquire new memories characterizes the early stages of the disease, whereas in later stages patients suffer from agnosia, aphasia and apraxia and long-term memory loss [30].

Despite the recent major advances regarding early detection and diagnosis of AD [31], currently no effective treatment exists to prevent, cure or halt the progression of AD [29]. Until now, available pharmacological therapies only provide symptomatic treatment. The most frequently prescribed medications consist of the *N*-methyl-D-aspartate (NMDA) receptor antagonist memantine, and acetylcholinesterase inhibitors such as donezepil, rivastigmine and galantamine [30]. These medications generally have a positive effect on cognitive abilities, but are only mildly and temporarily beneficial. Because of these limited therapeutic effects and the tremendous impact of AD on patients and caregivers, researchers are currently exploring new neuromodulatory techniques including DBS.

In AD histopathological changes can be found throughout the brain but with a predilection for the neuronal sites involved in memory and cognition. The various elements of the circuit of Papez and the nucleus basalis of Meynert have therefore been targeted for DBS in both preclinical and clinical studies [29, 32]. The rationale for DBS of certain structures within the circuit of Papez is to counteract the dysfunction of neuronal information processing caused by AD pathology. The theory behind DBS of the nucleus basalis of Meynert is to enhance the concentrations of acetylcholine in the target areas, analogous to the effect of acetylcholinesterase inhibitors, because cholinergic transmission is considered essential for cognitive performance [29].

In 2010, the results of a phase I trial of DBS for AD were published. Six patients with mild AD were implanted with bilateral electrodes in the fornix/hypothalamus (Figure 16.2) [33]. After 12 months of high-frequency stimulation with 130 Hz, 90 μs pulse width and 3.0–3.5 V, post-operative clinical and imaging data were

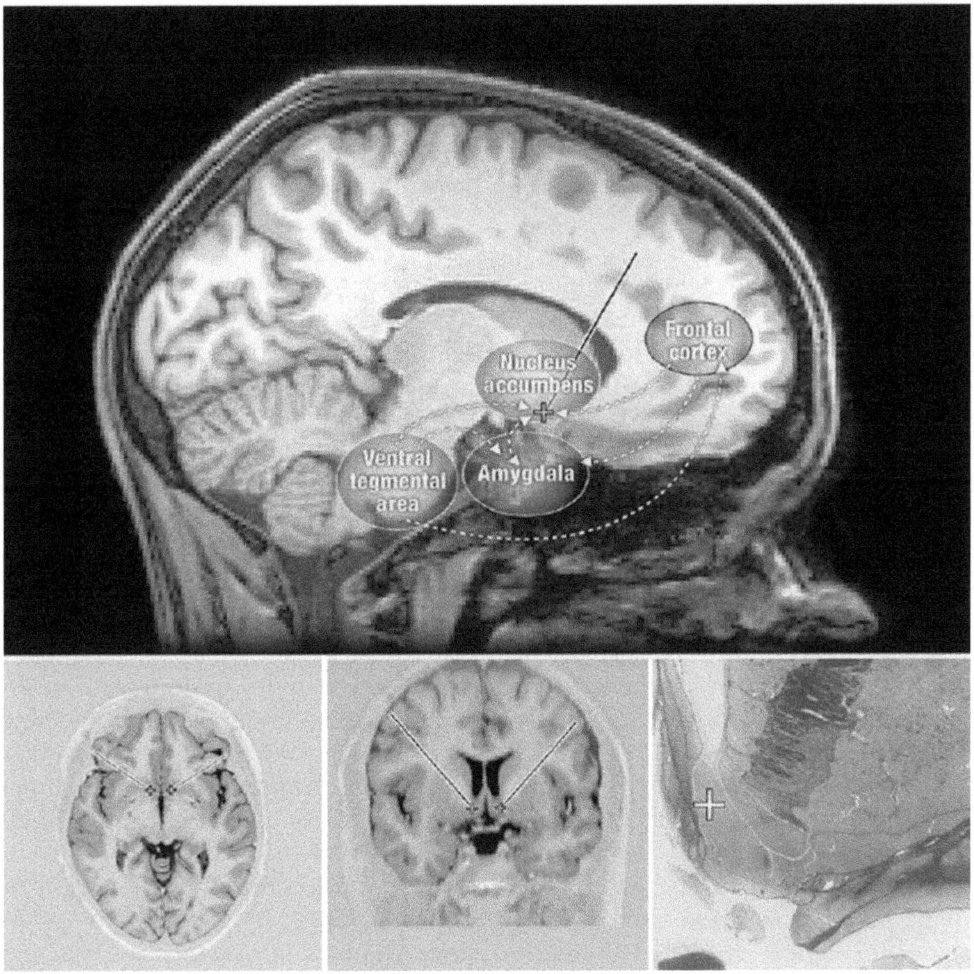

Figure 16.2 (Left) DBS electrode placement in the vicinity of the fornix in a sagittal MRI. (Right) Schematic representation of DBS electrode localization in a stereotactic atlas 3.5 mm from the midline. Source: Laxton *et al.* [33]. Reproduced with permission of Wiley.

compared with pre- and interoperative assessments. The authors found that forniceal DBS for AD could be performed safely and that the stimulation had strong biological effects in the dysfunctional brain areas: stimulation drove neuronal activity and caused a sustained increase in brain glucose metabolism. These effects were maintained after 12 months of continuous stimulation. However, the patients showed no clear clinical benefit [34]. In a single case study, a 71-year-old female with mild AD, who fulfilled the Diagnostic and Statistical Manual of Mental Disorders-IV criteria for AD for less than 2 years, bilateral fornix DBS has proven to stabilize memory scores. In particular, chronic stimulation with 130 Hz, 210 µs pulse width and 2.5 V resulted in stabilization of scores in the mini-mental state examination (MMSE), Alzheimer's Disease Assessment Scale – cognitive subscale (ADAS-cog) and Free and Cued Selective Reminding Test after 12 months follow-up [35].

In another study, a 74-year-old male patient, who had a 4-year history of progressive loss of recent memory and was diagnosed with mild-to-moderate AD, was implanted with unilateral DBS of the left nucleus basalis of Meynert. The stimulation parameters were medium frequency stimulation of 50 Hz, 210 μs, 3 V and cycling between 15 s on and 12 min off throughout the day and night. While no conclusion regarding therapeutic value could be drawn (due to the lack of neuropsychological tests), DBS had an effect on cerebral glucose metabolism. The patient's unstimulated contralateral hemisphere was used as a control to compare his pre- and post-operative fluorodeoxyglucose-positron emission tomography scans. In the right hemisphere, glucose metabolism in the frontal, temporal, parietal and occipital lobes decreased by 21, 24, 10 and 7.5%, respectively. In contrast, glucose use in the stimulated left hemisphere had decreased by only 12% in the frontal and 4.1% in the occipital lobe, remained stable in the parietal and was increased by 1.5% in the temporal lobe [36].

In addition to the memory circuit and the nucleus basalis of Meynert, the entorhinal cortex might also be considered as the potential target for DBS in memory-related disorders. In a human study with seven pharmacoresistant epilepsy patients, bilateral intracranial depth electrodes were implanted in the entorhinal cortex region. Stimulation was acute at a frequency of 50–130 Hz, 300–450 μs pulse width and 0.5–1.5 mA with a 5-s on/off cycle. Interestingly, stimulation resulted in an improved memory performance in a virtual spatial memory task in these patients [37].

The use of animal models plays a significant role in the evaluation of DBS target structures and efficacy [38]. In AD research, a number of animal studies have been performed to identify the most feasible stimulation targets in terms of clinical memory improvement. Based on the rodent memory circuit anatomy, various preclinical studies have applied DBS to the fornix, the anterior nucleus of the thalamus (ANT), the entorhinal cortex or the nucleus basalis of Meynert. Generally, an improvement in differential memory- and cognition-related tasks was observed [29].

Acute high-frequency stimulation of the forniceal region has shown to restore spatial memory performance in the object location task in a rat model of experimental dementia with high current densities and high and low frequencies [39]. Because the fornix consists of a bundle of myelinated fibres, the authors hypothesize that this effect is accomplished by driving the fornix activity, both orthodromically as well as antidromically [39–41].

As opposed to the acute effects observed with fornix stimulation, DBS of the ANT with 2.5 V, 130 Hz and 90 μs pulse width may induce long-term plastic changes. ANT stimulation increased memory performance in a delayed non-matching-to-sample task only 1 month after surgery, whereas a few days post-operatively the authors found no changes in memory scores [42]. Cognitive performance may be enhanced through DBS-induced restoration of disrupted hippocampal neurogenesis [42, 43]. However, an earlier study by the same group also found that ANT high-frequency stimulation with clinically relevant stimulation settings impaired spatial memory [40].

Like fornix stimulation, DBS (1 h at 130 Hz, 90 μs pulse width and 50 μA) of the entorhinal cortex in mice also showed improvements in spatial memory performance reflected by enhanced water maze scores. Six and a half weeks after surgery, behavioural improvement was accompanied by an observed increase in proliferation in the dentate gyrus, a hippocampal structure maintaining strong connections with the entorhinal cortex, as quantified by BrdU histochemistry [44]. BrdU is a thymidine analog which incorporates into newly synthesized DNA of replicating cells and because it was injected after entorhinal cortex DBS, the behavioural improvement of these rats can be linked to neurogenesis. Lastly, stimulation of nucleus basalis of Meynert in anaesthetized rats showed increased neural growth factor release [45]. This factor is essential for neuronal survival and maintenance and known to be locally down-regulated in AD [45, 46]. This effect, however, was only observed in adult but not in aged rats.

Overall, (limited) preclinical studies researching the feasibility of DBS for AD point to the fornix and entorhinal cortex as the most promising structures in terms of memory enhancement.

Disorders of consciousness

DBS is also under investigation as a treatment for consciousness disorders following traumatic brain injury. One of the first DBS reports originates from 1969, where stimulation of the basal pallidum and lateropolar thalamic nucleus led to a strong arousal response in a comatose patient [47]. In the following years, advances were made to distinguish between persistent vegetative state (PVS) and minimally conscious state (MCS). The MCS and PVS entail a different degree of environment awareness, communication capabilities and cortical functioning, whereby the MCS maintains a more advanced consciousness level [48]. This distinction proved to be essential in prognosis for recovery and outcome and possibly also for the putative DBS benefit [49].

The rationale for DBS of the thalamic nuclei and the reticular system originates from research of wakefulness and arousal which show that these structures play a key role [50, 51]. In addition, lesions of the intralaminar thalamic nuclei resulted in disorders of attention and consciousness, underlining the importance of these nuclei in maintaining consciousness [52].

In 1990, a trial was published in which eight PVS patients received chronic DBS of the mesencephalic reticular formation and/or nonspecific thalamic nuclei for 3–6 months. In 4 of 8 cases, the prolonged coma scale rose and three patients emerged from the PVS and were able to communicate at the end of the trial [53].

Cohadon and Richer [54] published the results of a series of 25 PVS patients receiving DBS of the centromedian–parafascicular complex during 12 h every day for 2 months. In 13 cases, an improvement in consciousness was attained, but even after 12 years follow-up all remained severely disabled or were deceased. Therefore, the authors questioned the practical usefulness of DBS in PVS.

Another study with a large cohort size included 26 patients (21 PVS and 5 MCS) [55]. The mesencephalic reticular formation (2 cases) or the centromedian–parafascicular complex (19 cases) was selected as target structures for PVS patients and the centromedian–parafascicular complex for all MCS patients. All patients were selected on the basis of specific electrophysiological criteria. The frequency of stimulation was mostly fixed at 25 Hz, while the intensity was set individually for each patient and was slightly higher than the threshold for inducing an arousal response. From the 21 PVS patients, 8 emerged from PVS and were able to communicate through some speech but remained bedridden. All the five MCS patients emerged from MCS following DBS and could return home and live with their families, although all but one remained bedridden and one required a wheelchair. A limitation of this study is that all patients were treated within 4–8 months after their incurred brain injury, which is within the 1-year accepted time frame of spontaneous recovery [49].

The best-known published case of DBS-induced improvements in consciousness disorders stems from 2007 [56]. In this case, a 38-year-old male who had been in MCS for over 6 years received DBS of the central thalamus. A 6-month double-blind crossover design turning the stimulation on and off was applied.

Final stimulation settings for each electrode were 100 Hz, right-side bipolar and left-side monopolar field with 4 V. The patient showed advances in responsiveness to commands, functional object use, intelligible vocalization and oral feeding. In this case, however, preoperatively the patient showed widely preserved brain structure and interactive behaviour such as visual pursuit and intermittently following commands, providing a clear substrate for further recovery. Therefore, the positive results of this case cannot be extrapolated to all MCS cases.

Correct diagnosis and assessment of consciousness level and brain function in a patient with a reduced consciousness level is challenging. In addition, quality-of-life-related questions and ethical aspects should be carefully considered in relation to research in comatose patients.

Schizophrenia

Schizophrenia is a severe disorder with a lifetime prevalence of 0.4% worldwide [57]. The onset of schizophrenia is early adulthood and it is often classified into positive and negative symptoms. Positive symptoms include delusions, hallucinations and disordered thoughts, while negative symptoms are characterized by poor emotional responses, lack of motivation and anhedonia [58]. The first line of treatment consists of antipsychotic medication, which can mainly reduce the positive symptoms of schizophrenia. However, about 20% of patients are resistant to standard antipsychotics and up to 75% of the patients experience recurrent relapse [59]. Consequently, the development of effective treatments for schizophrenia remains a major unmet need.

It has been well established that the symptoms are caused by a dysregulation of the mesolimbic dopaminergic pathways [59]. Therefore, the NAc and hippocampus have been suggested as targets for neurosurgical intervention in schizophrenia [60]. The underlying rationale is as follows: on the one side, hippocampal hyperactivity early in the course of the disease leads to excessive dopamine release. With DBS, this hyperactivity might be inhibited and dopamine levels modulated. The NAc, on the other hand, plays a role in the release of dopamine from the midbrain in response to hippocampal activation. Stimulating the NAc might stabilize dopamine release and result in therapeutic effects in schizophrenia [60].

Until now, only one case study was reported by Plewnia *et al.*, in which a 51-year-old woman with intractable OCD and residual symptoms of schizophrenia was treated with unilateral DBS of the right NAc [61]. Stimulation parameters were 130 Hz, 60 µs pulse width and 4.5 V. This patient showed a substantial reduction in obsessions and compulsions as well as an improvement in psychosocial functioning with DBS after 6 months, 1 year and 2 years follow-up. Besides this case study, no clinical evidence is available for the use of DBS in schizophrenia, but a clinical trial was recently launched in Canada and is currently recruiting patients (http://clinicaltrials.gov/show/NCT01725334).

Maternal exposure to infection during pregnancy has been suggested as an environmental risk factor for schizophrenia. In a rodent model of schizophrenia (established through prenatal methylazoxymethanol acetate administration), high-frequency stimulation of the ventral hippocampus with 130 Hz, 0.1 ms pulse width and 0.3 mA was able to normalize aberrant dopaminergic neuron activity and restore deficits in cognitive functioning [62].

In another rodent model of schizophrenia, pregnant rodents were injected with the viral mimic polyinosinic–polycitidilic acid (poly I:C) that leads to schizophrenia-like behavioural deficits in the adult offspring [63]. DBS was applied to regions of the cortico-basal ganglia-thalamocortical circuitry, whose dysfunction has been linked to schizophrenia. More specifically, DBS was applied to the medial prefrontal cortex (mPFC), dorsomedial thalamus, globus pallidus (GP, rodent equivalent to human GP externus), entopeduncular nucleus (rodent equivalent to human GP internus) or the STN. All rats were tested on pre-pulse inhibition (PPI) of the acoustic startle reflex. PPI reflects the ability of the nervous system to temporarily adapt to a strong stimulus when a preceding weaker signal is given and is a well-established cross-species phenomenon. A disrupted PPI response reveals the inability of an organism to filter out unnecessary information and is often seen in schizophrenia. The authors found that DBS with 130 Hz, 90 μs pulse width and 75 μA of the mPFC or 150 μA of the dorsomedial thalamus normalized PPI deficits. DBS of the GP also affected PPI, but results were less prominent [63].

Aggressiveness

Aggressiveness, directed against others, objects or one self, is difficult to capture in a particular disorder or in clearly defined diagnostic criteria. Aggression is often part of a range of different psychiatric disorders. In the fifth and most recent edition of the Diagnostic and Statistical Manual of Mental Disorders, aggression and other impulse disorders are described in a new chapter on Disruptive, Impulse-Control and Conduct Disorders covering diseases characterized by difficulties in emotional and behavioural self-control. In addition, aggressiveness is also part of personality disorders (antisocial personality), developmental disorders (attentional deficit and hyperactivity disorder) [64] and can occur after brain injury.

The treatment of aggressive behaviour is often not straightforward, as evidenced by the wide range of therapies and medications prescribed to patients. Pharmacological treatment includes antidepressants, anxiolytics, GABAergic mood stabilizers and anticonvulsive drugs. However, none seem to fully mitigate aggressive behaviour. Multiple drug regiments are often combined with various cognitive behavioural therapies focusing on relaxation and repressing aggressive impulses, unfortunately with limited success [65, 66].

From a neuroanatomical point of view, animal studies contributed to the discovery of key areas in the brain involved in aggressive behaviour. In this respect, electrical stimulation of the anterior hypothalamus in cats induced a generalized offensive behaviour including hissing and clawing directed towards carefully chosen cage mates, avoiding the more dominant animals. This hostility ceased when the stimulation was switched off [67]. Similar observations were made in experiments with non-human primates [67, 68].

Human electrophysiological data confirm the involvement of the posterior hypothalamus in aggression. A recent study recorded perioperative hypothalamic local field potentials from DBS electrodes implanted in the posterior hypothalamus in two patients. One of them was treated for pathological aggressiveness (43-year-old male; 160 Hz, 90 μs, 1.9 mA), and the other patient, a 31-year-old man treated for cluster headaches, was considered a control subject as this man was behaviourally normal with regard to aggressive behaviour (130 Hz, 90 μs, 2 mA). Comparison of the electrophysiological data showed increased low-frequency oscillations and reduced alpha activity in the posterior hypothalamus of the aggressive patient compared to the control patient. Moreover, clinically, the stimulation reduced the aggressive episodes of the aggressive patient by 70% [69]. Another region of the hypothalamus close to the posterior part is the ventral tuberal hypothalamus. This region was stimulated in a preclinical study using miniature pigs. The intention of this study was to evaluate the stimulation impact of ventral tuberal hypothalamic DBS, now under investigation as a DBS target for obesity treatment. Amongst other findings, the researchers noted clear transient aggressive behaviours related to the stimulation [70].

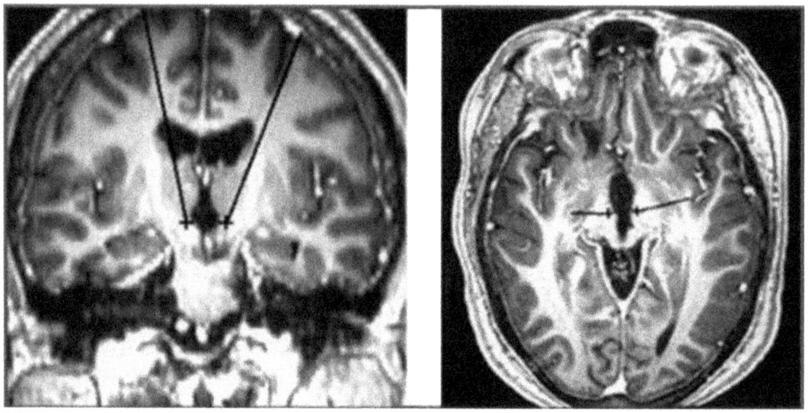

Figure 16.3 Reconstructed electrode trajectories towards the posterior hypothalamus superimposed on pre-operative coronal (**a**) and horizontal (**b**) MRI scans. Source: Kuhn *et al.* [71]. Reproduced with permission of Karger.

In another case study, bilateral DBS of the posterior hypothalamus (130 Hz, 90 μs, 1.5 V) completely eliminated self-mutilation in a brain-injured 22-year-old woman (Figure 16.3) [71]. In the same year, a report was published describing successful bilateral low-frequency stimulation of the medial portion of the posterior hypothalamus (15 Hz, 450 μs, 0.1 V) as a treatment for drug-resistant aggression in a 22-year-old male [72]. In a 2010 study, a 19-year-old patient suffering from intermittent explosive disorder was treated with DBS targeting the projections from the frontobasal cortex to the hypothalamus [73]. After determination of the ideal stimulation parameters (20 Hz, 360 μs, 2.0 V amplitude, 1 min on/off cycles), over the course of the 2-year follow-up she experienced a substantial decrease in the number of violent outbursts, a greatly improved quality of life. Interestingly, this case study notes that high-frequency stimulation induced defensive rage, whereas low-frequency settings achieved attenuation of the intermittent explosive symptomatology. This is in congruence with the above presented preclinical data in cats, where electrical stimulation of the hypothalamus also evoked rage and associated behaviour [67, 68].

To date, only two groups have reviewed the long-term outcomes of treating aggressive and disruptive behaviour by DBS of the posteromedial hypothalamus (PMH). Franzini and colleagues [74] reviewed a series of cases of PMH DBS, two of which are described above [71, 72]. All patients (aged 20–68 years, one female) suffered from refractory aggressive behaviour and some degree of mental retardation as a result of trauma, congenital toxoplasmosis, brain ischaemia or unknown origin. Patients were implanted with bilateral electrodes and most but not all received high-frequency stimulation (185 Hz, 60–90 μs, 1–3 V, varying current amplitude). In six of seven patients, DBS produced an immediate and marked improvement in aggressive behaviour, in some cases leading to a complete disappearance of violent outbursts. Other effects observed were a reduction of pharmacological therapy, prolongation of sleep duration and a decrease in epileptic seizure frequency. The beneficial effects of DBS were sustained during follow-up periods ranging from 1 to 9 years without any neurologic side effects. Similarly, Torres *et al.* [75] report an open-label study of seven patients suffering from intractable erethism, characterized by unprovoked aggression, hyperkinesia, destructive and self-aggressive behaviour. After implantation of PMH electrodes, behaviour was assessed using the Inventory for Client and Agency planning scale containing both self-directed and heteroaggression and asocial subscores. Behavioural improvement was observed in five of six patients throughout the 6- to 82-month follow-up. Stimulation parameters at the last follow-up visit varied between 130 and 185 Hz, 60 and 450 μs pulse width and 1.3 and 2.5 V.

Anorexia nervosa

Anorexia nervosa is a severe mental illness, characterized by abnormal eating behaviour, severe self-induced weight loss and psychiatric comorbidities [76]. It has been shown that pharmacological interventions including antipsychotics and antidepressants do not have an impact on weight gain [77]. Treatment usually consists of two phases: weight restoration followed by relapse prevention through psychotherapy [77]. Considering the high relapse rate of 30–50% under standard treatment as well as the vast number of morbidity and mortality cases [76], researchers are currently investigating novel therapies. Because anorexia nervosa is considered to be primarily a disorder of emotional processing, DBS has been proposed to be a potential tool to modulate limbic structures [78].

In a case study of depression, DBS improved comorbid anorexia nervosa. The patient was a 56-year-old female with severely disabling chronic recurrent depression suffering from anorexia since she was 17. DBS of the right subgenual cingulate area with intermittent stimulation, 2 min on and 1 min off, at 130 Hz, 91 μs pulse width and 5 mA was able to recover her eating disorder and the patient was able to maintain a BMI of 19.1 kg/m^2 for about 2 years [79]. Another case study described a 52-year-old female patient suffering from intractable OCD and anorexia nervosa. Unilateral DBS of the ventral capsule/ventral striatum of the left hemisphere with 120 Hz, 120 μs pulse width and 7.5 V led to an improvement in OCD symptoms and induced a BMI of about 19 kg/m^2. After adding another DBS electrode into the ventral caudate in an attempt to further improve symptoms, generalized anxiety, mood and OCD symptoms worsened, and she had a concurrent 6 kg weight loss. When this electrode was turned off, her symptoms improved again [80].

DBS to treat anorexia nervosa as a primary disorder has been the subject of two studies. Four young women with a BMI between 10 and 13.33 kg/m^2 were subjected to bilateral DBS of the NAc with 180 Hz, 90 μs pulse width and 6–8 V. All four patients suffered psychiatric comorbidities: three had OCD and one had generalized anxiety disorder. After 38 months of continuous stimulation, all patients showed an average weight gain of 65% and an average BMI of 18.4–22.1 kg/m^2 [81]. The second study is a phase I trial in which six female patients with refractory anorexia nervosa with comorbid depression, OCD or addiction received subcallosal cingulate DBS at 130 Hz, 90 μs pulse width and 5–7 V for 9 months (Figure 16.4). Before the surgery, the BMI of the patients was

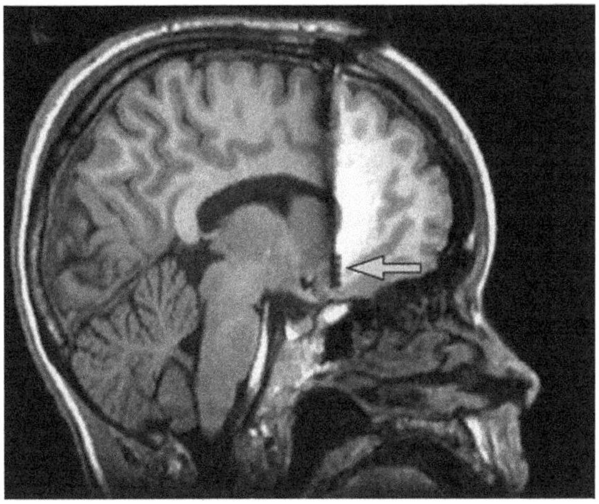

Figure 16.4 T1-weighted sagittal MRI showing DBS electrode (arrow) in the subcallosal cingulate area in an anorectic patient. Source: Lipsman *et al.* [82]. Reproduced with permission of Elsevier.

between 11.1 and 15.1 kg/m^2. After 9 months, half of the patients increased their BMI to 16–21 kg/m^2, while the remaining patients did not change from their historical baseline BMI [82].

Conclusion

Patients suffering from severe addiction, AD, schizophrenia, aggressive behaviour and anorexia have been subjected to DBS in either experimental case studies or in the context of phase I clinical trials. In the majority of the case reports, beneficial effects were found. Nevertheless, it is not yet possible to draw conclusions from these studies because the level of evidence is low. One common aspect of most of the abovementioned indications is that the rationale for stimulation involves a dysfunctional neural structure or circuit that can be modulated by DBS. For some indications, such as AD, the availability of adequate animal models seems to facilitate hypothesis-driven research, but in most of the emerging psychiatric indications the lack of valid animal evidence complicates their investigation in a preclinical setting.

Although the applicability of new psychiatric indications is being explored, we want to avoid the impression that severe psychiatric conditions can always be treated with DBS. Holding the dysfunction of a single structure or circuit responsible for complex and multifaceted psychiatric diseases such as schizophrenia or anorexia nervosa seems to be an oversimplification. Therefore, it is likely that the effectiveness of DBS will primarily consist of a reduction in specific symptoms linked to the neural site of modulation, rather than a global treatment.

A medical–ethical framework is an essential part of a research programme focusing on the surgical treatment of severe psychiatric conditions. In this respect, our concern is that the clinical application of DBS might be moving faster than the scientific evidence supporting or discouraging its application. Actually, the field is not in need for case reports of DBS delivered to 'exotic' brain regions; although case reports in general can be meaningful, new indications rather first need to be backed up by robust scientific evidence. This allows for well-designed clinical approaches [83].

We are witnessing the revival of neurosurgery for psychiatric illnesses and we have the feeling that, with the collaborative effort of neurosurgeons, psychiatrists, scientists and ethicists, we may change the 'negative' reputation of psychosurgery, originating from the experiences of the early and mid-20th century.

References

1 Hamani C, Temel Y Deep brain stimulation for psychiatric disease: contributions and validity of animal models. Sci Transl Med 4: 142rv148.
2 Nestler EJ, Barrot M, DiLeone RJ, Eisch AJ, Gold SJ, *et al.* (2002) Neurobiology of depression. Neuron 34: 13–25.
3 Krack P, Hariz MI, Baunez C, Guridi J, Obeso JA (2010) Deep brain stimulation: from neurology to psychiatry? Trends Neurosci 33: 474–484.
4 Temel Y, Blokland A, Steinbusch HW, Visser-Vandewalle V (2005) The functional role of the subthalamic nucleus in cognitive and limbic circuits. Prog Neurobiol 76: 393–413.
5 Temel Y, Hescham SA, Jahanshahi A, Janssen ML, Tan SK, *et al.* (2012) Neuromodulation in psychiatric disorders. Int Rev Neurobiol 107: 283–314.
6 Hasin DS, Stinson FS, Ogburn E, Grant BF (2007) Prevalence, correlates, disability, and comorbidity of DSM-IV alcohol abuse and dependence in the United States: results from the National Epidemiologic Survey on Alcohol and Related Conditions. Arch Gen Psychiatry 64: 830–842.
7 The EMI, Alonso J, Angermeyer MC, Bernert S, Bruffaerts R, *et al.* (2004) Prevalence of mental disorders in Europe: results from the European Study of the Epidemiology of Mental Disorders (ESEMeD) project. Acta Psychiatr Scand 109: 21–27.

8 Swift RM (1999) Drug therapy for alcohol dependence. N Engl J Med 340: 1482–1490.
9 Volkow ND, Wang G-J, Fowler JS, Tomasi D, Telang F (2011) Addiction: beyond dopamine reward circuitry. Proc Natl Acad Sci 108: 15037–15042.
10 Kuhn J, Bauer R, Pohl S, Lenartz D, Huff W, *et al.* (2009) Observations on unaided smoking cessation after deep brain stimulation of the nucleus accumbens. Eur Addict Res 15: 196–201.
11 Kuhn J, Lenartz D, Huff W, Lee S, Koulousakis A, *et al.* (2007) Remission of alcohol dependency following deep brain stimulation of the nucleus accumbens: valuable therapeutic implications? J Neurol Neurosurg Psychiatry 78: 1152–1153.
12 Muller UJ, Sturm V, Voges J, Heinze HJ, Galazky I, *et al.* (2009) Successful treatment of chronic resistant alcoholism by deep brain stimulation of nucleus accumbens: first experience with three cases. Pharmacopsychiatry 42: 288–291.
13 Zhou H, Xu J, Jiang J (2011) Deep brain stimulation of nucleus accumbens on heroin-seeking behaviors: a case report. Biol Psychiatry 69: e41–e42.
14 Kuhn J, Moller M, Treppmann JF, Bartsch C, Lenartz D, *et al.* (2014) Deep brain stimulation of the nucleus accumbens and its usefulness in severe opioid addiction. Mol Psychiatry 19: 145–146.
15 Ardouin C, Voon V, Worbe Y, Abouazar N, Czernecki V, *et al.* (2006) Pathological gambling in Parkinson's disease improves on chronic subthalamic nucleus stimulation. Mov Disord 21: 1941–1946.
16 Bandini F, Primavera A, Pizzorno M, Cocito L (2007) Using STN DBS and medication reduction as a strategy to treat pathological gambling in Parkinson's disease. Parkinsonism Relat Disord 13: 369–371.
17 Witjas T, Baunez C, Henry JM, Delfini M, Regis J, *et al.* (2005) Addiction in Parkinson's disease: impact of subthalamic nucleus deep brain stimulation. Mov Disord 20: 1052–1055.
18 Knobel D, Aybek S, Pollo C, Vingerhoets FJ, Berney A (2008) Rapid resolution of dopamine dysregulation syndrome (DDS) after subthalamic DBS for Parkinson disease (PD): a case report. Cogn Behav Neurol 21: 187–189.
19 Smeding HM, Goudriaan AE, Foncke EM, Schuurman PR, Speelman JD, *et al.* (2007) Pathological gambling after bilateral subthalamic nucleus stimulation in Parkinson disease. J Neurol Neurosurg Psychiatry 78: 517–519.
20 Lim SY, O'Sullivan SS, Kotschet K, Gallagher DA, Lacey C, *et al.* (2009) Dopamine dysregulation syndrome, impulse control disorders and punding after deep brain stimulation surgery for Parkinson's disease. J Clin Neurosci 16: 1148–1152.
21 Rouaud T, Lardeux S, Panayotis N, Paleressompoulle D, Cador M, *et al.* (2010) Reducing the desire for cocaine with subthalamic nucleus deep brain stimulation. Proc Natl Acad Sci USA 107: 1196–1200.
22 Baunez C, Dias C, Cador M, Amalric M (2005) The subthalamic nucleus exerts opposite control on cocaine and 'natural' rewards. Nat Neurosci 8: 484–489.
23 Uslaner JM, Yang P, Robinson TE (2005) Subthalamic nucleus lesions enhance the psychomotor-activating, incentive motivational, and neurobiological effects of cocaine. J Neurosci 25: 8407–8415.
24 Lardeux S, Baunez C (2008) Alcohol preference influences the subthalamic nucleus control on motivation for alcohol in rats. Neuropsychopharmacology 33: 634–642.
25 Liu HY, Jin J, Tang JS, Sun WX, Jia H, *et al.* (2008) Chronic deep brain stimulation in the rat nucleus accumbens and its effect on morphine reinforcement. Addict Biol 13: 40–46.
26 Knapp CM, Tozier L, Pak A, Ciraulo DA, Kornetsky C (2009) Deep brain stimulation of the nucleus accumbens reduces ethanol consumption in rats. Pharmacol Biochem Behav 92: 474–479.
27 Vassoler FM, Schmidt HD, Gerard ME, Famous KR, Ciraulo DA, *et al.* (2008) Deep brain stimulation of the nucleus accumbens shell attenuates cocaine priming-induced reinstatement of drug seeking in rats. J Neurosci 28: 8735–8739.
28 Henderson MB, Green AI, Bradford PS, Chau DT, Roberts DW, *et al.* (2010) Deep brain stimulation of the nucleus accumbens reduces alcohol intake in alcohol-preferring rats. Neurosurg Focus 29: E12.

29 Hescham S, Lim L, Jahanshahi A, Blokland A, Temel Y (2013) Deep brain stimulation in dementia-related disorders. Neurosci Biobehav Rev 37: 2666–2675.
30 Thies W, Bleiler L (2013) 2013 Alzheimer's disease facts and figures. Alzheimers Dement 9: 208–245.
31 Reiman EM (2014) Alzheimer's disease and other dementias: advances in 2013. Lancet Neurol 13: 3–5.
32 Laxton AW, Lozano AM (2013) Deep brain stimulation for the treatment of Alzheimer disease and dementias. World Neurosurg 80: S28.e21–S28.e28.
33 Laxton AW, Tang-Wai DF, McAndrews MP, Zumsteg D, Wennberg R, *et al.* (2010) A phase I trial of deep brain stimulation of memory circuits in Alzheimer's disease. Ann Neurol 68: 521–534.
34 Smith GS, Laxton AW, Tang-Wai DF, McAndrews MP, Diaconescu AO, *et al.* (2012) Increased cerebral metabolism after 1 year of deep brain stimulation in Alzheimer disease. Arch Neurol 69:1141–8.
35 Fontaine D, Deudon A, Lemaire JJ, Razzouk M, Viau P, *et al.* (2013) Symptomatic treatment of memory decline in Alzheimer's disease by deep brain stimulation: a feasibility study. J Alzheimers Dis 34: 315–323.
36 Turnbull IM, McGeer PL, Beattie L, Calne D, Pate B (1985) Stimulation of the basal nucleus of Meynert in senile dementia of Alzheimer's type. A preliminary report. Appl Neurophysiol 48: 216–221.
37 Suthana N, Haneef Z, Stern J, Mukamel R, Behnke E, *et al.* (2012) Memory enhancement and deep-brain stimulation of the entorhinal area. N Engl J Med 366: 502–510.
38 Hamani C, Temel Y (2012) Deep brain stimulation for psychiatric disease: contributions and validity of animal models. Sci Transl Med 4: 142rv148.
39 Hescham S, Lim LW, Jahanshahi A, Steinbusch HW, Prickaerts J, *et al.* (2013) Deep brain stimulation of the forniceal area enhances memory functions in experimental dementia: the role of stimulation parameters. Brain Stimul 6:72–7.
40 Hamani C, Dubiela FP, Soares JCK, Shin D, Bittencourt S, *et al.* (2010) Anterior thalamus deep brain stimulation at high current impairs memory in rats. Exp Neurol 225: 154–162.
41 Hamani C, McAndrews MP, Cohn M, Oh M, Zumsteg D, *et al.* (2008) Memory enhancement induced by hypothalamic/fornix deep brain stimulation. Ann Neurol 63: 119–123.
42 Hamani C, Stone SS, Garten A, Lozano AM, Winocur G (2011) Memory rescue and enhanced neurogenesis following electrical stimulation of the anterior thalamus in rats treated with corticosterone. Exp Neurol 232: 100–104.
43 Toda H, Hamani C, Fawcett AP, Hutchison WD, Lozano AM (2008) The regulation of adult rodent hippocampal neurogenesis by deep brain stimulation. J Neurosurg 108: 132–138.
44 Stone SS, Teixeira CM, Devito LM, Zaslavsky K, Josselyn SA, *et al.* (2011) Stimulation of entorhinal cortex promotes adult neurogenesis and facilitates spatial memory. J Neurosci 31: 13469–13484.
45 Hotta H, Kagitani F, Kondo M, Uchida S (2009) Basal forebrain stimulation induces NGF secretion in ipsilateral parietal cortex via nicotinic receptor activation in adult, but not aged rats. Neurosci Res 63: 122–128.
46 Cuello AC, Bruno MA, Allard S, Leon W, Iulita MF (2010) Cholinergic involvement in Alzheimer's disease. A link with NGF maturation and degradation. J Mol Neurosci 40: 230–235.
47 Hassler R, Ore GD, Dieckmann G, Bricolo A, Dolce G (1969) Behavioural and EEG arousal induced by stimulation of unspecific projection systems in a patient with post-traumatic apallic syndrome. Electroencephalogr Clin Neurophysiol 27: 306–310.
48 Malone Jr DA, Dougherty DD, Rezai AR, Carpenter LL, Friehs GM, *et al.* (2009) Deep brain stimulation of the ventral capsule/ventral striatum for treatment-resistant depression. Biol Psychiatry 65: 267–275.
49 Sen AN, Campbell PG, Yadla S, Jallo J, Sharan AD (2010) Deep brain stimulation in the management of disorders of consciousness: a review of physiology, previous reports, and ethical considerations. Neurosurg Focus 29: E14.
50 Moruzzi G, Magoun HW (1949) Brain stem reticular formation and activation of the EEG. Electroencephalogr Clin Neurophysiol 1: 455–473.
51 Purpura KP, Schiff ND (1997) The thalamic intralaminar nuclei: a role in visual awareness. Neuroscientist 3: 8–15.

52 Castaigne P, Lhermitte F, Buge A, Escourolle R, Hauw JJ, *et al.* (1981) Paramedian thalamic and midbrain infarct: clinical and neuropathological study. Ann Neurol 10: 127–148.
53 Tsubokawa T, Yamamoto T, Katayama Y, Hirayama T, Maejima S, *et al.* (1990) Deep-brain stimulation in a persistent vegetative state: follow-up results and criteria for selection of candidates. Brain Inj 4: 315–327.
54 Cohadon F, Richer E (1993) Deep cerebral stimulation in patients with post-traumatic vegetative state. 25 cases. Neurochirurgie 39: 281–292.
55 Yamamoto T, Katayama Y (2005) Deep brain stimulation therapy for the vegetative state. Neuropsychol Rehabil 15: 406–413.
56 Schiff ND, Giacino JT, Kalmar K, Victor JD, Baker K, *et al.* (2007) Behavioural improvements with thalamic stimulation after severe traumatic brain injury. Nature 448: 600–603.
57 McGrath J, Saha S, Chant D, Welham J (2008) Schizophrenia: a concise overview of incidence, prevalence, and mortality. Epidemiol Rev 30: 67–76.
58 Torres-Gonzalez F, Ibanez-Casas I, Saldivia S, Ballester D, Grandon P, *et al.* (2014) Unmet needs in the management of schizophrenia. Neuropsychiatr Dis Treat 10: 97–110.
59 Smith T, Weston C, Lieberman J (2010) Schizophrenia (maintenance treatment). Am Fam Physician 82: 338–339.
60 Mikell CB, McKhann GM, Segal S, McGovern RA, Wallenstein MB, *et al.* (2009) The hippocampus and nucleus accumbens as potential therapeutic targets for neurosurgical intervention in schizophrenia. Stereotact Funct Neurosurg 87: 256–265.
61 Plewnia C, Schober F, Rilk A, Buchkremer G, Reimold M, *et al.* (2008) Sustained improvement of obsessive-compulsive disorder by deep brain stimulation in a woman with residual schizophrenia. Int J Neuropsychopharmacol 11: 1181–1183.
62 Perez SM, Shah A, Asher A, Lodge DJ (2013) Hippocampal deep brain stimulation reverses physiological and behavioural deficits in a rodent model of schizophrenia. Int J Neuropsychopharmacol 16: 1331–1339.
63 Klein J, Hadar R, Götz T, Männer A, Eberhardt C, *et al.* (2013) Mapping brain regions in which deep brain stimulation affects schizophrenia-like behavior in two rat models of schizophrenia. Brain Stimul 6: 490–499.
64 Association AP (2013) Highlights of Changes from DSM-IV-TR to DSM-5. Arlington, VA: American Psychiatric Association.
65 Humble F, Berk M (2003) Pharmacological management of aggression and violence. Hum Psychopharmacol 18: 423–436.
66 Coccaro EF (2012) Intermittent explosive disorder as a disorder of impulsive aggression for DSM-5. Am J Psychiatry 169: 577–588.
67 Delgado JM (1986) Physical Control of the Mind: Toward a Psychocivilized Society. New York: Harper and Row.
68 Faria MA, Jr. (2013) Violence, mental illness, and the brain – A brief history of psychosurgery: Part 2 – From the limbic system and cingulotomy to deep brain stimulation. Surg Neurol Int 4: 75.
69 Rosa M, Franzini A, Giannicola G, Messina G, Altamura AC, *et al.* (2012) Hypothalamic oscillations in human pathological aggressiveness. Biol Psychiatry 72: e33–e35.
70 Ettrup KS, Sorensen JC, Rodell A, Alstrup AK, Bjarkam CR (2012) Hypothalamic deep brain stimulation influences autonomic and limbic circuitry involved in the regulation of aggression and cardiocerebrovascular control in the Gottingen minipig. Stereotact Funct Neurosurg 90: 281–291.
71 Kuhn J, Lenartz D, Mai JK, Huff W, Klosterkoetter J, *et al.* (2008) Disappearance of self-aggressive behavior in a brain-injured patient after deep brain stimulation of the hypothalamus: technical case report. Neurosurgery 62: E1182; discussion E1182.
72 Hernando V, Pastor J, Pedrosa M, Pena E, Sola RG (2008) Low-frequency bilateral hypothalamic stimulation for treatment of drug-resistant aggressiveness in a young man with mental retardation. Stereotact Funct Neurosurg 86: 219–223.
73 Maley JH, Alvernia JE, Valle EP, Richardson D (2010) Deep brain stimulation of the orbitofrontal projections for the treatment of intermittent explosive disorder. Neurosurg Focus 29: E11.
74 Franzini A, Broggi G, Cordella R, Dones I, Messina G (2013) Deep-brain stimulation for aggressive and disruptive behavior. World Neurosurg 80: S29 e11–S29 e24.
75 Torres CV, Sola RG, Pastor J, Pedrosa M, Navas M, *et al.* (2013) Long-term results of posteromedial

hypothalamic deep brain stimulation for patients with resistant aggressiveness. J Neurosurg 119: 277–287.

76 Guarda AS (2008) Treatment of anorexia nervosa: insights and obstacles. Physiol Behav 94: 113–120.

77 Bulik CM, Berkman ND, Brownley KA, Sedway JA, Lohr KN (2007) Anorexia nervosa treatment: a systematic review of randomized controlled trials. Int J Eat Disord 40: 310–320.

78 Oudijn M, Storosum J, Nelis E, Denys D (2013) Is deep brain stimulation a treatment option for anorexia nervosa? BMC Psychiatry 13: 277.

79 Israel M, Steiger H, Kolivakis T, McGregor L, Sadikot AF (2010) Deep brain stimulation in the subgenual cingulate cortex for an intractable eating disorder. Biol Psychiatry 67: e53–e54.

80 McLaughlin NC, Didie ER, Machado AG, Haber SN, Eskandar EN, *et al.* (2013) Improvements in anorexia symptoms after deep brain stimulation for intractable obsessive-compulsive disorder. Biol Psychiatry 73: e29–e31.

81 Wu H, Van Dyck-Lippens PJ, Santegoeds R, van Kuyck K, Gabriels L, *et al.* (2013) Deep-brain stimulation for anorexia nervosa. World Neurosurg 80: S29 e1–S29 e10.

82 Lipsman N, Woodside DB, Giacobbe P, Hamani C, Carter JC, *et al.* (2013) Subcallosal cingulate deep brain stimulation for treatment-refractory anorexia nervosa: a phase 1 pilot trial. Lancet 381: 1361–1370.

83 Temel Y, Lim LW (2013) Neurosurgical treatments of depression. Curr Top Behav Neurosci 14: 327–339.

CHAPTER 17

Vagus nerve stimulation: Introduction and technical aspects

Jared Pisapia and Gordon Baltuch

University of Pennsylvania Health System, Philadelphia, USA

Introduction

In 1997, the Food and Drug Administration (FDA) approved vagus nerve stimulation (VNS) as an adjunctive, non-pharmacological therapy for patients more than 12 years of age with medically refractory partial onset seizures [1]. Reports of unanticipated improvements in mood in epilepsy patients undergoing VNS, independent of improved seizure control [2], and the observation that multiple antiepileptic medications are also useful in the treatment of depression [3], raised the notion of VNS as a potential treatment option for major depressive disorder. Based on subsequent clinical trials, in 2005, the FDA approved VNS as an adjunctive long-term therapy for chronic or recurrent major depression (unipolar or bipolar) in patients more than 18 years of age who failed in at least four adequate antidepressant drug trials [4, 5]. Since its initial approval, more than 65 000 patients worldwide have safely undergone VNS for epilepsy or depression, and investigations continue into further indications for VNS in psychiatric disease.

Intermittent pulses arising from a generator implanted subcutaneously in the chest travel along a lead to electrodes wrapped around the vagus nerve in the neck. These signals then travel in an afferent manner via the vagus nerve to exert widespread brain effects. The purpose of this chapter is to review the development of VNS and to focus on technical aspects, including device components, surgical implantation and related complications. Clinical trials and the effectiveness of VNS in epilepsy, depression and other disorders will be discussed in Chapter 18.

Preclinical studies

Multiple animal studies beginning in the 1880s generated data to support the development of VNS and its implantation in humans. In early studies, VNS was found to desynchronize electrical activity [6] and reduce or eliminate chemically induced interictal epileptic events in the frontal cortex of cats [7]. It altered single-unit activity recordings in the basal ganglia of squirrel monkeys [8] and generated slow waves that were detected in the lateral frontal cortex of anaesthetized monkeys [4]. In 1985, Zabara inferred from these earlier studies that VNS could desynchronize electroencephalographic activity and theoretically reduce seizure activity [9]. He went on to show that VNS attenuated

Neuromodulation in Psychiatry, First Edition. Edited by Clement Hamani, Paul Holtzheimer, Andres M. Lozano and Helen Mayberg.

motor seizures that were induced by strychnine in dogs and that the beneficial effects of VNS outlasted the acute stimulation period [10]. Further animal studies by Zabara and others showed that VNS was associated with reduced seizure frequency [11–13]. Favourable safety and efficacy established in animal models led to the development of a programmable pulse generator and electrode for VNS in humans. Penry and Dean reported the first implanted VNS device for long-term seizure control in humans in 1988 [14].

Mechanism of VNS

The exact mechanism by which VNS reduces seizure activity or alters mood in humans remains unclear, although neuro-anatomic and neuro-chemical studies suggest several possibilities. The locus coeruleus is the largest population of noradrenergic neurons in the brain and receives projections from the nucleus of the solitary tract [15], which, in turn, receives afferent input from the vagus nerve. The vagus nerve also projects to the raphe nucleus, a major source of serotonin, the amygdala and other limbic structures [16]. Through direct or indirect anatomic connections, the vagus nerve has structural connections with several brain areas implicated in controlling mood [17].

In addition to a structural relationship between the vagus nerve and other brain regions involved in emotion, VNS results in chemical changes in these regions that are functionally significant. For instance, in rat studies, chronic VNS was associated with increased extracellular levels of serotonin in the dorsal raphe [18], and the pharmacologic destruction of serotonin or noradrenergic neurons resulted in the loss of anti-depressant VNS effects [19]. Similarly, in rat studies of VNS for epilepsy, VNS resulted in a sustained increase in norepinephrine over time [4], and norepinephrine depletion in the locus coeruleus completely abolished the seizure-reducing effect of VNS [20, 21]. Thus, VNS-induced changes in neurotransmitter systems may play a role in reducing seizures or modulating mood.

Imaging studies offer an additional approach to studying VNS mechanisms and documenting physiological changes in response to VNS. In patients with partial epilepsy, positron emission tomography (PET) studies showed that VNS affected several medial temporal and limbic structures [22, 23]. Furthermore, in chronic VNS for depression, PET scans showed a decline in resting brain activity in the ventromedial prefrontal cortex, which connects to the amygdala and other brain regions modulating emotion [24]. Other PET studies showed increased blood flow and an inferred increase in synaptic activity in the bilateral thalami in response to VNS. Thalamo-cortical relay neurons have broad synaptic projections that are known to influence cortical rhythms [25]. Therefore, for epilepsy, VNS may decrease seizure activity by increasing synaptic activity in the thalamus [26]. Although thalamic changes on positron emission topography have been noted in VNS for epilepsy, such changes have not been observed in VNS for depression. Instead, blood oxygenation level-dependent activity in various regions implicated in mood disorders and regulated by the vagus nerve increases bilaterally after VNS [23].

Device

VNS is currently carried out by the neurocybernetic prosthesis (NCP) system developed by Cyberonics (Houston, TX). The device consists of a generator (Figure 17.1), a stimulation lead (wire) and an electrode array that wraps around the vagus nerve (Figure 17.2). The generator consists of a lithium battery housed in a titanium shell. The generator is most commonly inserted in the left chest wall in a subcutaneous supra-muscular compartment. A stimulation lead is inserted into the generator

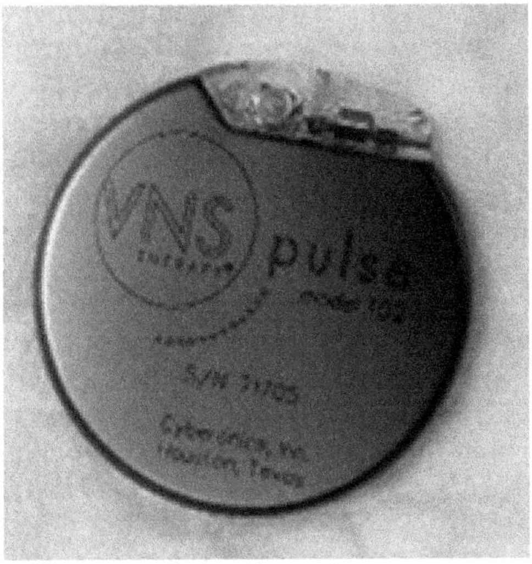

Figure 17.1 Implantable, programmable VNS pulse generator.

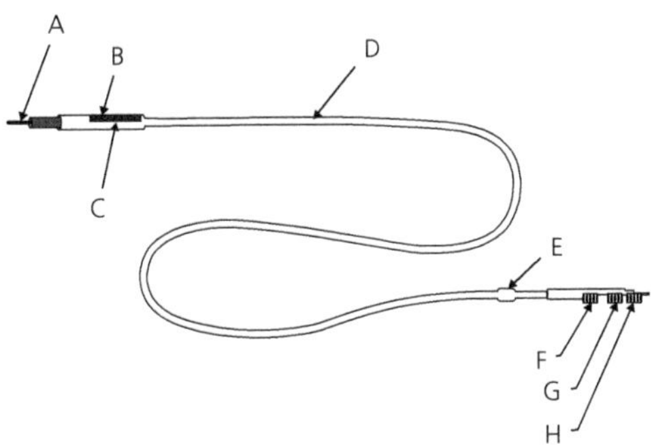

Figure 17.2 Stimulation lead with connector pin (A), lead connector (B), model number tag (C), lead body (D), electrode bifurcation (E), anchor tether (F), positive electrode, white suture (G), and negative electrode, green suture (H). Source: Adapted from VNS therapy physician's manual, with permission from Cyberonics, Inc. [27].

at the superior–lateral aspect and secured with a set of screws tightened by a hexagonal torque wrench. The silicone-insulated platinum iridium stimulation lead is 43 cm in length. Its other end is composed of an electrode array made up of three discrete helical coils, each with three loops that are placed around the vagus nerve. The

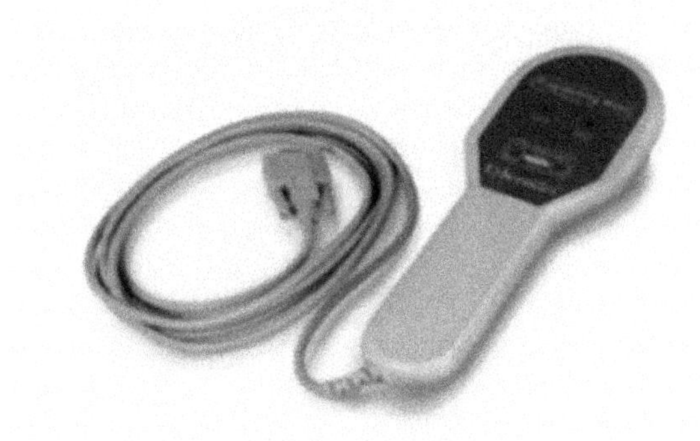

Figure 17.3 Hand-held programming wand transmits information between the VNS programming computer and the VNS pulse generator. Source: Adapted from VNS therapy physician's manual, with permission from Cyberonics, Inc. [27].

bottom coil serves as an anchoring tether to lend extra support to the construct when the neck is turned. Suture tails that extend from both sides of the helix are used to aid in manipulation of the coils without damaging the platinum contacts inside the middle loop of each helix [28].

The generator also contains an antenna that receives radiofrequency signals from an external programming wand (Figure 17.3). The internal antenna transfers the signals to a microprocessor that regulates the electrical output of the generator. The output may be programmed with respect to current, frequency, pulse width, stimulation on-time and stimulation off-time. In addition, a hand-held NCP magnet (Figure 17.4) facilitates real-time control of the device. In response to an aura or seizure onset, caregivers or patients may pass the magnet over the chest wall in order to trigger stimulation superimposed on baseline generator output, which may limit seizure onset or progression. In the case of VNS for depression or other psychiatric diseases, patients experiencing severe stimulation-induced side effects may pass the magnet over the device to temporarily turn off the system, with the system restarting when the magnet is removed [29].

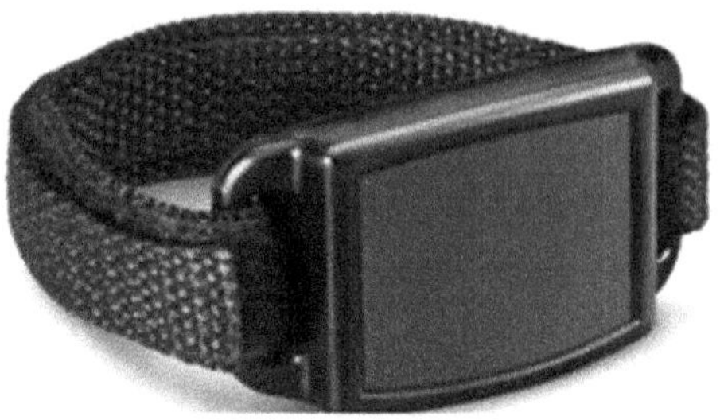

Figure 17.4 A magnet may be placed over the generator to trigger stimulation superimposed on baseline generator output, which may limit seizure onset or progression, or to temporarily stop the device, if stimulation-induced side effects are severe. Source: Adapted from VNS therapy physician's manual, with permission from Cyberonics, Inc. [27].

Surgical anatomy

An intimate understanding of the anatomy of the vagus nerve is useful not only for implantation of the VNS device but also for understanding complications arising from direct stimulation or nerve injury. The tenth cranial nerve, the vagus nerve, arises from several brainstem nuclei to exert a wide variety of effects. Efferent fibres arise from the nucleus ambiguous and innervate somatic muscles of the pharynx and larynx. Additional efferent fibres arise from the dorsal-motor nucleus and supply parasympathetic innervation to the heart, lungs and gastrointestinal tract [30]. Unilateral lesions of the dorsal-motor nucleus are rarely clinically significant and include dysarthria and hoarseness; however, bilateral lesions may produce life-threatening autonomic instability. Injury to the pharyngeal branches of the vagus nerve causes dysphagia, while lesion of the superior laryngeal nerve produces anaesthesia of the upper part of the pharynx and paralysis of the cricothyroid muscle, leading to a weak voice that is easily fatigable [26]. Eighty per cent of vagal fibres, however, are general somatic and special visceral afferents that project to the brain [31]. The vagus nerve carries sensory information from the mucosa of the oropharynx and upper gastrointestinal tract to the spinal nucleus of the trigeminal nucleus and from the thoracic and abdominal organs to the nucleus of the solitary tract [28].

The right vagus nerve preferentially innervates the sinoatrial node of the heart, whereas the left vagus nerve projects to the atrioventricular node [28]. Thus, the VNS electrode is usually applied on the left vagus nerve in order to avoid possible stimulation-induced bradycardia or asystole [32]; however, there are several reports suggesting the efficacy and safety of a right-sided approach as well [33–35]. Furthermore, the mid-cervical portion of the vagus nerve is chosen for lead application because this portion of the nerve is relatively free from branches. In contrast, the upper cervical portion gives off branches to the pharynx, carotid sinus, and superior and inferior cardiac branches leading to the cardiac plexus [28].

Pre-operative evaluation

For the treatment of seizure, VNS therapy is only considered for patients with epilepsy who have failed two or more adequate antiepileptic drug trials and for which surgery is contraindicated. For the treatment of depression, VNS is reserved for treatment-resistant major depression, which is defined as a failure to respond to four or more anti-depressant medication trials [36]. The surgical team discusses the risks and benefits of the procedure, including long-term outcomes, with all candidates.

Surgical implantation

We present the operative approach at our institution for implantation of the NCP system for VNS, although several variations on the technique exist [37–39]. The pulse generator is implanted in the left upper chest. A stimulation lead is tunnelled between a neck incision and a pocket in the left upper chest, where one end of the lead is connected to the generator. The other end of the lead, in the cervical region, contains electrodes that are placed on the vagus nerve. The overall position of the implanted device is shown in Figure 17.5. We perform VNS surgery under general anaesthesia, although implantation under regional blockade has been performed successfully. The patient is positioned supine, with the head

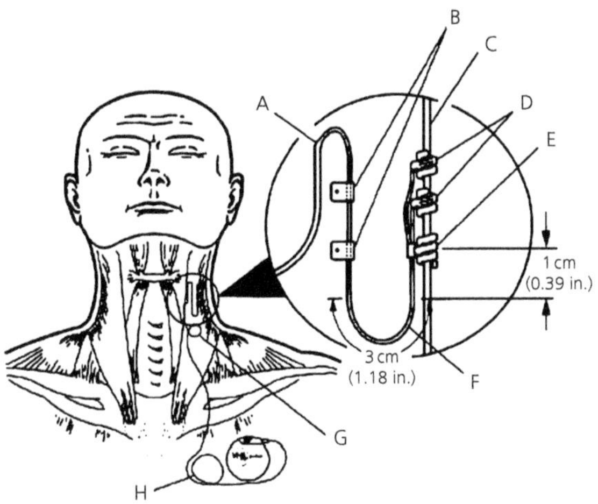

Figure 17.5 The stimulation lead (A) carries helical electrodes (D) and an anchor tether (E), which all wrap around the vagus nerve (C). For additional support, a strain relief bend (F) and a strain relief loop (G) are created in the neck. The lead is further secured with tie downs (B). Extra lead is coiled in the chest (H). Source: Adapted from VNS therapy physician's manual, with permission from Cyberonics, Inc. [27].

resting on a donut pillow and arms tucked at the sides. A rolled blanket or inflatable device may be placed between the shoulder blades to help extend the neck, and the head is rotated to the right side. The primary surgeon stands on the patient's left side, with his/her assistant directly across the operative table.

We prepare the generator site first. A longitudinal incision is made along the lateral aspect of the pectoralis major muscle, and blunt dissection is used to create a subcutaneous pocket large enough to accommodate the generator. Attention is then moved to the left cervical region. A linear skin incision is made in the left anterior neck region overlying the mid-body of the sternocleidomastoid muscle, corresponding to the level of the cricothyroid membrane. The incision is made transversely in a skin crease for cosmetic reasons. The platysma is opened parallel to its muscle fibres and held open by a vertically placed self-retaining retractor. Dissection is then carried out medial to the sternocleidomastoid muscle.

An NCP tunnelling device (Figure 17.6) sheathed within plastic tubing is inserted into the neck incision. The bullet-tip end of the tunneller is placed in the neck incision and passed subcutaneously over the clavicle and into the previously created chest wall pocket. The bullet tip is then unscrewed and removed. The tunneller is pulled back out through the neck incision, leaving behind the plastic cylinder that had sheathed the tunnelling device. The plastic sheath now extends through both the infra-clavicular chest incision and the neck incision. The free end of the stimulator

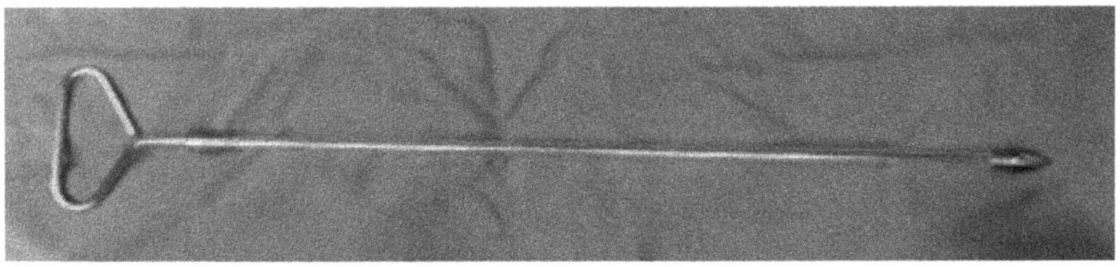

Figure 17.6 Tunneller device, with screw-on bullet tip (far right) and encased along its shaft by a transparent plastic sheath (middle).

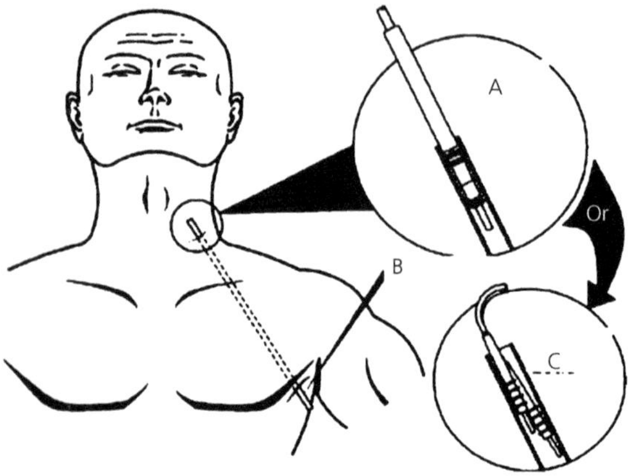

Figure 17.7 After the tunneller sleeve (B) is placed between the two incisions, the stimulation lead connector, either single-pin (A) or double-pin (C), is placed inside the end of the sleeve at the neck incision. The sleeve, along with the stimulation lead connector, is pulled from the chest incision, leaving the lead connector exiting the chest incision. Source: Adapted from VNS therapy physician's manual, with permission from Cyberonics, Inc. [27].

lead, which will attach to the generator, is securely placed inside the sheath at the neck incision. It is then drawn, along with the sheath, from the neck incision to the chest wall incision, until the stimulation lead completely exits the chest incision. The sheath is then removed through the chest incision, and the stimulation lead is connected to the generator. Tunnelling can be performed in either direction (Figure 17.7).

Attention is then turned back to the neck incision. The carotid sheath is exposed. The vagus nerve is usually found between the carotid artery and jugular vein in the posterior groove of the carotid sheath. Fine tip titanium forceps are used to coil the helical electrodes and the anchor tether around a 3–4 mm stretch of exposed nerve. A silicone sheet may be helpful to separate the nerve from the surrounding tissue during the procedure. The leads are placed on the left vagus nerve halfway between the clavicle and the mastoid process, where it is clear of branches, below the level at which the superior and inferior cervical cardiac branches separate from the vagus nerve. The leads in the chest are connected to the battery using a hexagonal screwdriver if not yet performed.

Next, a programming wand is introduced under sterile technique to the field. The wand is held over the generator as the neurologist or company representative performs the electrodiagnostic testing using a personal data assistant. Once data are obtained and the generator is working, one to two sutured tie-downs are placed after securing the anchor tether on the nerve to support the electrode and used to incorporate a 3-cm strain relief in the lead (Figure 17.4). The incisions are thoroughly irrigated and closed in layers. Patients may be discharged the same day at our institution.

Stimulation programming

Intra-operatively, the output current of the generator is usually set to zero and titrated upwards. Studies showed that frequencies over 50 Hz cause permanent damage to the vagus nerve [40]. Therefore, the FDA approved frequencies between 20 and 30 Hz; the most common starting parameters for the treatment of refractory epilepsy and depression are 20–30-Hz signal frequency, 500-μs pulse width, 30 s on-time and 5 min off-time [26]. In clinical trials of VNS for depression, the median current was 1.25 mA (range 0.25–2.25 mA), and the mean current was 1.27 mA [41]. A retrospective study noted an association between decreased depression scores and a low-strength/high-frequency (<1.5 mA/20 Hz) stimulation pattern as compared to a high-strength/low-frequency (>1.5 mA/15 Hz) setting [42]. In clinical practice, post-operative titration is based on individual patient response and tolerance at 2 weeks, at the discretion of the treating neurologist/psychiatrist [4, 26].

Battery change and system removal

Although rechargeable generators exist, most currently implanted generators are not rechargeable and must be replaced before losing power. The electrodes wrapped around the vagus nerve do not need to be removed in order to replace the generator, unless the stimulation lead is severed. In the event of device removal, the electrodes are usually left in place, except in the setting of deep infection. Several reports demonstrate successful removal of the electrodes, despite extensive fibrosis, without injury to the vagus nerve [43–45]. Newer generator versions provide an estimate of the service life of the battery, which is based on stimulation frequency and on-time. The battery life ranges from 1 to 16 years depending on the settings [27]. We perform battery revisions under conscious sedation. Bipolar cautery is generally avoided. Once a new battery is implanted, stimulation parameters are placed to minimal settings and increased over time, as if an original battery had been inserted.

Adverse events

Although VNS is generally well tolerated, adverse events may arise related to stimulation effects or the surgical procedure. The majority of adverse events come from the study of patients undergoing VNS for epilepsy. Stimulation-induced adverse events are usually transient and mainly occur at the time of initial calibration. Such symptoms may be mitigated or corrected with patient acclimation and further titration of settings. Stimulation-induced effects will be discussed in further detail in Chapter 18.

VNS for depression and other psychiatric disease is likely to have overlapping types of complications as in VNS for epilepsy, as well as some adverse events unique to patients with depression. In clinical studies assessing safety and efficacy of VNS, adverse events specific to the depression population included hypomania [46], attempted medication overdose, attempted or completed suicide, and worsening of depression [16, 41]. VNS has not been shown to negatively affect cognition, memory or attention; in fact, some studies have shown improvement in executive and psychomotor function after VNS for depression [47].

Other complications are structural in nature and relate to the surgery or device itself. At the time of initial intra-operative interrogation of the device, bradycardia and even complete heart block can occur in 0.1% of patients [48]. Severe bradycardia is treated with atropine and the device is turned off. Infection is the most common complication, estimated to occur in 3.5–7% of patients, with half being deep infections requiring device removal [49]. Treatment without removal of the device is a viable option in certain cases [50]. Interestingly, infection rates among paediatric patients may be slightly higher [51]. Voice alteration may occur with improper electrode placement or patient-inflicted traction injury due to device manipulation [52]. We place the device laterally in the chest to decrease the likelihood of self-inflicted injury. Electrode fracture and hardware failure have been reported in up to 16% of cases [49]. Some children may experience decreased respiratory airflow during sleep, which is managed with positive pressure treatment or variation in stimulation parameters [53].

VNS is a magnetic resonance imaging (MRI) conditional device, meaning that it is safe to perform MRI within a specified magnetic resonance environment [27]. MRI performed outside of specified parameters may result in excessive heating of lead electrodes, up to a 30°C increase in temperature, which can cause tissue injury or necrosis. Heating is especially likely to occur at the end of an exposed lead; thus, MRI should not be performed on patients with a fractured lead or one who is not connected to a generator. Additional potential risks include device reset, malfunction or damage. Under the specified MRI parameters, the VNS system is not expected to distort the MRI signal in the brain. Cyberonics only performed testing in closed scanners and therefore does not approve the use of open MRI scanners for VNS patients. Finally, the body region between C7 and T8, referred to as the exclusion region, is unsafe for direct MRI scanning, regardless of the parameters [27].

Conclusion

VNS is currently approved as an adjunctive therapy for the treatment of medically refractory epilepsy and treatment-resistant major depression. Compared to current anti-depressants, VNS addresses the issues of medication interaction (no additional medications), treatment compliance (implanted system) and safety in pregnancy (current does not spread to the foetus) [22]. The placement of the NCP device is generally considered a safe procedure, with the majority of side effects corrected by adjustment of stimulation parameters. In addition, the system can be removed safely and replaced if needed. Less invasive approaches, such as transcutaneous VNS, are currently investigational and do not have FDA approval at this time.

Investigations into new indications for VNS continue to expand. Recent studies suggest that VNS may inhibit systemic inflammation by suppressing pro-inflammatory cytokine production [54, 55]. Such findings have opened new lines of investigation to assess the effects of VNS in disease states such as colitis [56]. In addition, the use of VNS is being explored for the treatment of several neuropsychiatric diseases, including anxiety disorder, post-traumatic stress disorder, migraine and various pain syndromes [22].

References

1 Terry RS, Tarver WB, Zabara J. The implantable neurocybernetic prosthesis system. Pacing Clin Electrophysiol 1991 Jan;14(1):86–93.
2 Elger G, Hoppe C, Falkai P, Rush AJ, Elger CE. Vagus nerve stimulation is associated with mood improvements in epilepsy patients. Epilepsy Res 2000 Dec;42(2–3):203–210.
3 Yatham LN. Newer anticonvulsants in the treatment of bipolar disorder. J Clin Psychiatry 2004;65(Suppl 10):28–35.
4 Groves DA, Brown VJ. Vagal nerve stimulation: a review of its applications and potential mechanisms that mediate its clinical effects. Neurosci Biobehav Rev 2005 May;29(3):493–500.
5 Rush AJ, George MS, Sackeim HA, Marangell LB, Husain MM, Giller C, *et al.* Vagus nerve stimulation (VNS) for treatment-resistant depressions: a multicenter study. Biol Psychiatry 2000 Feb 15;47(4):276–286.
6 Bailey P, Bremer F. A sensory cortical representation of the vagus nerve with a note on the effects of low pressure on the cortical electrogram. J Neurophysiol 1938;1:405–412.
7 Zanchettia A, Wang SC, Moruzzi G. The effect of vagal afferent stimulation on the EEG pattern of the cat. Electroencephalogr Clin Neurophysiol 1952 Aug;4(3):357–361.
8 Radna RJ, MacLean PD. Vagal elicitation of respiratory-type and other unit responses in basal limbic structures of squirrel monkeys. Brain Res 1981 May 25;213(1):45–61.
9 Zabara J. Peripheral control of hypersynchronous discharge in epilepsy. Electroencephalogr Clin Neurophysiol 1985;S61:162.
10 Zabara J. Inhibition of experimental seizures in canines by repetitive vagal stimulation. Epilepsia 1992 Nov-Dec;33(6):1005–1012.
11 Woodbury DM, Woodbury JW. Effects of vagal stimulation on experimentally induced seizures in rats. Epilepsia 1990;31(Suppl 2):S7–S19.
12 Lockard JS, Congdon WC, DuCharme LL. Feasibility and safety of vagal stimulation in monkey model. Epilepsia 1990;31(Suppl 2): S20–S26.
13 Takaya H, Nii S, Kawaizumi F, Takahashi K. Enrichment of surfactant from its aqueous solution using ultrasonic atomization. Ultrason Sonochem 2005 Aug;12(6):483–487.

14 Penry JK, Dean JC. Prevention of intractable partial seizures by intermittent vagal stimulation in humans: preliminary results. Epilepsia 1990;31(Suppl 2):S40–S43.
15 Van Bockstaele EJ, Peoples J, Telegan P. Efferent projections of the nucleus of the solitary tract to peri-locus coeruleus dendrites in rat brain: evidence for a monosynaptic pathway. J Comp Neurol 1999 Sep 27;412(3):410–428.
16 Marangell LB, Rush AJ, George MS, Sackeim HA, Johnson CR, Husain MM, *et al*. Vagus nerve stimulation (VNS) for major depressive episodes: one year outcomes. Biol Psychiatry 2002 Feb 15;51(4):280–287.
17 Nemeroff CB, Mayberg HS, Krahl SE, McNamara J, Frazer A, Henry TR, *et al*. VNS therapy in treatment-resistant depression: clinical evidence and putative neurobiological mechanisms. Neuropsychopharmacology 2006 Jul;31(7): 1345–1355.
18 Manta S, El Mansari M, Debonnel G, Blier P. Electrophysiological and neurochemical effects of long-term vagus nerve stimulation on the rat monoaminergic systems. Int J Neuropsychopharmacol 2013 Mar;16(2):459–470.
19 Furmaga H, Shah A, Frazer A. Serotonergic and noradrenergic pathways are required for the anxiolytic-like and antidepressant-like behavioral effects of repeated vagal nerve stimulation in rats. Biol Psychiatry 2011 Nov 15;70(10):937–945.
20 Krahl SE, Clark KB. Vagus nerve stimulation for epilepsy: a review of central mechanisms. Surg Neurol Int 2012;3(Suppl 4):S255–S259.
21 Krahl SE, Clark KB, Smith DC, Browning RA. Locus coeruleus lesions suppress the seizure-attenuating effects of vagus nerve stimulation. Epilepsia 1998 Jul;39(7):709–714.
22 George MS, Nahas Z, Borckardt JJ, Anderson B, Burns C, Kose S, *et al*. Vagus nerve stimulation for the treatment of depression and other neuropsychiatric disorders. Expert Rev Neurother 2007 Jan;7(1):63–74.
23 Henry TR, Bakay RA, Votaw JR, Pennell PB, Epstein CM, Faber TL, *et al*. Brain blood flow alterations induced by therapeutic vagus nerve stimulation in partial epilepsy: I. Acute effects at high and low levels of stimulation. Epilepsia 1998 Sep;39(9):983–990.
24 Pardo JV, Sheikh SA, Schwindt GC, Lee JT, Kuskowski MA, Surerus C, *et al*. Chronic vagus nerve stimulation for treatment-resistant depression decreases resting ventromedial prefrontal glucose metabolism. Neuroimage 2008 Aug 15;42(2):879–889.
25 Steriade M, Contreras D. Relations between cortical and thalamic cellular events during transition from sleep patterns to paroxysmal activity. J Neurosci 1995;15:623–642.
26 Milby AH, Halpern CH, Baltuch GH. Vagus nerve stimulation for epilepsy and depression. Neurotherapeutics 2008 Jan;5(1):75–85.
27 Cyberonics I. VNS therapy physician's manual. 2013; Available at: http://dynamic.cyberonics.com/manuals/. Accessed 11 January 2013.
28 Baumgartner J, Gretchen V. Chapter 67: vagus nerve stimulation for intractable epilepsy. In: Winn H, editor. Youmans Neurological Surgery. Sixth ed. Philadelphia: Elsevier Saunders; 2011. p. 806–812.
29 Daban C, Martinez-Aran A, Cruz N, Vieta E. Safety and efficacy of vagus nerve stimulation in treatment-resistant depression. A systematic review. J Affect Disord 2008 Sep;110(1–2):1–15.
30 Brannagan T, Weimer L. Chapter 72: cranial and peripheral nerve lesions. In: Rowland L, Pedley T, editors. Merrit's Neurology. Eighth ed. Philadelphia: Lippincott Williams & Wilkins; 2010. p. 509–510.
31 George MS, Sackeim HA, Rush AJ, Marangell LB, Nahas Z, Husain MM, *et al*. Vagus nerve stimulation: a new tool for brain research and therapy. Biol Psychiatry 2000 Feb 15; 47(4):287–295.
32 Hancock JC, Hoover DB, Hougland MW. Distribution of muscarinic receptors and acetylcholinesterase in the rat heart. J Auton Nerv Syst 1987 Apr;19(1):59–66.
33 Navas M, Navarrete EG, Pascual JM, Carrasco R, Nunez JA, Shakur SF, *et al*. Treatment of refractory epilepsy in adult patients with right-sided vagus nerve stimulation. Epilepsy Res 2010 Jun;90(1–2):1–7.
34 Spuck S, Nowak G, Renneberg A, Tronnier V, Sperner J. Right-sided vagus nerve stimulation in humans: an effective therapy? Epilepsy Res 2008 Dec;82(2–3):232–234.
35 McGregor A, Wheless J, Baumgartner J, Bettis D. Right-sided vagus nerve stimulation as a treatment for refractory epilepsy in humans. Epilepsia 2005 Jan;46(1):91–96.

36 Aaronson ST, Carpenter LL, Conway CR, Reimherr FW, Lisanby SH, Schwartz TL, *et al.* Vagus nerve stimulation therapy randomized to different amounts of electrical charge for treatment-resistant depression: acute and chronic effects. Brain Stimul 2013 Jul;6(4): 631–640.
37 Reid SA. Surgical technique for implantation of the neurocybernetic prosthesis. Epilepsia 1990;31(Suppl 2):S38–S39.
38 Landy HJ, Ramsay RE, Slater J, Casiano RR, Morgan R. Vagus nerve stimulation for complex partial seizures: surgical technique, safety, and efficacy. J Neurosurg 1993 Jan;78(1):26–31.
39 Horowitz G, Amit M, Fried I, Neufeld MY, Sharf L, Kramer U, *et al.* Vagal nerve stimulation for refractory epilepsy: the surgical procedure and complications in 100 implantations by a single medical center. Eur Arch Otorhinolaryngol 2013 Jan;270(1):355–358.
40 Agnew WF, McCreery DB. Considerations for safety with chronically implanted nerve electrodes. Epilepsia 1990;31(Suppl 2):S27–S32.
41 Christmas D, Steele JD, Tolomeo S, Eljamel MS, Matthews K. Vagus nerve stimulation for chronic major depressive disorder: 12-month outcomes in highly treatment-refractory patients. J Affect Disord 2013 Sep 25;150(3): 1221–1225.
42 Muller HH, Kornhuber J, Maler JM, Sperling W. The effects of stimulation parameters on clinical outcomes in patients with vagus nerve stimulation implants with major depression. J ECT 2013 Sep;29(3):e40–e42.
43 O'Neill BR, Wilberger JE. Revision of vagal nerve stimulator electrodes through a posterior cervical triangle approach: technical note. Neurosurgery 2010 Dec;67(2 Suppl Operative):457–460.
44 MacDonald J, Couldwell WT. Revision of vagal nerve stimulator electrodes: technical approach. Acta Neurochir (Wien) 2004 Jun;146(6): 567–570; discussion 570.
45 Espinosa J, Aiello MT, Naritoku DK. Revision and removal of stimulating electrodes following long-term therapy with the vagus nerve stimulator. Surg Neurol 1999 Jun;51(6):659–664.
46 Rush AJ, Marangell LB, Sackeim HA, George MS, Brannan SK, Davis SM, *et al.* Vagus nerve stimulation for treatment-resistant depression: a randomized, controlled acute phase trial. Biol Psychiatry 2005 Sep 1;58(5):347–354.
47 Sackeim HA, Keilp JG, Rush AJ, George MS, Marangell LB, Dormer JS, *et al.* The effects of vagus nerve stimulation on cognitive performance in patients with treatment-resistant depression. Neuropsychiatry Neuropsychol Behav Neurol 2001 Jan;14(1):53–62.
48 Ali II, Pirzada NA, Kanjwal Y, Wannamaker B, Medhkour A, Koltz MT, *et al.* Complete heart block with ventricular asystole during left vagus nerve stimulation for epilepsy. Epilepsy Behav 2004 Oct;5(5):768–771.
49 Kahlow H, Olivecrona M. Complications of vagal nerve stimulation for drug-resistant epilepsy: a single center longitudinal study of 143 patients. Seizure 2013 Dec;22(10):827–833.
50 Air EL, Ghomri YM, Tyagi R, Grande AW, Crone K, Mangano FT. Management of vagal nerve stimulator infections: do they need to be removed? J Neurosurg Pediatr 2009 Jan; 3(1):73–78.
51 Smyth MD, Tubbs RS, Bebin EM, Grabb PA, Blount JP. Complications of chronic vagus nerve stimulation for epilepsy in children. J Neurosurg 2003 Sep;99(3):500–503.
52 Ramsay RE, Uthman BM, Augustinsson LE, Upton AR, Naritoku D, Willis J, *et al.* Vagus nerve stimulation for treatment of partial seizures: 2. Safety, side effects, and tolerability. First International Vagus Nerve Stimulation Study Group. Epilepsia 1994 May–Jun;35(3):627–636.
53 Hsieh T, Chen M, McAfee A, Kifle Y. Sleep-related breathing disorder in children with vagal nerve stimulators. Pediatr Neurol 2008 Feb;38(2):99–103.
54 Bonaz B, Picq C, Sinniger V, Mayol JF, Clarencon D. Vagus nerve stimulation: from epilepsy to the cholinergic anti-inflammatory pathway. Neurogastroenterol Motil 2013 Mar;25(3): 208–221.
55 Yamakawa K, Matsumoto N, Imamura Y, Muroya T, Yamada T, Nakagawa J, *et al.* Electrical vagus nerve stimulation attenuates systemic inflammation and improves survival in a rat heatstroke model. PLoS One 2013;8(2): e56728.
56 Sun P, Zhou K, Wang S, Li P, Chen S, Lin G, *et al.* Involvement of MAPK/NF-kappaB signaling in the activation of the cholinergic anti-inflammatory pathway in experimental colitis by chronic vagus nerve stimulation. PLoS One 2013 Aug 2;8(8):e69424.

CHAPTER 18

Vagus nerve stimulation for treatment-refractory depression

Charles R. Conway, Britt M. Gott and Naazia H. Azhar
Washington University School of Medicine in St. Louis, Department of Psychiatry, St. Louis, Missouri, USA

Introduction and rationale for VNS in treatment-refractory major depression (TRD)

In 2005, the United States Food and Drug Administration (U.S. FDA) approved vagus nerve stimulation (VNS) for the treatment of depression not responding to four or more adequate antidepressant trials [1]. This decision emerged from two large clinical trials [2–4] studying VNS in treatment-refractory depression (TRD), which demonstrated the antidepressant efficacy with sustained stimulation. Currently, despite this FDA approval, Medicare and Medicaid (as well as most private insurance companies) do not typically reimburse for VNS for TRD on the basis that the treatment remains unproven/experimental (discussed further in 'Future Directions'). Ongoing efforts are in progress to make VNS more accessible to those suffering from TRD.

Rationale for the use of VNS in TRD

VNS is also approved by the FDA for use in treatment-refractory epilepsy [1, 5]. The original idea that VNS might be efficacious in major depressive disorder (MDD) evolved from anecdotal clinical reports suggesting improvement in mood observed in VNS-implanted epilepsy patients. This prompted two prospective, open-label, pilot trials to assess for the effects of VNS on mood. The first [6] did a within-subjects and across subjects comparison of 20 VNS-implanted epilepsy patients and 20 epilepsy patients who were not implanted with VNS, but were receiving stable anticonvulsant medications. This study found a significant reduction in depression scores *within* the VNS-implanted subjects ($p=0.017$) but not a between-group difference, although one self-reported between-group comparison (Beck Depression Inventory) approached statistical significance ($p=0.07$). Interestingly, this observed decrease in depression scores occurred *independent of the VNS anti-seizure benefits*, suggesting potentially different mechanisms of action for epilepsy and depression. Significant limitations of this trial included the fact that, on average, the two groups were not depressed, and the VNS-implanted subjects had significantly more seizures per month than the control group. The second prospective, pilot trial [7] reported on a small group of 11 subjects receiving VNS for medication-refractory, partial onset seizures. Comparing baseline depression scores to 3 and 6 months of stimulation, this group found statistically significant differences on several depression measures at both time points. Those patients getting higher doses of

Neuromodulation in Psychiatry, First Edition. Edited by Clement Hamani, Paul Holtzheimer, Andres M. Lozano and Helen Mayberg.

current had greater antidepressant responses, although this difference did not achieve statistical significance ($p=0.1$). It is notable that the subjects in the study by Elger *et al.*, unlike those in the study by Harden *et al.*, did have mild clinical depression at baseline (mean Montgomery Asberg Depression Rating Scale score of 10.8). Like the study by Harden *et al.*, the antidepressant effects occurred independent of the anti-seizure effects.

Building on these findings, a group of psychiatrists conducted the first open-label study of VNS in TRD [2], which demonstrated preliminary positive findings (study details in the section 'Results of clinical trials'). These initial positive results prompted a larger, multi-centre, double-blind trial of VNS in TRD [4], which showed a trend towards separation from placebo. However, following 10 weeks of stimulation (including a 2 week period of increasing the current), there was no measurable difference noted. Importantly, results from the open-label extension phase of this trial did demonstrate a significant and robust response [3]. Further, similar parallel studies of 'treatment as usual' (psychiatrist treating TRD patients with equally severe MDD and allowed to use any available treatment, including electroconvulsive therapy (ECT)) demonstrated that VNS was superior to 'treatment as usual' [8].

How the VNS device applies current to the Vagus

The primary VNS device used in the US and Europe is the Neurocybernetic Prosthesis™ system (NCP; Cyberonics, Houston, TX). This device is an implantable, multi-programmable, battery-operated current generator that is typically implanted under the skin below the left clavicle (typically surgically accessed via the left axilla; Figure 18.1). A tunnelling device is used to move the electrical leads emanating from the device under the skin into the neck region. A second incision is made in the neck region for the attachment of the electrical leads to the vagus nerve. The bipolar lead is typically attached above the cardiac branch of the vagus.

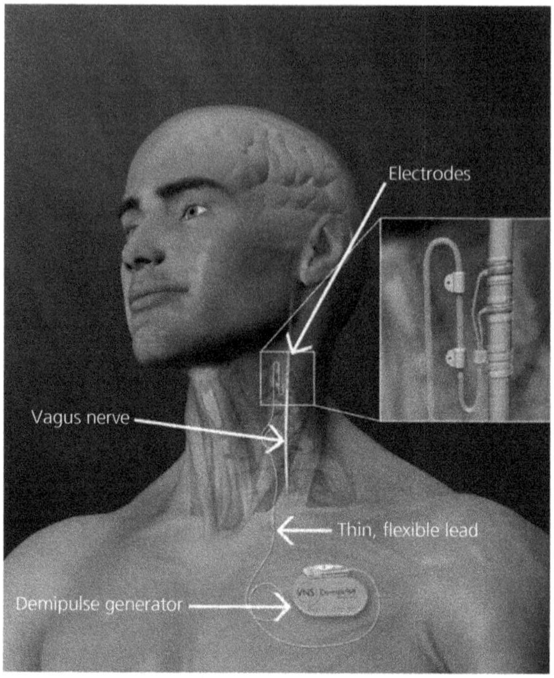

Figure 18.1 Illustration of the attachment of the VNS lead to the mid-cervical region of the left vagus nerve. The bipolar lead is coiled around the vagus in two adjacent regions with a tether attached to the surrounding fascia to prevent lead movement under tension. Source: Reproduced with permission of Cyberonics. (*See insert for colour representation of the figure.*)

The device delivers around-the-clock stimulation to the left vagus. It allows for the manipulation of multiple electrical stimulus parameters including current (milliamps, mA), pulse width (micrometers, μm), frequency (Hertz, Hz) and manipulation of duty cycle (time 'on' versus time 'off').

Animal studies, as well as extensive experience in humans, demonstrate that at the current levels at which clinical VNS is delivered, the vast majority of the stimulus is directed afferently (towards the brain). For this reason, most of the thoracic and abdominal organs subserved by the vagus (e.g. heart, lungs, gastrointestinal tract) are minimally affected by VNS. The more proximal/afferently located recurrent laryngeal nerve (which supplies the larynx) does frequently receive afferent stimulus; hence, approximately two thirds of patients do experience hoarseness/stridor during VNS stimulation (more details provided in the section 'Results of clinical trials' and Table 18.2).

The vagus nerve

The vagus nerve is the longest of the cranial nerves (the term 'vagus' comes from the Latin term 'vagi', which translates as 'wanderer') and provides afferent and efferent innervation to organs in the thoracic, abdominal and pelvic cavities including the heart, lungs, gastrointestinal tract as well as other abdominal organs. The vagus is composed of fibres with numerous functions including visceral sensory, visceral motor, somatic motor and somatic sensory functions [9]. It is composed largely of afferent type unmyelinated C-fibres (80%), which have lower stimulation thresholds that fortuitously allows low-current stimulation from VNS to primarily transmit upstream (and not towards efferent organs/regions, e.g. the heart, gastrointestinal tract).

Efferent vagus nerve fibres originate from medullary (brainstem) nuclei, which include the dorsal motor nucleus and the nucleus ambiguus. The majority of the afferent vagal fibres originate from two large ganglia located just inferior to the foramen magnum (nodose and jugular ganglia; [9, 10]). Further, there are special and general visceral afferent fibres, which carry gustatory and visceral sensory information to the brainstem. Finally, afferent vagal somatic sensory information is also relayed to the brainstem [11].

VNS electrical leads are surgically attached to the vagus nerve in the mid-inferior cervical region of the left vagus (Figure 18.1). In the neck, the vagus nerve is positioned between the internal jugular vein and carotid artery, all of which are enclosed in fascia (carotid sheath). The cervical vagus nerve is composed of multiple fibre types. The most common ones are the narrow, unmyelinated C-fibres, which have lower stimulation thresholds and are believed to be the primary nerve fibres activated during VNS [12]. With increases in current, VNS can also inadvertently activate myelinated vagal efferent fibres, which innervate the larynx and pharynx; this is manifested in the frequently observed vocal alteration/stridor observed with higher stimulation [13].

In humans, parasympathetic innervation of the heart is asymmetric, with the left vagus primarily innervating the sinoatrial node (responsible for establishing and maintaining heart rate) and the right vagus supplying the atria-ventricular node (responsible for controlling atrial-ventricular conduction; [14]). Hence, to prevent potential intracardiac conduction problems, the left vagus has been historically favoured for VNS. Studies assessing the effects of VNS on downstream vagal effector organs (e.g. gastrointestinal, pulmonary and cardiac systems) demonstrate that therapeutic left VNS has limited effects on these systems [15, 16]. However, to date, there have been no systematic studies on the effects of VNS in individuals with disease in these end-organ systems (e.g. congestive heart failure, pulmonary disease); hence, considerable caution is warranted with consideration of implanting VNS devices in individuals with these conditions. In particular, caution is advised in individuals who suffer from sleep apnoea (see section 'Results of clinical trials').

Afferent vagal pathways

The afferent vagal pathways in humans are very complex and not completely understood. What follows is a summary of those pathways, and a more complete description is provided in another review [17].

Afferent vagal fibres carry visceral sensory (pharnyx, larynx, thoracoabdominal organs), special sense (taste) and somatic sensory (small area of external ear) information. Afferent vagal fibres enter the brainstem at the level of the medulla, decussate and then synapse at several nuclei. For the purposes of VNS, the most critical pathway is the tractus solitarius, which terminates in the nucleus tractus solitarius (NTS; etc. [18–20]).

Ascending NTS fibres then project primarily to the pontine parabrachial nucleus (PBN); however, other projections synapse in other medullary and pontine nuclei, cerebellar regions and the periaqueductal grey. These NTS projections are believed to regulate respiration and pain. Hence, it is believed that the worsening of sleep apnoea observed with VNS may be a result of activation of these pathways [21]. In contrast, the periaqueductal grey region, believed to be critical in central pain modulation, may be responsible for the observed analgesic effects associated with VNS [22].

From a mood regulation standpoint, perhaps the most critical NTS projections are to brainstem nuclei (medulla and pons) critical in regulating biogenic amines associated with mood. The NTS projects to both the pontine locus ceruleus (primary brainstem site for noradrenergic nuclei) and the medullary and pontine raphe nuclei (primary brainstem regions for serotonergic nuclei; [23]). Although little is known about how VNS affects these systems in humans, animal models of VNS in MDD suggest that chronic, but not acute, VNS leads to enhanced autonomous firing of both the locus ceruleus and the dorsal raphe nuclei [24].

Afferent vagal projections to the thalamus and cerebrum

Afferent vagal information travels to higher brain regions (thalamus and cerebrum) via several pathways; however, the majority of information travels via multi-synapse pathways [17, 25]. The most common pathway involves NTS projections to the pontine PBN; however, some NTS fibres bypass the NTS [10, 17, 26] sending projections to several regions known to be important in major depression including the hypothalamus, thalamus, nucleus accumbens, amygdala and the stria terminalis.

The PBN serves as a brainstem 'relay station' for incoming gustatory and other autonomic information. Afferent vagal projections emerging from the PBN project to multiple upstream/cortical regions [17, 27] including the hypothalamus, thalamus, anterior insula, lateral prefrontal cortex, amygdala (central and basolateral nuclei), infralimbic cortex and other cortical regions [28–31]. The insular cortex has projections that communicate with more rostral cortical regions (orbital and ventrolateral prefrontal cortex) and also indirectly communicate with the medial prefrontal cortex [31, 32]. These connections may be critical in VNS effects on major depressive disorder. Many of these regions have been observed to undergo changes in VNS functional human neuroimaging studies in both depression and epilepsy [33–35].

Many clinicians have observed that VNS is associated with increased alertness. This may be as a result of PBN projections to the medial reticular formation. The reticular formation is associated with numerous central nervous system functions including alertness, generation of sleep waves and slow sleep electroencephalography waves [36, 37]. Malow *et al.* [38] demonstrated that epilepsy patients with VNS demonstrated improved diurnal alertness with VNS, which was not related to anti-seizure effects.

Results of clinical trials

There have been five clinical trials (several with extension phases) that have examined the efficacy of VNS in TRD [2–4, 39–43]. All of these trials were longitudinal with open-label, observational periods. Two had an initial randomized, double-blind period [3, 4, 39], and one of those was a dose-finding trial [39]. These trials have been summarized in Table 18.1. All of the studies except one [39]

Table 18.1 Summary of clinical trials of VNS in adults with treatment-refractory depression.

	Sample size	Age (mean)	% MDD	% Bipolar	Duration	TRD definition (# of failed AD trials)	Study design	Results	Comments
Rush *et al.* [2]	60	46.8	70	30	12 weeks	2	Open, acute-phase, pilot, multisite	Response rate of 40% by HRDS-28 and CGI, 50% by MADRS, 17% remission rate	Different stimulation parameters (low, medium, high)
Marangell *et al.* [41]	30	46.8	70	30	12 months	2	Open, naturalistic, follow-up	Response rate sustained (40–46%) and remission rate significantly increased (17–29%) $p=0.045$	
Nahas *et al.* [42]	59	46.8	73	27	24 months	2	Open, naturalistic, follow-up	Response rate 42% after 2 years; remission rate 22% after 2 years	
Rush *et al.* [4]	222	46.5	90	10	10 weeks	2; ≤6	Double-blind, controlled, American multisite	No statistically significant difference in response rate active vs. sham VNS (15.2 vs. 10%) at 10 weeks	
Rush *et al.* [3]	205	46.3	90	10	12 months	2; ≤6	Open-label follow-up after 12 weeks	Cumulative increase observed in MDD response rates (HRDS-24) over sustained stimulation, up to 30% response at 1 year	
Schlaepfer *et al.* [43]	74	47.4	73	27	12 months	2; ≤6	Open-label, uncontrolled, European multisite	Response rate 53% after 1 year; remission rate 33% after 1 year	
Bajbouj *et al.* [40]	74	47.4	73	27	24 months	2; ≤6	Open, naturalistic, follow-up	Response rate 53% and remission rate 38.9% sustained at 2 years	
Aaronson *et al.* [39]	331	47.9	78	22	50 weeks	≥4	Double blind, randomized dose-finding, multisite	Higher dosing predicted a greater *sustained* antidepressant effect at 1 year. Amount of charge delivered over time correlated with degree of AD response	
Christmas *et al.* [44][a]	13	47.3	100	0	12 months	≥4	Open, uncontrolled	Response rate of 30.8% in chronic, unipolar severe TRD subgroup	

Abbreviations: HRDS, Hamilton Rating Scale for Depression; CGI, clinical global impression; MADRS, Montgomery Åsberg Depression Rating Scale; VNS, vagus nerve stimulation; MDD, major depressive disorder; AD, antidepressant; TRD, treatment-resistant depression.

[a] Refers to new subgroup not included elsewhere.

defined treatment resistance as having failed at least two adequate trials of antidepressants from different classes during the current depressive episode.

The first trial [2] assessed the safety and efficacy of VNS in TRD to estimate the degree and timing of antidepressant effects and to determine if a randomized study of antidepressant efficacy was warranted. For this study, and in all other described studies (except Aaronson *et al.* [39]), VNS was implanted and the stimulation was delayed for 2 weeks post-surgical recovery. Then, the VNS device was turned on with initial stimulation parameters of output current: 0.25 mA, frequency: 20 or 30 Hz, pulse width: 500 ms and a duty cycle of 30 s 'on' every 5 min. There were gradual increases permitted in the output current, and the parameter settings were made based on patient tolerance. After 1 month, the parameters were fixed for the initial phase. Based on a 50% drop in the 28-item Hamilton Depression Rating Scale (HRDS-28) score, this proof-of-concept study demonstrated a high response rate (40%) and a 17% remission rate with 10 weeks of VNS. Given that TRD is so severe and disabling, this response rate was promising and it suggested the importance of doing larger, double-blind prospective trials.

Subjects receiving VNS from this original pilot trial were followed up for 1 and 2 years respectively [41, 42], which showed sustained benefits of VNS. After 1 year, the percentage of responders was about the same (40% 1 month; 46% 1 year, $p = 0.317$) and the remission rate increased (17% 1 month; 29% 1 year, $p = 0.045$); [41]. After 2 years, the response rate was found to be 42% and the remission rate 22% [42]. These sustained response and remission rates are notable, because most studies of TRD, including those involving ECT, have demonstrated very high relapse rates [45, 46]. Further, these extension studies supported that VNS in TRD was very well tolerated. All of the aforementioned studies were limited by the absence of a control group; however, they supported the need for a prospective, double-blind, controlled study of VNS in TRD.

In the first and only true prospective, double-blind, controlled study to date of VNS in TRD, 235 subjects were implanted with VNS devices, but only half ($n = 112$) had active treatment for the first 12 weeks, while the others received sham VNS (device implanted, but not activated; [4]). This trial defined treatment response as a 50% reduction in the 24-item Hamilton Rating Scale for Depression (HRDS-24). Following stimulation of 10 weeks duration (including 2 weeks to increase the output current), the results showed no significant difference ($p = 0.251$) in response rate between active VNS (15.2%) and sham VNS (10%). Although the primary outcome was HRSD-24, a secondary depression measurement scale, the 30-item Inventory of Depression Symptomatology – Self Report (IDS-SR 30), did show a significant difference between the control and treatment group at 10 weeks ($p = 0.032$). Importantly, this study [4] provided vagus stimulation for only 10 weeks. Several other clinical outcome studies [39, 40] and neuroimaging studies [34, 47, 48] have demonstrated that the antidepressant efficacy effects of VNS likely come about as a result of *sustained* vagal stimulation. These studies support that the majority of patients likely require between 6 and 9 months of vagal stimulation before an antidepressant response is achieved. Notably, this phenomenon of improved cumulative clinical outcomes with increased stimulation duration has also been observed in VNS studies in refractory epilepsy [5].

Why there was such a large difference in the 10 week, open-label pilot study response [2] (~40% response rate) and the double-blind, multi-centre trial response [4] (15.2% response rate) is not clear. Besides the more obvious possible reason (open-label, observer bias), the original pilot study [2] was conducted at only four sites, which may have allowed more careful individual patient selection, which is likely critical in determining the response rate.

Following the 10 week, double-blind study, Rush *et al.* conducted an open-label extension of the acute stimulation trial, which followed the same TRD subjects for an additional 42 weeks. During this extension, considerably more flexibility was allowed in adjusting the electrical parameters and concurrent medications [3]. Using the HRDS-24 as the primary measure, this study demonstrated a significant reduction in HRDS-24 score per month ($p < 0.001$). At 1 year of stimulation, this extension achieved an overall response rate of 27.2% and a remission rate of 15.8%. As noted previously, a cumulative increase in response rate was observed over time: at 3 months, 15% had responded; at 6 months, approximately 18%; at 9 months, approximately 25%; and at 12 months, approximately 30%.

A large-scale, open-label, extended duration European study of VNS in TRD was also conducted using a similar protocol. Similar to the findings of the open-label study by Rush *et al.* [3], Schlaepfer *et al.* [43] found that there was a cumulative increase in the number of patients responding to VNS (as measured by the HRSD-24) after 3, 6, 9 and 12 months of VNS. After 1 year of VNS, this group had a response rate of 53% and a remission rate of 33% [43]. Notably, the median time to respond in this trial was 9 months. Further, a sustained response was again observed with 44% of patients in the study showing response and an absence of relapse in the first year. An extension study [40] found that the response and remission rates persisted at 2 years.

Why were the response rates in the European study [43] considerably higher than those seen in either the open-label US trial [2] or the double-blind US trial [4]? As detailed in the comparative analysis [43], the European trial TRD subjects appeared to be markedly less sick on numerous measures including fewer depressive episodes, lower duration of current depressive episode, fewer failed antidepressant trials, less severe baseline depression scores and less exposure to electroconvulsive treatment. Hence, the European trial's greater response rate may be attributable to a less severely depressed population than the first US trial [2].

How do VNS antidepressant response rates compare with other standard MDD treatments? In an effort to study this, George *et al.* [8] conducted a parallel naturalistic trial examining the antidepressant response rates for 'treatment as usual' (TAU, any treatment, including ECT, deemed appropriate for patients suffering from TRD). Critically, this trial selected patients who were equally treatment resistant (i.e. equivalent number of failed antidepressant trials, depression duration, etc.) as those in Rush *et al.* [3, 4]. This study demonstrated a significantly higher response rate at 1 year (21.1% for VNS+TAU; 11.6% for TAU; $p=0.029$) and significantly higher remission rate at 1 year (15.0% for VNS+TAU; 3.6% for TAU; $p=0.006$). This study, although compelling, was limited by the lack of subject randomization, that is, George *et al.* were comparing a separate, but equivalently depressed, population to a similar population in a separate study. Observed differences between the samples were controlled for in the analyses, but other potential differences could not be controlled for due to the lack of randomization.

To further extrapolate the effectiveness of VNS to severely depressed patients, Christmas *et al.* [44] isolated the response rates of two small subgroups of participants with particularly severe (failing ≥4 adequate treatment trials) and chronic (≥2 years in the current major depressive episode) unipolar TRD. The authors selected patients with specific TRD severity and chronicity who were treated in an open-label clinical trial of VNS in Europe ($n=28$, D03 database [43]) and separately a small sample ($n=13$) of 'consecutive (TRD patients) who received VNS for chronic, unipolar TRD in Dundee.' Following treatment in the European subset of patients, the response rate at 12 months was 35.7% (defined as a

50% drop in HRDS-17 in both groups). In the smaller sample, the 12 month response rate was 30.8%. Despite the absence of a control group and the inclusion of open-label studies only, the overall response rates in these selective samples suggest an encouraging response to treatment. In this sample of two separate cohorts of highly chronic, severe unipolar TRD, the response to VNS is consistent with a more heterogeneous depressed population sample as shown in other studies.

Only one clinical trial has addressed the issue of whether differences in electrical parameters play a role in VNS antidepressant efficacy in TRD [39]. There are four modifiable electrical parameters available with standard implantable VNS. These include current (milliamps, mA), pulse width (microseconds), frequency (Hertz, Hz) and duty cycle (amount of stimulation time 'on' (seconds) vs. time 'off' (minutes)). Instead of using the standard parameters, Aaronson *et al.* [39] randomized subjects to one of three different dosing groups: 'low', 'medium' and 'high'. The doses differed in pulse width and current; however, the groups had identical duty cycles (30 s 'on', 5 min 'off') and pulse frequencies (20 Hz). This trial had an acute phase (first 22 weeks) and a long-term phase (subsequent 28 weeks). The acute phase had 'fixed' parameters (same parameters held for entire duration of the phase); however, the long-term phase allowed for upward dose titration. This dose-finding trial found no significant difference in acute-phase efficacy between stimulus dose cohorts, that is, the higher dose acute-phase parameter groups showed higher numerical, but not statistical, antidepressant efficacy rates than the lower dose groups. The study did further demonstrate VNS efficacy in TRD: all three dosing cohorts had improvement in depression, which continued into the long-term phase. Importantly, an analysis of total charge delivered per day showed that the higher the total charge, the greater the improvement in depressive symptoms ($r=-0.21$; $p<0.001$). Further, at the conclusion of the long-term phase, the 'medium' and 'high' dose cohorts were less likely to have a depressive relapse, suggesting a clinical advantage to higher dosing in order to improve sustained antidepressant VNS response in TRD [39]. For this reason, it is clinically advisable to maximize the current output when doing initial VNS dose titration (as discussed in the section 'Clinical use of VNS in TRD').

Berry *et al.* [49] conducted a meta-analysis of six trials using a Bayesian hierarchical model. This group found that VNS TRD response rates increased over the duration of stimulation; further, the analysis demonstrated that TRD patients receiving VNS were more likely to respond than those receiving TAU alone, using both the Montgomery Åsberg Depression Rating Scale (MADRS; odds ratio = 3.19, 95% confidence interval: 2.12, 4.66) and the Clinical Global Inventory-Improvement scale (CGI-I; odds ratio = 7.00, 95% confidence interval: 4.63, 10.83).

In sum, there have been several VNS TRD efficacy trials, which demonstrate that a significant percentage of TRD patients respond to VNS. Critically, most patients do not respond immediately but rather after several months of sustained stimulation. The response rate in depression after VNS treatment ranges from 30 to 53% [3, 39, 43]. The findings for stimulation parameters in VNS support the importance of providing maximally tolerated higher charge to achieve the highest and the most sustained effect in TRD [39].

Side effects and contraindications for VNS therapy in TRD patients

Side effects and adverse events associated with VNS in TRD

There are currently more than 74 000 individuals in 70 countries implanted with VNS devices (estimated ~74 000 for epilepsy and

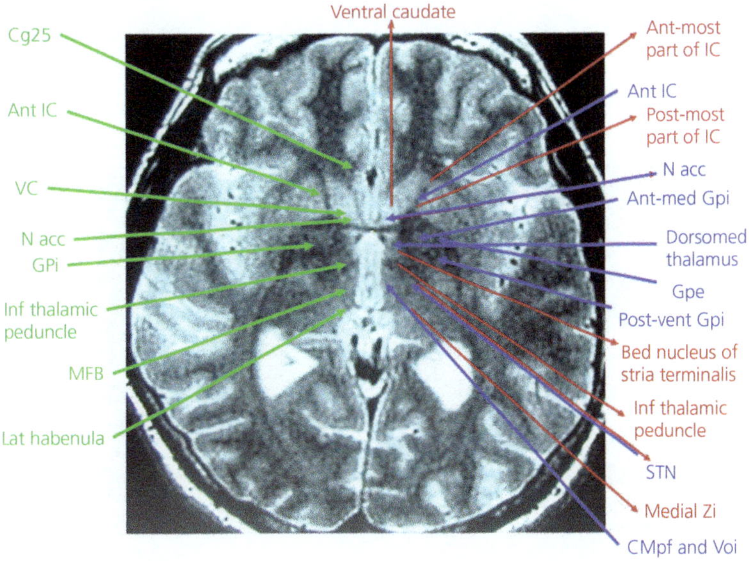

Figure 1.1 Published brain targets submitted to DBS for depression (green) OCD (red), and Tourette (blue). Some targets are overlapping between these three conditions. Note: Not all targets are visible on this axial slice at the level of anterior–posterior commissural plane. Ant-med, anteromedial; Ant-most, anteriormost; Cg25, Cingulum area 25; CMPf, centre median parafascicular nucleus of thalamus; Dorsomed, dorsomedial; GPe, globus pallidus externus; GPi, globus pallidus internus; IC, internal capsule; Inf, inferior; Lat, lateral; MFB, medial forebrain bundle; N acc, Nucleus accumbens; Post-most, posteriormost; Post-vent, posteroventral; STN, subthalamic nucleus; VC, ventral caudate; Voi, nucleus ventralis oralis internus of thalamus; Zi, zona incerta.

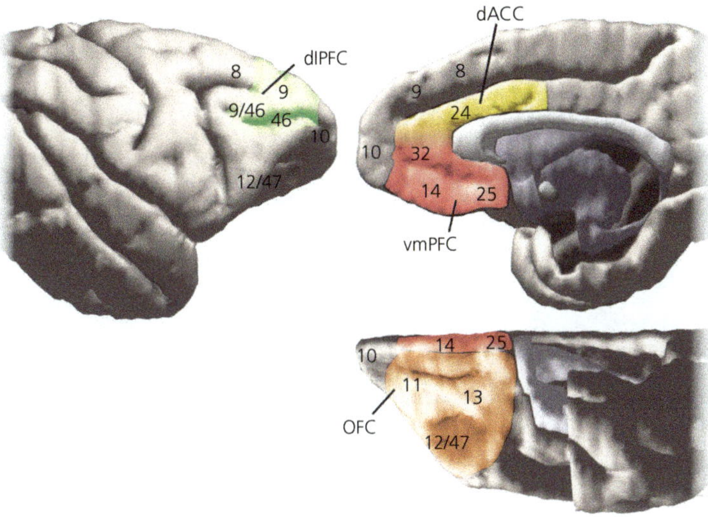

Figure 3.1 Schematic illustrating key PFC regions associated with OCD, addiction, depression and schizophrenia, displayed on the macaque brain. dACC = yellow; DLPFC = green; OFC = orange; vmPFC = red. Source: From Haber and Behrens [1]. Reproduced with permission of Elsevier.

Neuromodulation in Psychiatry, First Edition. Edited by Clement Hamani, Paul Holtzheimer, Andres M. Lozano and Helen Mayberg.

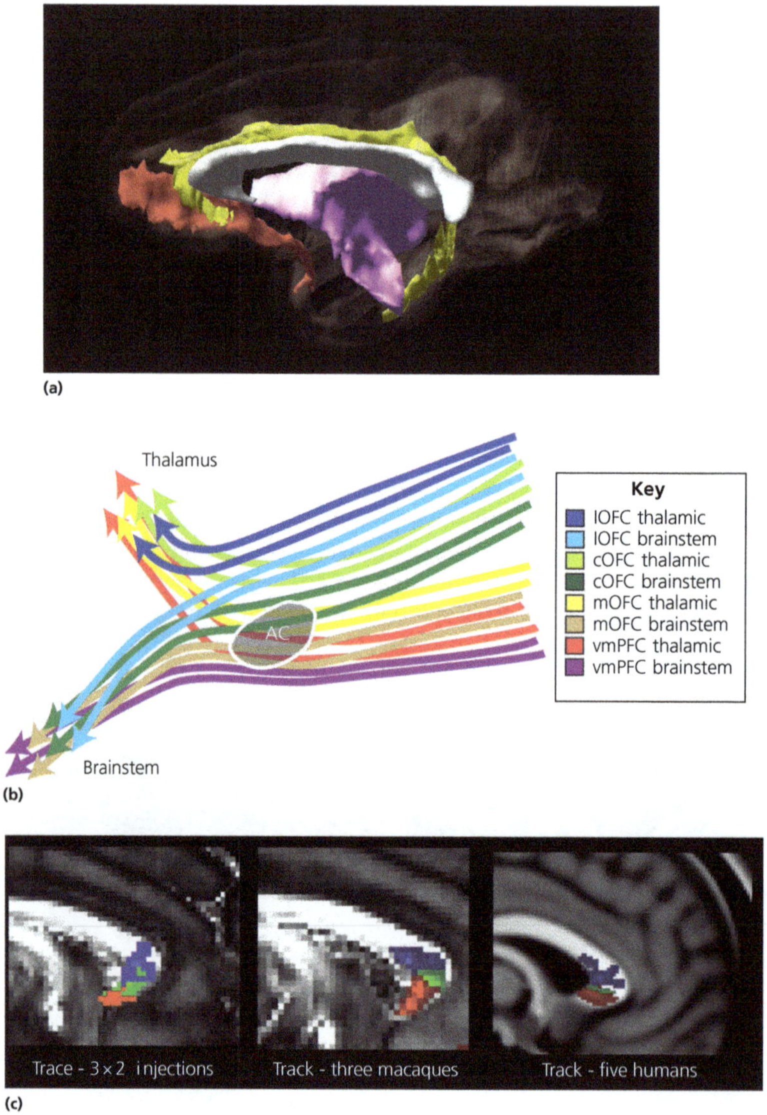

Figure 3.2 WM pathways central to psychiatric disorders. (**a**) 3D renderings of the CC (white), UF (red), ALIC (purple) and CB (yellow) in the monkey brain. (**b**) In the ALIC, vmPFC fibres travel ventral to mOFC fibres, which are ventral to cOFC fibres, which are ventral to lOFC fibres. Each set of axons splits into two bundles in the ALIC: the dorsal bundle travels to the thalamus, while the ventral bundle continues to the brainstem. Adapted from Ref. 101. (**c**) The ventral–dorsal gradient in vPFC fibres in the CC, as seen in monkey tracing (left), monkey dMRI (middle) and human dMRI (right) studies. Source: From Jbabdi et al. [102]. Reproduced with permission of Society for Neuroscience.

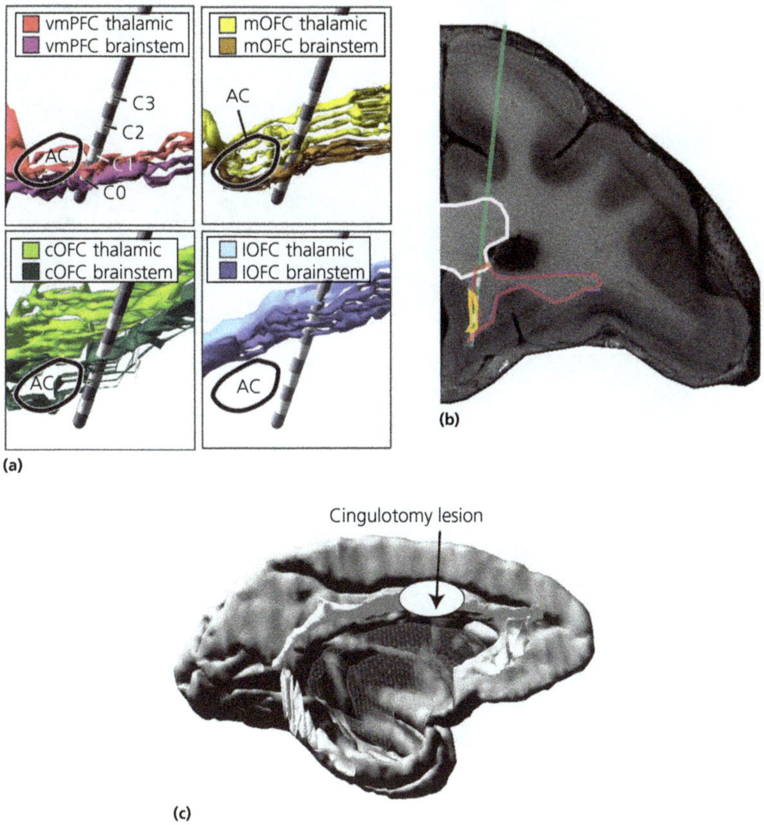

Figure 3.3 WM pathways central to neuromodulatory interventions for psychiatric disorders. (**a**) Each contact on the ALIC electrode intersects a unique set of vmPFC, mOFC, cOFC and lOFC fibres. Adapted from Ref. 101. (**b**) The subcallosal DBS electrode intersects the UF (red), CB (yellow) and CC (white). Adapted from Ref. 117. (**c**) The cingulotomy lesion intersects the dACC and the WM of the anterior portion of the dorsal CB. Source: From Heilbronner and Haber [117]. Reproduced with permission of Society for Neuroscience.

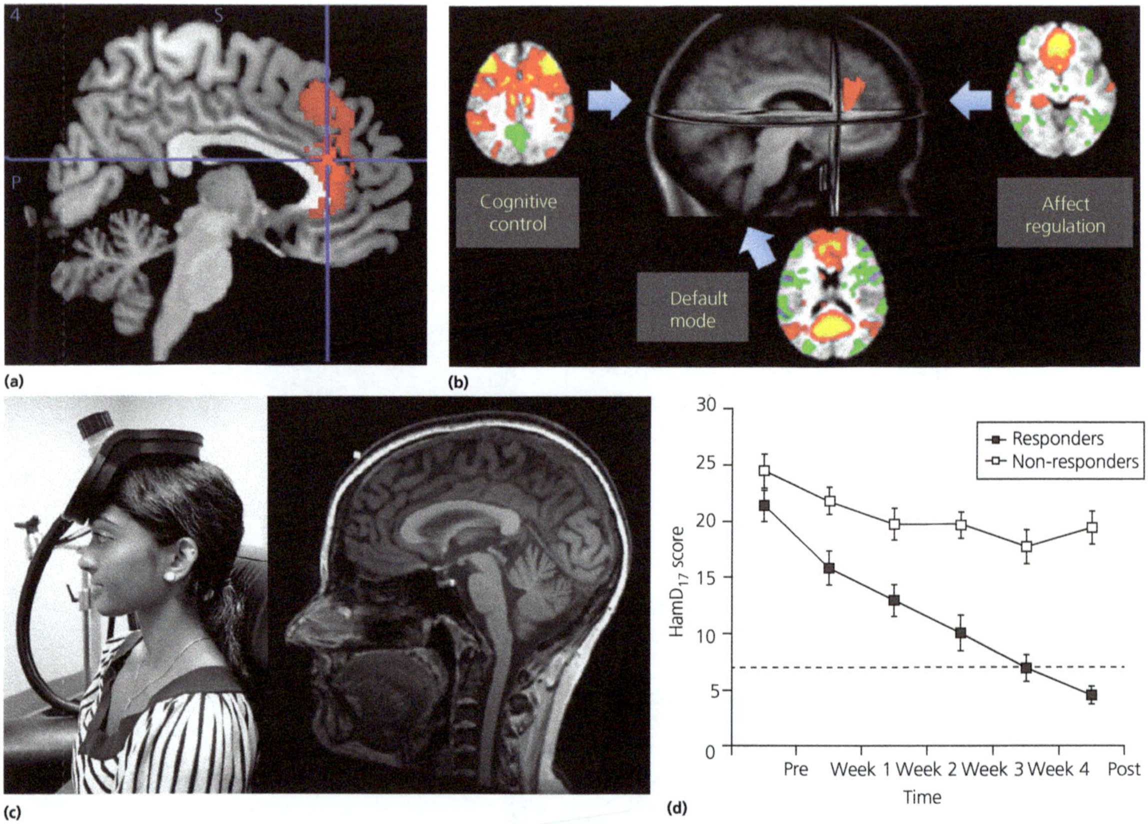

Figure 4.3 Use of MRI in preclinical identification of stimulation targets. (**a**) VBM meta-analyses identified the DMPFC as a region of consistent grey matter volume reduction in major depressive disorder. Source: From Bora et al. [59]. Reproduced with permission of Elsevier. (**b**) rs-fMRI studies also identified the DMPFC as a 'dorsal nexus' region in major depressive disorder, where networks for cognitive control, affect regulation and the 'default mode' intersected. Source: From Adapted from Sheline et al. [60]. Copyright PNAS. (**c**) These findings prompted the development of techniques for applying rTMS to the DMPFC under MRI guidance for the treatment of major depression. (**d**) As suggested by the preclinical work, rTMS of the DMPFC achieved remission in >40% of patients with major depression. Source: c and d reprinted by permission of Elsevier from Downar et al. [45]. Copyright 2013 by the Society of Biological Psychiatry.

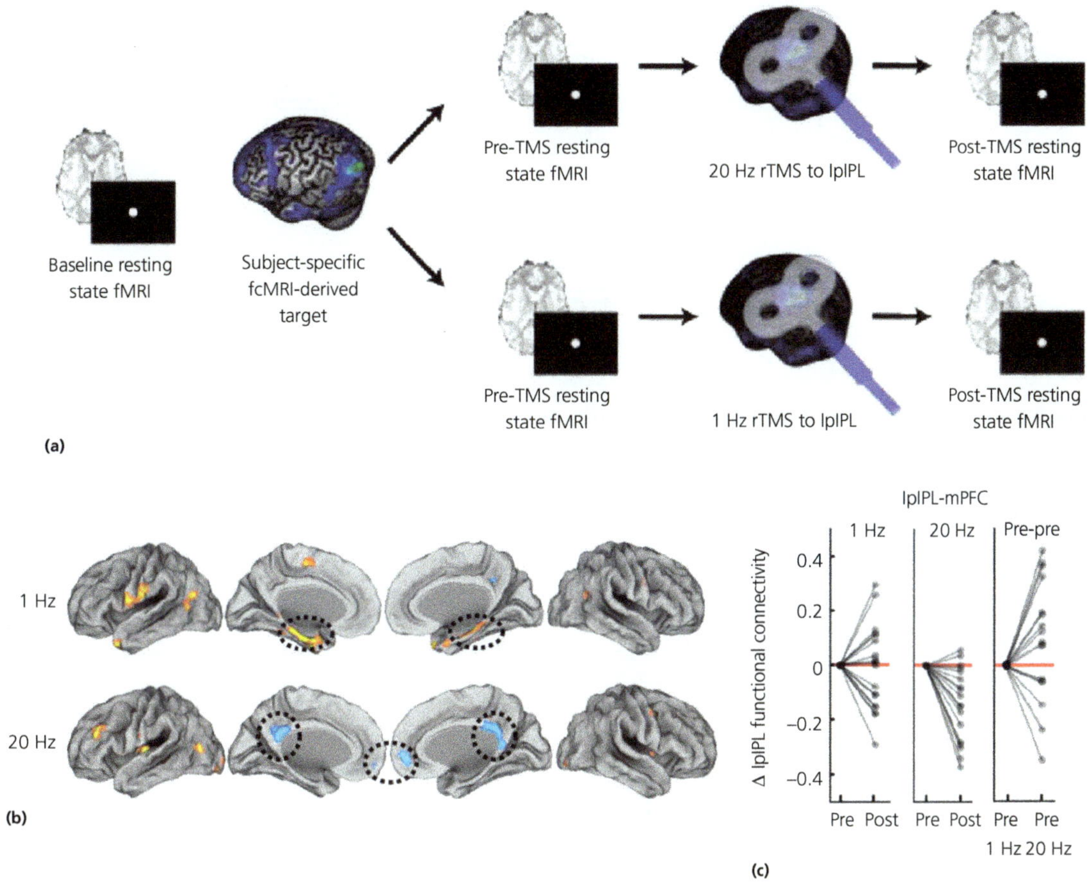

Figure 4.5 Use of MRI in characterizing effects of neuromodulation. (**a**) Eldaief et al. [110] used rs-fMRI to localize the default-mode network in individual subjects. They then applied either 1or 20 Hz rTMS to the left posterior IPL node of this network, using the peak activation coordinate in each subject. (**b**) Comparison of resting-state functional connectivity to the left posterior IPL, on fMRI scans obtained pre- and post-rTMS, revealed that 1 and 20 Hz rTMS produced distinct patterns of increases (orange) or decreases (blue) in whole-brain connectivity to the seed region, thus characterizing the effects of rTMS at the network level. (**c**) Inspection of individual subjects' changes in connectivity between two regions of the default-mode network (the IPL and the MPFC) revealed considerable inter-individual variability in both the magnitude and direction of effect for 1 Hz stimulation. Effects of 20 Hz stimulation were more consistent in direction but still variable in magnitude across subjects. Source: From Eldaidef et al. [110]. Reproduced with permission of PNAS.

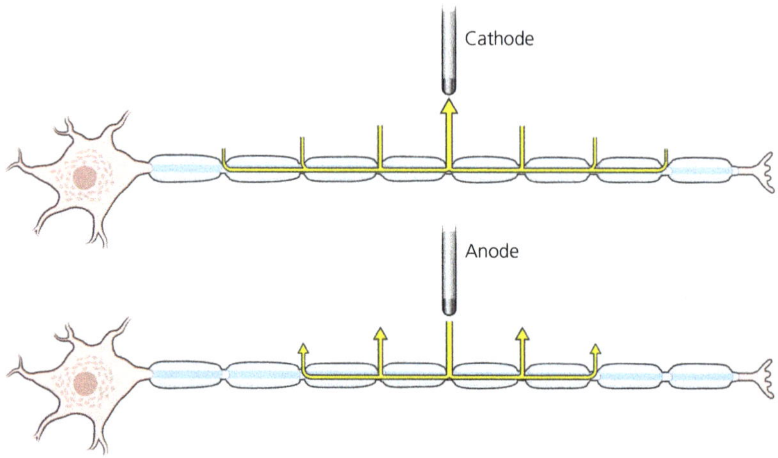

Figure 6.1 Current flow under cathodic and anodic stimulation. Under cathodic stimulation, the highest currents flow outward through the closest nodes of Ranvier, while under anodic stimulation, the opposite process occurs. Source: Illustration by David Schumick, BS, CMI. Reprinted with the permission of the Cleveland Clinic Center for Medical Art & Photography. Copyright 2014.

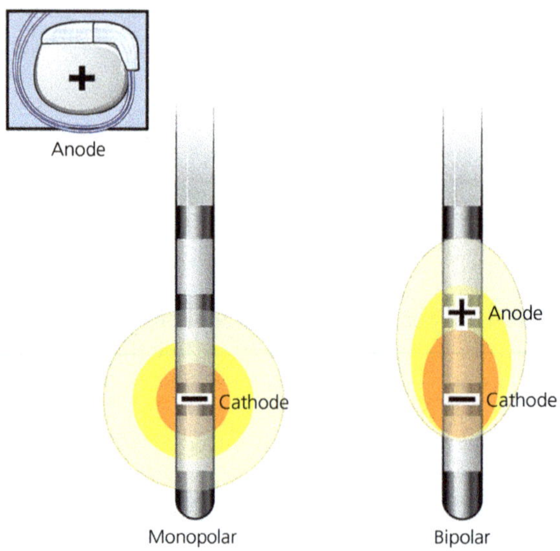

Figure 6.3 Schematic representation of the electrical field generated by different cathode–anode configurations. Monopolar configuration: one (or more) contact is set as the cathode and the pulse generator case is set as the anode. Bipolar stimulation: two contacts (or more) are activated, one as cathode and the other as anode. Source: Illustration by David Schumick, BS, CMI. Reprinted with the permission of the Cleveland Clinic Center for Medical Art & Photography. Copyright 2014.

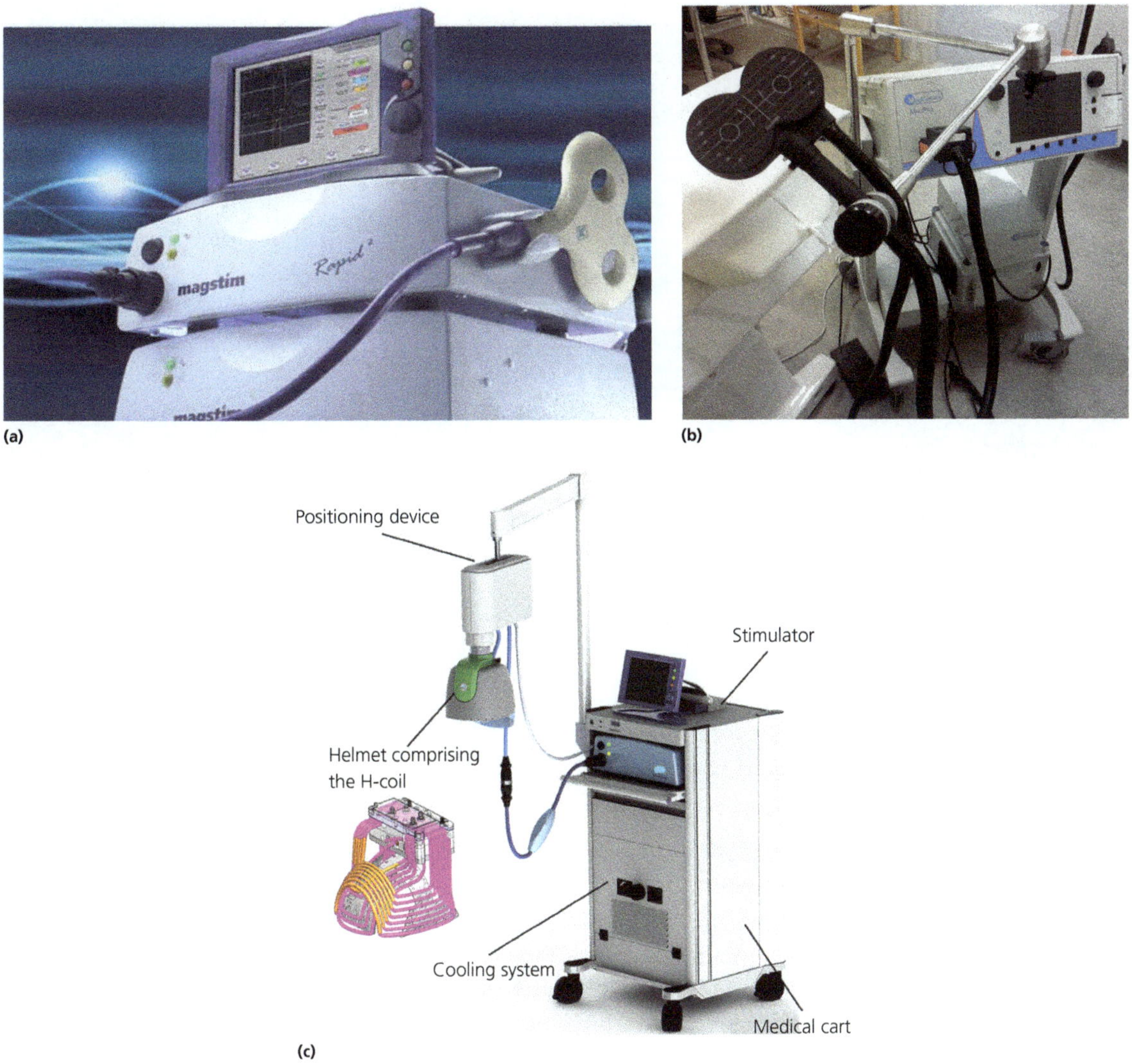

Figure 8.12 Images of TMS devices and coils. (**a**) Magstim Rapid² stimulator and 70 mm figure-8 coil. (**b**) MagVenture MagPro stimulator and C-B60 Butterfly coil. (**c**) Brainsway deep TMS system and H1 coil.

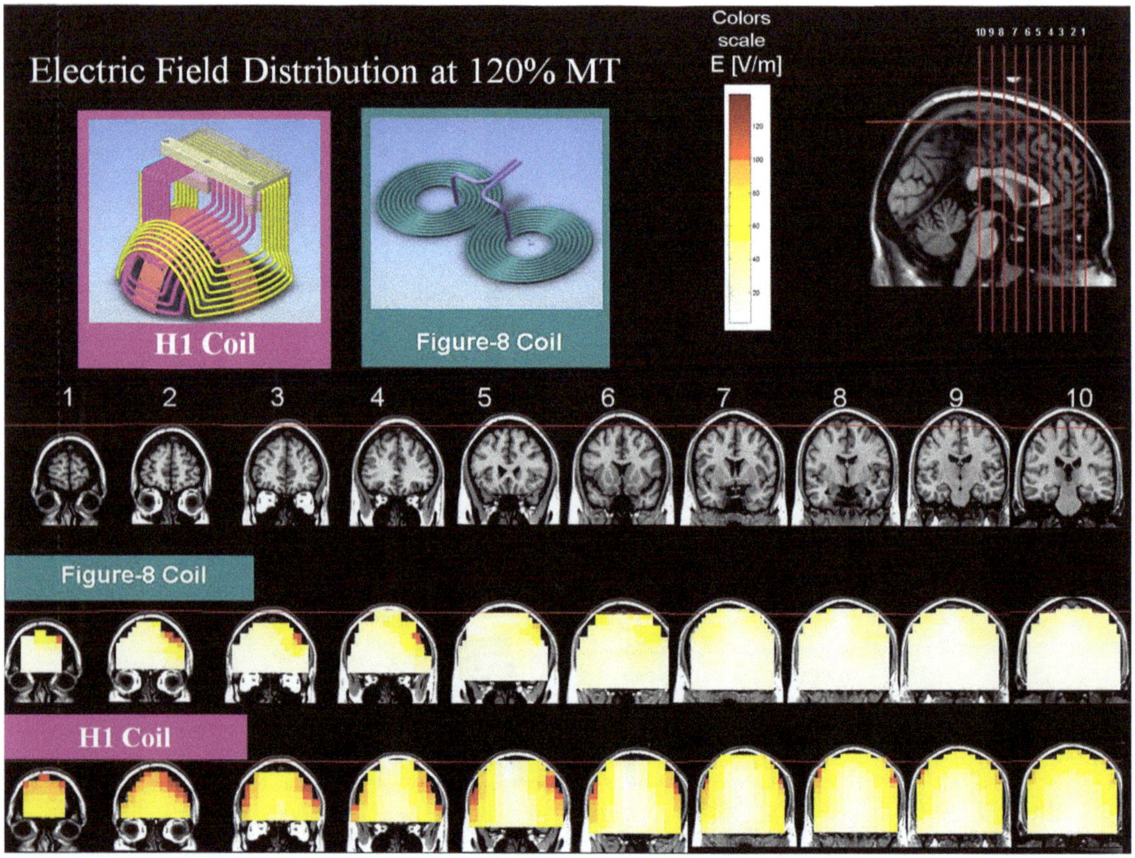

(a)

Figure 8.13 Coloured field maps indicating the electrical field absolute magnitude in each pixel over coronal slices 1 cm apart. The red pixels indicate field magnitude above the threshold for neuronal activation, which was set to 100 V/m. (**a**) Maps for a figure-8 coil and deep TMS H1 coil. The field maps are adjusted for stimulator power output level required to obtain 120% of the hand motor threshold for each coil, at a depth of 1.5 cm. (**b** and **c**) Maps for the 90 mm circular coil (**b**) and the deep TMS H7 coil (**c**). The field maps are adjusted for stimulator power output level required to obtain 100% of the leg motor threshold for each coil, at a depth of 3 cm.

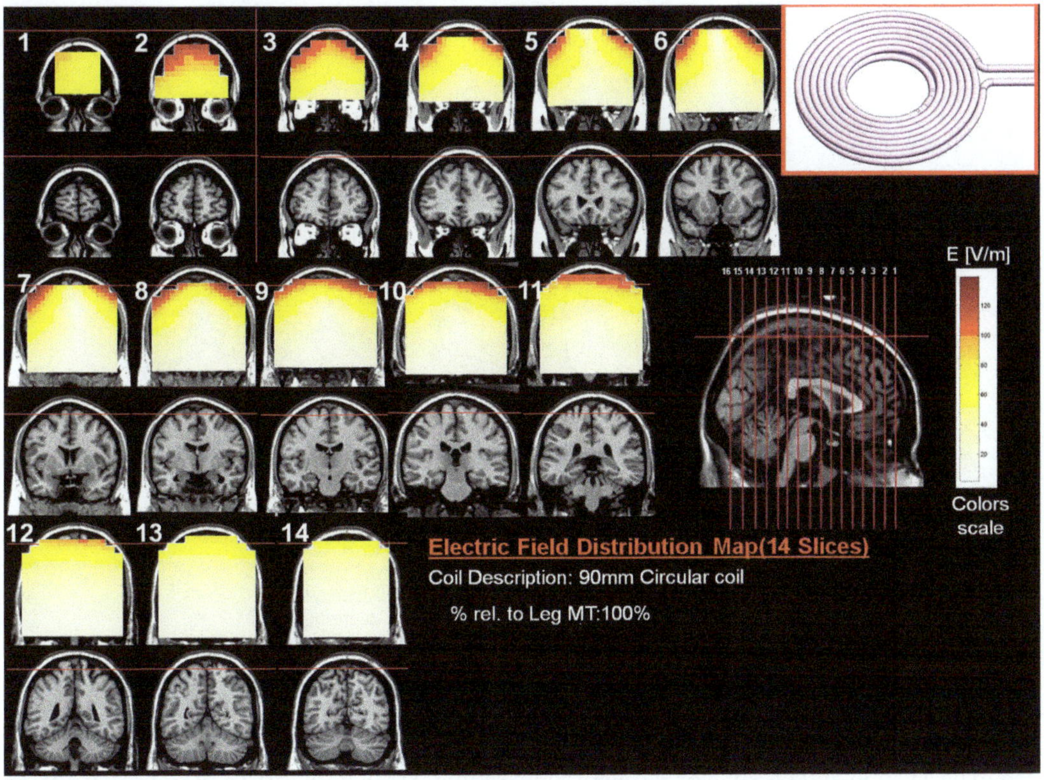

(b)

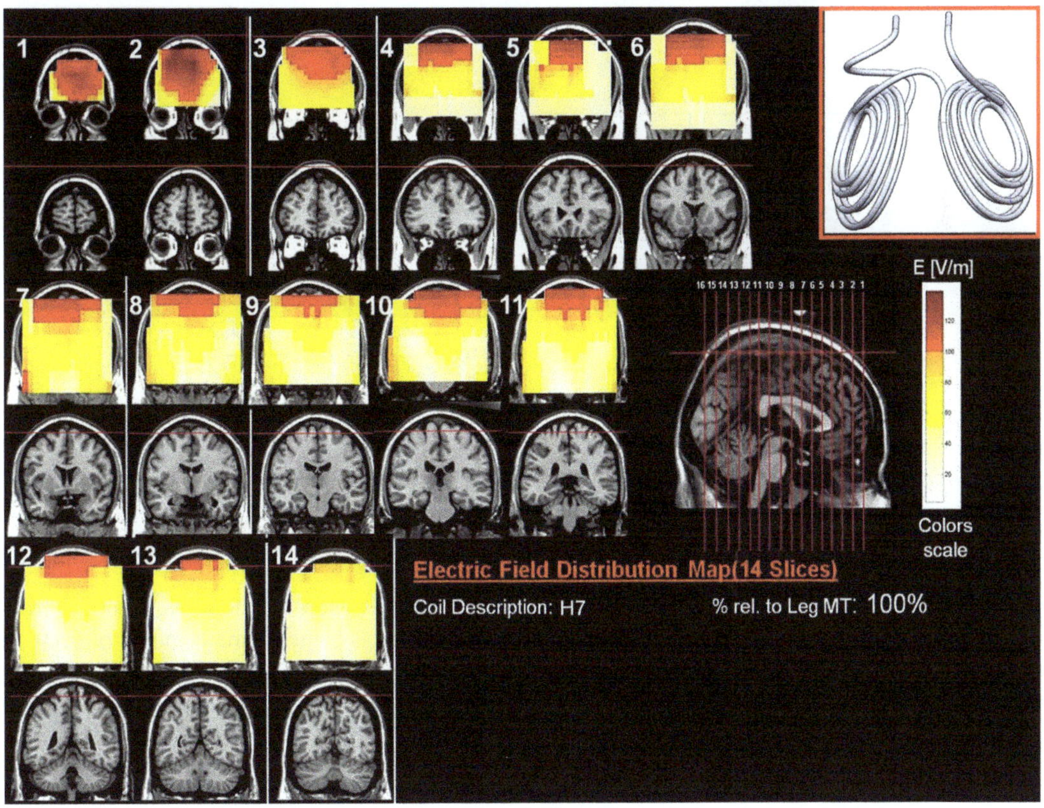

(c)

Figure 8.13 (Continued)

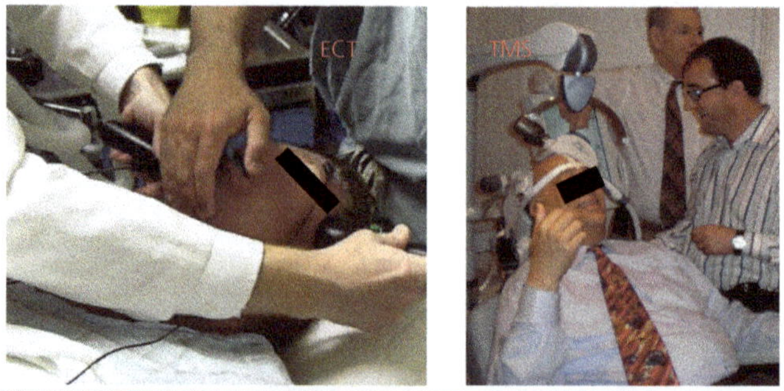

Comparison	ECT	TMS
Anaesthesia?	Yes	No
Seizure?	Yes	No*
Intended population	Severe depression, psychotic subtype	Moderate depression
Setting	ECT suite	Office

Figure 9.2 Comparison of ECT and TMS. In contrast to ECT, TMS does not require anaesthesia, can be given at subconvulsive levels, is not indicated for psychotic or catatonic subtypes of depression and does not need to be given in an ECT suite or recovery room setting. *TMS does carry a risk of seizure at dosages in excess of safety guidelines.

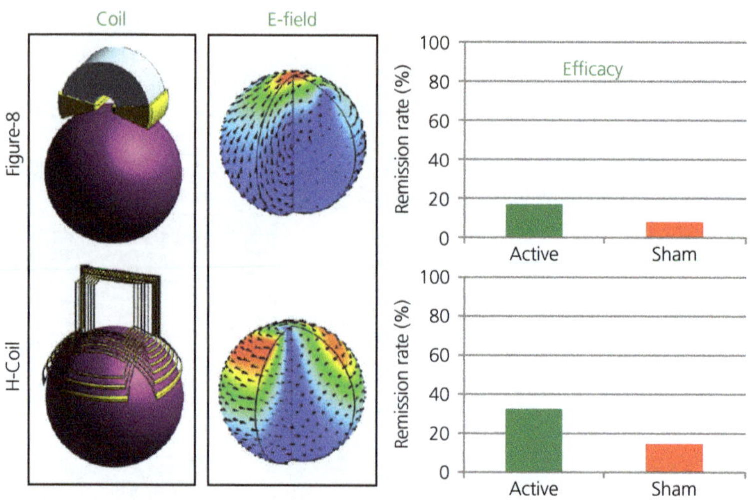

Figure 9.3 TMS coils approved by the FDA for the treatment of depression. Top row: Neuronetics iron-core figure-8 coil. Bottom row: Brainsway H-coil. Left column depicts finite element model of each coil, overlaid on a five concentric spherical model of the head. Middle column: E-field simulation. Right column: efficacy of active and sham TMS from the pivotal trial leading to FDA approval. Source: Adapted from Deng *et al.* [5] and O'Reardon *et al.* [3] and FDA 510K 122288.

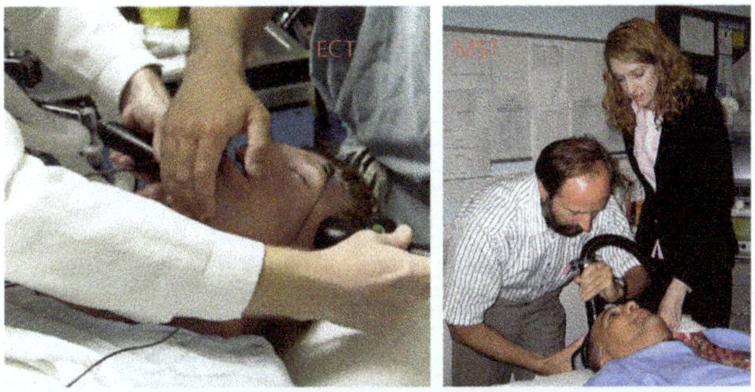

Comparison	ECT	MST
Means of induction	Electrical	Magnetic
Scalp preparation?	Yes	No
Tissue impedance?	Yes	No
Site of stimulation	Diffuse	Focal

Figure 9.4 Comparison of ECT and MST. In contrast to ECT, MST uses electromagnetic induction to trigger the seizure. Scalp preparation is not required as no electricity is applied directly to the scalp. Magnetic induction is not affected by tissue impedance from the scalp or skull. MST is relatively more focal than ECT.

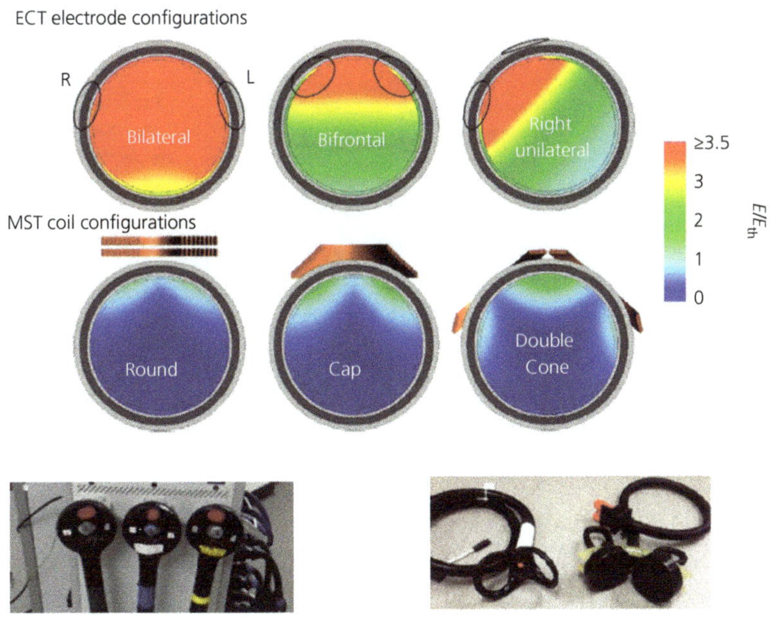

Figure 9.5 Finite element modelling of electric field strength induced in a five-concentric spherical model of the head by ECT (top row) and MST (bottom row) configurations. Adapted from Deng *et al.* [9]. Photo insert on left shows MagStim Theta Round coil switcher box allowing rapid coil swapping between trains. Photo insert on right shows Magstim Double Cone coil for MST on left and MagVenture Twin-Coil on right. Both deliver a field distribution similar to the double-cone configuration.

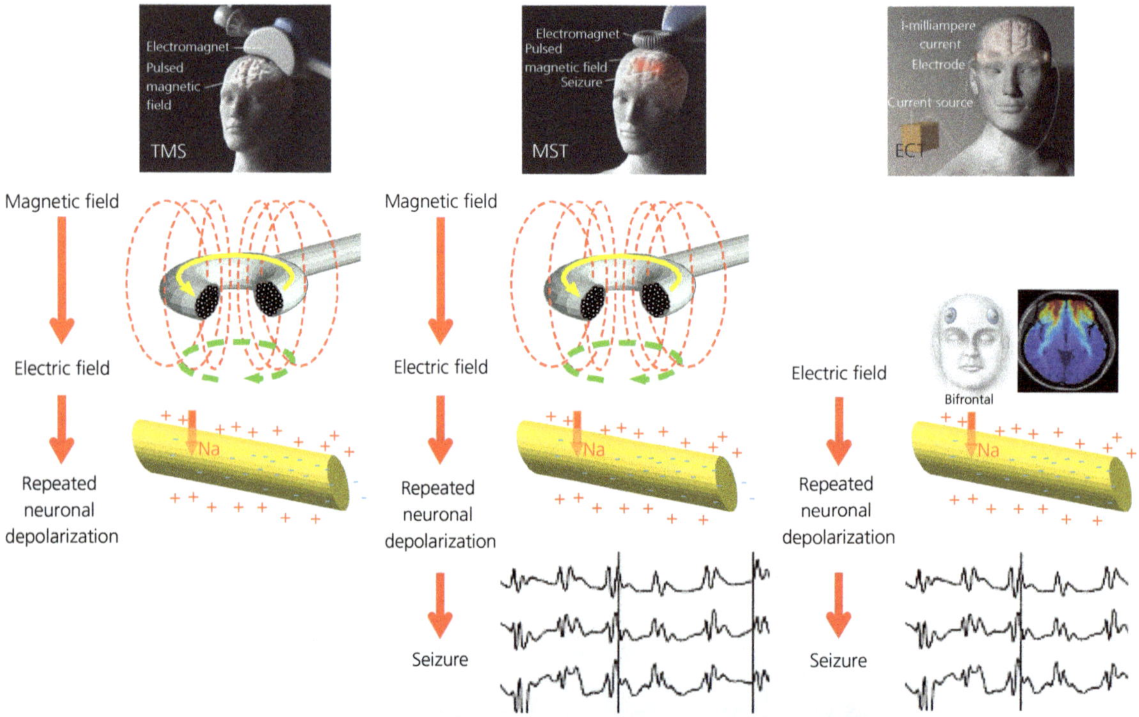

Figure 9.6 Comparative mechanisms of TMS, MST and ECT. TMS and MST share the application of a magnetic field. TMS, MST and ECT all involve the repeated application of an electric field, which induces repeated neuronal depolarization. In the case of MST and ECT, this results in deliberate seizure induction. TMS can induce a seizure at sufficiently high dosage, and this is a known potential side effect.

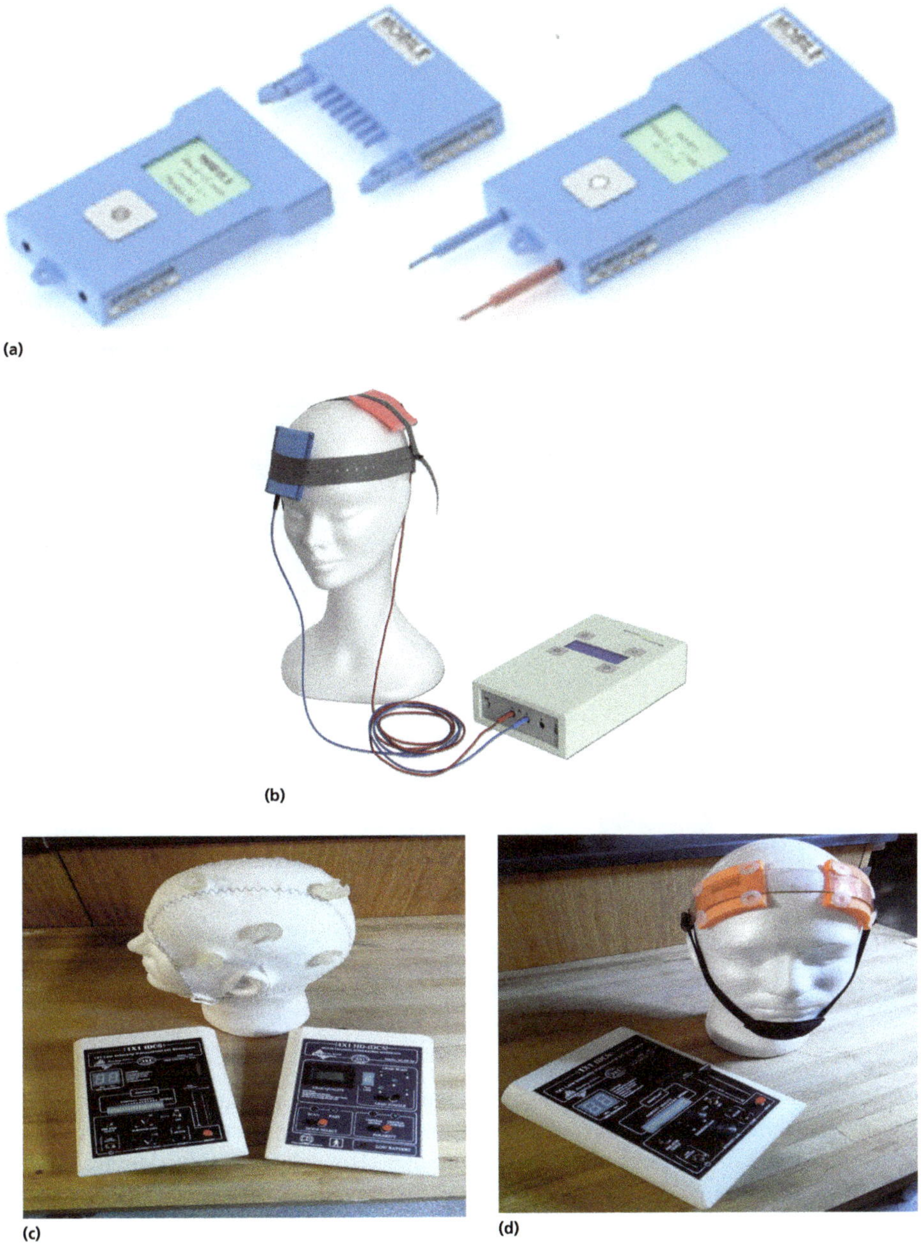

Figure 11.1 Examples of commercial tDCS devices. All devices are composed by a power generator (batteries) and electrodes that are placed over the scalp. (**a**) 'Mobile' tDCS device of Neuroconn™ DC-stimulator, presenting increased portability, due to its low size. (**b**) Neuroconn™ device, one 'standard' tDCS device used in clinical research. The electrodes and the sponges placed over the scalp are illustrated. (**c**) Soterix™ 1-1 and 4×1 (high-definition) tDCS devices, also 'standard' tDCS devices used in clinical research. (**d**) Soterix™ device with EASYstraps™ (headbands) and EASYpads™ (sponges). Source: Reproduced with permission of neuroConn and Copyright Soterix Medical.

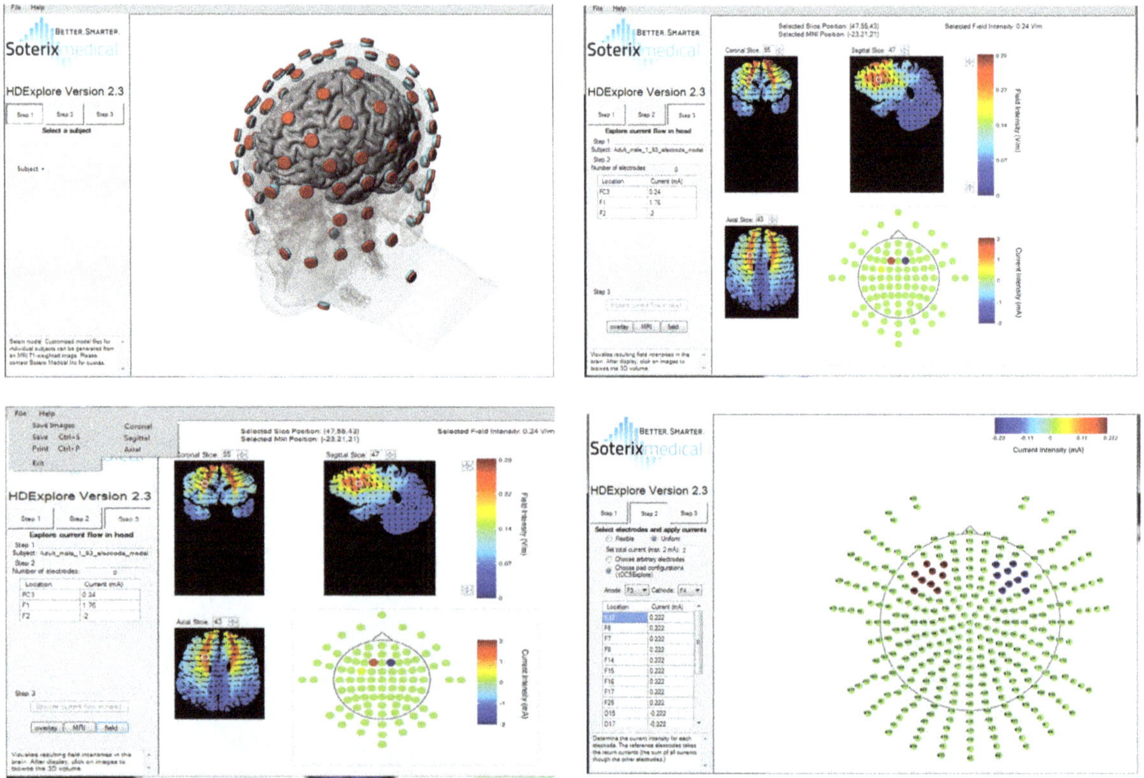

Figure 11.3 Software used for tDCS modelling studies. The dots in the phantoms' head represent possible spots for electrode placement. The software simulates current density under the anode and the cathode according to the placement of the electrodes. Source: Images provided by Soterix Medical.

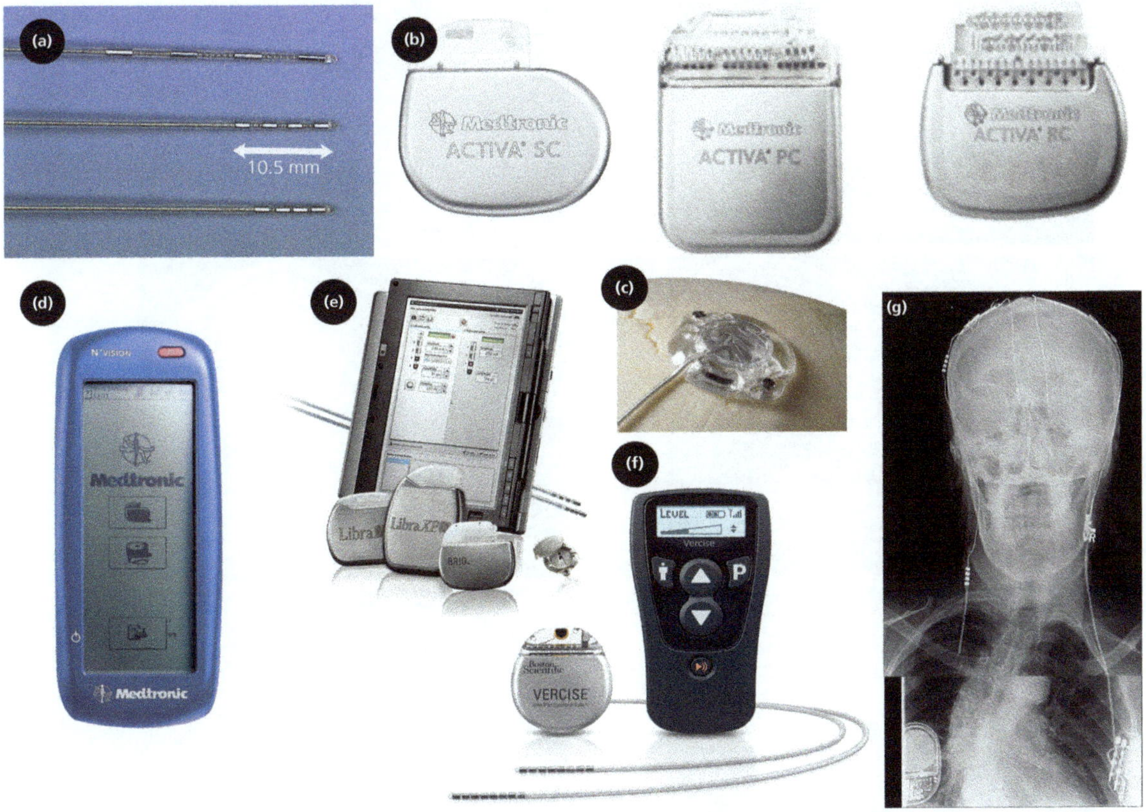

Figure 13.2 Deep brain stimulation equipment. (**a**) DBS leads of different configurations. The contacts of the bottom two leads are 1.5 mm long cylinders, separated by 1.5 mm (middle lead) or 0.5 mm (bottom lead). The upper electrode array has larger contacts (3.0 mm) and wider spacing (3.0 mm) adapted for use in the anterior internal capsule (e.g. for OCD; in the United States, this is the only use for which this lead is approved by the FDA, under a HDE). (**b**) Internal pulse generators (IPGs) are primary cell (left and middle) or rechargeable (right), and either single channel (left) or dual-channel (middle, right). (**c**) StimLoc ring for anchoring the DBS lead to the bone and covering the burr hole. (**d**) IPGs are programmed telemetrically. Source: a–d reproduced with permission of Medtronic. (**e**) St. Jude Medical also offers single (left) and dual-channel (centre, right) IPGs, as well as a dual-channel rechargeable IPG (right); depicted also are the DBS electrodes, and the burr-hole anchoring device. Source: Reproduced with permission of St Jude Medical. (**f**) Boston Scientific offers a dual-channel rechargeable IPG, and DBS leads with eight closely spaced contacts. Source: Reproduced with permission of Roshini Jain. (**g**) X-ray showing bilateral DBS leads, extension cables connected in the head (left side of figure) and neck (right side of figure), and IPGs. In fact, the latter is a poor location for the DBS-to-extension connection to be located, which predisposes to breakage, which occurred with a previous right extension cable where the connection was in the neck (left side of figure).

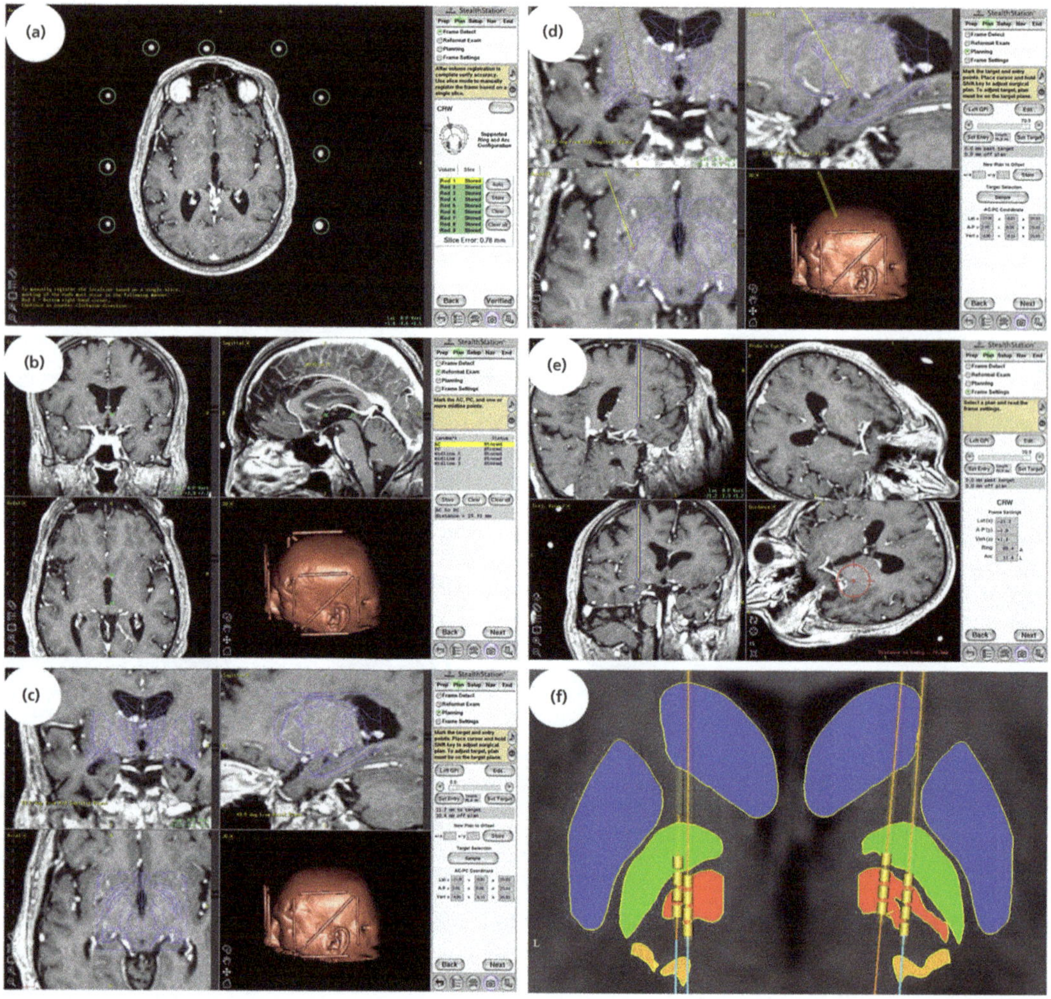

Figure 13.3 Stereotactic planning of DBS electrodes. Images from the Stealth Framelink software (Medtronic), showing the stages of planning a DBS electrode insertion. (**a**) The contrast-enhanced MRI is performed after affixing the stereotactic frame base ring (in this case a CRW Stereotactic System, Integra). The locations of the fiducial bars (9 circled points) is noted by the software, to register the brain MRI space to the physical space of the frame allowing transformations of brain targets to the instrument holder. (**b**) The locations of the anterior commissure (AC) and posterior commissure (PC), and the line connecting them, provide a consistent internal reference for a 3D space in which common functional stereotactic targets such as the basal ganglia can be targeted. Here AC and PC are noted in the software for targeting with respect to the AC–PC line (synonymous with a so-called Talairach space). The 3D reconstruction of the fiducial localizer box is seen in the bottom right corner. (**c**) Most software programs allow a digital version of the classic Schaltenbrand and Wahren (or other) atlas to be co-registered to the patient's MRI scan via AC/PC coordinates, to aid in so-called indirect targeting. Here the target in the globus pallidus (red dot) has been selected based on its relationship to the AC–PC line and the atlas. (**d**) The entry point is chosen to provide a rational trajectory for the DBS lead (i.e. here proceeding rostrally through the globus pallidus) and to avoid critical neurovascular structures. This image shows the trajectory on coronal (upper left), sagittal (upper right) and axial (bottom left) images; in each plane the oblique trajectory is out-of-plane. (**e**) The path is in 'trajectory' views that depict the whole trajectory in one plane allowing easy visualization of veins and arteries and the ventricle that may lay in the path. (**f**) Planning can include a depiction of the location of the DBS lead(s) with respect to brain structures. In this case, we have used our proprietary software (OneTrack) to depict a coronal trajectory view of the basal ganglia in a patient-specific fashion, allowing us to see the location of the DBS leads with respect to the globus pallidus in this patient who underwent bilateral anteromedial and posterolateral globus pallidus DBSs for Tourette Syndrome. Source: Courtesy of K. Mewes, Emory University.

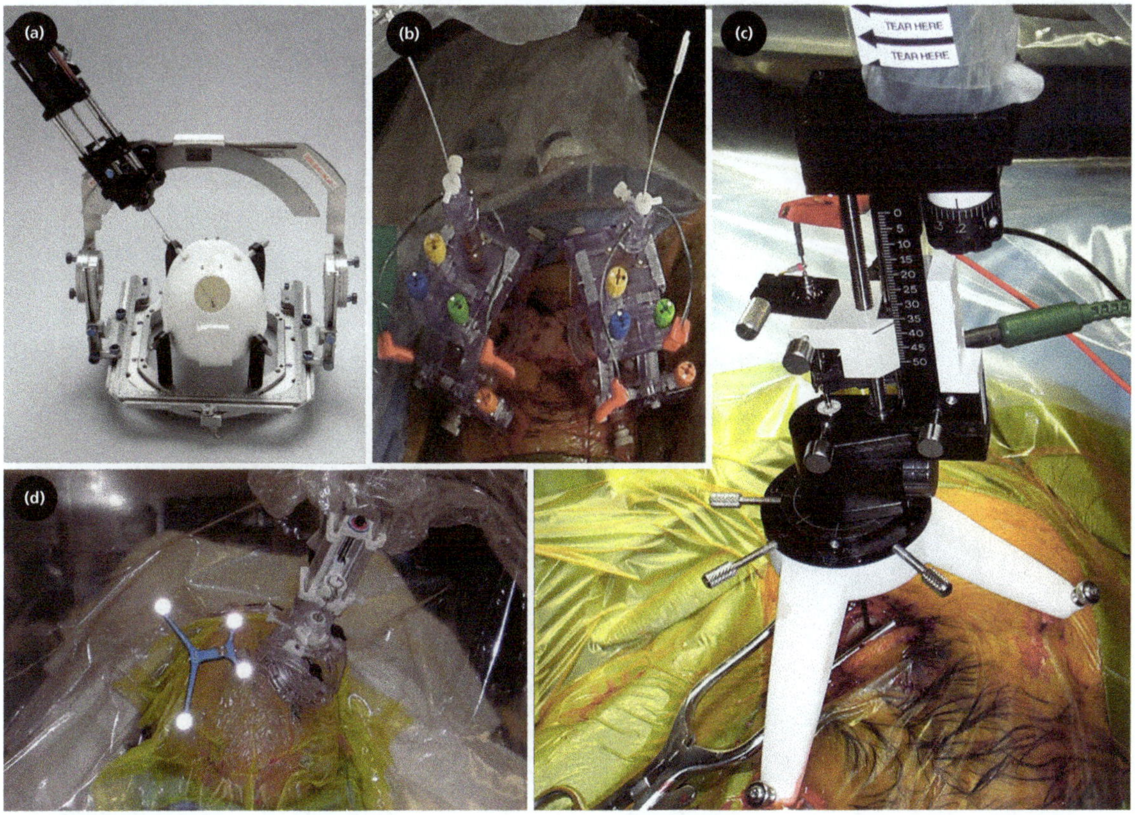

Figure 13.4 Classic and modern stereotactic devices. Classic frames, such as the CRW (**a**, Integra), incorporate the fiducials into the stereotactic device using an attached localizer (see Figure 13.1b) during imaging to relate and transform the brain imaging (MRI, CT) space to the physical frame space. The relationship, yielding frame coordinates for adjusting the instrument holder (stereotactic arc, as shown), is calculated using software or by direct measurement on X-ray, CT and/or MRI. Newer stereotactic devices use different approaches. The microTargeting platform (**c**, Fred Haer Corp.) physically separates the imaging fiducials from the frame. The fiducials are physically attached to the patient's head before CT and MRI imaging and the trajectory is planned on proprietary software. An acrylic stereotactic platform is custom-manufactured (white tripod in **c**) that attaches to the fiducials, instantiating in physical space the imaging-planned trajectory (the picture shows the microelectrode drive attached to the platform). The NexFrame (**d**, Medtronic) also separates the fiducials from the frame. A CT is performed with fiducials attached and co-registered to an MRI for trajectory planning. In the operating room, the relationship of the imaging fiducials to the NexFrame, a plastic stereotactic device affixed atop the burr hole, is calculated by software after detection of their location in physical space using a camera to visualize reflective balls (seen in picture attached to the stereotactic device). The Clearpoint Smartframe (**b**, MRI Interventions) utilizes a fiducial cannula prefilled with gadolinium. The stereotactic device is affixed to the patient in the MRI scanner, and the relationship of the cannula (physical space) to the brain space is determined with an MRI. The software calculates the necessary adjustments to align the attached tower containing the fiducial cannula to the planned trajectory, which are made using four coloured knobs. The DBS is inserted through the fiducial cannula, as shown.

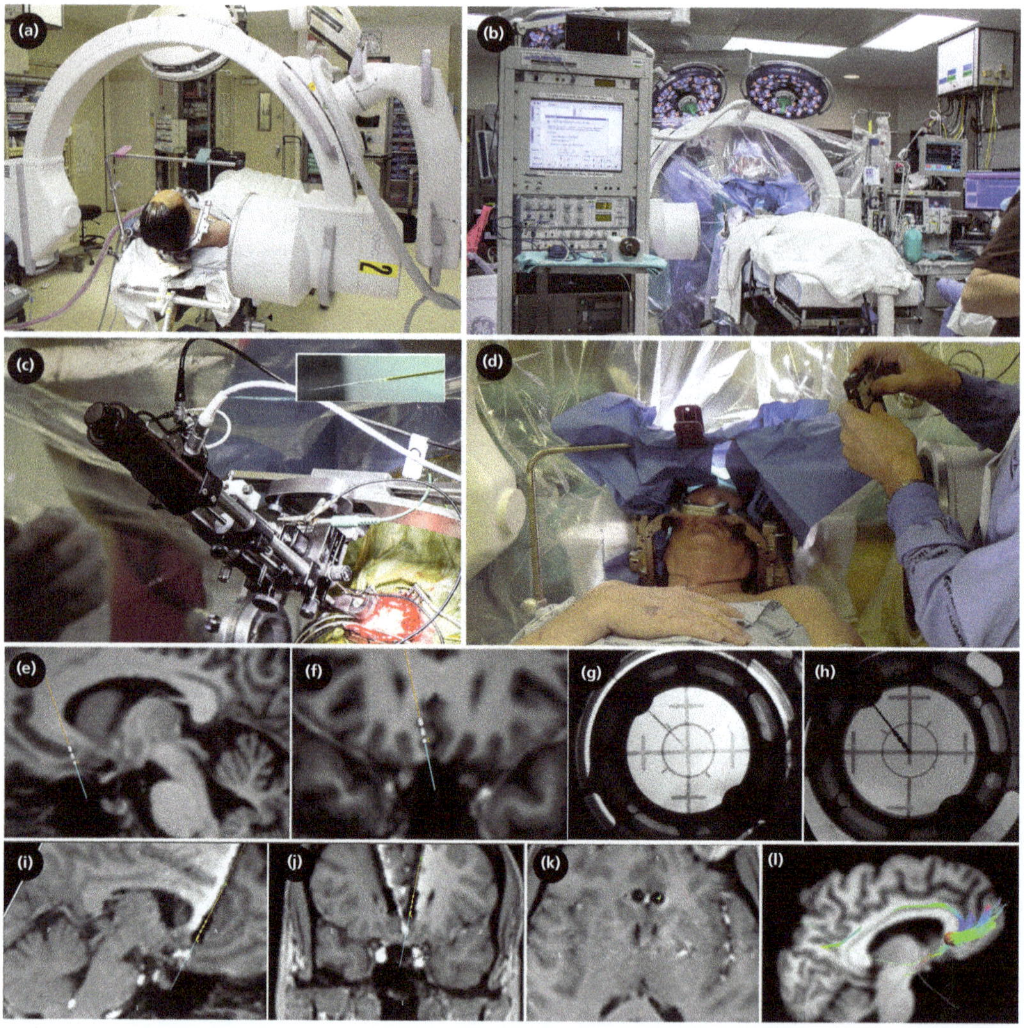

Figure 13.5 DBS insertion in the operating room, using microelectrode and/or stimulation mapping. In procedures performed in the OR, the patient is positioned comfortably supine (**a**), in this case with a CRW frame affixed to the table (in NexFrame and microTargeting platform cases, the head is held in a cervical collar rather than affixed to the table). For radiological control, a C-arm is positioned for lateral fluoroscopy (**a** and **b**): by alignment through the middle of the frame it provides stereotactic accuracy feedback in the sagittal plane (anterior/posterior and superior/inferior) but does not indicate medial/lateral accuracy (**g** and **h**). In contrast, 3D imaging with CT or MRI provides radiological control in all three planes (see Figure 13.6). The surgeon remains behind a sterile clear drape (**b**) to maintain sterility while still being able to monitor the patient, who may remain awake during some or all of the procedure. The MER equipment is seen to the left in (**b**). The microelectrode is driven in by an electric microdrive (**c**, Axon Instruments) controlled by the operator; the high-impedance microelectrode is inset in (**c**). Thus, a physiological map of the target area is developed and overlain upon the MRI scan (**e**, sagittal; **f**, coronal; in this case using our proprietary OneTrack software). Radiological accuracy is checked by lateral fluoroscopy (**g**). Following microelectrode mapping (if used), the DBS is inserted through the same cannula and the accuracy checked (**h**). Stimulation mapping to check for clinical benefits and/or side effects is performed in the awake patient (**d**). After affixing the lead to the skull, post-operative imaging (MRI and/or CT) is performed, and the image can be overlain upon the intraoperative map depicted in the OneTrack software (**i**, sagittal; **j**, coronal; **k**, axial) to check for accurate implantation and to guide post-operative programming decisions with respect to contact(s) utilized for stimulation. **(l)** DTI of white matter pathways, in this case of the subgenual cingulate region, can aid in targeting as well, and may one day – in combination with 3D radiological control (see Figure 13.6) – obviate the need for microelectrode mapping. (OneTrack images – courtesy of K. Mewes, Emory University; DTI image – courtesy of K. Choi and H. Mayberg, Emory University).

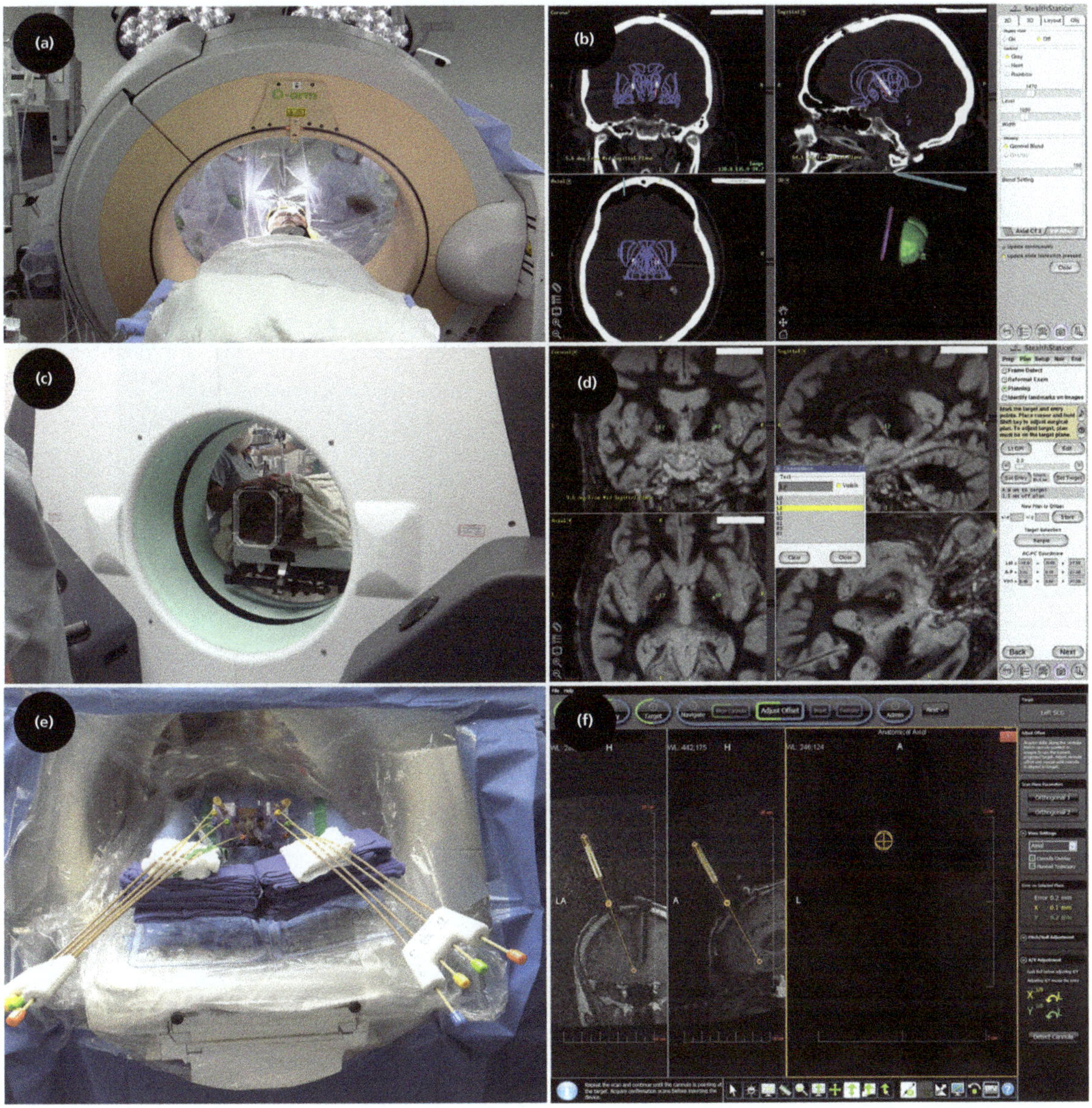

Figure 13.6 Three-dimensional (3D) radiological control. 3D radiological control is the gold standard for ascertaining final DBS implantation accuracy and is the *best* when it occurs intraoperatively when adjustments can more easily be made than post-operatively (**a**). Several options are available at present. The O-arm (Medtronic) is a flat-panel cone-beam CT scanner that provides both intraoperative lateral and anterior/posterior fluorography as well as 3D CT scanning (**b**) (albeit with somewhat less resolution that traditional fan-beam CT). It can be used for determining intraoperative accuracy by co-registration to the pre-operative MRI using the Stealth neuronavigational workstation. Source: a and b are courtesy of K. Holloway, Medical College of Virginia. True fan-beam intraoperative CT scanning is available using the Bodytom (**c**) or the smaller Ceretom (Samsung Neurologica). The intraoperative CT scans can similarly be co-registered to the pre-operative MRI using neuronavigational software (e.g. Stealth, **d**). Source: c and d are courtesy of F. Ponce, Barrow Neurological Institute. Surgery can be performed in the MRI suite (**e**), or in the operating room using an intraoperative MR unit. In this case, DBS insertion is performed after aligning the stereotactic device (e.g. Clearpoint as shown in **e** and **f**, MRI Interventions) and checking insertion accuracy with a ceramic stylet inserted through a peel-away sheath. Any inaccuracies are immediately seen on the MRI scan and can be adjusted before closure.

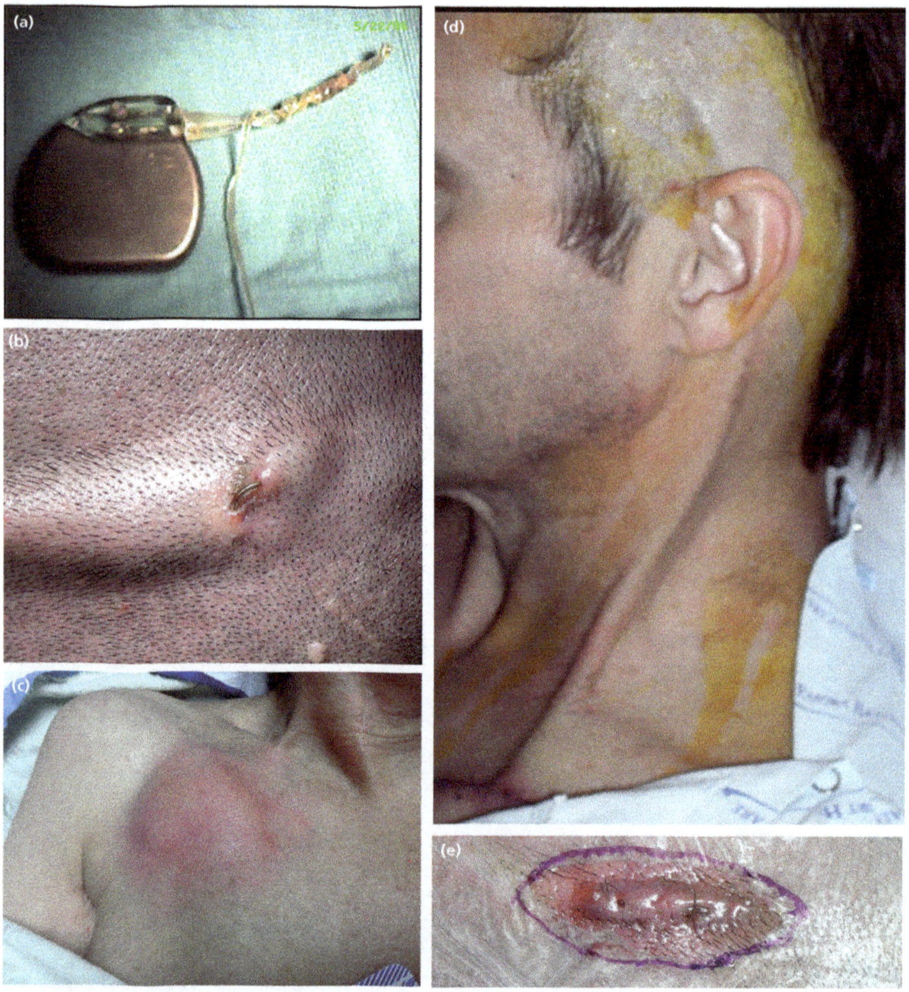

Figure 13.7 Some complications of DBS. (**a**) A case of 'twiddling': the patient rotated the IPG over and over until the tension on the wires caused them to break. This presented in a manner typical for lead or extension wire fracture, with loss of benefit and high impedance of the system detected during programming, prompting intraoperative investigation. (**b**) Erosions of the hardware through the skin can be infected, or sterile as in this case of erosion due to a loop of the DBS lead. The skin in fact has healed below the wire so that it comes out and goes back into the skin. This was repaired surgically without requiring removal. Infected systems often present with cellulitis (**c**); in many cases this can be treated with antibiotics alone, if no fluid collection has developed that envelopes and permeates the hardware. In the latter circumstance, all exposed hardware almost invariably needs to be removed and replaced at a later date. Less clear is the circumstance shown in E, a chronic erosion. We perform complete debridement of the affected region, which usually cultures positively, and rotate a scalp advancement with the assistance of plastic surgery colleagues; this is effective approximately 50% of the time for chronic erosions. Bowstringing is another hardware-related complication (**e**), due to a hypertrophic scar capsule forming around the extension wires. This tethers the DBS-to-extension wire connection to the IPG, although the extension wire within the capsule is freely mobile. Removing the extension wire is not sufficient: the picture shows the appearance in this patient *after* the wire had been removed. In these extreme cases, severing the scar capsule at four or five places releases the tension band and mitigates the tethering.

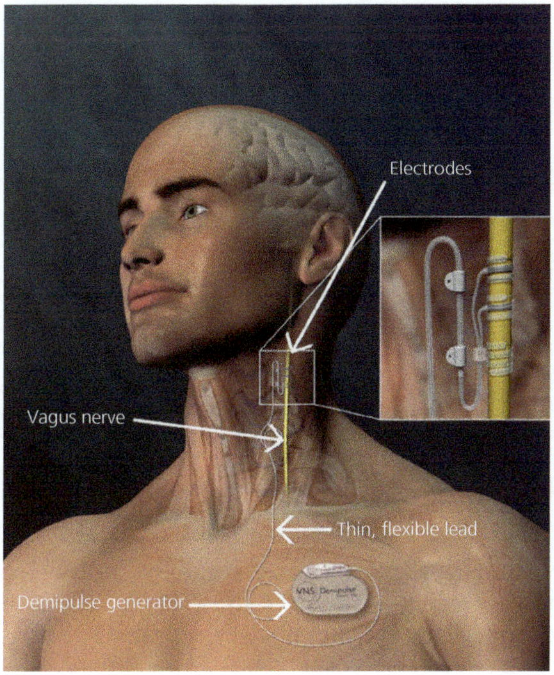

Figure 18.1 Illustration of the attachment of the VNS lead to the mid-cervical region of the left vagus nerve. The bipolar lead is coiled around the vagus in two adjacent regions with a tether attached to the surrounding fascia to prevent lead movement under tension. Source: Reproduced with permission of Cyberonics.

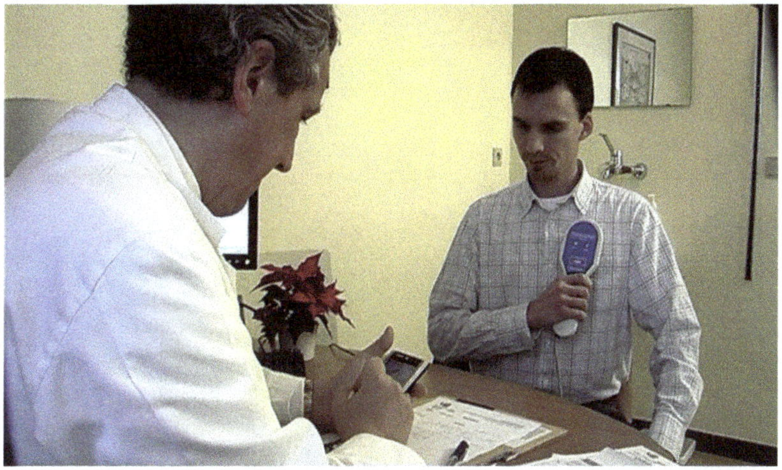

Figure 18.2 Demonstration of the use of the programming wand and handheld programmer. The wand is positioned directly over the device. Using a handheld programming device, the VNS generator can be assessed for circuit integrity (stimulus being successfully transmitted to vagus nerve) as well as programming the electrical parameters being delivered during VNS. Source: Reproduced with permission of Cyberonics.

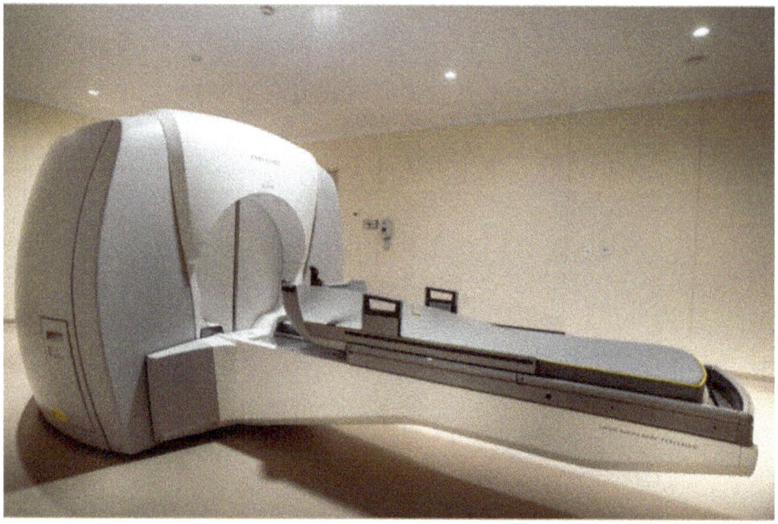

Figure 19.2 Gamma Knife Perfexion® last model installed in the HCor (Hospital do Coração) neuroscience in Sao Paulo, Brazil. This model can be called 'Plus' with the addition of a cone beam computed tomography at the entrance of the device to check the patient's position and target.

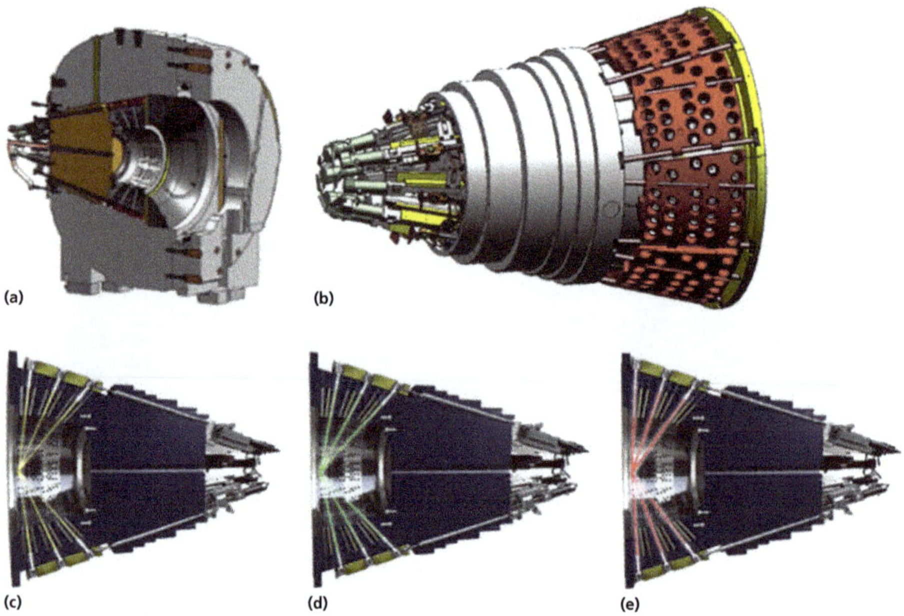

Figure 19.3 Conic collimation system of the GK Perfexion. Notice in (**a**) demonstration of the cross section of the device showing the three main sectors of the collimator, with the motor capable to move the sectors, the site for location of the sources and the helmet with the pores of three different sizes, 4, 8 and 16 mm in diameter. (**b**) Shows a complete view of the device, including motors, and (**c**), (**d**) and (**e**) demonstrate the radiation with the three collimations.

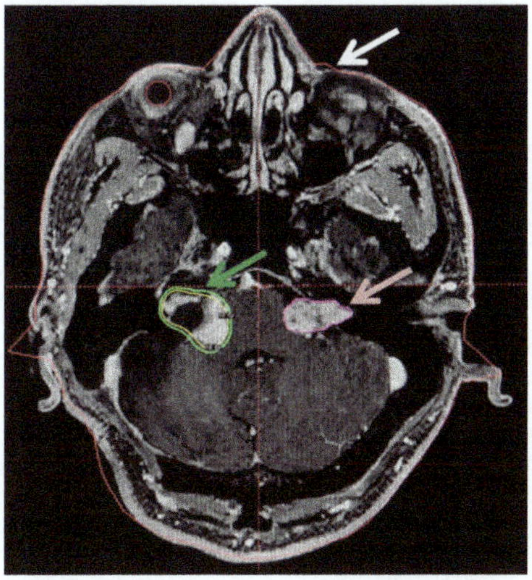

Figure 19.4 Steps of planning; T1 MRI image with 1 mm thickness obtained days before the procedure fused to a CT on the day of the procedure with the patient having the stereotactic frame for definition of coordinates. The CT also provides the automatic contour of the patient's head; notice the white arrow showing the red line contouring the image, which defines the surface of the patient for calculation of beam attenuation. The tumour on the right of the figure demonstrated the segmentation of the lesion, which was contoured with the automatic tools of the software, determining the volume of the lesion (pink arrow). The green arrow demonstrates the multiple-isocentre-depicted isodoseline. It conforms to a partially removed acoustic neuroma in the neurofibromatosis patient. Notice the two lines, yellow and green, representing the 12 Gy and the 10 Gy lines, respectively.

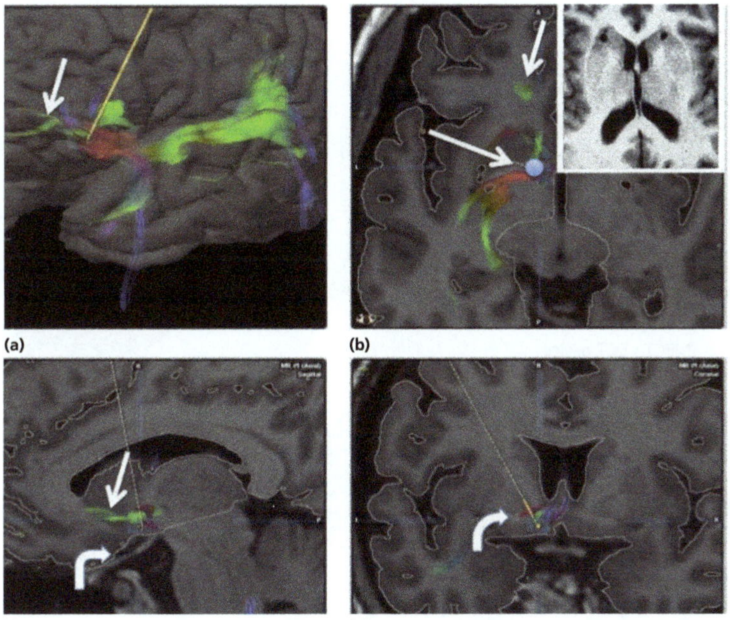

Figure 19.6 Notice the fibres in the direction of the frontal lobe that are interrupted by the capsulotomy (white arrows). (**a**) 3D visualization of fibretracking from the anterior limb of the internal capsule with spread of fibres to the frontal area, and also to the temporal lobe and associated areas in the temporo-parietal region (**b**). Depth of the intended lesion to achieve the shell of the accumbens (large arrow) The inset in the upper right shows an example of an ideal radiofrequency lesion between the putamen and caudate. Courtesy of Dr. Marwan Hariz. (**c**) Sagittal view showing the safe distance of target to the optic nerve (curve arrow). (**d**) Relationship of the posterior portion of the lesion that should not extend to the anterior commissure, which is approximately 20 mm posterior to the centre of the lesion (fibretracking produce by Dr. Mark Sedrak in our group).

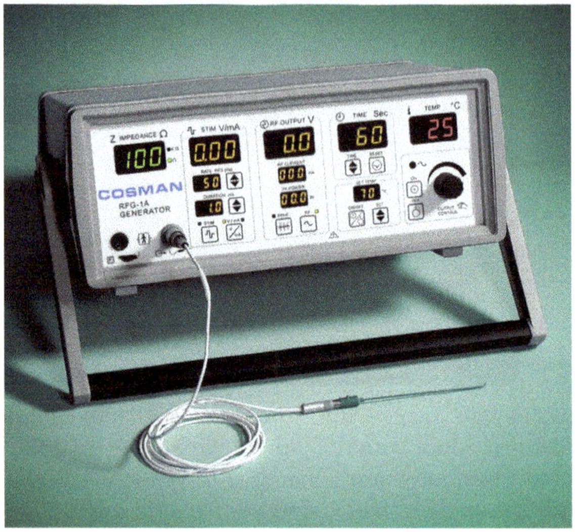

Figure 21.1 A modern RF generator. The Cosman RFG-1A generator is shown, which includes real-time impedance and temperature monitoring, stimulation capability, automatic temperature control and freehand output control capability. Also shown is a lesioning electrode with built-in thermocouple. Source: Cosman Medical, Inc.

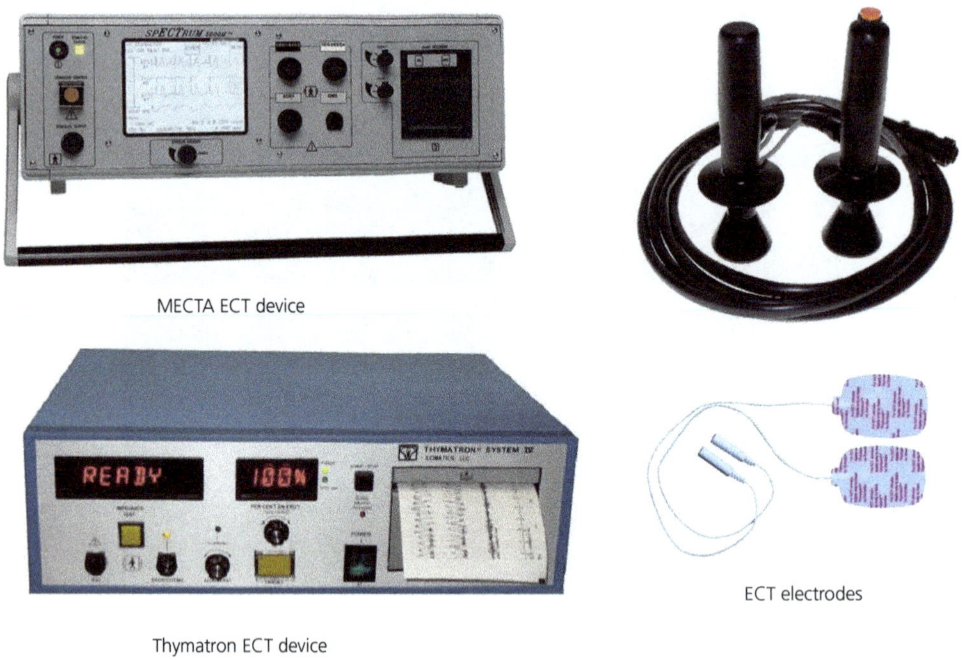

Figure 23.2 ECT device and electrodes. Source: Top left image used with permission of MECTA Corporation; bottom left and right images used with permission of Somatics, LLC.

~4000 for TRD; 2014 data provided by Cyberonics, Houston, TX, USA). With this considerable clinical exposure, a large amount of safety data has been accrued regarding the safety and tolerability of VNS [50, 51]. The safety profile in refractory epilepsy has been well described [5]. With extensive clinical trials, considerable safety and tolerability data has also been collected in TRD. Fortunately, many of the studies of VNS in TRD have used a standardized system of recording adverse events (AEs), the Coding Symbols for Thesaurus of Adverse Reaction Terms [52], to measure AEs occurring throughout VNS treatment. Across nine treatment trials (including seven longer term extensions), the most commonly reported AEs due to stimulation are outlined in Table 18.2. These AEs were generally similar to those in previous studies of epilepsy [5]. A small percentage were related to the implantation of the VNS devise itself, that is, pain or infection at the incision site (0.4–30% of patients) or incision site reaction (<10%). If reported, however, pain or irritation would generally dissipate in the subsequent 2 weeks. The most common AEs that were possibly, probably, or definitely related to treatment stimulation were hoarseness, voice alternation, throat pain, shortness of breath, general pain and neck pain. These events occurred during stimulation and were overall mild and well tolerated. A small percentage reported rashes or paraesthesias, which also shortly subsided.

Similar to the acute-phase side effect profile, longitudinal extensions of TRD trials recorded the most common AEs post-device implantation (1–2 years later) such as voice alteration, shortness of breath, increased cough, difficulty swallowing, nerve pain and neck pain. These symptoms were again typically reported as mild and occurred only during stimulation. A significant decrease in the severity of these adverse symptoms was typical.

Serious AEs (SAEs) related to VNS implantation or stimulation occurred at an overall low rate. There were two reported instances of cardiac SAEs (asystole and bradycardia) during surgery [4]. Likely related to implantation, there was one instance each of leg pain, deep venous thrombophlebitis and infection. Very rare, singular cases that could possibly be related to VNS stimulation involved back pain, appendicitis and central nervous system toxicity. Out of more than 580 total patients actively treated with VNS for TRD across all studies, there were 90 (estimated incidence 14%) reported AEs related to worsened depression, 32 (<10%) suicide attempts and 13 (<5%) instances categorized as either agitation, panic, emergence of manic symptoms or dysphoria. This, in part, could be due to either concomitant medication withdrawal [2], previous history of suicide attempts or the inclusion of patients with bipolar disorder (every trial besides one). Six patients (or <1% overall) committed suicide, one incidence occurring after receiving 5 weeks of VNS treatment [3]. Seven participants with worsening depression were in an acute-phase sham group [4]. Across all studies, including seven with outcomes at 1 year or more, there were only 12 (<3%) reports of study discontinuation specifically due to VNS-related AEs. In reviewing the AEs associated with VNS, it is critical to keep in mind that the population treated is the 'sickest of the sick' as related to major depression. Many of these patients have failed numerous medication/psychotherapy trials and have previous suicide histories.

In all, assessing the combined clinical trial experience of VNS in TRD, as well as the very low AE incidence and dropout rates observed in these trials, evidence suggests that VNS is exceptionally well tolerated in TRD.

Contraindications for VNS in TRD

Limited contraindications exist for VNS in TRD: short wave, microwave or therapeutic ultrasound diathermy cannot be performed with the implanted device [50]. There are

Table 18.2 Most commonly reported adverse events related to stimulation from clinical trials of VNS in adults with treatment-refractory depression (*numbers represent % of the participants*).

	Rush *et al.* [2]	**Marangell *et al.* [41]**	**Nahas *et al.* [42]**	**Rush *et al.* [4]**	**Rush *et al.* [3]**	**Schlaepfer *et al.* [43]**	**Bajbouj *et al.* [40]**	**Aaronson *et al.* [39]**	**Christmas *et al.* [44]**
			3 months; 24 months	Active; *Sham*	3 months; 12 months	3 months; 12 months		Low; High	
Voice alteration/ hoarseness	53	21	60; 27	68; *38*	58; 54	63; 55	25	64; 76	46
Shortness of breath/dyspnoea	17	7	15; 8	23; *14*	14; 16	10; 10		30; 34	
Neck pain	17	7	22; 13	21; *10*	16; 13	7; –		11; 18	
Increased cough	13	–		29; *9*	24; 6	26; 3		24; 25	15
General pain	20	–			6; 6	20; –	11	25; 42	
Difficulty swallowing/ pharyngitis	23	3		21; *11*	13; 4	6; 3		17; 17	8
Throat pain	27								23
Headache	30	3			5; 4	3; 2		17; 19	
Neuralgia						3; 55			
Laryngismus				11; *2*	10; 5	–; –			
Nausea	7	3				1; 2		14; 8	
Paraesthesia				16; *10*	11; 4	1; –		28; 35	
Number of Participants	30 implanted	28 available of 30	3 mos (*n*=59), 12 mos (*n*=54), 24 mos (*n*=53)	235 implanted; active VNS (*n*=119), *sham* (*n=116*)	209 available of 235	74 implanted 3 mos (*n*=70), 6 mos (*n*=61), 9 mos (*n*=54), 12 mos (*n*=60)	49 available of 74	331 total: low (*n*=111); medium (*n*=107); high (*n*=113) dose	13 new implanted
Comments		9 month maintenance phase of Rush [2]			9 months maintenance of Rush *et al.* [4]	Unchanged dose acute phase: 3 months; then 9 months of altered dose	Naturalistic follow up of Schlaepfer [43]	22 weeks acute phase; 50 weeks randomized into dosage groups	

important limitations to the use of whole body magnetic resonance imaging (MRI) with VNS, and patients who may need future MRI assessment (e.g. patients with histories of severe bone degeneration or cancer) may need to evaluate this contraindication when considering VNS implantation. The FDA-approved MRI options are outlined by the VNS device manufacturer [53]. VNS is not suggested for patients with damage to the left vagus nerve or those with severe pulmonary and cardiac disease. Because stimulation can lead to an onset of sleep apnoea, those with obstructive sleep apnoea may experience increased apnoeic events. The latest safety information is available at http://us.cyberonics.com/important-safety-information. Lastly, concurrent ECT treatment showed no complications when the VNS device was turned 'off' [42].

Clinical use of VNS in TRD

Indications for use of VNS in TRD

On 15 July 2005, the US FDA approved VNS for use in TRD, with the following guidelines: (i) patients with TRD must be 18 years of age or older and (ii) patients will be required to have failed at least four adequate antidepressant medication trials and/or ECT. The FDA elaborated on prescribing/treatment guidelines for VNS in TRD: VNS is not intended to be used as a first-line treatment, even in patients with severe depression; the treatment should be prescribed and monitored only by physicians who have specific training and expertise in managing TRD and managing the VNS device (programming and altering electrical parameters). The device should only be implanted by surgeons who are trained in surgeries of the carotid sheath and who have received specific training in the implantation of the VNS device. The FDA guidelines for using VNS in TRD are summarized on their website [1].

Where VNS falls in the TRD treatment hierarchy is a subject to some debate. Technically, following the FDA-approved guidelines, any patient who has failed four selective serotonin reuptake inhibitor (SSRI) trials would be an acceptable VNS candidate. In our opinion, this VNS threshold is too low. It is the practice of our clinic to first ensure that VNS candidates have failed very aggressive pharmacotherapy trials. We typically prefer that TRD patients fail at least four antidepressants (more typically more than six), one of which is either ECT or a monoamine oxidase inhibitor. In general, we prefer these four antidepressant trials be from different antidepressant classes (e.g. SSRIs, tricyclic antidepressants, dual (serotonin-norepinephrine) reuptake inhibitors); preferably, the antidepressant has had adequate trial duration (minimum of 8 weeks at the effective dose range). A reasonable guideline to assist with determination of an adequate trial is the Antidepressant Treatment History Form [46].

An advantageous aspect of VNS in the TRD population is that once implanted, the patient can subsequently receive additional available antidepressant treatment (e.g. augmentation with pharmacotherapies, ECT, rTMS), with perhaps the exception of deep brain stimulation. Our clinic has successfully treated patients with combined ECT and VNS with positive outcomes.

Managing the patient undergoing VNS

Setting reasonable expectations

Because of the novel nature of VNS in treating major depressive disorder, it is critical to set reasonable expectations for the TRD patient. As discussed below, patients should be aware that the majority of VNS response in TRD occurs well into treatment (typically following 6–12 months of stimulation). Hence, patients should be told in advance not to expect a 'quick fix', that is, the process will be gradual and occurs over many months of stimulation.

Surgical procedure

In general, the implantation procedure is done on an outpatient basis. The entire procedure (including VNS therapy generator implantation and attachment of the lead to left vagus nerve) takes about 1.5–2 h. Details of the procedure are described in a different chapter of this book. The procedure has a very low complication rate.

Post-operative recovery

Because of limited pain and swelling that occur at the incision sites, a waiting period of at least 2 weeks post-implantation is recommended before initiation of VNS therapy stimulation.

Titration of VNS charge delivery

Since the advent of VNS therapy for TRD, there has been much debate about the 'optimal' VNS stimulation parameters. What follows is a summary of the Washington University/St. Louis University VNS experience informed by the existing literature:

There are five electrical parameters that can be modified in VNS using the handheld wand attached to a programmable handset. The handheld wand is placed over the skin above the VNS generator as shown in Figure 18.2. A handheld programming device is attached to the wand that allows the programmer to check device integrity and modify electrical parameters.

The modifiable electrical parameters involved in VNS include output current (milliamps, mA), current frequency (Hertz, Hz), pulse width (microseconds, µs) and duty cycle (time 'on' versus time 'off').

For titrating VNS in TRD, the clinician must first take into account patient comfort. Our experience has taught us that certain trends are observed with regard to dose titration. First, there are great degrees of differing tolerability among patients receiving VNS for TRD; in general, the tolerable maximal current used in TRD is likely lower than that tolerated in refractory epilepsy (our experience is that most TRD patients can tolerate an output current of 1.25–1.5 mA, but some much less). A subset of patients tolerate very low output currents only (as low as 0.5 mA), whereas others can tolerate much higher output current (2.0 mA or above). Consistent with the epilepsy literature, our experience suggests that patients' tolerance to VNS increases with time, that is, there is an adaptation that occurs over time with greater exposure to VNS. For this reason, we recommend *very gradual, small dose*

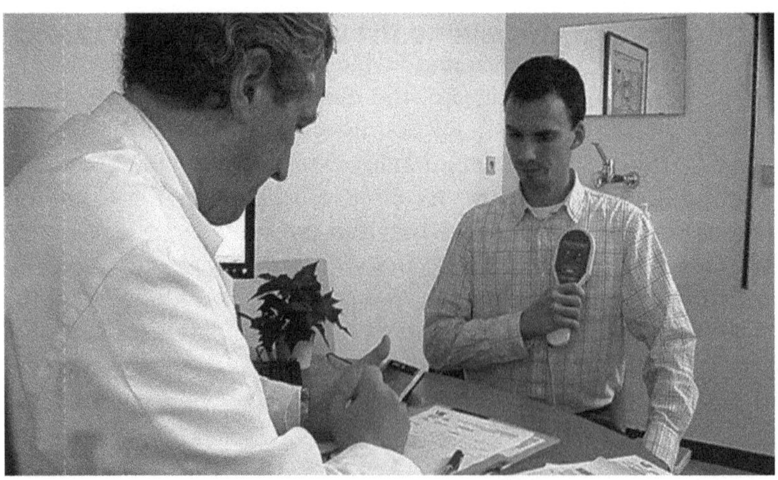

Figure 18.2 Demonstration of the use of the programming wand and handheld programmer. The wand is positioned directly over the device. Using a handheld programming device, the VNS generator can be assessed for circuit integrity (stimulus being successfully transmitted to vagus nerve) as well as programming the electrical parameters being delivered during VNS. Source: Reproduced with permission of Cyberonics. (*See insert for colour representation of the figure.*)

increases. Additionally, experience has also demonstrated that certain stimulation parameters are more frequently associated with pain or discomfort. In particular, frequencies above 20 Hz and pulse widths greater than 250 µs are avoided during initial titrations, as we have found these to be more frequently associated with patient discomfort.

An obvious question evolving from VNS use in TRD follows: is more current more efficacious? Based on our current knowledge, the answer would be a guarded 'yes'. As described in the section 'Results of clinical trials' of this Chapter, Aaronson *et al.* [39] reported on a VNS 'dose finding' study in TRD. Although this study had limitations, it demonstrated that TRD patients receiving higher stimulation parameters did *not* have greater short-term antidepressant efficacy; however, they did have *greater sustained efficacy* (i.e. better 1-year outcomes). For this reason, we recommend titrating to the highest tolerable output current during the initial titration period.

In summary, our experience, and that of many users of VNS in TRD, is to start with low-frequency (20 Hz), low pulse width (250 µs) and a 'standard' duty cycle of 30 s 'on' and 5 min 'off'. We typically use the first two to three office visits to titrate up to a tolerable dose with a period of observation of 20–30 min between upward output current titrations.

Example Titration

<u>Office Visit #1</u>: Initiate with the following parameters:

Frequency: 20 Hz, pulse width (250 µs), duty cycle: 30 sec 'on' and 5 min 'off'. Start with an output current of 0.25 mA and have the patient sit in the waiting room for 20–25 min to allow the device to cycle—four to five times to assess patient tolerability. If the patient tolerates these settings without pain/discomfort/side effects, we will increase the output current by another 0.25 mA (to 0.50 mA), followed by another 20–25 min observation. This is repeated a third time on the first office visit with a final first visit output current (assuming patient tolerates this) of 0.75 mA. If at any time during the upward titration the patient experiences pain/discomfort/side effects, we decrease the output current by 0.25 mA to the previously tolerated level. We then have the patient return in 1 week and re-attempt to increase the output current by at least 0.25 mA.

<u>Office Visit #2</u>: Frequency: 20 Hz, pulse width (250 µs), duty cycle: 30 s 'on' and 5 min 'off'; output current 0.75 mA. Similar to Visit #1, we increase the output current by 0.25–1.0 mA and observe the patient while the device cycles—four to five times; during this process, we ask the patient if they are experiencing any pain/discomfort/side effects. This is repeated—one to two more times during this visit.

Some clinicians will be much more aggressive with their upward titration (increasing by current output increments >0.25 mA); however, we have observed that a more gradual titration allows for greater final output currents and greater patient comfort.

When to make further parameter adjustments

Evidence from clinical and neuroimaging studies [3, 34, 47] strongly suggest that response to VNS in TRD typically occurs over the course of many months. As was described in the open-label extension of the large US multi-centre trial, the response rates (i.e. a 50% drop in standard MDD measures) appear to increase most precipitously at 6–12 months. For this reason, we believe that once the maximally tolerated output current (during original titration) is achieved, it is wise to maintain these parameters for at least 12 months.

If the patient is having partial/incomplete/no response to treatment, our experience suggests that increasing the amount of charge delivered over time has the greatest influence on antidepressant outcome. This can be achieved by either increasing the amount of 'on' time or decreasing the amount of 'off' time between charge deliveries. The VNS therapy user guide, which accompanies the VNS programming system, details the allowable percentage on time/duty cycle. A duty cycle in excess of 50% 'on' time equal to or greater than 'off' time is not recommended.

It should be noted that increasing the amount of charge delivered in a given time span will also more rapidly decrease battery life, so this step should be reserved for situations in which standard parameter settings have not proven successful.

What constitutes a good VNS response in TRD?

Studies of chronic VNS in TRD (see section 'Results of clinical trials') suggest a wide response range of clinical responses of VNS in TRD. The largest longitudinal, multi-centre study of VNS in TRD suggested that the 12 month responses could be grossly categorized into three response ranges. Approximately one third of the patients have a clear-cut antidepressant response, which could include those who have achieved remission (essentially minimal depressive symptoms). A second group of approximately one-third of the subjects have achieved a significant and clinically meaningful response (i.e. their depressive scores did not drop below 50% from baseline, but dropped by 25–40%). This group may benefit from additional parameter modulation and potential augmentation from other therapies. Another approximately one third appears to have little/no response to VNS.

It is difficult to determine the degree to which a lower percentage improvement in depression score translates into an improvement in quality of life. This is partly true because these studies have differing baseline depression scores (i.e. a 25% improvement from a higher score represents a lesser change in depressive symptomatology). In general, our practice is to counsel prospective patients that the existing VNS data in TRD suggest the one third superb response, one third limited but clinically meaningful response and one third no response.

Finally, many patients receiving VNS describe improvements in mood and daily functioning that may not be easily detected in standard antidepressant measures. Many patients who do not experience remission of TRD describe that VNS places a 'floor' on how severe their depressive episodes are, that is, they still experience depressive episodes, but these episodes are not perceived as severe or disabling as before. Along these same lines, we have observed several patients who thought they were not benefiting from VNS and requested their devices be turned off, only to find that once off, they experienced a worsening of their perceived depressive state and requested their devices be turned back on.

The future of VNS in TRD

Currently, accessibility to VNS for TRD in the United States and Europe is limited.

Despite the US FDA approval of VNS for TRD in July of 2005, the United States Committee on Medicare and Medicaid Services (CMS) made a no-reimburse decision for VNS in TRD in May of 2007. The arguments used in this determination included: (i) a lack of a clear definition (within the field of psychiatry) of what defines 'treatment-resistance' and (ii) the opinion that the existing clinical evidence in 2007 did not support clinical efficacy (i.e. the treatment remained 'experimental'). This decision has had a profoundly negative effect on the availability of VNS in TRD, as private medical insurance companies have fallen in step with CMS and are denying patients access to this care. Essentially, only in rare instances are those who need VNS for TRD able to obtain medical insurance reimbursement for the procedure.

Since the time of this decision, several additional clinical trials [39, 40, 43], summarized in the section 'Results of clinical trials', meta-analyses and medical economic studies [49], as well as functional neuroimaging studies

[47, 54], have been completed that further support the efficacy of VNS in TRD. Ongoing efforts from science, industry and patients and their families are currently underway to reconsider this decision regarding reimbursement.

Future research directions

Pre-implantation prediction of response in VNS

Because VNS is a permanent and invasive treatment, any method that would allow improved likelihood of treatment efficacy would potentially decrease the rate of implantation without an antidepressant response. With this in mind, Conway *et al.* [54] conducted a study using ^{18}fluorodeoxyglucose positron emission tomography (FDG-PET) to determine if baseline (pre-treatment) metabolic brain activity predicted the eventual antidepressant outcomes. This group found that higher baseline (pre-treatment) orbitofrontal cortex cerebral metabolic activity and lower anterior insular cortex cerebral metabolic activity correlated strongly with eventual antidepressant response. This finding suggests the possibility that based on different patterns of cerebral metabolic activity, not all cases of TRD are the same, that is, certain patterns may be more likely to respond to VNS. Additional, larger scale studies in VNS treatment response patterns are needed.

Transcutaneous, non-invasive VNS

The external acoustic meatus, in particular the tragus, has extensive sensory innervation provided by the auricular branch of the vagus nerve [11]. Hence, theoretically, one could enhance affective neural signaling in the vagus via electrical stimulation of this region.

Early study of the effects of electrical, transcutaneous auricular stimulation demonstrated reproducible sensory-evoked potentials (measured from the scalp). Since then, Kraus *et al.* [55], using a measure of affective state and blood oxygen–dependent functional MRI (BOLD fMRI), studied the effects of transcutaneous electrical auricular stimulation in non- depressed, healthy subjects. Using a single-blind, placebo-controlled study and real-time BOLD fMRI, they were able to demonstrate that a limited series of transcutaneous auricular stimulations applied to the tragus led to increased feelings of well-being. Further, this group also found that electrical stimulation of the tragus, but not the ear lobe, was associated with robust BOLD-signal decreases in limbic brain regions, including the amygdala, hippocampus and parahippocampal gyrus. Increased activation was seen in the insula, precentral gyrus and the thalamus. This proof of concept study has several significant limitations, including the fact that the stimulations were very brief (three 30 s stimulations separated by 2 min) and that the subjects were not clinically depressed. To date, no large-scale transcutaneous vagal nerve stimulation studies have been reported in clinically depressed populations. A small proof of concept of transcutaneous vagus nerve stimulation in treatment-refractory epilepsy demonstrated a reduction of seizure frequency in a subset of patients; however, this study lacked a placebo-controlled group [56].

References

1 Food and Drug Administration. VNS Therapy System – P970003s050. U.S. Department of Health and Human Services; 2005 [updated 09/04/2013, accessed 02/07/2014]. Available from: http://www.fda.gov/MedicalDevices/ProductsandMedicalProcedures/DeviceApprovalsandClearances/Recently-ApprovedDevices/ucm078532.htm (accessed on 27 June 2015).

2 Rush AJ, George MS, Sackeim HA, Marangell LB, Husain MM, Giller C, *et al.* Vagus nerve stimulation (VNS) for treatment-resistant depressions: a multicenter study. Biol Psychiatry. 2000;47(4):276–86.

3 Rush AJ, Sackeim HA, Marangell LB, George MS, Brannan SK, Davis SM, *et al.* Effects of 12 months of vagus nerve stimulation in treatment-resistant depression: a naturalistic study. Biol Psychiatry. 2005;58(5):355–63.

4 Rush AJ, Marangell LB, Sackeim HA, George MS, Brannan SK, Davis SM, *et al.* Vagus nerve stimulation for treatment-resistant depression: a randomized, controlled acute phase trial. Biol Psychiatry. 2005;58(5):347–54.
5 Morris GL, 3rd, Mueller WM. Long-term treatment with vagus nerve stimulation in patients with refractory epilepsy. The Vagus Nerve Stimulation Study Group E01-E05. Neurology. 1999;53(8):1731–5.
6 Harden CL, Pulver MC, Ravdin LD, Nikolov B, Halper JP, Labar DR. A pilot study of mood in epilepsy patients treated with vagus nerve stimulation. Epilepsy Behav. 2000;1(2):93–9.
7 Elger G, Hoppe C, Falkai P, Rush AJ, Elger CE. Vagus nerve stimulation is associated with mood improvements in epilepsy patients. Epilepsy Res. 2000;42(2–3):203–10.
8 George MS, Rush AJ, Marangell LB, Sackeim HA, Brannan SK, Davis SM, *et al.* A one-year comparison of vagus nerve stimulation with treatment as usual for treatment-resistant depression. Biol Psychiatry. 2005;58(5):364–73.
9 Nieuwenhuys R, Voogd J, van Huijzen C. The Human Central Nervous System: A Synopsis and Atlas. 3rd ed. Berlin: Springer-Verlag; 1988.
10 Parent A. Carpenter's Human Neuroanatomy. 9th ed. Baltimore: Williams & Wilkins; 1996.
11 Peuker ET, Filler TJ. The nerve supply of the human auricle. Clin Anat. 2002;15(1):35–7.
12 Foley JO, DuBois FS. Quantitative studies of the vagus nerve in the cat. I. The ratio of sensory to motor fibers. J Comp Neurol. 1937;67(1): 49–67.
13 Ben-Menachem E. Vagus nerve stimulation, side effects, and long-term safety. J Clin Neurophysiol. 2001;18(5):415–8.
14 San Mauro MP, Patronelli F, Spinelli E, Cordero A, Covello D, Gorostiaga JA. Nerves of the heart: a comprehensive review with a clinical point of view. Neuroanatomy. 2009;8:26–31.
15 Binks AP, Paydarfar D, Schachter SC, Guz A, Banzett RB. High strength stimulation of the vagus nerve in awake humans: a lack of cardiorespiratory effects. Respir Physiol. 2001; 127(2–3):125–33.
16 Banzett RB, Guz A, Paydarfar D, Shea SA, Schachter SC, Lansing RW. Cardiorespiratory variables and sensation during stimulation of the left vagus in patients with epilepsy. Epilepsy Res. 1999;35(1):1–11.
17 Henry TR. Therapeutic mechanisms of vagus nerve stimulation. Neurology. 2002;59(6 Suppl 4):S3–14.
18 Beckstead RM. An autoradiographic examination of corticocortical and subcortical projections of the mediodorsal-projection (prefrontal) cortex in the rat. J Comp Neurol. 1979;184(1): 43–62.
19 Kalia M, Sullivan JM. Brainstem projections of sensory and motor components of the vagus nerve in the rat. J Comp Neurol. 1982;211(3): 248–65.
20 Rhoton AL, Jr., O'Leary JL, Ferguson JP. The trigeminal, facial, vagal, and glossopharyngeal nerves in the monkey. Afferent connections. Arch Neurol. 1966;14(5):530–40.
21 Malow BA, Edwards J, Marzec M, Sagher O, Fromes G. Effects of vagus nerve stimulation on respiration during sleep: a pilot study. Neurology. 2000;55(10):1450–4.
22 Kirchner A, Birklein F, Stefan H, Handwerker HO. Left vagus nerve stimulation suppresses experimentally induced pain. Neurology. 2000;55(8):1167–71.
23 Saper CB, editor. Diffuse Cortical Projection Systems: Anatomical Organization and Role in Cortical Function. Bethesda: American Physiological Society; 1987.
24 Dorr AE, Debonnel G. Effect of vagus nerve stimulation on serotonergic and noradrenergic transmission. J Pharmacol Exp Ther. 2006; 318(2):890–8.
25 Agostoni E, Chinnock JE, De Daly MB, Murray JG. Functional and histological studies of the vagus nerve and its branches to the heart, lungs and abdominal viscera in the cat. J Physiol. 1957;135(1):182–205.
26 Beckstead RM, Morse JR, Norgren R. The nucleus of the solitary tract in the monkey: projections to the thalamus and brain stem nuclei. J Comp Neurol. 1980;190(2):259–82.
27 Saper CB, Loewy AD. Efferent connections of the parabrachial nucleus in the rat. Brain Res. 1980;197(2):291–317.
28 Bester H, Bourgeais L, Villanueva L, Besson JM, Bernard JF. Differential projections to the intra-

laminar and gustatory thalamus from the parabrachial area: a PHA-L study in the rat. J Comp Neurol. 1999;405(4):421–49.
29 Carmichael ST, Price JL. Sensory and premotor connections of the orbital and medial prefrontal cortex of macaque monkeys. J Comp Neurol. 1995;363(4):642–64.
30 Krout KE, Loewy AD. Parabrachial nucleus projections to midline and intralaminar thalamic nuclei of the rat. J Comp Neurol. 2000;428(3):475–94.
31 Saleem KS, Kondo H, Price JL. Complementary circuits connecting the orbital and medial prefrontal networks with the temporal, insular, and opercular cortex in the macaque monkey. J Comp Neurol. 2008;506(4):659–93.
32 Ongur D, Price JL. The organization of networks within the orbital and medial prefrontal cortex of rats, monkeys and humans. Cereb Cortex. 2000;10(3):206–19.
33 Conway CR, Sheline YI, Chibnall JT, George MS, Fletcher JW, Mintun MA. Cerebral blood flow changes during vagus nerve stimulation for depression. Psychiatry Res. 2006;146(2):179–84.
34 Nahas Z, Teneback C, Chae JH, Mu Q, Molnar C, Kozel FA, *et al.* Serial vagus nerve stimulation functional MRI in treatment-resistant depression. Neuropsychopharmacology. 2007;32(8):1649–60.
35 Henry TR, Bakay RA, Votaw JR, Pennell PB, Epstein CM, Faber TL, *et al.* Brain blood flow alterations induced by therapeutic vagus nerve stimulation in partial epilepsy: I. Acute effects at high and low levels of stimulation. Epilepsia. 1998;39(9):983–90.
36 Herbert H, Moga MM, Saper CB. Connections of the parabrachial nucleus with the nucleus of the solitary tract and the medullary reticular formation in the rat. J Comp Neurol. 1990;293(4):540–80.
37 Cox CL, Huguenard JR, Prince DA. Nucleus reticularis neurons mediate diverse inhibitory effects in thalamus. Proc Natl Acad Sci U S A. 1997;94(16):8854–9.
38 Malow BA, Edwards J, Marzec M, Sagher O, Ross D, Fromes G. Vagus nerve stimulation reduces daytime sleepiness in epilepsy patients. Neurology. 2001;57(5):879–84.
39 Aaronson ST, Carpenter LL, Conway CR, Reimherr FW, Lisanby SH, Schwartz TL, *et al.* Vagus nerve stimulation therapy randomized to different amounts of electrical charge for treatment-resitant depression: acute and chronic effects. Brain Stimul. 2013;6(4):631–40.
40 Bajbouj M, Merkl A, Schlaepfer TE, Frick C, Zobel A, Maier W, *et al.* Two-year outcome of vagus nerve stimulation in treatment-resistant depression. J Clin Psychopharmacol. 2010;30(3):273–81.
41 Marangell LB, Rush AJ, George MS, Sackeim HA, Johnson CR, Husain MM, *et al.* Vagus nerve stimulation (VNS) for major depressive episodes: one year outcomes. Biol Psychiatry. 2002;51(4):280–7.
42 Nahas Z, Marangell LB, Husain MM, Rush AJ, Sackeim HA, Lisanby SH, *et al.* Two-year outcome of vagus nerve stimulation (VNS) for treatment of major depressive episodes. J Clin Psychiatry. 2005;66(9):1097–104.
43 Schlaepfer TE, Frick C, Zobel A, Maier W, Heuser I, Bajbouj M, *et al.* Vagus nerve stimulation for depression: efficacy and safety in a European study. Psychol Med. 2008;38(5):651–61.
44 Christmas D, Steele JD, Tolomeo S, Eljamel MS, Matthews K. Vagus nerve stimulation for chronic major depressive disorder: 12-month outcomes in highly treatment-refractory patients. J Affect Disord. 2013;150(3):1221–5.
45 Dunner DL, Rush AJ, Russell JM, Burke M, Woodard S, Wingard P, *et al.* Prospective, long-term, multicenter study of the naturalistic outcomes of patients with treatment-resistant depression. J Clin Psychiatry. 2006;67(5):688–95.
46 Sackeim HA, Prudic J, Devanand DP, Decina P, Kerr B, Malitz S. The impact of medication resistance and continuation pharmacotherapy on relapse following response to electro convulsive therapy in major depression. J Clin Psychopharmacol. 1990;10(2):96–104.
47 Conway CR, Chibnall JT, Gebara MA, Price JL, Snyder AZ, Mintun MA, *et al.* Association of cerebral metabolic activity changes with vagus nerve stimulation antidepressant response in treatment-resistant depression. Brain Stimul. 2013;6(5):788–97.

48 Pardo JV, Sheikh SA, Schwindt GC, Lee JT, Kuskowski MA, Surerus C, *et al.* Chronic vagus nerve stimulation for treatment-resistant depression decreases resting ventromedial prefrontal glucose metabolism. Neuroimage. 2008;42(2):879–89.
49 Berry SM, Broglio K, Bunker M, Jayewardene A, Olin B, Rush AJ. A patient-level meta-analysis of studies evaluating vagus nerve stimulation therapy for treatment-resistant depression. Med Devices (Auckl). 2013;6:17–35.
50 Cyberonics Inc. Important Safety Information. Houston, TX; 2003. http://us.cyberonics.com/important-safety-information (accessed 27 June 2015).
51 Rush AJ, Siefert SE. Clinical issues in considering vagus nerve stimulation for treatment-resistant depression. Exp Neurol. 2009;219(1):36–43.
52 Food and Drug Administration. COSTART: Coding Symbols for Thesaurus of Adverse Reaction Terms. In: US Department of Health and Human Services, Center for Drug Evaluation and Research. 5th ed. Rockville, MD: Center for Drugs and Biologics; 1995.
53 Cyberonics Inc. Cyberonics Receives FDA Approval for Expansion of MRI Use With VNS Therapy® Systems. [Press Release]: Acquire Media; 2011 [accessed 02/07/2014]. Available from: http://ir.cyberonics.com/releasedetail.cfm?ReleaseID=619246 (accessed on 27 June 2015).
54 Conway CR, Chibnall JT, Gangwani S, Mintun MA, Price JL, Hershey T, *et al.* Pretreatment cerebral metabolic activity correlates with antidepressant efficacy of vagus nerve stimulation in treatment-resistant major depression: a potential marker for response? J Affect Disord. 2012;139(3):283–90.
55 Kraus T, Hosl K, Kiess O, Schanze A, Kornhuber J, Forster C. BOLD fMRI deactivation of limbic and temporal brain structures and mood enhancing effect by transcutaneous vagus nerve stimulation. J Neural Transm. 2007;114(11): 1485–93.
56 Stefan H, Kreiselmeyer G, Kerling F, Kurzbuch K, Rauch C, Heers M, *et al.* Transcutaneous vagus nerve stimulation (t-VNS) in pharmacoresistant epilepsies: a proof of concept trial. Epilepsia. 2012;53(7):e115–8.

CHAPTER 19

Gamma Knife radiosurgery: Introduction and technical aspects

Alessandra A. Gorgulho[1,2] and Antônio A.F. De Salles[2]

[1] *HCOR Neuroscience Center, São Paulo, Brazil*

[2] *University of California Los Angeles, Los Angeles, USA*

Introduction

The idea of focusing external beam radiation to concentrate dose to pathology and spare the peripheral structures appeared in the literature in 1906. It was described by Kohl only 18 years after the discovery of X-rays. During the following years, the idea evolved with spiral converging beams, pendulum-directed beams and finally rigid hemispheric attached beam directed with stereotactic precision [1]. It was Lars Leksell, a functional neurosurgeon at Karolinska University in Stockholm, Sweden, who integrated the stereotactic precision with the penetrating capability and the radiobiological effect of the X-ray beam. As widely described, Leksell attached an X-ray tube to his stereotactic frame and delivered radiosurgery to the first patient submitted to the technique, targeting the trigeminal ganglion for the treatment of trigeminal neuralgia. The term 'radiosurgery' was coined [2]. This was actually the first application of photon radiosurgery.

Proton beam radiosurgery became popular in the 1960s for its sharp dose distribution properties and the possibility to modulate and stop the penetration of the beam inside of the target. Dr. Leksell explored the proton sharp property, but not the modulatory property, at the cyclotron in Uppsala. Although possible to treat patients with the proton beam, it proved to be too expensive and not amenable to the hospital setting at that time. This hindered the possibility of treating large number of patients and perfecting the technology. Few facilities existed in the world at the time capable of using the proton beam for therapeutic purposes.

Radiosurgery evolved during the last half of the last century linked to the explosion of imaging techniques [3]. While dependent on ventriculography, cysternography and angiography, the applications of radiosurgery were largely limited to the pathologies visualized by these techniques. Functional applications were based on principles of functional neurosurgery localization, for example using the anterior commissure (AC) and posterior commissure (PC) seen by ventriculography to guide targeting. Meckel's cave contrast material injection and cysternography provided visualization of targets such as the trigeminal ganglion in the Meckel's cave and the acoustic neuroma's prominence in the cerebello-pontine angle, previously not seen in plain skull radiographs [4, 5].

Neuromodulation in Psychiatry, First Edition. Edited by Clement Hamani, Paul Holtzheimer, Andres M. Lozano and Helen Mayberg.

The inception of the Gamma Knife

Dr. Leksell experienced the need of a device capable of treating a large number of patients, with precision and being amenable to the hospital setting. He went back to the principle of the cobalt unit, then widely used in radiotherapy, to devise the first commercially available dedicated radiosurgery device. In 1968, Leksell and Larsson developed the first Gamma Knife (GK) Unit in Sweden. Larsson was a medical physicist dedicated to develop GK and to treat patients with this technique for many decades [6]. The unit was housed in a private setting at the Queen Sophia Hospital (Sophiahemmet) in Stockholm; in 1982, this Unit was transferred to the University of California Los Angeles (Figure 19.1), being the first GK Unit in the United States.

The remarkable results obtained with the GK Unit treatment of arteriovenous malformations (AVMs), starting in 1972, impressed the neurosurgical community, which realized the potential of the technique as a solution for treatment of these formidable lesions. Angiography provided the visualization of AVMs, making them the classic application of radiosurgery [7]. The build-up of radiosurgery applications with the introduction of structural diseases such as acoustic neuromas and AVMs increased the demand for affordable radiosurgery devices throughout the world. Two more units where installed before the complete popularization of the GK, one in Sheffield, UK, and the other in Buenos Aires, Argentina. Together with the Stockholm Unit, the Sheffield and the Buenos Aires units served the world until a new unit came to the University of Pittsburgh in 1987 in the United States [8]. During the early 1980s, there were less than 10 radiosurgery devices serving the world's population: four gamma units and a few heavy particle beam facilities. Linac radiosurgery was therefore developed to popularize

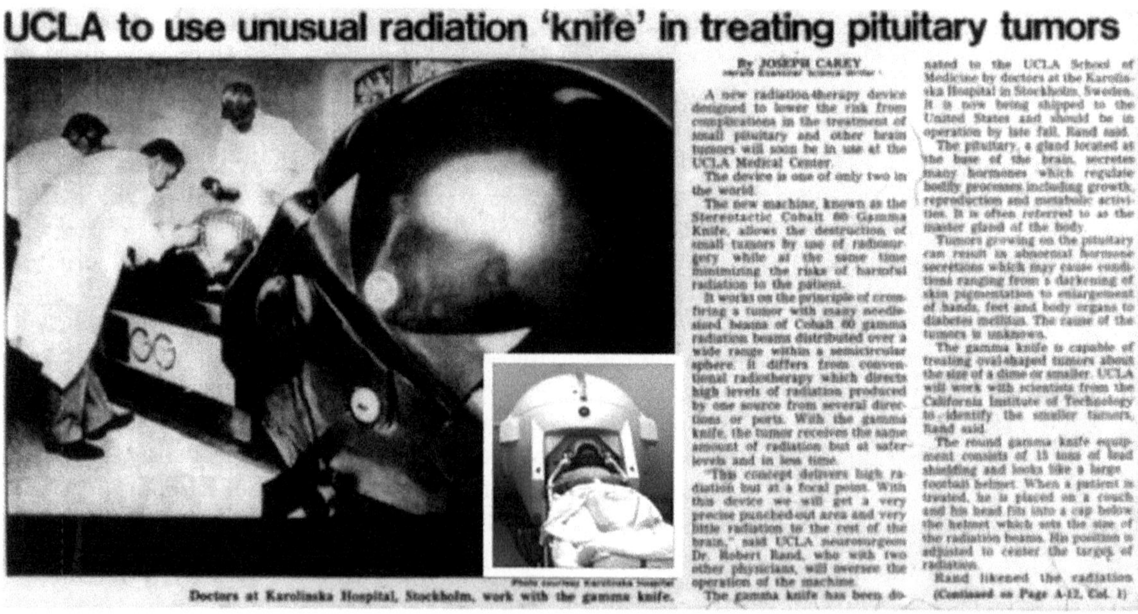

UCLA to use unusual radiation 'knife' in treating pituitary tumors

By JOSEPH CAREY

A new radiation-therapy device designed to lower the risk from complications in the treatment of small pituitary and other brain tumors will soon be in use at the UCLA Medical Center.

The device is one of only two in the world.

The new machine, known as the Stereotactic Cobalt 60 Gamma Knife, allows the destruction of small tumors by use of radiosurgery while at the same time minimizing the risks of harmful radiation to the patient.

It works on the principle of cross-firing a tumor with many needle-sized beams of Cobalt 60 gamma radiation beams distributed over a wide range within a semicircular sphere. It differs from conventional radiotherapy which directs high levels of radiation produced by one source from several directions or ports. With the gamma knife, the tumor receives the same amount of radiation but at safer levels and in less time.

"This concept delivers high radiation but at a focal point. With this device we will get a very precise punched-out area and very little radiation to the rest of the brain," said UCLA neurosurgeon Dr. Robert Rand, who with two other physicians, will oversee the operation of the machine.

The gamma knife has been donated to the UCLA School of Medicine by doctors at the Karolinska Hospital in Stockholm, Sweden. It is now being shipped to the United States and should be in operation by late fall, Rand said.

The pituitary, a gland located at the base of the brain, secretes many hormones which regulate bodily processes including growth, reproduction and metabolic activities. It is often referred to as the master gland of the body.

Tumors growing on the pituitary can result in abnormal hormone secretions which may cause conditions ranging from a darkening of skin pigmentation to enlargement of hands, feet and body organs to diabetes mellitus. The cause of the tumors is unknown.

The gamma knife is capable of treating oval-shaped tumors about the size of a dime or smaller. UCLA will work with scientists from the California Institute of Technology to identify the smaller tumors, Rand said.

The round gamma knife equipment consists of 15 tons of lead shielding and looks like a large football helmet. When a patient is treated, he is placed on a couch and his head fits into a cap below the helmet which sets the size of the radiation beams. His position is adjusted to center the target of radiation.

Rand likened the radiation

(Continued on Page A-12, Col. 1)

Doctors at Karolinska Hospital, Stockholm, work with the gamma knife.

Figure 19.1 The first Gamma Knife (GK) built by Dr. Leksell was donated to the UCLA to be used by the stereotactic neurosurgeon Dr. Robert Rand. The physicist Dr. Gene Holly treated the first patient at the UCLA in 1983 with Dr. Rand and Dr. Michael Selch. This GK was painted white, treating the first patient with the GK in the United States (inset). Only two GKs existed at that time in the world.

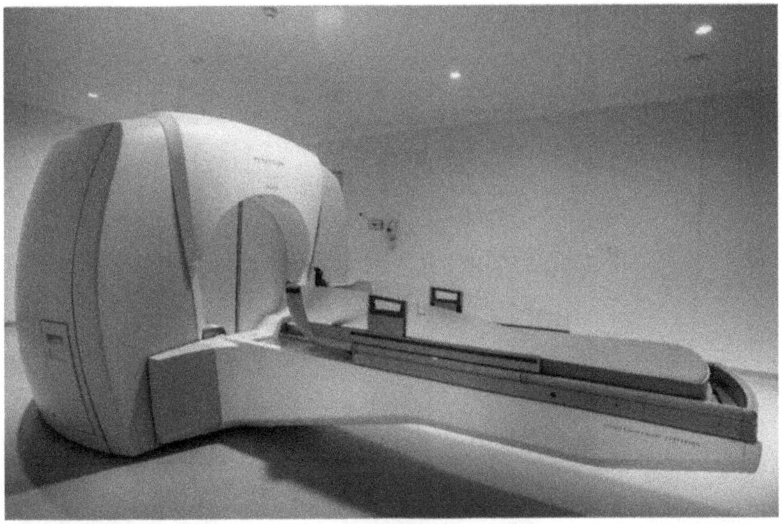

Figure 19.2 Gamma Knife Perfexion® last model installed in the HCor (Hospital do Coração) neuroscience in Sao Paulo, Brazil. This model can be called 'Plus' with the addition of a cone beam computed tomography at the entrance of the device to check the patient's position and target. (*See insert for colour representation of the figure.*)

stereotactic radiosurgery to every hospital capable of treating cancer patients with conventional radiation therapy, leading three decades later to the movement of whole body stereotactic radiosurgery [3, 9].

The GK evolved to be the only dedicated radiosurgery device for intracranial lesions, competing favourably among neurosurgeons with the various linear accelerator adaptations, when using single dose of radiation. The appearance of computerized imaging in the 1970s and 1980s amplified radiosurgery applications, creating the demand for dedicated devices throughout the world [5]. Several models of GK represent the evolution of the machine to its state now called commercially as Perfexion® (Figure 19.2).

Collimation system

The ^{60}Cobalt decay to ^{60}Ni inputs a half-life of 5.26 years to the cobalt sources adapted to the GK. It is this very decay, however, that produces the gamma rays that are collimated to the patient's lesion to achieve the desired biological effect. Gamma rays of 1.17 and 1.33 MeV are grouped by three different collimation sizes available in the GK Perfexion to automatically take advantage of modulation and shaping capabilities [10]. The previous collimation system of the models U, B and C, which was dependent on four exchangeable helmets with four different sizes of apertures (4, 8, 14, 18 mm) with manual plugging and placement, was replaced by a single dynamic conic helmet. This new collimation system is capable of movement throughout three different apertures (4, 8, 16 mm), as well as plugging them strategically to modulate and shape the dose distribution (Figure 19.3), as desired to optimize the intensity of radiation to the lesion and decrease it towards the surrounding structures (Table 19.1). The cumbersome process of hoisting the collimators every time that the size of the isocentre was changed, serving to delay and bring possible errors to the procedure, is now bypassed in the GK Perfexion [11, 12].

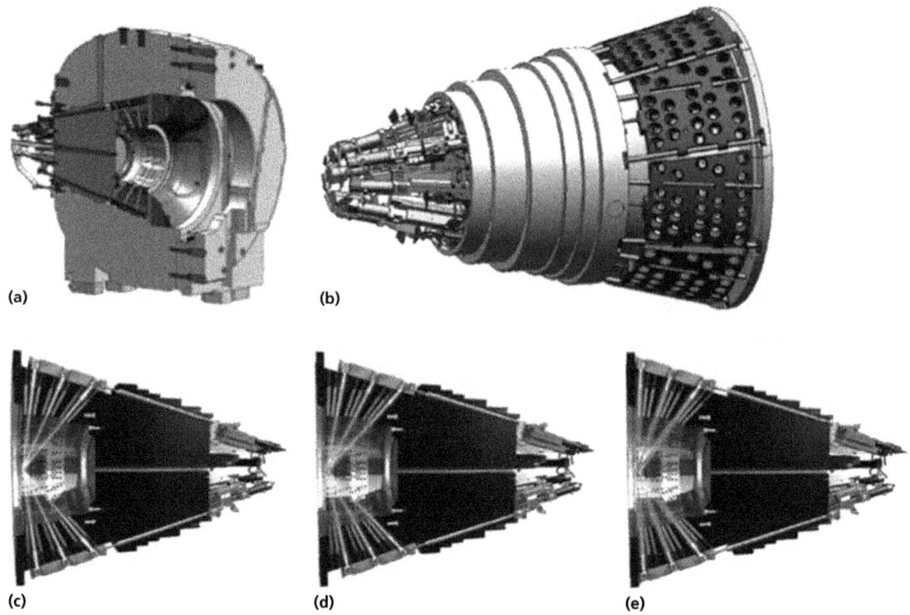

Figure 19.3 Conic collimation system of the GK Perfexion. Notice in **(a)** demonstration of the cross section of the device showing the three main sectors of the collimator, with the motor capable to move the sectors, the site for location of the sources and the helmet with the pores of three different sizes, 4, 8 and 16 mm in diameter. **(b)** Shows a complete view of the device, including motors, and **(c)**, **(d)** and **(e)** demonstrate the radiation with the three collimations. (*See insert for colour representation of the figure.*)

Table 19.1 Evolution of gamma unit models – technical and economical demands.

Gamma Knife (GK) U	I – Pioneer: functional neurosurgery (^{60}Co 179 sources) II – Initial applications for morphological radiosurgery
GK B	I – Initial worldwide demand: devices for large-scale treatment and diversity of histology and applications II – Economical pressure: replacement of sources at ± 7 years interval (^{60}Co 201 sources) became possible.
GK C	I – Computer integration allowing initial efforts of robotization II – Computerized treatment plan – replacement of Kula planning – Expediting the number of patients treated daily.
GK Perfexion	I – Full robotization decreasing possibility of human error II – Maximization of collimator interplay for conformality and treatment speed. Replacement of four hemispherical helmets of apertures in millimeters (4, 8, 14, 18) each by one conical helmet with apertures in millimeters (4, 8, 16) capability, sectors accepting exposure of different number of the ^{60}Co 192 sources available. The GK Perfexion Plus brings imaging check capabilities at the time of the treatment.

Robotic capabilities

All movements of the system, patient and collimation are completely robotized and controlled by the GK Perfexion panel based on the radiosurgery plan. The computer driving the machine enforces all the numbers obtained during planning, including coordinates (couch), number of isocentres, size of collimation and weight of each 'shot' (conic helmet). The only operator intervention is the positioning of the patient in relation to the machine and the angle of flexion/extension of the patient's head, which allows for three positions. An error in this setting makes the computerized control reject the setting, thereby not delivering the treatment until the error is corrected. One also is capable of modifying the height of the couch manually to improve the patient's cervical comfort. The robotic couch moves in the *x*, *y* and *z* stereotactic coordinate directions in concert with the collimation to deliver the treatment. This has immensely expedited the treatment of patients and decreased the possibility of human error. Busy services are able to treat more than 10 patients per day during normal working hours when the process of treatment is well streamlined, that is, placement of stereotactic frame, imaging acquisition, imaging transfer and fusion, treatment planning and finally placement of the patient in the machine, treatment delivery and discharge of the patient, given that the cobalt 60 source is new.

Flow of patient treatment

Patients are treated as outpatients after acquisition of the magnetic resonance imaging (MRI) dedicated for the treatment. They are asked to come to the GK department in a fasting state. The day before the procedure, they are advised to wash their heads with an antiseptic shampoo. The risks of the procedure are discussed and the patients sign the informed consent understanding the implications of the radiation, including immediate, delayed and long-lasting effects, as well as the purpose of the procedure, that is slow and long-lasting effect of radiation. Patients are instructed to continue taking their usual medications for the disease being treated, since radiation effects are delayed. Radiation's peak of action occurs between 6 and 18 months after delivery even though immediate radiation action on cells start at the moment of treatment. They receive a dose of steroids to mitigate immediate effects of radiation and to minimize the peri-orbital oedema caused by the placement of the stereotactic frame.

Placement of the stereotactic frame

The patients are prepared sterile in the forehead and occipital region using a topical anaesthetic cream followed by injection of 5 cc of mixed Lidocaine/Marcaine and sodium bicarbonate in each stereotactic frame pin site. The frame is applied strategically with the care of including the pathology inside of the stereotactic space. The compatibility of the stereotactic frame placement with all hardware attachments of the GK is checked. Measurements of the head surface are acquired with a plastic stick helmet, as well as the measurements of the stereotactic hardware for input in the Gamma Plan for calculation of beam attenuation. The patient is transferred for computed tomography (CT) scan for the stereotactic image acquisition to be merged with the previously obtained MRI. The contour of the patient's head obtained based on the CT scan can be used instead of the manual measurements previously obtained to calculate the attenuation of the beams.

Treatment planning

The treatment planning now available, the Gamma Plan, takes advantage of a fully computerized system to combine three different collimation sizes available in an interplay of isocentre's weight and strategic position to conform the volume of radiation, as exquisitely as possible, to the volume shape of the lesions/target. The planning takes into consideration the location of the lesion with the strategy of smaller collimation in the proximity of the most eloquent areas of the brain, sparing of function and allowing concentration of dose in areas of the tumour where it is desired to cause the most treatment effect. Yomo *et al.* investigated the dose distribution with the GK novel collimation system in a randomized group of patients and arrived at the conclusion that the dose planning capabilities of the GK Perfexion on a cohort of vestibular schwannomas demonstrated a better conformity and energy distribution, with better cochlear sparing and without any particular drawback. In addition, there is an improvement in peripheral dose gradient in larger lesions [13], confirming the initial observations of Régis *et al.* [11] The translation of this to improved outcomes awaits clinical studies.

Indexes were developed to objectively measure the radiosurgery planning quality [14–16].

$$\text{Conformity index}\ (\text{CI}) = \frac{\text{PIV}}{\text{TV}}$$

$$\text{Paddick Conformity Index}\ (\text{PCI}) = \frac{\text{TV}_{\text{PIV2}}}{\text{TV} \times \text{PIV}}$$

$$\text{Gradient Index}\ (\text{GI}) = \frac{(\text{PIV}_{50\%})}{\text{PIV}}$$

Where CI is Conformity Index, TV is target volume, PIV is prescription isodose volume and GI Gradient Index.

Dosimetry

The main dosimetric characteristic of radiosurgery is to deliver a high dose of radiation to the target tissue and low radiation dose to the normal tissue in the periphery of the lesion. This can be accomplished when multiple fields converge to a point called isocentre. The isocentre is generally placed strategically to have the radiation volume completely cover the lesion. However, the maximum radiation point, due to the pass point characteristics of converging beams, is usually situated slight superiorly to the isocentre, when planning intracranial radiosurgery. This occurs because the entrance of the multiple pencil beans is from the top of the head, bringing the 'hot spot' to a site slightly above the isocentre.

The imposed limitation of the radiosurgery technique by the beam is the volume of normal tissue immediately adjacent to the lesion that, together with the lesion volume, receives a certain dose of radiation leading to increased risk of radiation-induced complications. This is the area, outside the lesion, where the multiple fields (beams) partially overlap [17]. As the target volume increases, the intermediate volume area also enlarges, meaning that more volume of normal parenchyma is encompassed by higher doses of radiation. This is why target volume in radiosurgery is suggested to be no greater than 3 cm (~12.6 cc). The target volume also impacts in the shaping capabilities of radiosurgery.

Functional lesion considerations

Prescribing to a point

Sharp and well-circumscribed lesions that disconnect pathways or ablate nuclei are the goals of this application. The prescription dose for functional neurosurgery is by convention and by tradition to the isocentre. This means that 100% of the dose (= maximal dose) is prescribed to a target point, that is, prescribed to the isocentre. The radiation prescription dose is the same as the maximal dose when prescribing to the maximum [18]. The fall-off distance, that is, the volume of tissue receiving at least 50% of the dose is proportional to the diameter of the aperture. The application of this concept is nicely seen during the targeting of the root entry zone in trigeminal neuralgia with the 4 mm field.

The diameter of the 50% isodoseline (IDL) is 4 mm. This also determines the use of the lesion used for other functional applications, such as movement disorders and psychiatric disorders [19–25].

The placement of the isocentre while planning radiosurgery for trigeminal neuralgia relies on the IDL to determine the distance of the isocentre to the brainstem. The dose distributions in trigeminal neuralgia exemplify well the concept of prescribing to a point in GK radiosurgery, the dose touching the brainstem represents the percentage of the absolute dose coined by the IDL chosen.

Prescribing to a volume

Volumetric and well-conformal dose distribution for modifying the function of the irradiated target tissue by either rendering the cells of a tumour apoptotic or modifying the firing pattern of a seizure focus or causing repair reaction in the vasculature of an AVM is the goal of this application. Seizure focus represents an excellent example of prescription to a volume. It is becoming apparent that one is able to change the firing pattern of cells in a seizure focus and still maintain the integrity of the tissue. This is possible due to the effects of radiation in the cell make-up, tissue blood supply and the changes in the cell ability to produce neurotransmitters [26]. The threshold of cell firing in the seizure focus can be increased without inducing radiation necrosis in the tissue [27]. What is not quite defined is the ideal dose, either single or fractions of radiation. Regis *et al.* have accumulated important experience on the effects of single-dose radiation to control seizure focus, either due to a hypothalamic hamartoma with gelastic seizures or due to typical temporal lobe epilepsy [28, 29]. Here is an excellent example of shaping the radiation to a volume in the internal portion of the hypothalamic hamartoma, keeping the fall-off of dose inside of the lesion and experiencing remarkable control of seizure episodes [30]. The volume of the epileptic focus or lesion to be treated is covered by the prescribed dose, that is the absolute dose of prescription is the one that most completely (specificity) and most conformably covers the target (conformity) (Figure 19.4).

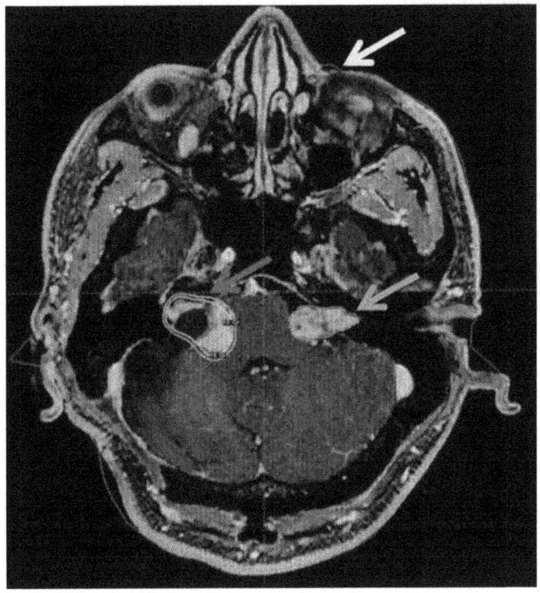

Figure 19.4 Steps of planning; T1 MRI image with 1 mm thickness obtained days before the procedure fused to a CT on the day of the procedure with the patient having the stereotactic frame for definition of coordinates. The CT also provides the automatic contour of the patient's head; notice the white arrow showing the red line contouring the image, which defines the surface of the patient for calculation of beam attenuation. The tumour on the right of the figure demonstrated the segmentation of the lesion, which was contoured with the automatic tools of the software, determining the volume of the lesion (pink arrow). The green arrow demonstrates the multiple-isocentre-depicted isodoseline. It conforms to a partially removed acoustic neuroma in the neurofibromatosis patient. Notice the two lines, yellow and green, representing the 12 Gy and the 10 Gy lines, respectively. (*See insert for colour representation of the figure.*)

Considerations of volumetric dosimetry

The simplest dose distribution is achieved with a single collimator radiosurgery plan. However, limited radiosurgery targets can be optimally treated with cones. Examples are lesions to targets such as the trigeminal nerve and the thalamus, perfectly round metastases/primary tumours or small and round AVMs are amenable to a single isocentre plan. All other lesions do not carry a shape amenable to be covered with a single isocentre without spreading too much radiation to the surrounding brain.

Considering a brain metastasis or a small round glioma, it is desirable to cover the gross contrast-enhancing lesion or gross target volume (GTV) with some margin, usually 1 or 2 mm. This may account for micro-dissemination of malignant cells surrounding the area defined by the contrast enhancement. This volume is called clinical target volume (CTV). Besides the CTV, one should account for the uncertainties of the radiation delivery process, which, at best, considering any technique approaches 2 mm [31]. The final irradiated volume, defined as the CTV plus usually 2 mm margins, is named the PTV (planned target volume). The minimal radiation dose considered to be clinically safe and effective is prescribed to the PTV. The dose that adequately covers the target is named prescription radiation dose. Usually, in GK radiosurgery, the prescription IDL is low, 50% or even lower. This means that the maximal dose is 50% larger than the dose at the periphery of the lesion, according to whether the prescription was to the 50% or lower IDL, respectively (Figure 19.4). The example in Figure 19.4 shows prescription to the 50% IDL, in yellow.

Radiation dose fall-off

The dose fall-off in the GK radiosurgery is very steep. This defines the attractiveness of the method, allowing for high radiation dose collimation inside the target with very fast radiation dose fall in the normal brain surrounding the target. The dose fall-off varies according to the aperture size and the multiple isocentre technique. This area of radiation fall-off is called the penumbra. Considering the dosimetric consequences of penumbra is important because this radiation quantity may be still sufficiently high to cause toxicity in the eloquent structure neighbouring the lesion such as brainstem, motor strip or the optic nerve. On the other hand, at the margin of a complex lesion, the fall-off dose may be still effective to control tumour growth, although under-dosed in relation to the remaining lesion volume.

In the context of skull base lesions abutting the optic apparatus or the brainstem, it is unwise to deliver the same radiation dose prescribed to the lesion to these eloquent structures. Although it may be attractive to cover the lesion with additional safety margins, the risks of radiation-induced damage are not justifiable. In these situations, one possible approach is to slightly under-dose the boundary of the lesion touching the eloquent structure to allow the fall-off of the dose to occur inside of the lesion, and not start in the border of the lesion, avoiding in this way a substantial dose outside of the contrast-enhancing limits. Another strategy is to resort fractions of radiation to completely cover the lesion.

Homogeneity

The tailored addition of tri-dimension margins to the GTV, according to surrounding structure constrains, and the interplay of weighting and plugging of apertures aiming an asymmetrical dose fall-off around a lesion bring the concept of homogeneity and intensity modulation to discussion. This is a very controversial aspect of the radiation plan.

In order to accomplish conformity to an irregular shape, multiple isocentres are agglomerated leading to an overlap of many spherical volumes. The volumes where the prescription dose of isolated isocentres intersects constitute a 'hot spot'. The number of hot spots in the PTV increases as the number of isocentres in the plan increases, due to increased overlap. The plans are built to allow the minimal difference between the radiation prescribed to cover the periphery of the lesion and maximal doses within the lesion; therefore, prescription to higher IDL tends to be desirable [32]. The steeper fall-off of a dose distribution is observed within the segment of the curve between the 50 and 90% IDL. Mathematical simulations of different IDL prescription strategies for the same plan show the advantage of sparing the surrounding normal tissue when prescribing to the highest IDL. Although homogeneity is suggested to be mathematically advantageous, its translation into better clinical outcomes after radiosurgery remains to be proven. Unfortunately, a randomized clinical trial having IDL as the main endpoint variable, and balancing the randomization for all others covariates playing an important prognostic role, is unlikely practical.

Volume shaping techniques

Initially, the available instrumentation to deliver high doses of radiation to deep structures without spreading high doses to the normal brain was through multiple isocentres based in four helmets, 4, 8, 14 and 18mm. Plugging of beans was a painstaking proposition. Now, with the automation of interplay of 4, 8 and 16mm aperture of the GK Perfexion, the process is seamless, allowing plugging, weighing and automatic optimization of the plan with sparing of structures at risk using just the clicks of a computer. Plotting the combination of conforming tools provides high conformity to very irregularly shaped lesions with high specificity. Arrangement of the proper optimal isocentre and collimator size for achieving conformity in complex lesions is an art. Practitioners may take hours to be satisfied with a plan. Although modern software has automated the simulation of the best arrangements, it still requires time and judgement from the medical radiosurgery team to make the final decision.

Imaging for radiosurgery

The success of the treatment planning and delivery of radiation, and therefore of the radiosurgery procedure, hinges in the quality of the imaging permitting the visualization of the pathology and anatomy to be spared, or targeted definition in cases of functional procedures. Sequences of MRI and addition of CT for correction of distortions and calculation of attenuation of beans make the system completely devoid of the need of human reading of the numbers, therefore avoiding the most common error in the procedure. This makes safety and reproducibility a hallmark of the procedure.

MRI distortion is a reality and can happen for multiple reasons, because of poor calibration of the machine, common in radiological units not linked to stereotactic services, and due to the presence of metal in the patient's clothes, teeth, hair, etc. Therefore, strict care needs to be taken while obtaining images to input in the Gamma Plan®. Now that image fusion is promptly obtained without the difficulty of the early years [33], acquisition of a stereotactic CT immediately before the procedure, with the patient with the stereotactic frame, provides for most reliable stereotactic coordinates and correction of the distortions that can hamper the quality of the GK surgery. This also allows for the convenience of obtaining the MRI days before the procedure and the CT, a faster acquisition image, with fewer issues of claustrophobia, movement issues and possible distortions, on the day of the procedure. To improve quality of the fusion, a CT post-contrast is recommended, using the vascular structures seen in the CT and MRI, as well as the patient's lesion, if capturing gadolinium and iodine contrast, as an assurance of perfect image merge [34].

Clinical applications

As suggested in Table 19.2, GK radiosurgery is indicated for the great majority of tumours involving the encephalon, either as a first form of therapy or as a complement to a partial resection. It is also commonly applied

Table 19.2 Minimal quality of imaging and sequences for treatment planning.

Pituitary tumours:	Coronal T1 – 1 mm tck, n/g, n/c.
	Coronal T1 – 1 mm tck, n/g, w/c, w/fs.
	Coronal T2 – 2 mm tck n/g.
	Axial T1 v/a – 1 mm tck, n/g, w/c, w/fs, whole brain
Meningiomas	Axial T2 – 1 mm tck, n/g, w/fs
Cranial base and orbit:	Axial and coronal T1 – 1 mm tck, w/c, w/fs.
	Axial T1 v/a – 1 mm tck, n/g, w/c, w/fs, whole brain.
Cranial base lesions	Axial T2 – 1 mm tck, n/g
Clivus chordoma	Sagittal and axial T1 – 1 mm tck, n/g, w/c, w/fs
Lymphoma, etc.:	Axial T1 v/a – 1 mm tck, n/g, w/c, w/fs, whole brain
Acoustic neuromas:	Axial 3D CISS/FIESTA – 0.8 mm tck, mastoid a/q.
	Axial and coronal T1 – 1 mm tck, w/c, n/g.
	Axial T1 v/a – 1 mm tck, n/g, w/c, w/fs, whole brain.
Trigeminal neuralgia:	Axial CISS/FIESTA – 0.4 mm tck
	Axial T1 v/a – 1 mm tck, n/g, w/c, w/fs, whole brain.
AVMs:	Digital angiography 2D or 3D, when needed.
	Axial T1 v/a – 1 mm tck, n/g, w/c, w/fs, whole brain.
	Axial T2 – 2 mm tck, whole brain.
	MRA – whole brain.
	CTA – whole brain.
Metastases:	Axial T1 v/a – 1 mm tck, n/g, w/c, w/fs, whole brain.
	Axial, sagittal, coronal a/q with double dose of contrast.
Primary brain tumours:	Axial T1 v/a – 1 mm tck, n/g, w/c, w/fs, whole brain.
	Axial T2 v/a – 2 mm tck.
Functional procedures:	T2 – volumetric fast spin echo recovery through basal ganglia Axial T1 v/a – 1 mm tck, n/g, w/c, w/fs, whole brain.
Stereotactic CT:	Axial a/q, 1 mm tck, n/c and w/c, whole brain.

tck, thickness, n/g: no gap, n/c: no contrast, w/c: with contrast, w/fs: with fat saturation, v/a: volumetric acquisition. a/q: acquisition; AVM, Arteriovenous malformation. All slabs must be of at least 6 cm span, encompassing completely the lesion for a proper imaging fusion and anatomical landmarks visualization. Notice that all pathologies need a volumetric acquisition of whole brain with contrast and without gantry tilt. All patients undergo CT for stereotactic localization and with contrast for better fusion based on vascular structures.

in the recurrence setting after a partial resection. Several of the tumour indications are controversial when a resection is possible. This is because of the inability of the GK procedure to provide timely decrease of mass effect and histological confirmation. However, due to the evolution of the imaging techniques, lesions are diagnosed before they lead to neurological deficits due to mass effect, which requires surgery. Moreover, the great majority of the lesions are diagnosed with a certainty of histology due to its aspect on MRI, CT and positron emission tomography. There is an increased acceptance in the neurosurgical and radiation oncology community to treat patients without histological confirmation, by relying on the imaging aspect of the lesions.

Penetration worldwide

Patients' appeal for a more comfortable treatment, avoidance of large surgeries and reliability of the treatment and prognosis was met by radiosurgery. Progressively, the treatment of the patient does not depend on the manual skills of a person, but on the intellectual and mathematical expertise of a team of specialists dedicated to provide the most reliable and comfortable care for the patient. This development worldwide based on the mushrooming of the computer technology permitted the introduction of robotized medicine and the GK is a prototype of this approach, relying exclusively on computer capability to deliver treatment. The indication and the management of the patient are still dependent on the doctor's expertise, mostly when tumour-causing mass effects and medical therapy are unable to provide the cure and relief from suffering expected by the patient.

As GK provided this immediate population need, it received immediate acceptance in the developed world and has marched progressively through the countries in development, as resources became available. Up to now, more than 700 000 patients have been treated by the technology and the numbers are increasing in exponential fashion (Figure 19.5).

Technical aspects of specific treatment planning

Obsessive compulsive disorder

The target for obsessive-compulsive disorder (OCD) has been in the anterior limb of the internal capsule, as determined by the head of the caudate medially and the putamen laterally [35, 36]. It has evolved from the midpoint of the internal capsule as one sees it in the coronal MRI scan to the most inferior portion of the capsule in the proximity of the nucleus accumbens [37]. It became apparent over the years of experience by the groups of Karolinska University and Brown University that as the target was brought ventrally, the results improved [38, 39]. Sheehan *et al.* suggest placement of the 50% IDL at the most ventral portion of the internal capsule [37]. Recently, a randomized trial performed by a Brazilian group showed that this rationale might hold true [40]. Studies are under way to confirm this hypothesis.

The GK capsulotomy calls for a 4-mm collimator aimed to the anterior limb of the internal capsule on each side. It is planned to be located 19–21 mm anterior to the AC on the intercommissural plane. This approximately corresponded to the midputaminal point. T1- and T2-weighted MRI demonstrates precisely the mid-putaminal point of the anterior limb of the capsule. The most ventral portion of the 50% IDL reaches the most ventral portion of the internal capsule. Doses in the literature have varied from 140 to 200 Gy [37, 38, 40]; therefore, 70–100 Gy reaches the shell of the accumbens at the base of the IC. (Figure 19.6). Konziolka *et al.* showed consistent lesions in the internal capsule using two isocentres of 4 mm, while trying to obtain an oval-shaped

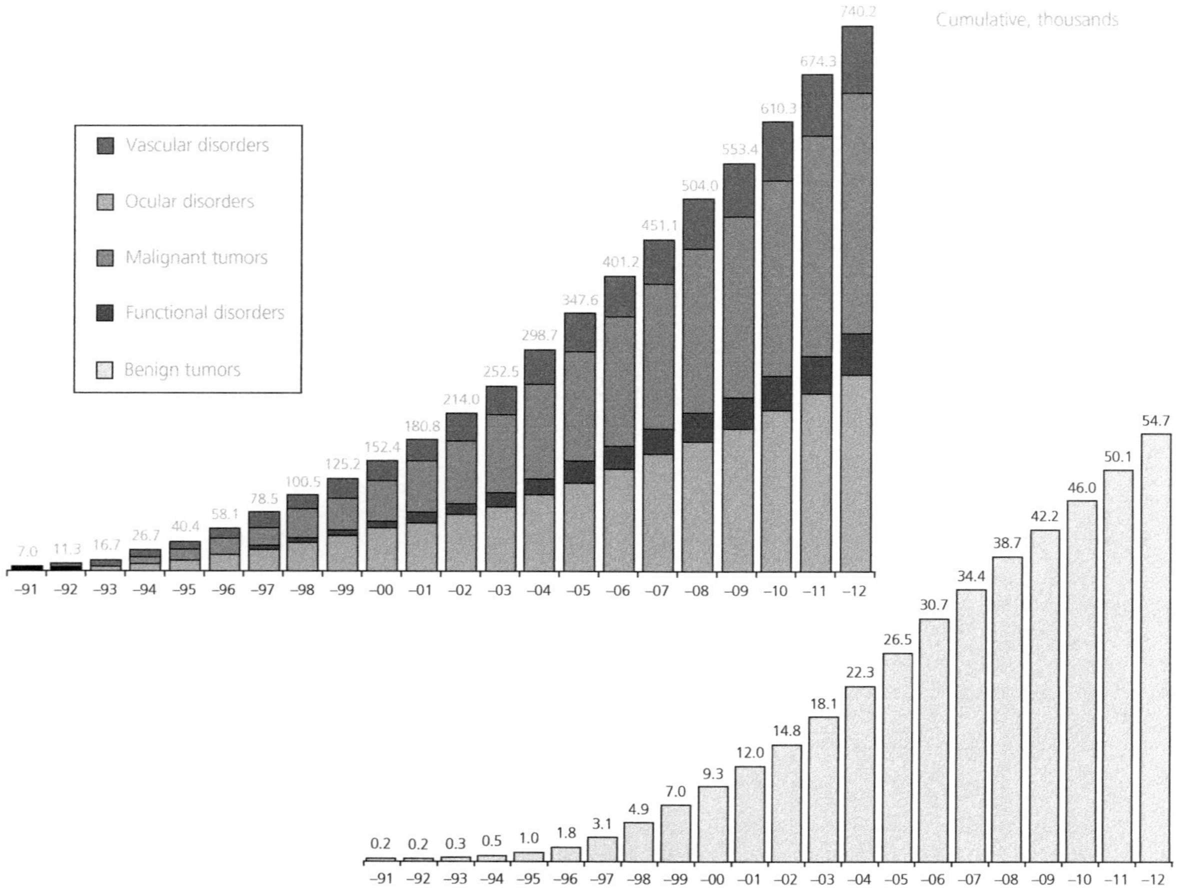

Figure 19.5 More than 740 000 patients were treated using the Leksell GK worldwide in 2012. Upper left graph shows the cumulative by thousands of patients treated until 2012 separated by classification of the application, vascular, ocular disorders, malignant tumours, functional disorders and benign tumours, as the reader looks from the top of the bars to their bases. Notice the growing applications in malignant disease, as well, mostly represented by metastatic diseases. Also, there is a growing number of applications in functional disorders over the last 20 years. This is represented in the lower right graph. Trigeminal neuralgia represents the bulk of the functional applications, 47 000 of the 50 000 treated worldwide. Source: Leksell Gamma Knife Society.

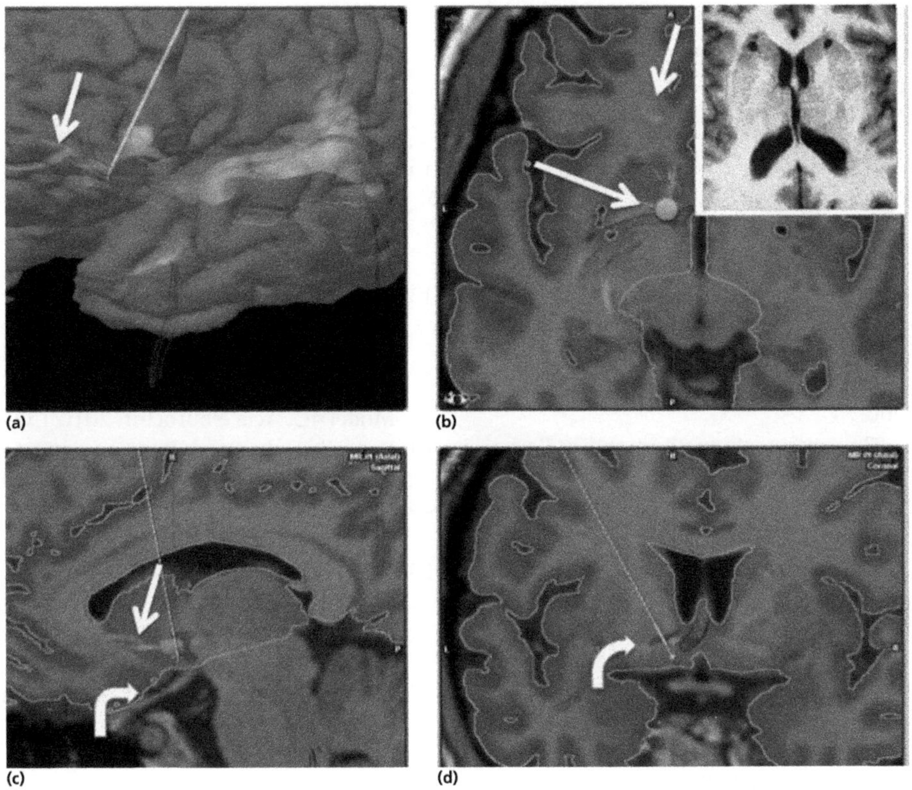

Figure 19.6 Notice the fibres in the direction of the frontal lobe that are interrupted by the capsulotomy (white arrows). **(a)** 3D visualization of fibretracking from the anterior limb of the internal capsule with spread of fibres to the frontal area, and also to the temporal lobe and associated areas in the temporo-parietal region **(b)**. Depth of the intended lesion to achieve the shell of the accumbens (large arrow) The inset in the upper right shows an example of an ideal radiofrequency lesion between the putamen and caudate. Courtesy of Dr. Marwan Hariz. **(c)** Sagittal view showing the safe distance of target to the optic nerve (curve arrow). **(d)** Relationship of the posterior portion of the lesion that should not extend to the anterior commissure, which is approximately 20 mm posterior to the centre of the lesion (fibretracking produce by Dr. Mark Sedrak in our group). (*See insert for colour representation of the figure.*)

lesion of 48 mm^3 with its most inferior extension in the ventral portion of the internal capsule. The doses used in their study were 140 and 150 Gy.

Conclusion

Modern GK radiosurgery offers ease of treatment planning and delivery with patient's comfort as an important goal. The stereotactic frame is still necessary, either with the traditional bonny fixation using pins attached to the frontal and occipital region or with a relocatable mouthpiece vacuum fixation device. A mask-based system is also being developed in conjunction with an on-board cone beam CT. It is possible to perform hypofractionation with the GK at this time, either with the relocatable frame or keeping the patient with the frame attached to the skull for the days of treatment. Oncoming developments in the GK-plus® will expand; it is unquestionable that the GK technique has reached a well-defined success and place in the neurosurgical management of neuropsychiatric conditions.

References

1 Holly FE. Radiosurgery Equipment: Physical Principles, Precision, Limitations. In De Salles AAF, Goetsch SJ (eds.): Stereotactic Surgery and Radiosurgery. Medical Physics Publishing Corporation, Madison, Wisconsin, 1993, pp 185–200.
2 Leksell L. The stereotaxic method and radiosurgery of the brain. Acta Chir Scand. 1951;102:316.
3 De Salles AAF, Gorgulho A, Agazaryan N. Linear Accelerator Radiosurgery: technical aspects. In Youmans Neurologic Surgery. 67th edition, 3rd volume, Elsevier, Amsterdam, The Netherlands, 2011 pp 2622–2632.
4 Gorgulho AA, Warren I, De Salles AAF. General Imaging Modalities: Basic Principles. In Gildenberg P, Tasker R, Lozano A (eds.): Text Book of Stereotactic and Functional Neurosurgery (2nd edn., chapter 17, 251–268). Springer, Berlin, 2009.
5 De Salles AA, Gorgulho AA, Pereira JL, McLaughlin N. Intracranial stereotactic radiosurgery: concepts and techniques. Neurosurg Clin N Am. 2013 Oct;24(4):491–8.
6 Leksell L. Stereotaxis and Radiosurgery. An Operative System. Charles C Thomas, Publisher, Springfield, 1971 pp 47–52.
7 Steiner L, Leksell L, Greitz T, Forster DMC, Backlund EO. Stereotaxic radiosurgery for cerebral arteriovenous malformations. Report of a case. Acta Chir Scand. 1972;138:459–64.
8 Lunsford LD, Flickinger J, Lindner G, Maitz A. Stereotactic radiosurgery of the brain using the first United States 201 cobalt-60 source gamma knife. Neurosurgery. 1989 Feb;24(2):151–9.
9 Betti O, Derechinsky V. Multiple-beam stereotaxic irradiation. Neurochirurgie. 1983;29(4):295–8
10 Bhatnagar JP, Novotny J Jr, Huq MS. Dosimetric characteristics and quality control tests for the collimator sectors of the Leksell Gamma Knife(®) Perfexion(TM). Med Phys. 2012 Jan;39(1):231–6.
11 Régis J, Tamura M, Guillot C, Yomo S, Muraciolle X, Nagaje M, Arka Y, Porcheron D. Radiosurgery with the world's first fully robotized Leksell Gamma Knife PerfeXion in clinical use: a 200-patient prospective, randomized, controlled comparison with the Gamma Knife 4C. Neurosurgery. 2009 Feb;64(2):346–55.
12 De Salles AAF, Gorgulho A, Selch M, De Marco J, Agazaryan N. Radiosurgery from the brain to the spine: 20 years experience. Acta Neurochir Suppl. 2008;101:163–8.
13 Yomo S, Tamura M, Carron R, Porcheron D, Régis J. A quantitative comparison of radiosurgical treatment parameters in vestibular schwannomas: the Leksell Gamma Knife Perfexion versus Model 4C. Acta Neurochir. 2010;152:47–55.
14 Paddick I. A simple scoring ratio to index the conformity of radiosurgical treatment plans. Technical Note. J Neurosurg. 2000;93(Suppl 3):219–22.
15 Lomax NJ, Scheib SG. Quantifying the degree of conformity in radiosurgery treatment planning. Int J Radiat Oncol Biol Phys. 2003;55(5):1409–19.
16 Knöös T, Kristensen I, Nilsson P. Volumetric and dosimetric evaluation of radiation treatment plans: radiation conformity index. Int J Radiat Oncol Biol Phys. 1998;42(4):1169–76.
17 Kooy HM, Bellerive MR, Loefler JS. In Philip L. Gildenberg, Ronald R. Tasker (eds.): Text Book of Stereotactic and Functional Neurosurgery. McGraw-Hill Companies, New York, 1998, pp 687–704.
18 Leksell L. Cerebral radiosurgery. I. Gammathalanotomy in two cases of intractable pain. Acta Chir Scand. 1968;134(8):585–95.
19 Friehs GM, Park MC, Goldman MA, Zerris VA, Norén G, Sampath P. Stereotactic radiosurgery for functional disorders. Neurosurg Focus. 2007;23(6):E3. Review.
20 Elias WJ, Huss D, Voss T, Loomba J, Khaled M, Zadicario E, Frysinger RC, Sperling SA, Wylie S, Monteith SJ, Druzgal J, Shah BB, Harrison M, Wintermark M. A pilot study of focused ultrasound thalamotomy for essential tremor. N Engl J Med. 2013 Aug 15;369(7):640–8.
21 Kondziolka D, Flickinger JC, Lunsford LD. Stereotactic radiosurgery for epilepsy and functional disorders. Neurosurg Clin N Am. 2013 Oct;24(4):623–32.
22 Frighetto L, De Salles AAF, Cabatan-Awang C, Ford J, Solberg T, Selch MT. Linear accelerator

thalamotomy. Surg Neurol. 2004 Aug;62(2): 106–13.

23 Wintermark M, Huss DS, Shah BB, Tustison N, Druzgal TJ, Kassell N, Elias WJ. Thalamic connectivity in patients with essential tremor treated with MR imaging-guided focused ultrasound: in vivo fiber tracking by using diffusion-tensor MR imaging. Radiology. 2014 Mar 9:132112.

24 Sedrak M, Gorgulho A, Frew A, Behnke E, De Salles A, Pouratian N. Diffusion Tensor imaging (DTI) and colored fractional anisotropy (FA) mapping of the ventralis intermedius (VIM) nucleus of the thalamus. Neurosurgery. 2011 Nov;69(5):1124–9.

25 Frighetto L, Bizzi J, Annes RD, Silva Rdos S, Oppitz P. Stereotactic radiosurgery for movement disorder. Surg Neurol Int. 2012;3(Suppl 1): S10–6.

26 De Salles AAF, Melega WP, Lacan G, Steele LH, Solberg TD. Radiosurgery with a 3 mm collimator in the subthalamic nucleus and substantia nigra of the vervet monkey. J Neurosurg. 2001;95:990–7.

27 Sun B, De Salles AAF, Medin P, Solberg T, Hoebel B, Felder-Allen M, Wie C-W, Ackerman R. Reduction of hippocampal-kindled seizure activity in rats by stereotactic radiosurgery. Exp Neurol. 1998;154:691–5.

28 Regis J, Bartolomei F, Rey M, Haayashi M, Chauvel M, Peragut JC. Gamma knife surgery for mesial temporal lobe epilepsy. J Neurosurg. 2000;93(Suppl 3):141–6.

29 Régis J, Scavarda D, Tamura M, Villeneuve N, Bartolomei F, Brue T, Morange I, Dafonseca D, Chauvel P. Gamma knife surgery for epilepsy related to hypothalamic hamartomas. Semin Pediatr Neurol. 2007 Jun;14(2):73–9. Review

30 Selch MT, Gorgulho A, Mattozo C, Solberg TD, Cabatan-Awang C, DeSalles AA. Linear accelerator stereotactic radiosurgery for the treatment of gelastic seizures due to hypothalamic hamartoma. Minim Invasive Neurosurg. 2005 Oct;48(5):310–4.

31 Ma L, Nichol A, Hossain S, Wang B, Petti P, Vellani R, Higby C, Ahmad S, Barani I, Shrieve DC, Larson DA, Sahgal A. Variable dose interplay effects across radiosurgical apparatus in treating multiple brain metastases. Int J Comput Assist Radiol Surg. 2014;9:1079–86.

32 Goetsch SJ, De Salles AAF, Solberg TD, Holly E, Selch T, Bajada CL. Treatment Planning for Stereotactic Radiosurgery. In De Salles AAF, Goetsch SJ (eds.): Stereotactic Surgery and Radiosurgery. Medical Physics Publishing Corporation, Madison, Wisconsin, 1993, pp 277–91.

33 De Salles AAF, Asfora WT, Abe M, Kjelberg RN. Transposition of target information from the magnetic resonance and CT-scan images to the conventional x-ray stereotactic space. Appl Neurophysiol. 1987;50:23–32.

34 Jonker BP. Image fusion pitfalls for cranial radiosurgery. Surg Neurol Int. 2013;4(4):123–8.

35 Leksell L, Backlund EO. Radiosurgical capsulotomy – a closed surgical method for psychiatric surgery. Lakartidningen. 1978 Feb 15; 75(7):546–7.

36 Leksell L, Herner T, Leksell D, Persson B, Lindquist C. Visualisation of stereotactic radiolesions by nuclear magnetic resonance. J Neurol Neurosurg Psychiatry. 1985 Jan;48(1):19–20.

37 Sheehan JP, Patterson G, Schlesinger D, Xu Z. Gamma knife surgery anterior capsulotomy for severe and refractory obsessive-compulsive disorder. J Neurosurg. 2013;119:1112–8.

38 Ruck C, Karlsson A, Steele D, Edman G, Meyerson BA, Ericson K, Nyman H, Asberg M, Svanborg P. Capsulotomy for obsessive-compulsive disorder. Long-term follow-up of 25 patients. Arch Gen Psychiatry. 2008;65(8):914–22.

39 Lippitz B, Mindus P, Meyerson BA, Kihlstrom L, Lindquist C. Lesion topography and outcome after thermocapsulotomy or gamma knife capsulotomy for obsessive-compulsive disorder: relevance of the right hemisphere. Neurosurgery. 1999;44(3):452–60.

40 Lopes A, Greenberg B, Noren G, Canteras MM, Busatto GF, de Mathis ME, Taub A, D'Alcante CC, Hoexter MQ, Gouvea FS, Cecconi JP, Gentil AF, Ferrão YA, Fuentes D, de Castro CC, Leite CC, Salvajoli JV, Duran FL, Rasmussen S, Miguel EC. Treatment of resistant obsessive-compulsive disorder with ventral capsular/ventral striatal gamma capsulotomy: a pilot prospective study. J Neuropsychiatry Clin Neurosci. 2009;21(4): 381–92.

CHAPTER 20

Gamma knife surgery: Clinical results

Antonio Carlos Lopes, Marcelo Batistuzzo, Andre Felix Gentil, Marcelo Queiroz Hoexter and Euripedes Constantino Miguel
University of São Paulo Medical School, São Paulo, Brazil

Introduction

Ablative neurosurgery has been employed for decades in the treatment of severe mental disorders. Gamma Knife (GK) radiosurgery is one of these ablative treatment modalities, which consists in the production of actinic lesions after the focalization of hundreds of collimated beams of gamma rays derived from ^{60}Cobalt seeds in preselected brain targets. Albeit a traditional procedure, GK radiosurgery continues to be not only an alternative to deep brain stimulation (DBS) but also potentially the first indication in some selected psychiatric refractory patients. The procedure has been evolving to define targets progressively smaller, more precise and effective, but with a reduced profile of side effects.

Historical background and operative techniques

The first stereotactic neurosurgical procedures in humans were performed by Spiegel and Wycis in the United States in 1947. Two years later, Leksell in Sweden and Tailarach in France independently reported the use of different instruments for human stereotactic operations. Among these very first functional neurosurgical techniques, capsulotomy by thermocoagulation (bilateral lesions of the anterior limb of the internal capsule) was investigated for the treatment of severe psychiatric disorders. Later, in 1953, Leksell conducted the first radiosurgical capsulotomy, using 300 kV X-rays (Leksell *et al.*, 1955 cited in Ref. 1).

Since then, different anatomical targets have been chosen for different indications. The anterior limb of the internal capsule (i.e. the anterior capsulotomy technique) remained an important target for treating obsessive-compulsive disorder (OCD) and anxiety disorders, especially in Europe. In the United States, the cingulotomy technique, which is characterized by lesions at the anterior cingulum, was employed for treating depression and OCD [2–5], while in Britain, lesions of the substantia innominata (in subcaudate tractotomy) or a combination of subcaudate tractotomy and cingulotomy (the limbic leucotomy technique) were developed for treating depression, OCD and anxiety [6–8].

In 1976, the first GK capsulotomy was conducted at the Karolinska Institutet [9]. Their experience, accrued in almost four decades of performing GK procedures for psychiatric disorders, reveals important technical differences between their first and the last series of patients. This heterogeneity must be carefully

Neuromodulation in Psychiatry, First Edition. Edited by Clement Hamani, Paul Holtzheimer, Andres M. Lozano and Helen Mayberg.

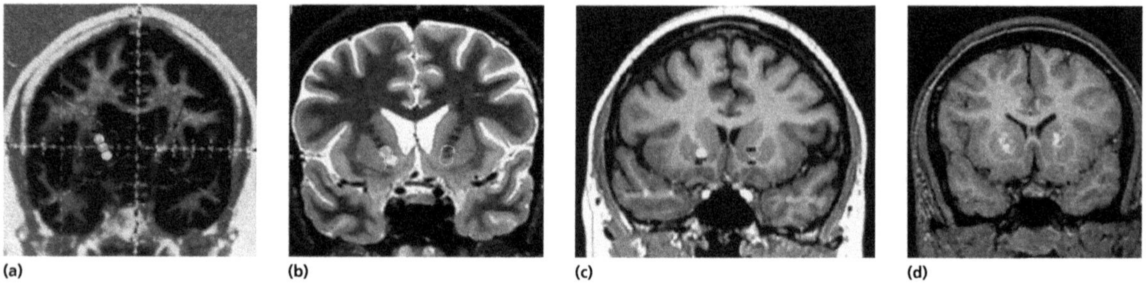

Figure 20.1 Different types of Gamma Knife lesions for psychiatric patients. **(a)** Original target for gamma capsulotomy (triple bilateral lesions with 4 mm collimators). **(b)** Gamma ventral capsulotomy (double-shot bilateral lesions). **(c)** single-shot Gamma ventral capsulotomy. **(d)** Gamma Knife limbic leucotomy targets.

weighed when analysing efficacy and safety profiles. In the 1970s, lesions were almost rectangular in shape, with an anterior-posterior diameter of 3 mm and a transverse diameter ranging from 5 to 11 mm [10, 11]. With the employment of 4 and 8 mm round collimators, lesion geometry significantly changed and the number of isocentres on each hemisphere also varied considerably (Figure 20.1). While some patients received three bilateral 4-mm shots, others received only two bilateral shots, and, in a few subjects, single shots were performed using the large 8-mm collimators. Radiation doses also varied, as new technologies became available: while the median of 100% isodoses of the first series of patients was 160 Gy (doses ranging from 80 to 180 Gy), it increased to 200 Gy with the development of modern GK devices.

In parallel to the Swedish experience, researchers at Brown University in the United States proposed changes to the original anterior capsulotomy technique in 2001. At first, they employed only bilateral single-shot, mid-ventral lesions at the anterior limb of the internal capsule using 4-mm collimators and a standard dose of 180 Gy [12]. However, the patients only improved after the association of additional ventral shots adjacent to the nucleus accumbens. This double-shot technique was termed 'ventral capsular/ventral striatal gamma capsulotomy', or simply 'gamma ventral capsulotomy' (GVC) (Figure 20.1).

In a collaborative study between the University of São Paulo, Brazil and Brown University, Lopes *et al.* in 2009 described the results of a pilot study with bilateral double-shot GVC for the treatment of five OCD refractory patients [13]. Based on the favourable results, a double-blind randomized controlled trial was conducted in 16 additional patients [14]. The surgical technique was the same as the one described in the pilot study (180 Gy, double-shot lesions with 4-mm collimators at the ventral internal capsule). Efficacy and safety are described below.

Similar to the original Brown University study, researchers at the University of Pittsburgh in 2011 reported their experience with GVC, this time with a lower dose (160 Gy) [15]. Furthermore, in a recent study by Sheehan *et al.* in 2013, five OCD patients who refused to receive DBS were operated with a single-shot GVC [16]. However, instead of targeting the mid-capsular isocentres, only the most ventral portion of the internal capsule was chosen (see Figure 20.1). Patients received either 140 Gy ($n=3$) or 160 Gy ($n=2$), delivered trough 4-mm collimators [16].

Nevertheless, contrary to the tendency of making smaller and fewer lesions, a group from Mexico in 2006 reported their experience with 10 patients treated with either single or combined GK lesions in the cingulum and internal capsule using multiple isocentres (Figure 20.1) [17].

Indications

Ablative neurosurgical procedures may be offered for the treatment of specific neuropsychiatric disorders. OCD, major depressive disorder (MDD), anxiety disorders and Tourette syndrome (TS) are the main indications. To date, GK radiosurgery has data supporting its use only in OCD and anxiety disorders. These procedures are restricted to the most severe and highly impaired patients, with a history of lack of response to several medications and psychotherapy.

A single study has described the use of GK for treating severely aggressive patients [17]. This is not considered an indication for radiosurgery. Indeed, using ablative surgeries for treating severe aggressive behaviours remains controversial [18, 19].

Ethical issues

Given that radiosurgical interventions have been conducted for different psychiatric disorders, it is fundamental that the dissemination of this technology be done by following strict ethical norms. In addition, each country has its specific rules and regulations that must be strictly followed. Only the most treatment-refractory and disabled patients should be selected for surgery. Furthermore, GK radiosurgery must be carried out only after a patient has given fully informed consent. Thus, it is always preferable to select patients who have their decision-making capacities preserved. Patients must also be informed that they have the right to halt their participation in this type of procedure.

An independent review panel should always be formed to check that a patient has truly understood the possible benefits and risks involved in the surgical interventions. Additionally, it can also ascertain that the surgical patients have met the inclusion and exclusion criteria for a GK study. If possible, this independent committee should be formed, at least, by an independent psychiatrist, a neurologist and a member of the patient organizations.

Selection criteria for surgical interventions

Selection criteria

The first gamma capsulotomy studies did not appropriately describe their inclusion and exclusion criteria. However, in spite of relative differences in their selection process, studies of GK for OCD or anxiety disorders that were published in the last decade share some similar inclusion criteria. Briefly, a history of chronic symptoms for at least 5 years, severe and disabling symptoms, refractoriness to many different treatments and the capacity of providing consent form are common features. There is also recent evidence that different preoperative symptoms (specially hoarding) might be associated with a worse clinical outcome after the interventions, making a case for systematic screening of symptom profiles in candidates for ablative surgery [20, 21]. Except for two studies, most of them did not explicitly describe their exclusion criteria [13, 14].

Efficacy and safety

By the time of the first GK capsulotomies, specific psychopathological rating scales were not available, and global improvement instruments (such as the Pippard scale and the similar ones) were the only efficacy ratings applied. Only after the 1990s did studies systematically employ specific batteries to measure obsessive-compulsive symptoms (such as the Yale-Brown Obsessive Compulsive Scale – Y-BOCS), anxiety (Beck Anxiety Scale, or the Brief Scale for Anxiety) and depression (Beck Depression Inventory and the Montgomery–Åsberg Depression Rating Scale).

In one of the first studies showing the results of GK capsulotomy in psychiatry, Rylander in 1978 reported that three of five (60%) OCD patients and two of four (60%) chronic anxiety subjects showed global improvements, after a median of 5 and 6 months of follow-up, respectively (Table 20.1) [9]. Although there were no adverse cognitive or emotional complications, including personality changes, other side effects secondary to the surgical procedure were not described. Further, technical details of the surgical procedure, such as the number of isocentres, radiation doses and sizes of the lesions, were not provided in their publication.

Later, Mindus *et al.*, in 1987, described seven chronic anxiety disorder patients who received gamma capsulotomy: three of them had a primary diagnosis of panic disorder with agoraphobia, three patients had generalized anxiety disorder and one suffered from social phobia [10]. Global improvements were shown in five of seven patients, after a median of 7 years. On the other hand, side effects secondary to radiosurgery were not reported. Most subjects were irradiated by the cross-firing of collimated, narrow (3 × 5 mm) beams of ^{60}Co gamma radiation, with a median dose of 160 Gy. Although the same technique was employed in all patients, in the two cases with a poor response, magnetic resonance imaging scans failed to identify clear, bilateral lesions.

The first systematic description of side effects after GK capsulotomy came from Kihlström *et al.*, in 1995 [22]. Eleven patients were followed up for a period of 33–41 post-operative months. Nine patients received a very high dose of radiation – 200 Gy, with at least three isocentres (four isocentres in one patient), using 4-mm round collimators. The other two subjects received a dose of 160 Gy, with either one single-shot, 8-mm collimators, or three shots, 4-mm collimators. Four out of eleven (36.4%) patients were described as being 'clinically improved'. However, only the five OCD patients showed some reduction of symptoms, whereas the remaining patients with non-OCD anxiety disorders had unsatisfactory results. In terms of safety, five of nine patients who were exposed to 200 Gy of gamma radiation presented meaningful side effects in the long-term follow-up, especially headaches and symptoms of frontal lobe syndrome, especially apathy, fatigue, loss of initiative and sometimes disinhibited behaviours. The authors clearly recommended that only one single or two isocentres with 4-mm collimators should be employed in future studies.

Attempts to predict good response to GK surgery came from Lippitz *et al.*, in 1999, who reanalysed the data obtained from OCD patients who underwent gamma capsulotomy between 1976 and 1989 [11]. Seven of ten (70%) subjects had a minimum of 50% improvement in the Comprehensive Psychopathological Rating Scale-Obsessive-Compulsive subscale or in the Yale-Brown Obsessive-Compulsive Scale scores. Good treatment responses were associated with lesions at a circumscribed region of the right anterior limb of the internal capsule. Conversely, lesions located elsewhere were associated with poor outcomes, especially those located in the more anterior part of the internal capsule.

Almost 10 years later, Rück *et al.* assessed the records of all OCD patients who received either thermocapsulotomy or gamma capsulotomy between 1988 and 2000 [23]. Nine subjects had been submitted to GK surgery. Four (44.4%) and five (55.5%) of the nine patients achieved a minimum of 35% reduction of their original Y-BOCS scores at post-operative month 12, or at their last follow-up visits, respectively. Moreover, both 12-month and last follow-up Y-BOCS scores, as well as depression and anxiety ratings, were significantly lower when compared to those at the baseline. However, frontal lobe dysfunction, as measured by the Execution, Apathy and Disinhibition (EAD) scale, was strikingly high in all of the patients who had received very high doses of radiation (200 Gy in 3 isocentres, $n=3$) or multiple radiosurgical procedures ($n=1$).

As described above, Rasmussen, in 2001, employed smaller lesions with the GVC technique [12]. Fifteen patients received single-shot lesions. However, after 8 months of follow-up, only one patient had improved clinically, and additional ventral shots were then performed in 13 of the original 15 patients. After 1 year of follow-up, 5 of 13 patients had globally improved with this double-shot approach. Since then, 55 patients have been operated on at Brown University (Greenberg, pers. comm.).

Lopes *et al.*, in 2009, described the results of their pilot study, using the original Brown University double-shot GVC in the treatment of refractory OCD [13]. The same treatment response criteria that were employed in pharmacological trials were used to assess the efficacy in this study, as defined by a minimum of 35% reductions in Y-BOCS scores and Clinical Global Impression ratings '1' (very much improved) or '2' (much improved) [24]. Subjects were also assessed in terms of depression/anxiety symptoms and neuropsychological and personality measures, along multiple follow-up visits. Furthermore, side effects were investigated by a specific rating instrument. In terms of efficacy, two (40%) and three (60%) of five subjects were treatment responders at post-operative months 12 and 48, respectively. Their mean Y-BOCS scores dropped from 32.2 (severe symptoms) to 20.2 (moderate symptoms). However, one patient did show worsened OCD symptoms after surgery, possibly due to an atypical reaction to the effects of radiation, characterized by the development of smaller than expected actinic lesions after GK. Depression and anxiety symptoms decreased in the majority of patients. As for side effects, most were transient, such as headaches, nausea, vertigo, weight changes, post-operative throat swelling, 1-day haematuria, local dermatitis and discrete pain on the scalp. To the investigators' surprise, no post-operative adverse neuropsychological or personality deficits were observed.

Employing the same GVC technique, Kondziolka *et al.*, in 2011, reported that a smaller dose of radiation could also be effective [15]. Three patients received either 140 Gy ($n=2$) or 150 Gy ($n=1$). Two of them had a primary diagnosis of OCD, while one subject suffered from severe skin picking disorder (SPD – a grooming disorder with compulsive behaviours, but usually not associated with obsessions). In a mean follow-up of 42 months, average Y-BOCS scores dropped from 37.3 to 16.3, a 55% improvement. Of the three subjects included, the one with SPD had the highest substantial improvement. Reasons to explain this finding as well as how a patient without obsessions could have had such a high Y-BOCS score remain unclear. Only one patient had neuropsychological assessments after surgery, which suggests a normal frontal lobe performance, despite signs of impulsivity and perseveration [15, 25].

Similar to the original Brown University study, Sheehan *et al.*, in 2013, operated on five OCD patients who refused to receive DBS, using single-shot GVC [16]. Four of the five patients (80%) had their Y-BOCS scores reduced by a median of 61%. Adverse events were not systematically described, but 'no adverse events' were described in three patients in a long-term follow-up.

Until recently, there were no double-blind, randomized controlled trials of GK for the treatment of mental disorders, which precluded evidence-based conclusions regarding efficacy and safety of this radiosurgical procedure. However, one study has filled this literature gap [14]. Lopes *et al.* in 2014 randomized 16 OCD patients into two treatment groups, in a double-blind fashion: eight patients received sham GVC (ST group), while eight subjects were treated with actual GVC surgery (ATa group). To ensure the blinding, all patients were sedated throughout the radiosurgical procedure and a sham Cobalt chamber was attached to the original GK

Table 20.1 Main studies of Gamma Knife radiosurgery in psychiatry and their characteristics.

Study	Design	Surgical technique	Target	Dose	Isocentres	Collimators	Sample size	Main diagnosis
Rylander [9]	Case series	Capsulotomy	ALIC	ND	ND	ND	9	Obsessive + anxiety symptoms [5], chronic anxiety and phobic symptoms [4]
Mindus *et al.* [10]	Case series	Capsulotomy	ALIC	120 Gy (1 pt.), 152 Gy (1 pt.), 160 Gy (5 pt.)	–	Rectangular: Narrow (3 × 5 mm) beams	7	PDA (3), GAD [3], SP [1]
Kihlström *et al.* [22]	Case series	Capsulotomy	ALIC	160 Gy (2 pt.), 200 (9 pt.)	One bilateral (1 pt.), 3 bilateral (9 pt.), 4 bilateral (1 pt.)	Round 4 mm (10 pt.), 8 mm (1 pt.)	11	OCD [5], GAD or phobias [6]
Lippitz *et al.* [11]	Case series	Capsulotomy	ALIC	120 Gy, 180 Gy	ND	Both rectangular (narrow 3 × 5–11 mm beams) and round 4–8 mm	13, but only 9 with complete data	OCD [13]
Rück *et al.* [23]	Case series	Capsulotomy	ALIC	180 Gy (4 pt.), 200 Gy (5 pt.)	One or three bilateral	4 mm (9 pt.)	9	OCD
Lopes *et al.* [13]	Case series	Ventral capsulotomy	Ventral border ALIC	180 Gy (5 pt.)	Two bilateral	4 mm (5 pt.)	5	OCD
Kondziolka *et al.* [15]	Case series	Ventral capsulotomy	Ventral border ALIC	140 Gy (2 pt.), 150 Gy (1 pt.)	Two bilateral	4 mm (3 pt.)	3	OCD (2 pt.), skin picking disorder (1 pt.)

Comorbidities	Mean age at surgery	Mean years of disorder	Genders	Inclusion/ exclusion criteria	Efficacy	Adverse events	Mean maximum period of follow-up
Not clearly stated	40	16	7 female, 2 male	ND	OC symptoms: 3/5 improved; anxiety: 2/4 improved	ND	5 months
ND	40.1	16.1	5 female, 2 male	Poorly defined	Global improvement: 5/7 (71.4%) patients	ND	ND
ND	41.4	ND	4 female, 7 male	Poorly defined	Clinical improvement: 4 of 11 (36.4%) patients	Headaches, signs of frontal lobe syndrome (apathy, fatigue, loss of initiative, occasional disinhibition)	36.9 months (MRI)
ND	41.7	ND	5 female, 5 male	Poorly defined	Clinical improvement: 7 of 10 (70%) patients	ND	ND
Not clearly stated	43.9	ND	ND	Poorly defined	Significant YBOCS reductions: 4 of 9 (44%) pt. in 1 yr; 5 of 9 (55%) pt. at last FU	Apathy (2 pt.), memory problems (1 pt.), executive dysfunction (1 pt.), urinary incontinence (1 pt.), seizures (1 pt.), sexual dysinhibition (1 pt.)	11.4 years
Major depression (3 pt.), anxiety disorders (2 pt.), alcohol abuse (1 pt.), clusters B (1 pt.) and C (2 pt.) personality disorders.	35	17.4	3 female, 2 male	Well defined	Significant YBOCS reductions + global improvement: 2 of 5 (40%) pt. in 1 yr; 3 of 5 (60%) pt. at last FU	Most common: Episodic headaches (3 pt.), light-headedness/vertigo (4 pt.), weight changes (4 pt.), nausea/vomiting (2 pt.), insomnia (3 pt.), mood and anxiety changes (4 pt.).	48 months
ND	43.7	27.7	2 female, 1 male	Well defined inclusion criteria only	Significant YBOCS reductions: 2 of 3 (67%) pt. at last FU	ND	41.7 months

(continued)

Table 20.1 (Continued)

Study	Design	Surgical technique	Target	Dose	Isocentres	Collimators	Sample size	Main diagnosis
Sheehan *et al.* [16]	Case series	Ventral capsulotomy	Ventral border ALIC	140 Gy (3 pt.), 160 Gy (2 pt.)	One bilateral	4 mm (5 pt.)	5	OCD
Lopes *et al.* [14]	Double-blind, randomized trial	Ventral capsulotomy	Ventral border ALIC	180 Gy (16 pt.)	Two bilateral	4 mm (16 pt.)	16	OCD
Del Valle *et al.* [17]	Case series	Capsulotomy (5 pt.), limbic leucotomy (4 pt.) or subcaudate tractotomy (1 pt.)	ALIC, anterior cingulum, substantia inomminata?	ND	ND	ND	10	Schizoaffective disorder with aggressive behaviors (3 pt.), OCD (3 pt.), organic mental disorder with impulsiveness (2 pt.), Asperger and Tourette syndromes (1 pt.), major depression (1 pt.)

ALIC, anterior limb of the internal capsule; FU, follow-up; GAD, generalized anxiety disorder; MRI, magnetic resonance imaging; ND, not described; OC, obsessive-compulsive; OCD, obsessive-compulsive disorder; PDA, panic disorder with agoraphobia; SP, social phobia, YBOCS, Yale-Brown Obsessive Compulsive Scale score.

equipment. Masking was also warranted in the treatment planning. Furthermore, the only contact of the operative team (a neurosurgeon, a physicist, a radiotherapist and a nurse) with the patient, while under sedation, was during the surgical procedure. Blinded raters provided assessments of all patients during 12 months of follow-up. Two of eight patients (25%) who had received the active procedure improved during the blinded phase of the study, but none of the sham GVC patients improved. After blinding was broken, four of the original eight patients in the sham GVC group were treated with active radiosurgical procedure (the ATb group). In the long-term follow-up, five of the eight patients

Comorbidities	Mean age at surgery	Mean years of disorder	Genders	Inclusion/ exclusion criteria	Efficacy	Adverse events	Mean maximum period of follow-up
Depresion [1], anorexia nervosa [1]	36.8	20	2 female, 3 male	Well defined	Significant YBOCS reductions: 4 of 5 (80%) pt. at last FU	None? Not systematically described	24 months (median)
Major depression (12 pt.), anxiety disorders (8 pt.), alcohol abuse/ dependence (2 pt.), clusters A (2 pt.), B (2 pt.) and C (12 pt.) personality disorders.	32.1 (intervention group), 34.1 (sham group)	16.4 (intervention group), 17.1 (sham group)	6 female, 10 male	Well defined	Significant YBOCS reductions + global improvement: 3 of 8 (38%) pt. in intervention group, versus 0 of 8 pt. in sham group; 5 of 8 (63%) pt. at long term FU in intervention group	Episodic headaches (4 pt.), nausea/ vomiting (6 pt.), weight/appetite changes (6 pt.), transient skin paresthesia (8 pt.), insomnia (2 pt.), mania (2 pt.), asymptomatic brain cyst (1 pt.)	55.2 months
OCD? Impulse control disorder? Refractory anxiety? Mental retardation?	28.2	ND	4 female, 6 male	Poorly defined	All patients improved aggressive or impulsive behaviours? OCD and depression improved?	Poorly described	ND

(62.5%) from the active GVC group and two of the four ATb group patients (50%) were treatment responders. Most adverse events were relatively mild and transient (episodic headaches, nausea, weight changes), However, an excessive radionecrotic reaction, followed by a brain cyst, was observed in one patient. This subject developed delirium and confabulation for a few days, accompanied by cognitive changes for 5 months. Other associated adverse events included mania (in two patients) and episodic impulsive behaviours (binge-eating, compulsive buying, dipsomania). Nevertheless, there were no persistent adverse neuropsychological changes in a long-term follow-up.

In spite of the relatively low incidence of severe adverse events, brain cyst development secondary to an abnormal radionecrotic tissue reaction is probably the most troublesome complication of radiosurgery. At Brown University, 3 of 55 patients who underwent GVC ultimately developed delayed brain cysts few years after the original procedure (Rasmussen, pers. comm.). One of those three patients required open stereotactic surgical cyst drainage to correct neurological symptoms.

The exact understanding of the relationship between the model of the Leksell GK (LGK) equipment employed and cyst formation is not known. More than half of the patients in the Brown University study were treated with the LGK model U installed in Providence in March 1992 (Norén, pers. comm.). No adverse radiation-induced reaction occurred in any of those patients. The remaining patients were treated with LGK model C (installed in December 2000) with cyst formation in three cases. Model C has the same source distribution as LGK model B and consequently an identical isodose configuration of the shots of radiation. However, the source distribution and, as a result, the isodose configuration differ markedly when compared with those of model U, especially for isodose levels below 50%, which may well explain the zero incidence of adverse reactions in patients treated with that model. In the Brazilian study, one patient first developed a symptomatic abnormal radionecrotic reaction (brain oedema), months before the advent of a delayed brain cyst. No neurological symptoms were associated with the cyst. Of note, all Brazilian patients were treated in an LGK model B. Regarding the newest LGK equipment (Perfexion, launched in 2006), the helmet configuration and source geometry are quite different from those of the earlier LGK models. However, despite these significant technical differences, according to the manufacturer, the isodose configuration of the Perfexion was the same as for the LGK models B and C. Future studies should carefully address the outcome differences based on the model of the LGK equipment employed.

Factors determining individual radiosensitivity and radioresistance are still poorly understood, and most of the data in the literature are derived from studies of arteriovenous malformations and brain tumours [26–28]. Intrinsic brain tissue factors, such as the radiation damage repair rate, and extrinsic factors, such as medications with radioprotective effects, might play a role in radiosensitivity or radioresistance [29]. It is known that the post-radiosurgery lesion is dependent on dose, volume and dose rate.

When compared to similar radiosurgical procedures, papers published over the past few years on GK thalamotomies found no instance of development of cyst at or close to the target [30–35]. The overall incidence of complications using this technique ranged between 5 and 10% [30, 31, 33, 34]. In the recently published thalamotomy papers, the maximum dose was not similar, but lower, in all reports, usually 130–140 Gy [31, 34]. The highest dose at one centre was 165 Gy [35]. All thalamotomies were performed using a single 4 mm shot. No reference to GK model with regard to the outcome of thalamotomies currently was found to be available.

The lack of cyst development in the recent study by Sheehan *et al.* using single-shot, 4-mm isocentres and a maximum radiation doses of 140–160 Gy should be received with interest [16]. The continued follow-up of their treated OCD patients might be of relevance to a deeper understanding of or lack of cyst formation, especially if they add more observations and cases over time.

A better understanding of the potentially serious complication of cyst formation will be essential in determining the interest in and usefulness of this procedure in the future. Forthcoming studies of GK in psychiatry should explore the effects of radiation dose, dose rate, lesion volume and radiosensitivity.

Neuropsychological changes

Several studies have addressed the cognitive effects of radiotherapy [36], as well as the neuropsychological outcomes after GK for brain tumours, metastases or arteriovenous malformations [36, 37]. However, there are only a few studies describing this issue in psychiatry.

In their 2008 article, Rück *et al.* reported the outcomes of OCD patients treated with thermocapsulotomy ($n=16$) or gamma capsulotomy ($n=9$) [23]. Neuropsychological instruments were applied in 23 patients, in a mean follow-up of 11 years, comparing the average post-operative group performance with the standard population norms. Patients showed deficits in many cognitive domains at long-term follow-ups, especially in executive functions and verbal fluency, when compared with the general population. Of note, pre- and post-operative neuropsychological assessments were available for only seven subjects (two of them with a radiosurgical procedure). Executive functions (as assessed by the Wisconsin Card Sorting Test) and attention (Digit Span scores) were impaired after 11 years of follow-up, but the most pronounced changes were observed in one patient who was received single-shot GK with 8-mm collimators. The main shortcoming of this study was the comparison with population-based scores. Since severe OCD patients usually do worse in neuropsychological tests when compared with normal controls, these subjects might have been already cognitively impaired even before radiosurgery. Furthermore, the patients were not similar in terms of type of surgery (thermocapsulotomy versus gamma capsulotomy), number of repeated surgical interventions and collimator sizes.

Trying to address this issue, Batistuzzo *et al.* in Brazil studied 17 refractory OCD patients who were evaluated before and 1 year after GVC [38]. All subjects were assessed in terms of intellectual functioning, attention, verbal and visuospatial memory, spatial perception, executive functions and motor functioning. In the pilot phase, qualitative analyses of five patients suggested post-operative improvements in attention, vocabulary, learning, abstract reasoning and memory measures [39]. Later on, another 12 patients from the double-blind trial of GVC were added, for a total sample of 17 OCD subjects. At 1 year of follow-up, within-group comparisons revealed improvements in attention, vocabulary, intellectual functioning (mainly on performance IQ), visuospatial memory, executive functioning and motor skills. Moreover, it is noteworthy that no impairments in any of the neuropsychological domains, on average, were observed at 12 months of follow-up [38]. However, as described above, one patient developed radionecrotic-induced cognitive changes at 8 months of follow-up, with attention deficits and signs of perseverations and confabulation. These symptoms were reversed in a few days with the use of corticosteroids, but memory changes remained for 5 months.

A qualitative comparison of these data with those from the study by Ruck *et al.* suggests that a larger lesion (4 mm collimators, bilateral doses of 180–200 Gy, three isocentres) at the internal capsule could have a negative impact on cognition, whereas smaller lesions (4 mm collimators, bilateral doses of 180 Gy, one or two isocentres) may be beneficial to neuropsychological functions after surgery. As a limitation of these studies, although comprehensive neuropsychological assessments were made, they did not cover all the possible cognitive domains. Thus, the impact of radiosurgical procedures on some 'hidden' neuropsychological functions might have been potentially not measured.

To summarize, unlike DBS and even thermolesion surgeries, the number of publications regarding cognitive changes secondary to GK in mental disorders is small. Furthermore, as stated above, studies are different in terms of neuropsychological instruments, lesion size, radiation dose and localization of the targets.

Therefore, it is premature to draw definite conclusions about the neuropsychological effects of GK in the cognition of psychiatric patients. Smaller lesion volumes at well-defined locations are likely associated with no deleterious neuropsychological changes.

Comparative pros and cons of GK and DBS for treating mental disorders

GK radiosurgery precludes trephination. This is the main advantage of this surgical technique, as long as central nervous system bleeding and infections (which are the most severe and permanent complications of DBS) are prevented from occurring. However, the delayed effects of radiation, and consequently, their associated adverse events, can sometimes be observed in the brain several years after a GK intervention. Furthermore, the brain lesions produced by radiosurgery are irreversible, which can be either an advantage or a disadvantage to a psychiatric patient. For example, GK capsulotomy can usually maintain its efficacy for several years. Conversely, unexpected changes in the neurostimulation parameters of the DBS equipment may sometimes happen in the post-operative follow-up, and this may lead to symptom relapse, such that the neurostimulator will need adjustment to regain its efficacy. On the other hand, sometimes, unexpected aberrant radionecrotic tissue reactions may develop in GK surgery, which can lead to late, permanent complications of radiosurgery (such as brain cyst). Comparatively, the adverse events of stimulation with DBS can be reversed by changes in the stimulation parameters.

Another important difference between GK and DBS is the relative time course for initial clinical response, which is usually delayed in GK (ranging from 6 to 9months in GVC for OCD, for example), while DBS-associated symptom improvements can be observed 4–12weeks after VC/VS DBS, or 2–12weeks after other DBS techniques [14, 40–45]. The long-term efficacy of GK and DBS seems to be equivalent among studies. However, in terms of evidence-based medicine, there is only one double-blind, randomized controlled trial of GK in psychiatry, while few randomized trials of DBS surgery for psychiatric patients have been published so far, especially for the treatment of OCD.

There are no studies comparing GK and DBS in terms of financial costs and patient burden. Nevertheless, the total costs involved in conducting a radiosurgical procedure are usually lower than their equivalent DBS counterparts. Moreover, depending on the specific DBS technique that is employed, battery replacements (as in the non-rechargeable neurostimulators) may be more frequently needed and thus require additional surgical interventions every few years. As for GK, re-operations are uncommon and should be restricted to those few patients who show radioresistance to a first radiosurgical intervention.

Conclusion

New technical refinements have allowed GK radiosurgery to maintain its indication as a treatment for severe and refractory mental disorders, especially OCD. Experience accrued so far indicates that it is probably as efficacious as DBS.

The latest studies suggest that, for disorders such as OCD, smaller lesion volumes, ventral targets and lower total radiation doses have been associated with a smaller incidence of severe advents events, while continuing to be effective. However, GK remains an irreversible surgical procedure, meaning that it should only be employed for the most untreatable psychiatric patients, in specialized GK facilities, committed to long-term neurosurgical psychiatric follow-up.

References

1 Kondziolka D. Functional radiosurgery. Neurosurgery. 1999 Jan;44(1):12–20; discussion 20–2.
2 Ballantine HT, Bouckoms AJ, Thomas EK, Giriunas IE. Treatment of psychiatric illness by stereotactic cingulotomy. Biol Psychiatry. 1987 Jul;22(7):807–19.
3 Steele JD, Christmas D, Eljamel MS, Matthews K. Anterior cingulotomy for major depression: clinical outcome and relationship to lesion characteristics. Biol Psychiatry. 2008 Apr 1; 63(7):670–7.
4 Dougherty DD, Baer L, Cosgrove GR, Cassem EH, Price BH, Nierenberg AA, *et al*. Prospective long-term follow-up of 44 patients who received cingulotomy for treatment-refractory obsessive-compulsive disorder. Am J Psychiatry. 2002 Feb;159(2):269–75.
5 Sheth SA, Neal J, Tangherlini F, Mian MK, Gentil A, Cosgrove GR, *et al*. Limbic system surgery for treatment-refractory obsessive-compulsive disorder: a prospective long-term follow-up of 64 patients. J Neurosurg. 2013 Mar;118(3):491–7.
6 Knight G. Stereotactic tractotomy in the surgical treatment of mental illness. J Neurol Neurosurg Psychiatry. 1965 Aug;28:304–10.
7 Hodgkiss AD, Malizia AL, Bartlett JR, Bridges PK. Outcome after the psychosurgical operation of stereotactic subcaudate tractotomy, 1979–1991. J Neuropsychiatry Clin Neurosci. 1995; 7(2):230–4.
8 Kelly D, Mitchell-Heggs N. Stereotactic limbic leucotomy – a follow-up study of thirty patients. Postgrad Med J. 1973 Dec;49(578):865–82.
9 Rylander G. Försök med gammakapsulotomi vid ångest- och tvångsneuroser. Lakartidningen. 1978;75(7):547–9.
10 Mindus P, Bergström K, Levander SE, Norén G, Hindmarsh T, Thuomas KA. Magnetic resonance images related to clinical outcome after psychosurgical intervention in severe anxiety disorder. J Neurol Neurosurg Psychiatry. 1987 Oct;50(10):1288–93.
11 Lippitz BE, Mindus P, Meyerson BA, Kihlström L, Lindquist C. Lesion topography and outcome after thermocapsulotomy or gamma knife capsulotomy for obsessive-compulsive disorder: relevance of the right hemisphere. Neurosurgery. 1999 Mar;44(3):452–8; discussion 458–60.
12 Rasmussen SA. Anterior gamma capsulotomy for intractable OCD. Proceedings of the fifth International Obsessive Compulsive Disorder Conference. Sardinia, Italy; 2001.
13 Lopes A, Greenberg B, Norén G, Canteras M, Busatto G, de Mathis M, *et al*. Treatment of resistant obsessive-compulsive disorder with ventral capsular/ventral striatal gamma capsulotomy: a pilot prospective study. J Neuropsychiatry Clin Neurosci. 2009;21(4):381–92.
14 Lopes AC, Greenberg BD, Canteras MM, Batistuzzo MC, Hoexter MQ, Gentil AF, *et al*. Gamma ventral capsulotomy for obsessive-compulsive disorder: a randomized clinical trial. JAMA Psychiatry. 2014 Sep 1;71(9):1066–76.
15 Kondziolka D, Flickinger JC, Hudak R. Results following gamma knife radiosurgical anterior capsulotomies for obsessive compulsive disorder. Neurosurgery. 2011 Jan;68(1):28–32; discussion 23–3.
16 Sheehan JP, Patterson G, Schlesinger D, Xu Z. Gamma Knife surgery anterior capsulotomy for severe and refractory obsessive-compulsive disorder. J Neurosurg. 2013 Nov;119(5): 1112–8.
17 Del Valle R, de Anda S, Garnica R, Aguilar E, Perez-Pastenes M. Psychiatric radiosurgery with Gamma Knife. Salud Ment. 2006;29(1): 18–27.
18 White R, Williams S. Amygdaloid neurosurgery for aggressive behaviour, Sydney, 1967–1977: societal, scientific, ethical and other factors. Australas Psychiatry. 2009;17(5):410–6.
19 Lévêque M, Weil AG, Régis J. Surgery for aggressive behavior disorder. Stereotact Funct Neurosurg. 2013;91(3):198–200.
20 Rück C, Larsson KJ, Mataix-Cols D. Predictors of medium and long-term outcome following capsulotomy for obsessive–compulsive disorder: one site may not fit all. Eur Neuropsychopharmacol. 2012 Jun;22(6):406–14.
21 Gentil AF, Lopes AC, Dougherty DD, Rück C, Mataix-Cols D, Lukacs TL, *et al*. Hoarding symptoms and prediction of poor response to limbic system surgery for treatment-refractory obsessive-compulsive disorder. J Neurosurg. 2014 Jul;121(1): 123–30.

22 Kihlström L, Guo WY, Lindquist C, Mindus P. Radiobiology of radiosurgery for refractory anxiety disorders. Neurosurgery. 1995 Feb;36(2):294–302.
23 Rück C, Karlsson A, Steele JD, Edman G, Meyerson BA, Ericson K, *et al.* Capsulotomy for obsessive-compulsive disorder: long-term follow-up of 25 patients. Arch Gen Psychiatry. 2008 Aug;65(8):914–21.
24 Pallanti S, Quercioli L. Treatment-refractory obsessive-compulsive disorder: methodological issues, operational definitions and therapeutic lines. Prog Neuropsychopharmacol Biol Psychiatry. 2006 May;30(3):400–12.
25 Kondziolka D, Hudak R. Management of obsessive-compulsive disorder-related skin picking with gamma knife radiosurgical anterior capsulotomies: a case report. J Clin Psychiatry. 2008 Aug;69(8):1337–40.
26 Foroughi M, Kemeny AA, Lehecka M, Wons J, Kajdi L, Hatfield R, *et al.* Operative intervention for delayed symptomatic radionecrotic masses developing following stereotactic radiosurgery for cerebral arteriovenous malformations – case analysis and literature review. Acta Neurochir (Wien). 2010 May;152(5):803–15.
27 Pan H-C, Sheehan J, Stroila M, Steiner M, Steiner L. Late cyst formation following gamma knife surgery of arteriovenous malformations. J Neurosurg 2005 Jan;102(Suppl):124–7.
28 Yeung AH, Sughrue ME, Kane AJ, Tihan T, Cheung SW, Parsa AT. Radiobiology of vestibular schwannomas: mechanisms of radioresistance and potential targets for therapeutic sensitization. Neurosurg Focus. 2009 Dec;27(6):E2.
29 Kondziolka D, Lunsford LD, Flickinger JC. The radiobiology of radiosurgery. Neurosurg Clin N Am. 1999 Apr;10(2):157–66.
30 Young RF, Li F, Vermeulen S, Meier R. Gamma Knife thalamotomy for treatment of essential tremor: long-term results. J Neurosurg. 2010 Jun;112(6):1311–7.
31 Kooshkabadi A, Lunsford LD, Tonetti D, Flickinger JC, Kondziolka D. Gamma Knife thalamotomy for tremor in the magnetic resonance imaging era. J Neurosurg. 2013 Apr;118(4):713–8.
32 Duma CM. Movement disorder radiosurgery – planning, physics and complication avoidance. Prog Neurol Surg. 2007;20:249–66.
33 Ohye C, Higuchi Y, Shibazaki T, Hashimoto T, Koyama T, Hirai T, *et al.* Gamma Knife thalamotomy for Parkinson disease and essential tremor: a prospective multicenter study. Neurosurgery. 2012 Mar;70(3):526–35; discussion 535–6.
34 Lim S-Y, Hodaie M, Fallis M, Poon Y-Y, Mazzella F, Moro E. Gamma Knife thalamotomy for disabling tremor: a blinded evaluation. Arch Neurol. 2010 May;67(5):584–8.
35 Friehs GM, Norén G, Ohye C, Duma CM, Marks R, Plombon J, *et al.* Lesion size following Gamma Knife treatment for functional disorders. Stereotact Funct Neurosurg. 1996;66(Suppl 1):320–8.
36 Armstrong CL, Gyato K, Awadalla AW, Lustig R, Tochner ZA. A critical review of the clinical effects of therapeutic irradiation damage to the brain: the roots of controversy. Neuropsychol Rev. 2004 Mar;14(1):65–86.
37 Laack NN, Brown PD. Cognitive sequelae of brain radiation in adults. Semin Oncol. 2004 Oct;31(5):702–13.
38 Batistuzzo M, Hoexter M, Taub A, Cesar R, Gentil A, Joaquim M, *et al.* Visuospatial memory improvement after gamma ventral capsulotomy in treatment refractory obsessive-compulsive disorder patients. Neuropsychopharmacol Off Publ Am Coll Neuropsychopharmacol 2015 Jul;40(8):1837–45.
39 Taub A, Lopes A, Fuentes D, Carina D, de Mathis M, Canteras M, *et al.* Neuropsychological outcome of ventral capsular/ventral striatal gamma capsulotomy for refractory obsessive-compulsive disorder: a pilot study. J Neuropsychiatry Clin Neurosci. 2009;21(4):393–7.
40 Goodman WK, Foote KD, Greenberg BD, Ricciuti N, Bauer R, Ward H, *et al.* Deep brain stimulation for intractable obsessive compulsive disorder: pilot study using a blinded, staggered-onset design. Biol Psychiatry. 2010 Mar 15;67(6):535–42.
41 Denys D, Mantione M, Figee M, van den Munckhof P, Koerselman F, Westenberg H, *et al.* Deep brain stimulation of the nucleus accumbens for treatment-refractory obsessive-compulsive disorder. Arch Gen Psychiatry. 2010 Oct;67(10):1061–8.
42 Greenberg BD, Gabriels LA, Malone DA, Rezai AR, Friehs GM, Okun MS, *et al.* Deep brain

stimulation of the ventral internal capsule/ventral striatum for obsessive-compulsive disorder: worldwide experience. Mol Psychiatry. 2010 Jan;15(1):64–79.

43 Huff W, Lenartz D, Schormann M, Lee S-H, Kuhn J, Koulousakis A, *et al.* Unilateral deep brain stimulation of the nucleus accumbens in patients with treatment-resistant obsessive-compulsive disorder: outcomes after one year. Clin Neurol Neurosurg. 2010 Feb;112(2):137–43.

44 Abelson JL, Curtis GC, Sagher O, Albucher RC, Harrigan M, Taylor SF, *et al.* Deep brain stimulation for refractory obsessive-compulsive disorder. Biol Psychiatry. 2005 Mar 1;57(5):510–6.

45 Nuttin BJ, Gabriels L, van Kuyck K, Cosyns P. Electrical stimulation of the anterior limbs of the internal capsules in patients with severe obsessive-compulsive disorder: anecdotal reports. Neurosurg Clin N Am. 2003 Apr;14(2):267–74.

CHAPTER 21

Radiofrequency lesions: Introduction and technical aspects

Seth F. Oliveria, Kristopher G. Hooten and Kelly D. Foote
University of Florida, Gainesville, USA

Introduction

Contemporary ablative psychiatric neurosurgical procedures use modern stereotactic techniques to create precise lesions in brain locations that are chosen based on the best available scientific evidence. These procedures are reserved for treatment of severe, intractable and incapacitating mental disorders in individuals who fail conservative therapies. Although the practice of psychiatric neurosurgery is often compared to the crude procedures from the historical era of psychosurgery such as the freehand prefrontal lobotomy, the contrast is actually quite stark. Unlike psychosurgical procedures that were performed relatively indiscriminately, current ablative procedures are typically performed at only a few highly specialized centres after a multidisciplinary committee has reviewed each case carefully. Crucially, the safety of modern stereotactic lesioning is dramatically improved such that major complications are rare. Further, the field has trended towards minimally invasive approaches, which are often performed under local anaesthesia and are typically well tolerated by patients.

Similar to neurosurgical interventions for epilepsy, psychiatric neurosurgical interventions can provide unique insight into human brain function and dysfunction. Many stereotactic neurosurgical procedures rely upon microelectrode recording (MER) for accurate targeting within the brain. This technique provides a fortuitous opportunity to record from individual neurons along the chosen trajectory to the target in awake, behaving individuals. Additionally, rapid progress is occurring in several areas relevant to psychiatric neurosurgery, including functional and structural brain imaging, neurophysiology, neuroanatomy and implantable device development. In combination, these techniques provide novel tools for hypothesis-driven investigation of the structure and function of normal and pathological neuronal circuitry in the human brain, and they will ultimately improve therapeutic applications for future patients suffering from mental disorders.

There are several modalities available to generate ablative brain lesions for the treatment of psychiatric conditions, and deep brain stimulation (DBS) represents an emerging therapy for nondestructive psychiatric neuromodulation. Nevertheless, the most extensive experience to date for generating stereotactic lesions in the brain has been with the use of radiofrequency lesioning (RFL) to thermocoagulate brain tissue. Radiofrequency (RF) ablation became the most popular modality because of its

Neuromodulation in Psychiatry, First Edition. Edited by Clement Hamani, Paul Holtzheimer, Andres M. Lozano and Helen Mayberg.

compatibility with stereotactic systems and its capability to create well-circumscribed, temperature-controlled lesions with excellent target control [1, 2]. In modern neurosurgical practice, this technique uses standard magnetic resonance imaging (MRI) stereotaxis to place the tip of a RF electrode at a precise location within the brain, where a RF lesion generator can be used to accurately create a lesion of the desired size and shape. In this chapter, we will introduce the most commonly performed stereotactic brain RFL procedures for psychiatric indications. We will also provide a detailed discussion of the technical aspects of stereotactic brain RFL surgery.

Neuroanatomic basis for RFL in psychiatric conditions

Stereotactic RFL for mental disorders involves the disruption of carefully selected anatomic circuits within the frontal lobe. In a simplified model, there are five parallel frontal lobe circuits [3–5]. Each circuit originates from frontal lobe cortex and projects topographically to a defined striatal target. The *dorsolateral circuit* is involved with executive function and projects from the lateral anterior frontal lobe to the dorsolateral caudate head; the *orbitofrontal circuit* is responsible for frontal modulation of limbic activity and projects from the inferolateral prefrontal cortex to medial caudate and nucleus accumbens; the *anterior cingulate circuit* mediates motivated behaviour and projects from the anterior cingulate gyrus to the ventromedial caudate, ventral putamen, nucleus accumbens and olfactory tubercle; the *motor circuit* is responsible for voluntary motor function and originates in the supplementary motor area, premotor cortex, motor cortex and somatosensory cortex and projects to the putamen; finally, the *oculomotor circuit* participates in voluntary eye movement and projects from the frontal eye fields to the body of the caudate nucleus. From the striatum, information remains segregated within topographically arranged parallel circuits as it travels to the pallidum and substantia nigra, on to the thalamus and ultimately back to the frontal cortex to form a closed loop.

It is important to recognize that frontal circuit disruption can itself result in abnormal behavioural syndromes. Most notably, dorsolateral circuit lesions cause executive dysfunction, orbitofrontal circuit lesions cause disinhibitive personality changes and anterior cingulate circuit lesions can cause apathy. Psychiatric conditions are being increasingly well understood as disorders of frontal lobe circuitry in which some pathological neuronal activity results in a characteristic disruption of function in the frontal behavioural network. The goal of selective RFL is, therefore, to identify and interrupt a pathological signal that is disrupting the normal function of the network.

Psychiatric indications for RFL

Obsessive-compulsive disorder (OCD) is a condition in which individuals experience persistent intrusive obsessions and engage in ritualistic compulsive behaviours. Both obsessions and compulsions typically evoke significant anxiety for the individual. Dysfunctional activity is thought to occur within the orbitofrontal and anterior cingulate corticostriatal–thalamocortical circuitry in patients with OCD [6–9]. In OCD patients, functional neuroimaging suggests that there is hyperactivity within these circuits, and structural neuroimaging has demonstrated abnormal connectivity within the cingulate and anterior limb of the internal capsule [6, 8, 10–13]. Reports also suggest that focal lesions in the frontal cortex and basal ganglia can cause OCD [10, 14]. Standard treatment for this condition involves cognitive behavioural therapy and selective serotonin reuptake inhibitors. However, 20–40% of patients remain refractory to standard therapy [6, 15, 16]. Evidence of pathological frontal lobe corticostriatal–thalamocortical circuitry in OCD underlies the treatment rationale for ablative procedures that disrupt communication between the striatum and the anterior cingulate and/or the orbitofrontal areas. Severe intractable OCD is one of the most frequently performed and well-studied psychiatric indications for stereotactic brain RFL. OCD has been treated with anterior cingulotomy, anterior capsulotomy, subcaudate tractotomy and limbic leucotomy, each of which will be discussed further below. Considering the typical severity and the intractable nature of this disorder in patients who ultimately undergo the procedure, the reported efficacy is quite good: ranging from 40% of patients with permanent improvement to 73% at least 'much improved' [17–19].

There are much smaller series investigating the use of stereotactic brain ablation for non-obsessional anxiety disorders. The pathophysiological underpinnings for anxiety disorders are less well understood but are also thought to involve dysfunction of the frontal–subcortical and limbic–subcortical circuits. Rück *et al.* [17] have reported the largest cohort of 26 patients undergoing ablative procedures for non-obsessional anxiety disorders, who were treated with bilateral anterior capsulotomy [17].

Tourette's syndrome (TS) is characterized by motor and vocal tics that typically begin in childhood or early adolescence and is often associated with impulse control problems and attention deficits. OCD is also frequently present in these individuals, and there is considerable overlap between these two conditions. Indeed, functional neuroimaging demonstrates that, similar to OCD, TS patients also demonstrate hyperactivity in frontal subcortical areas, supporting the hypothesis that these circuits are disinhibited in both conditions [10, 20]. Thus, similar lesional approaches have been performed for TS to those listed above for OCD. Additionally, Hassler and Dieckmann [21] classically performed thalamotomy of the centromedial parafascicular complex, an area that has more recently become a promising target for DBS therapy for TS [21].

Major depression is a common and potentially incapacitating mental illness that can be lethal if unsuccessfully treated due to high suicide rates in this patient population. Functional neuroimaging has demonstrated abnormal brain activity in the medial prefrontal cortex, particularly the rostral portion of the anterior cingulate cortex (ACC) in patients with major depression when compared with normal controls [22–26]. Anterior cingulotomy disrupts connections to the striatum and limbic system via the cingulate bundle and is an established treatment option for both major depression and bipolar disorder once non-invasive treatment strategies have been exhausted [23, 27].

Intractable aggression is a more controversial indication for ablative brain lesioning. The amygdala is an important component of the limbic circuit that is important for emotional learning, regulation and planning and is considered to be central to the development of aggressive behaviour. Kluver and Bucy in 1939, among others, found that temporal lobectomy and amygdalectomy had a taming effect in monkeys and cats [28–31]. Terzian and Ore [32] were able to achieve similar results in humans, and subsequently Narabayashi *et al.* [33] reported a large series of amygdalotomies for severe aggression [32, 33]. However, this procedure has largely fallen out of favour in the past three decades both because the taming effect of amygdalotomy heralds back to the era of psychosurgery and because available neuropharmacological options have improved. While several surgical approaches and lesioning modalities, including RFL, can be used together to generate lesions within the amygdala, they are seldom performed in modern neurosurgical practice and thus will not be considered further in this chapter.

General principles of stereotactic brain RFL

RF energy was first introduced to functional neurosurgery in 1953. It is a low-voltage, high-frequency form of electrical energy capable of producing small, discrete, homogeneous necrotic lesions by heating tissue [34]. Before creating brain lesions via RF heating, a general understanding of the physics involved is required [1, 2]. An RF generator applies electrical current that is transferred through a cable to the lesion-producing active electrode. A receiving, dispersive electrode pad is placed on the patient and connected back to the generator by a cable to complete the electrical circuit. Modern generators contain a built-in impedance monitor, dual temperature monitors and a microprocessor controller with multiple functions that allow the functional neurosurgeon to safely stimulate and/or generate precise lesions within the brain [1, 2]. An example of a modern RF generator is pictured in Figure 21.1.

The lesioning (active) electrode is made up of a conducting metal with an insulated shaft and an exposed, uninsulated electrode tip. The underlying concept of RF thermocoagulation is that voltage applied at the tip of the lesioning electrode creates an oscillating electric field with the RF defined by the generator. Lower frequencies can have stimulating effects upon neural elements, thus frequencies above 250 kHz are used in the brain to generate lesions [35]. Charged ions in the tissue near the electrode tip are induced to move at the same frequency as the RF-generated electric field, thus causing frictional heating to occur. The current amplitude governs the resulting tissue temperature, which can be estimated by measuring the temperature at the electrode tip [1, 2, 36]. While reversible neural damage has been demonstrated between 42 and 44°C, the temperature must be elevated above 45°C to create an irreversible lesion in the brain [37]. Once tissue temperature reaches the lesioning threshold, a central zone of coagulated necrosis forms with a surrounding zone of vasogenic

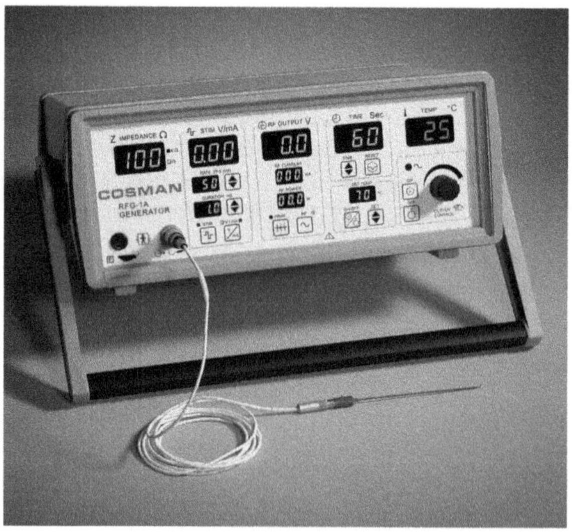

Figure 21.1 A modern RF generator. The Cosman RFG-1A generator is shown, which includes real-time impedance and temperature monitoring, stimulation capability, automatic temperature control and freehand output control capability. Also shown is a lesioning electrode with built-in thermocouple. Source: Cosman Medical, Inc. (*See insert for colour representation of the figure.*)

oedema [38]. During the lesioning process, the electrode temperature must be closely monitored to both ensure the desired lesion effect and avoid the point of boiling at 100°C, in which gas formation and tissue searing can occur [1, 2, 39].

If the electrode temperature is held constant during the lesion process, the lesion size will increase until it reaches a limit, which is referred to as the equilibrium lesion size [1, 2, 40]. For a given temperature, this typically occurs after 30–60 s. Lesion size generally increases with increasing uninsulated electrode tip size and electrode tip temperature [1, 2, 41]. It is thus important to choose the appropriate size and shape of the electrode to create the desired target lesion. Commercially available electrodes for brain RF vary in size ranging from 0.7 to 2.1 mm in diameter by 2 to 10 mm in length (Figure 21.2). If necessary, custom electrodes for specific targets and/or lesion sizes can also be engineered [42]. In addition to the size of the electrode tip and the temperature, the surrounding tissue physical properties and blood flow can affect the size and shape of a lesion. For example, the conductive properties of cerebrospinal fluid (CSF) differ from those of the brain tissue and may therefore distort the size or shape of a lesion performed in close proximity to a ventricular or pial surface [43]. Lesioning can be easily tested in vitro using media such as albumin solutions, but given the known physical properties of the tissue, the lesion size can also be mathematically modelled and simulated [43–46]. Because of the variables described above, a careful study of the target and the desired lesioning size is recommended, so that a lesion can be planned based on the predicted coagulation zone at the set temperature and time before any treatment is attempted. The lesion may also be 'shaped' to the target structure by making multiple lesions, either along a single track or multiple adjacent tracks [47–50]. Dr. Cosman summarizes the process of lesion making in the brain in four basic rules presented in Table 21.1 [1, 2].

When performing an RF ablation, accurate targeting is of the utmost importance both to avoid damage to surrounding structures and to maximize therapeutic efficacy [51, 52]. Techniques such as intraoperative MER, intraoperative electrode stimulation, atlas-based mapping and computer modelling can be performed to improve stereotactic accuracy prior to lesioning. Improvements in MRI technology are providing increasingly detailed anatomic

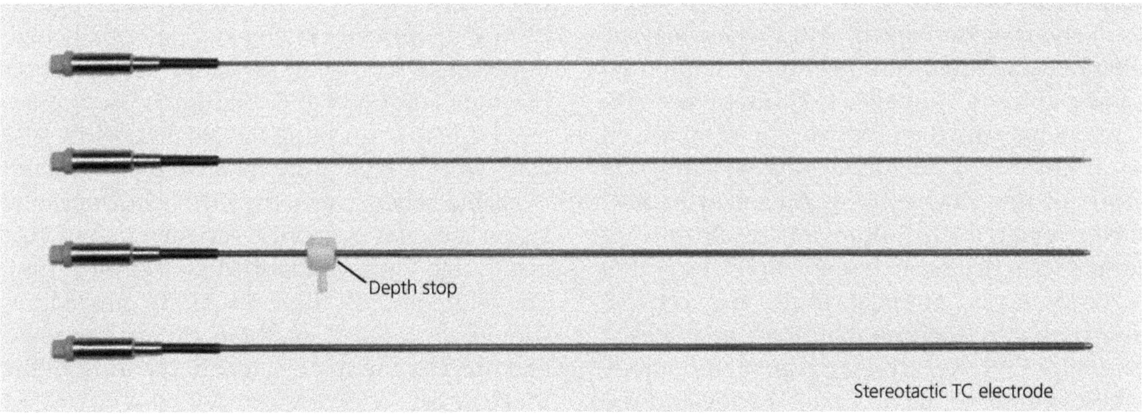

Figure 21.2 Modern RF lesioning electrodes. Cosman Stereotactic TC Electrodes have an insulated shaft except for an uninsulated electrode tip. They are available in a variety of standard shaft lengths, diameters and tip lengths. The exposed tip has a rounded end and a built-in thermocouple temperature sensor for thermal monitoring of the RF lesion process. Source: Cosman Medical, Inc.

Table 21.1 Cosman's rules of radiofrequency (RF) lesioning.

Rule 1	The RF current heats the tissue, and the tissue in turn heats the RF electrode.
Rule 2	Temperature is the basic lesioning parameter and should be measured. The measurement of electrode tip temperature is directly related to the tissue temperature and lesion size.
Rule 3	It is desirable to hold the proper tip temperature for 30–60 s to achieve the equilibrium size.
Rule 4	For consistent lesioning, the proper electrode size and tip temperature should be chosen.

information as well, and can be coupled with digital brain atlases that can be deformed to match a specific patient's anatomy, making accurate direct targeting techniques possible for some procedures [53, 54]. New high-resolution MRI sequences have been developed, such as the fast grey matter acquisition T1 inversion recovery (FGATIR) developed at the University of Florida, to improve resolution of deep brain structures for stereotactic planning [55]. Typical direct targeting procedures involve first identifying and defining the target on magnetic resonance (MR) images relative to the stereotactic frame [56]. Alternatively, non-stereotactic MR images may be obtained and fused with stereotactic computed tomography (CT) images [57]. Frameless stereotaxy may also be used, but the comparison to frame-based techniques is beyond the scope of this chapter [58]. Advances in MRI have resulted in improved resolution of target structures, such that direct targeting is becoming a more accurate and reliable alternative to traditional indirect, atlas-based targeting [59]. Regardless of the methodology employed, targeting accuracy is critical to the performance of successful ablative procedures and the functional neurosurgeon should use all available tools to maximize surgical safety and efficacy.

DBS has become an accepted treatment for movement disorders and is being investigated for neuropsychiatric indications. It is possible that DBS may ultimately replace the lesioning procedures for the majority of neuropsychiatric disorders [50, 60–65]. The conceptual advantage of DBS over lesioning is that it is adjustable, theoretically reversible, preserves structures for potential future therapies and appears to have a lower side effect profile [50, 60, 66–68]. In certain instances, patients implanted with DBS devices may require removal of their electrode because of infection or scalp erosion, or they may be losing efficacy of chronic stimulation. For these patients, a therapeutic radiofrequency (RF) lesion can be generated by connecting an RF lesion generator to their existing DBS lead prior to explantation [39, 69, 70]. The technical aspects of this procedure are similar to standard RF ablation, with the exception that a bipolar technique is employed and no temperature information from the site of lesion generation is available. The active electrode cable is connected to the DBS contact that is positioned at the target (i.e. the electrode contact used for stimulation), and the reference cable is connected to an adjacent electrode on the DBS lead. Available clinical and experimental data support initiating RF lesioning via DBS electrodes at a low amplitude, such as 25 mA, because of varying and potentially high impedances in order to avoid temperatures reaching 100°C [39, 69]. Caution must be exercised when performing RF ablation with DBS leads since temperature measurements are not available when using the DBS electrode and lesion size has a greater variability than that achievable with standard RFL electrodes [69]. The endpoint of these lesioning procedures should be guided by their clinical response and development of side effects during the procedures.

Several factors may contribute to the choice of anaesthesia during RF lesioning procedures. Classical ablative procedures for movement disorders were performed with awake patients so that real-time clinical effects could be evaluated intraoperatively to produce optimal results [71]. For many psychiatric indications, however, clinical endpoints cannot be fully assessed until several months post-operatively. Therefore these procedures may be performed awake with local anaesthesia alone, under general anaesthesia or with a combination of local anaesthesia and intravenous sedation [27, 72, 73]. This is a multi-factorial decision that is ultimately specific to the surgeon, procedure and the patient. It should be noted, however, that the use of intraoperative sedation may detrimentally affect the quality and utility of intraoperative MER.

As mentioned previously, there are many alternative methods for radiofrequency (RF) ablation for brain neuromodulation, which are listed in Table 21.2. Many of these methods are more extensively discussed in other chapters of this book.

Table 21.2 Alternatives methods of brain neuromodulation for psychiatric disorders.

Deep brain stimulation	Chronic stimulation, reversible, invasive
Vagal nerve stimulation	Chronic stimulation, reversible, invasive
Radiation/radiosurgery	Lesion producing, non-reversible, non-invasive
Focused ultrasound	Lesion producing, non-reversible, non-invasive
Cryogenics	Lesion producing, non-reversible, invasive
Chemical ablation	Lesion producing, non-reversible, invasive
Mechanical lesioning	Lesion producing, non-reversible, invasive
Laser ablation techniques	Lesion producing, non-reversible, invasive
RF ablation	Lesion producing, non-reversible, invasive
Direct current stimulation	Transcranial, non-invasive
Electroconvulsive therapy	Transcranial, non-invasive
Magnetic stimulation	Transcranial, non-invasive

RFL procedures for psychiatric indications

Anterior cingulotomy

The ACC comprises a rostral emotion region, an intermediate cognition region and a posterior motor region [3, 23, 74, 75]. The cingulate bundle is a white matter pathway associated with this cortical structure that runs predominantly in the anterior-posterior direction and communicates with the limbic system and the anterior cingulate–basal ganglia thalamocortical circuit. The targets for cingulotomy are the supracallosal fibres of the cingulate bundle that contribute to the Papez circuit as well as a focal portion of the rostral ACC itself [72].

The surgical technique for anterior cingulotomy is similar to all stereotactic brain RFL procedures for psychiatric indications and will be considered in detail. MRI-guided stereotaxis is performed with either a MRI-compatible stereotactic headframe or a preoperative MRI fused to a CT of the head that is obtained with a headframe in place. Gadolinium-enhanced T1-weighted images are used for stereotactic planning, which includes the following steps: (i) identification of the target within the cingulate gyri bilaterally; frequently quoted target coordinates are calculated bilaterally for a point in the ACC 2–2.5 cm posterior to the tip of the frontal horn of the lateral ventricle, 7 mm lateral to the midline and 1 mm above the roof of the ventricles bilaterally (Figure 21.3); (ii) identification of the ideal electrode trajectory through the brain to minimize the procedural risk of haemorrhage or damage to normal brain structures; careful attention is paid to avoid vascular structures, including cortical vessels, sulci and ventricular surfaces; and (iii) identification of the location for burr hole placement, again emphasizing safety by choosing a location centred over a gyrus that is devoid of cortical vessels [27]. In some instances, an additional lesion is planned lateral to the ACC location to further lesion the underlying cingulate bundle. Once planning is

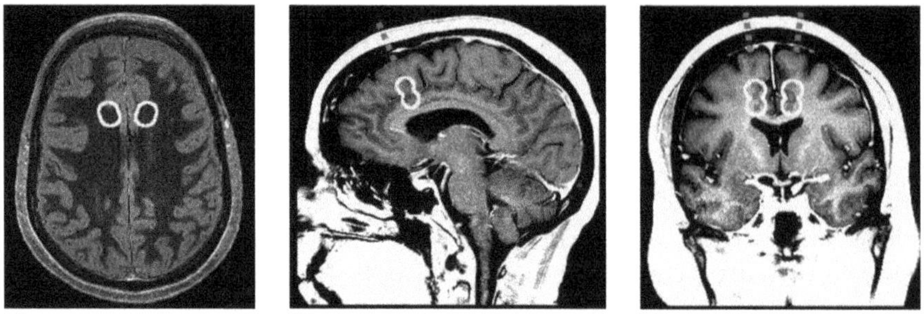

Figure 21.3 Anterior cingulotomy. **(a)** Axial Fast Grey Matter Acquisition T1 Inversion Recovery (FGATIR), **(b)** sagital T1-weighted, gadolinium-enhanced and **(c)** coronal T1 gadolinium-enhanced brain magnetic resonance images demonstrating the typical target, entry point and trajectory for an anterior cingulotomy. The dashed line indicates approximate electrode trajectory and the white circles indicate the approximate extent of lesion generation. The approximate target for an anterior cingulotomy is defined as a point in the ACC that is 2–2.5 cm posterior to the tip of the frontal horn of the lateral ventricle (out of the plane of the figure), 7 mm from the midline and 1 mm above the roof of the ventricles bilaterally. The total final cingulotomy lesion is approximately 2 cm in height and 8–10 mm in diameter.

complete, a burr hole is made at the desired locations bilaterally, and the dura and pia are incised and coagulated to achieve stringent haemostasis. The entry point is typically near Kocher's point, in the vicinity of the coronal suture and at least 2 cm lateral to midline. At this point, the stereotactic arc is mated to the frame on the patient's head to specify the planned entry point and trajectory through the brain to reach the desired target. MER can then be performed to improve three-dimensional localization along the chosen electrode track by identifying the upper and lower cortical banks of the cingulate gyrus, the cingulate bundle and the corpus callosum intraoperatively prior to lesion placement [77]. MER data can delineate cell-rich areas, corresponding to grey matter of the upper and lower banks of the cingulate gyrus, from areas devoid of action potentials that correspond to the myelinated fibres of the cingulate bundle and the corpus callosum. After the ideal target is elucidated via MER, radiofrequency (RF) thermolesioning is performed by inserting an electrode with a 10 mm uninsulated tip to the target coordinates and heating to achieve an equilibrium lesion. The electrode is then withdrawn 10 mm along the same track and a second lesion is created with the same parameters to achieve a total cingulotomy lesion of approximately 2 cm in height and 8–10 mm in diameter. If applicable, the arc can then be adjusted laterally and the electrode reinserted for cingulate bundle lesioning. The procedure is then repeated on the contralateral side, noting the possibility that subtle brain shift can occur and affect stereotactic targeting on the second side. To avoid brain shift, we recommend opening the dura only after both burr holes have been made to minimize CSF loss on the initial operative side. Once lesioning is complete and meticulous haemostasis is confirmed, the scalp is closed in two layers. While the intent of this procedure is to create a focused cingulotomy, patients with an insufficient clinical response may undergo a second procedure months later to create a more extensive lesion and/or to add a bundle lesion if this was not performed initially.

Anterior capsulotomy

The general principles of surgical technique are similar to those described above for anterior cingulotomy. The Karolinska group, which has extensive experience with this

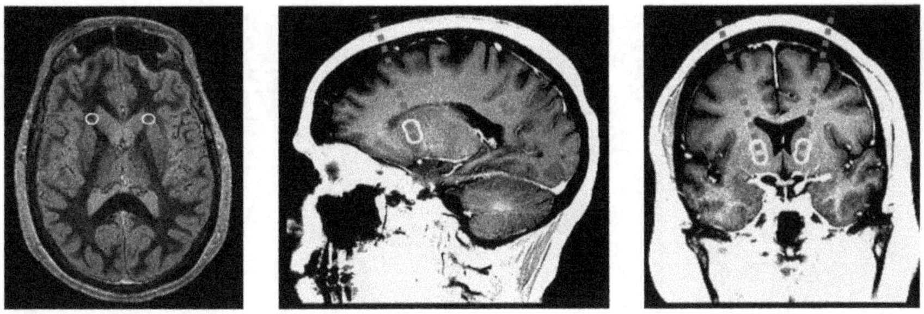
(a) (b) (c)

Figure 21.4 Anterior capsulotomy. Format is as in Figure 21.3. The target for anterior capsulotomy is defined by a point roughly halfway between the anterior commissure and the tip of the frontal horn of the lateral ventricle within the anterior internal capsule. The total final capsulotomy lesion is approximately 2 cm in height and 8–10 mm in diameter.

procedure, localizes the target by identifying the mid-point between the anterior commissure and the tip of the frontal horn of the lateral ventricle [17]. This places the lesion approximately 2 cm anterior to the anterior commissure (Figure 21.4). MER can be used to establish the three-dimensional positioning of the electrode track relative to the striatum and nucleus accumbens. Once optimal positioning is established, an RF electrode is inserted to the target coordinates. Using either a monopolar electrode with an 8–10 mm uninsulated tip or a bipolar electrode with an inter-electrode distance of 6–8 mm, successive ablations are performed along the electrode trajectory to generate a final capsulotomy lesion of approximately 2 cm in height and 8–10 mm in diameter. The procedure is then repeated on the contralateral side.

Subcaudate tractotomy

Subcaudate tractotomy targets the substantia innominata just inferior to the head of the caudate nucleus in the ventromedial frontal lobe, to disrupt frontolimbic fibres that connect the posterior orbitofrontal cortex to the structures including the cingulate gyrus, amygdala, hypothalamus and thalamus [6, 78, 80–82, 84]. It has been postulated that, at least for OCD, subcaudate tractotomy disrupts dysfunctional nucleus accumbens modulation of the amygdalo-basal ganglia-prefrontal circuitry [79, 82]. Again, the general surgical procedure is similar to that for cingulotomy and capsulotomy as described above. The target for subcaudate tractotomy is typically defined as 10 mm anterior, 10 mm superior and 6–14 mm lateral to the tuberculum sellae [82–84]. However, in comparison to the procedures described above, the trajectory for electrode insertion is performed at a more acute angle, such that the burr hole is usually placed just above the frontal sinus. By withdrawing the electrode and generating sequential lesions along this trajectory, the final cumulative lesion of 20–30 mm will have its long axis directed towards the frontal pole (Figure 21.5). Similar results can be achieved with either short (e.g. 2 mm) or long (e.g. 10 mm) uninsulated electrode tips by accordingly adjusting the number of sequential lesions that are generated along the electrode track. A second parallel lesion is performed approximately 8 mm lateral to the first track to fully disrupt the white matter within the subcaudate region. The procedure is repeated contralaterally prior to closure. Extra attention should be paid to cosmesis because of the location of the burr holes on the forehead. For example, low-profile burr hole covers can be considered to repair prominent skull defects. MER is not generally utilized during this procedure

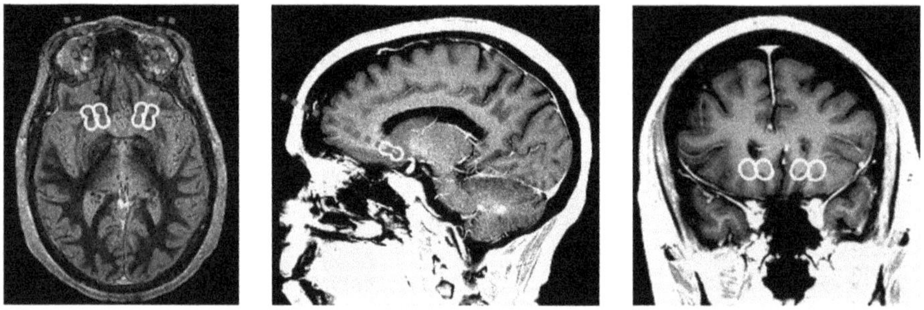

Figure 21.5 Subcaudate tractotomy. Format is as in Figure 21.3. The target for subcaudate tractotomy is defined as a point approximately 10 mm anterior, 10 mm superior and 6–14 mm lateral to the tuberculum sellae. The final cumulative lesion is 20–30 mm along its long axis, which is directed towards the frontal pole. A second parallel lesion is performed approximately 8 mm lateral to the first track to fully disrupt the subcaudate white matter.

since the electrode trajectory is exclusively within white matter after entering the brain.

Limbic leucotomy

Finally, limbic leucotomy is a term used to describe the combined use of both subcaudate tractotomy and anterior cingulotomy within the same procedure. This dual lesion technique is performed in order to achieve more significant functional outcomes by disrupting both the frontolimbic structures via subcaudate tractotomy and the Papez circuit via anterior cingulotomy. This procedure was first performed and reported by Kelly and colleagues in 1973, although the frontal lesions generated in this series were smaller than the conventional subcaudate tractotomy described above [72, 78, 85–88]. In modern neurosurgical practice, limbic leucotomy may be considered as an extension of either a subcaudate tractotomy or an anterior cingulotomy when partial or unsustained benefit is observed following the initial procedure.

Conclusions

Application of stereotactic RFL for the treatment of psychiatric disorders has dramatically improved the selectivity and accuracy of brain lesioning compared with historical freehand procedures performed in the era of psychosurgery. Most notably, these procedures can be performed safely and effectively with a low risk of major complications. Additionally, these surgeries are minimally invasive and have very low expected post-operative morbidity.

Current translational research holds the promise of increased application and improved efficacy for future neuromodulatory psychiatric neurosurgical procedures. Research efforts are currently focused upon understanding frontal–basal ganglia–thalamic circuitry as well as the effect of surgical manipulation of the components of this neural network. Tools to study the functional connectivity of white matter bundles such as diffusion tensor imaging and functional MRI are steadily improving and becoming increasingly available, permitting comparisons between conventional non-human primate fibre tracing and *in vivo* human data [78]. Additionally, multiple novel tools (high-resolution structural MRI, optogenetics, etc.) for the characterization of both normal and pathological functional neurocircuitry are rapidly expanding our understanding of the functional neural networks that determine human behaviour. Finally, investigational use of DBS for psychiatric disorders in brain structures that are targeted by ablative procedures will most certainly grant additional insight towards improved interventions for frontal lobe dysfunction. Together, the synthesis of this information will enable more effective frontal circuitry neuromodulation with more tailored, selective procedures to treat specific subsets of patients suffering from psychiatric illness.

References

1 Cosman ER. Radiofrequency lesions. In: Gildenberg PL, Tasker RR, editors. Stereotactic and Functional Neurosurgery. New York: McGraw-Hill; 1996. p. 973–86.
2 Cosman ER, Cosman BJ. Radiofrequency lesion – making in the nervous system. In: Wilkins RH, Regachary SS, editors. Neurosurgery. 3. New York: McGraw-Hill; 1984. p. 2490–8.
3 Mega MS, Cummings JL. Frontal-subcortical circuits and neuropsychiatric disorders. The Journal of Neuropsychiatry and Clinical Neurosciences. 1994;6(4):358–70.
4 Tekin S, Cummings JL. Frontal-subcortical neuronal circuits and clinical neuropsychiatry: an update. Journal of Psychosomatic Research. 2002; 53(2):647–54.
5 Mashour GA, Walker EE, Martuza RL. Psychosurgery: past, present, and future. Brain Research. Brain Research Reviews. 2005;48(3): 409–19.
6 Patel SR, Aronson JP, Sheth SA, Eskandar EN. Lesion procedures in psychiatric neurosurgery. World Neurosurgery. 2013;80(3–4):S31 e9–16.
7 Modell JG, Mountz JM, Curtis GC, Greden JF. Neurophysiologic dysfunction in basal ganglia/ limbic striatal and thalamocortical circuits as a pathogenetic mechanism of obsessive-compulsive disorder. The Journal of Neuropsychiatry and Clinical Neurosciences. 1989;1(1):27–36.
8 Saxena S, Brody AL, Maidment KM, Dunkin JJ, Colgan M, Alborzian S, *et al.* Localized orbitofrontal and subcortical metabolic changes and predictors of response to paroxetine treatment in obsessive-compulsive disorder. Neuropsychopharmacology. 1999;21(6):683–93.
9 Szeszko PR, MacMillan S, McMeniman M, Chen S, Baribault K, Lim KO, *et al.* Brain structural abnormalities in psychotropic drug-naive pediatric patients with obsessive-compulsive disorder. The American Journal of Psychiatry. 2004;161(6):1049–56.
10 Anderson CA, Arciniegas DB. Neurosurgical interventions for neuropsychiatric syndromes. Current Psychiatry Reports. 2004;6(5):355–63.
11 Cannistraro PA, Makris N, Howard JD, Wedig MM, Hodge SM, Wilhelm S, *et al.* A diffusion tensor imaging study of white matter in obsessive-compulsive disorder. Depression and Anxiety. 2007;24(6):440–6.
12 McGuire PK, Bench CJ, Frith CD, Marks IM, Frackowiak RS, Dolan RJ. Functional anatomy of obsessive-compulsive phenomena. The British Journal of Psychiatry. 1994;164(4):459–68.
13 Rauch SL, Jenike MA. Neurobiological models of obsessive-compulsive disorder. Psychosomatics. 1993;34(1):20–32.
14 Berthier ML, Kulisevsky J, Gironell A, Heras JA. Obsessive-compulsive disorder associated with brain lesions: clinical phenomenology, cognitive function, and anatomic correlates. Neurology. 1996;47(2):353–61.
15 Pallanti S, Quercioli L. Treatment-refractory obsessive-compulsive disorder: methodological issues, operational definitions and therapeutic lines. Progress in Neuro-Psychopharmacology & Biological Psychiatry. 2006;30(3):400–12.
16 Rasmussen SA, Eisen JL. The epidemiology and clinical features of obsessive compulsive disorder. The Psychiatric Clinics of North America. 1992;15(4):743–58.
17 Rück C, Andreewitch S, Flyckt K, Edman G, Nyman H, Meyerson BA, *et al.* Capsulotomy for refractory anxiety disorders: long-term follow-up of 26 patients. The American Journal of Psychiatry. 2003;160(3):513–21.
18 Herner T. Treatment of Mental Disorders with Frontal Stereotaxic Thermo Lesions: A Follow-Up Study of 116 Cases. Copenhagen, Munksgaard. 1961.
19 Burzaco J. Stereotactic surgery in the treatment of obsessive-compulsive neurosis. In: Perris C, Struwe G, Jansson B, editors. Biological Psychiatry. Amsterdam: Elsevier/North-Holland; 1981. p. 1103–9.
20 Segawa M. Neurophysiology of Tourette's syndrome: pathophysiological considerations. Brain & Development 2003;25(Suppl 1):S62–9.
21 Hassler R, Dieckmann G. Stereotaxic treatment of tics and inarticulate cries or coprolalia considered

as motor obsessional phenomena in Gilles de la Tourette's disease. Revue Neurologique. 1970; 123(2):89–100.
22 Ebmeier KP, Donaghey C, Steele JD. Recent developments and current controversies in depression. Lancet. 2006;367(9505):153–67.
23 Steele JD, Christmas D, Eljamel MS, Matthews K. Anterior cingulotomy for major depression: clinical outcome and relationship to lesion characteristics. Biological Psychiatry. 2008; 63(7):670–7.
24 Steele JD, Currie J, Lawrie SM, Reid I. Prefrontal cortical functional abnormality in major depressive disorder: a stereotactic meta-analysis. Journal of Affective Disorders. 2007;101(1–3):1–11.
25 Steele JD, Lawrie SM. Segregation of cognitive and emotional function in the prefrontal cortex: a stereotactic meta-analysis. NeuroImage. 2004; 21(3):868–75.
26 Drevets WC. Functional anatomical abnormalities in limbic and prefrontal cortical structures in major depression. In: Uylings HBM, Van Eden CG, De Bruin JPC, Feenstra MGP, Pennartz CMA, editors. Progress in Brain Research. 126. London: Elsevier Science; 2006. p. 413–31.
27 Spangler WJ, Cosgrove GR, Ballantine HT, Jr., Cassem EH, Rauch SL, Nierenberg A, *et al.* Magnetic resonance image-guided stereotactic cingulotomy for intractable psychiatric disease. Neurosurgery. 1996;38(6):1071–6; discussion 6–8.
28 Kluver H, Bucy PC. Preliminary analysis of functions of the temporal lobes in monkeys. 1939. The Journal of Neuropsychiatry and Clinical Neurosciences. 1997;9(4):606–20.
29 Mpakopoulou M, Gatos H, Brotis A, Paterakis KN, Fountas KN. Stereotactic amygdalotomy in the management of severe aggressive behavioral disorders. Neurosurgical Focus. 2008;25(1):E6.
30 Thomson AF, Walker AE. Behavioral alterations following lesions of the medial surface of the temporal lobe. Folia Psychiatrica, Neurologica et Neurochirurgica Neerlandica. 1950;53(2): 444–52.
31 Schreiner L, Kling A. Behavioral changes following rhinencephalic injury in cat. Journal of Neurophysiology. 1953;16(6):643–59.
32 Terzian H, Ore GD. Syndrome of Kluver and Bucy; reproduced in man by bilateral removal of the temporal lobes. Neurology. 1955;5(6):373–80.
33 Narabayashi H, Nagao T, Saito Y, Yoshida M, Nagahata M. Stereotaxic amygdalotomy for behavior disorders. Archives of Neurology 1963;9:1–16.
34 Sweet WH, Mark VH. Unipolar anodal electrolytic lesions in the brain of man and cat; report of five human cases with electrically produced bulbar or mesencephalic tractotomies. AMA Archives of Neurology and Psychiatry. 1953;70(2):224–34.
35 Alberts WW, Wright EW, Jr., Feinstein B, Gleason CA. Sensory responses elicited by subcortical high frequency electrical stimulation in man. Journal of Neurosurgery. 1972;36(1):80–2.
36 Alberts WW, Wright EW, Jr., Feinstein B, Von Bonin G. Experimental radiofrequency brain lesion size as a function of physical parameters. Journal of Neurosurgery. 1966;25(4):421–3.
37 Brodkey JS, Miyazaki Y, Ervin FR, Mark VH. Reversible heat lesions with radiofrequency current. A method of stereotactic localization. Journal of Neurosurgery. 1964;21:49–53.
38 Dieckmann G, Gabriel E, Hassler R. Size, form and structural peculiarities of experimental brailesions obtained by thermocontrolled radiofrequency. Confinia Neurologica. 1965;26(3):134–42.
39 Strickland BA, Jimenez-Shahed J, Jankovic J, Viswanathan A. Radiofrequency lesioning through deep brain stimulation electrodes: a pilot study of lesion geometry and temperature characteristics. Journal of Clinical Neuroscience. 2013;20(12):1709–12.
40 Cosman ER, Nashold BS, Ovelman-Levitt J. Theoretical aspects of radiofrequency lesions in the dorsal root entry zone. Neurosurgery. 1984;15(6):945–50.
41 Goldberg SN. Radiofrequency tumor ablation: principles and techniques. European Journal of Ultrasound. 2001;13(2):129–47.
42 Nashold BS, Jr., el-Naggar AO, Ovelmen-Levitt J, Abdul-Hak M. A new design of radiofrequency lesion electrodes for use in the caudalis nucleus DREZ operation. Technical note. Journal of Neurosurgery. 1994;80(6):1116–20.
43 Johansson JD, Loyd D, Wardell K, Wren J. Impact of cysts during radiofrequency lesioning in deep brain structures – a simulation and in vitro study. Journal of Neural Engineering. 2007;4(2):87–95.
44 Moringlane JR, Koch R, Schafer H, Ostertag CB. Experimental radiofrequency (RF) coagulation with computer-based on line monitoring of temperature and power. Acta Neurochirurgica. 1989;96(3–4):126–31.

45 Eriksson O, Backlund EO, Lundberg P, Lindstam H, Lindstrom S, Wardell K. Experimental radiofrequency brain lesions: a volumetric study. Neurosurgery. 2002;51(3):781–7; discussion 7–8.
46 Eriksson O, Wardell K, Bylund NE, Kullberg G, Rehncrona S. In vitro evaluation of brain lesioning electrodes (Leksell) using a computer-assisted video system. Neurological Research. 1999;21(1):89–95.
47 Baron MS, Vitek JL, Bakay RA, Green J, Kaneoke Y, Hashimoto T, *et al.* Treatment of advanced Parkinson's disease by posterior GPi pallidotomy: 1-year results of a pilot study. Annals of Neurology. 1996;40(3):355–66.
48 Vitek JL, Bakay RA, Hashimoto T, Kaneoke Y, Mewes K, Zhang JY, *et al.* Microelectrode-guided pallidotomy: technical approach and its application in medically intractable Parkinson's disease. Journal of Neurosurgery. 1998;88(6): 1027–43.
49 Lozano A, Hutchison W, Kiss Z, Tasker R, Davis K, Dostrovsky J. Methods for microelectrode-guided posteroventral pallidotomy. Journal of Neurosurgery. 1996;84(2):194–202.
50 Starr PA, Vitek JL, Bakay RA. Ablative surgery and deep brain stimulation for Parkinson's disease. Neurosurgery. 1998;43(5):989–1013; discussion 1013–5.
51 Amirnovin R, Williams ZM, Cosgrove GR, Eskandar EN. Experience with microelectrode guided subthalamic nucleus deep brain stimulation. Neurosurgery. 2006;58(1 Suppl):ONS96–102; discussion ONS96–102.
52 Chen SY, Lee CC, Lin SH, Hsin YL, Lee TW, Yen PS, *et al.* Microelectrode recording can be a good adjunct in magnetic resonance image-directed subthalamic nucleus deep brain stimulation for parkinsonism. Surgical Neurology. 2006; 65(3):253–60; discussion 260–1.
53 Pinsker MO, Volkmann J, Falk D, Herzog J, Alfke K, Steigerwald F, *et al.* Electrode implantation for deep brain stimulation in dystonia: a fast spin-echo inversion-recovery sequence technique for direct stereotactic targeting of the GPI. Zentralblatt für Neurochirurgie. 2008;69(2):71–5.
54 Chakravarty MM, Sadikot AF, Germann J, Bertrand G, Collins DL. Towards a validation of atlas warping techniques. Medical Image Analysis. 2008;12(6):713–26.
55 Sudhyadhom A, Haq IU, Foote KD, Okun MS, Bova FJ. A high resolution and high contrast MRI for differentiation of subcortical structures for DBS targeting: the Fast Gray Matter Acquisition T1 Inversion Recovery (FGATIR). NeuroImage. 2009;47(Suppl 2):T44–52.
56 Simon SL, Douglas P, Baltuch GH, Jaggi JL. Error analysis of MRI and leksell stereotactic frame target localization in deep brain stimulation surgery. Stereotactic and Functional Neurosurgery. 2005;83(1):1–5.
57 Liu X, Rowe J, Nandi D, Hayward G, Parkin S, Stein J, *et al.* Localisation of the subthalamic nucleus using Radionics Image Fusion and Stereoplan combined with field potential recording. A technical note. Stereotactic and Functional Neurosurgery. 2001;76(2):63–73.
58 Holloway KL, Gaede SE, Starr PA, Rosenow JM, Ramakrishnan V, Henderson JM. Frameless stereotaxy using bone fiducial markers for deep brain stimulation. Journal of Neurosurgery. 2005;103(3):404–13.
59 Schlaier J, Schoedel P, Lange M, Winkler J, Warnat J, Dorenbeck U, *et al.* Reliability of atlas-derived coordinates in deep brain stimulation. Acta Neurochirurgica. 2005;147(11):1175–80; discussion 80.
60 Tasker RR. Deep brain stimulation is preferable to thalamotomy for tremor suppression. Surgical Neurology. 1998;49(2):145–53; discussion 53–4.
61 Cosyns P, Gabriels L, Nuttin B. Deep brain stimulation in treatment refractory obsessive compulsive disorder. Verhandelingen – Koninklijke Academie voor Geneeskunde van België. 2003;65(6):385–99; discussion 99–400.
62 Nuttin B, Gybels J, Cosyns P, Gabriels L, Meyerson B, Andreewitch S, *et al.* Deep brain stimulation for psychiatric disorders. Neurosurgery Clinics of North America. 2003;14(2):xv–xvi.
63 Lozano AM, Mayberg HS, Giacobbe P, Hamani C, Craddock RC, Kennedy SH. Subcallosal cingulate gyrus deep brain stimulation for treatment-resistant depression. Biological Psychiatry. 2008;64(6):461–7.
64 Deep-Brain Stimulation for Parkinson's Disease Study Group. Deep-brain stimulation of the subthalamic nucleus or the pars interna of the globus pallidus in Parkinson's disease. The New England Journal of Medicine 2001;345(13):956–63.
65 Hung SW, Hamani C, Lozano AM, Poon YY, Piboolnurak P, Miyasaki JM, *et al.* Long-term outcome of bilateral pallidal deep brain

stimulation for primary cervical dystonia. Neurology. 2007;68(6):457–9.
66 Schuurman PR, Bosch DA, Bossuyt PM, Bonsel GJ, van Someren EJ, de Bie RM, *et al.* A comparison of continuous thalamic stimulation and thalamotomy for suppression of severe tremor. The New England Journal of Medicine. 2000;342(7):461–8.
67 Krack P, Hamel W, Mehdorn HM, Deuschl G. Surgical treatment of Parkinson's disease. Current Opinion in Neurology. 1999;12(4):417–25.
68 Koller WC, Pahwa R, Lyons KE, Albanese A. Surgical treatment of Parkinson's disease. Journal of the Neurological Sciences. 1999; 167(1):1–10.
69 Oh MY, Hodaie M, Kim SH, Alkhani A, Lang AE, Lozano AM. Deep brain stimulator electrodes used for lesioning: proof of principle. Neurosurgery. 2001;49(2):363–7; discussion 7–9.
70 Marras C, Zorzi G, Lenardi C, Rizzi M, Messina G, Alimehmeti R, *et al.* Deep brain stimulation electrode used for radiofrequency lesion of the globus pallidus internus in dystonia. Stereotactic and Functional Neurosurgery. 2009;87(6):348–52.
71 Warnke PC. Deep brain stimulation surgery under general anaesthesia with microelectrode recording: the best of both worlds or a little bit of everything? Journal of Neurology, Neurosurgery and Psychiatry. 2014;85:1063.
72 Christmas D, Matthews K, Eljamel MS. Neurosurgery for mental disorder. The British Journal of Psychiatry 2004;185:173–4; author reply 4.
73 Hassenbusch SJ, Pillay PK, Barnett GH. Radiofrequency cingulotomy for intractable cancer pain using stereotaxis guided by magnetic resonance imaging. Neurosurgery. 1990;27(2):220–3.
74 Bush G, Luu P, Posner MI. Cognitive and emotional influences in anterior cingulate cortex. Trends in Cognitive Sciences. 2000;4(6):215–22.
75 Mega MS, Cummings JL. The cingulate and cingulate syndromes. In: Trimble MR, Cummings JL, editors. Contempory Behavioural Neurology. Oxford: Butterworth-Heinemann; 2004. p. 189–214.
76 Ballantine HT, Jr., Bouckoms AJ, Thomas EK, Giriunas IE. Treatment of psychiatric illness by stereotactic cingulotomy. Biological Psychiatry. 1987;22(7):807–19.
77 Richter EO, Davis KD, Hamani C, Hutchison WD, Dostrovsky JO, Lozano AM. Cingulotomy for psychiatric disease: microelectrode guidance, a callosal reference system for documenting lesion location, and clinical results. Neurosurgery. 2004;54(3):622–8; discussion 8–30.
78 Greenberg BD, Gabriels LA, Malone DA, Jr., Rezai AR, Friehs GM, Okun MS, *et al.* Deep brain stimulation of the ventral internal capsule/ventral striatum for obsessive-compulsive disorder: worldwide experience. Molecular Psychiatry. 2010;15(1):64–79.
79 Sturm V, Lenartz D, Koulousakis A, Treuer H, Herholz K, Klein JC, *et al.* The nucleus accumbens: a target for deep brain stimulation in obsessive-compulsive- and anxiety-disorders. Journal of Chemical Neuroanatomy. 2003;26(4):293–9.
80 Knight G. Stereotactic tractotomy in the surgical treatment of mental illness. Journal of Neurology, Neurosurgery and Psychiatry. 1965;28:304–10.
81 Knight G. 330 cases of restricted orbital cortex undercutting. Proceedings of the Royal Society of Medicine. 1960;53:728–32.
82 Woerdeman PA, Willems PW, Noordmans HJ, Berkelbach van der Sprenkel JW, van Rijen PC. Frameless stereotactic subcaudate tractotomy for intractable obsessive-compulsive disorder. Acta Neurochirurgica. 2006;148(6):633–7; discussion 7.
83 Cosyns P, Caemaert J, Haaijman W, van Veelen C, Gybels J, van Manen J, *et al.* Functional stereotactic neurosurgery for psychiatric disorders: an experience in Belgium and The Netherlands. Advances and Technical Standards in Neurosurgery 1994;21:239–79.
84 Kim MC, Lee TK, Choi CR. Review of long-term results of stereotactic psychosurgery. Neurologia Medico-Chirurgica. 2002;42(9):365–71.
85 Kelly D. Therapeutic outcome in limbic leucotomy in psychiatric patients. Psychiatria, Neurologia, Neurochirurgia. 1973;76(5):353–63.
86 Kelly D, Mitchell-Heggs N. Stereotactic limbic leucotomy – a follow-up study of thirty patients. Postgraduate Medical Journal. 1973;49(578): 865–82.
87 Kelly D, Richardson A, Mitchell-Heggs N. Stereotactic limbic leucotomy: neurophysiological aspects and operative technique. The British Journal of Psychiatry. 1973;123(573):133–40.
88 Kelly D, Richardson A, Mitchell-Heggs N, Greenup J, Chen C, Hafner RJ. Stereotactic limbic leucotomy: a preliminary report on forty patients. The British Journal of Psychiatry. 1973;123(573):141–8.

CHAPTER 22

Ablative procedures in psychiatric neurosurgery

David Huie, Joshua P. Aronson and Emad N. Eskandar
Massachusetts General Hospital, Boston, USA

Introduction

The advent of frontal leucotomy/lobotomy in 1936 marked the beginnings of modern neurosurgical intervention for psychiatric disorders [1]. Pioneered by neurologist Egas Moniz and neurosurgeon Pedro Almeida Lima, the goal of the operation was to sever white matter tracts within the frontal lobes, first by injection of alcohol directly into the brain and later using the leucotome. Despite the lack of evidence demonstrating the safety and efficacy of the procedure, and immediate controversy regarding its use, frontal lobotomy gained widespread application. In the United States, more than 20 000 lobotomies were performed by 1951, largely through the work of psychiatrist Walter Freeman and neurosurgeon James Watts [2]. Moniz was awarded the 1949 Nobel Prize in Physiology or Medicine 'for his discovery of the therapeutic value of leucotomy in certain psychoses' [3]. Despite a lack of controlled trials evaluating lobotomy and its significant side effects including seizures, personality change and loss of functional independence, it was not until the advent of chlorpromazine as a satisfactory medical alternative that frontal lobotomy fell out of use.

The introduction of stereotaxis helped bring about a revival in psychiatric neurosurgery. Use of stereotaxis in psychosurgical operations allowed surgeons to access specific brain structures with minimal disruption of the surrounding tissue and make accurate, discrete lesions within the brain. This, along with further technological advancements such as the development of functional imaging and physiological recording, permitted the significant refinement of psychiatric neurosurgical technique. A timeline of notable advancements in the field of psychosurgery may be seen in Figure 22.1.

In this chapter, we will first discuss several of the psychiatric disorders currently treated with neurosurgical intervention, with emphasis on the functional circuitry that is disrupted in each condition. We will continue with a discussion of the neurosurgical techniques currently employed to treat these conditions, describing the areas targeted for ablation and reviewing procedural outcomes as reported in the literature.

Depression

Major depressive disorder (MDD) is one of the most common mood disorders and is a leading cause of functional impairment and mortality. The World Health Organization identifies

Neuromodulation in Psychiatry, First Edition. Edited by Clement Hamani, Paul Holtzheimer, Andres M. Lozano and Helen Mayberg.

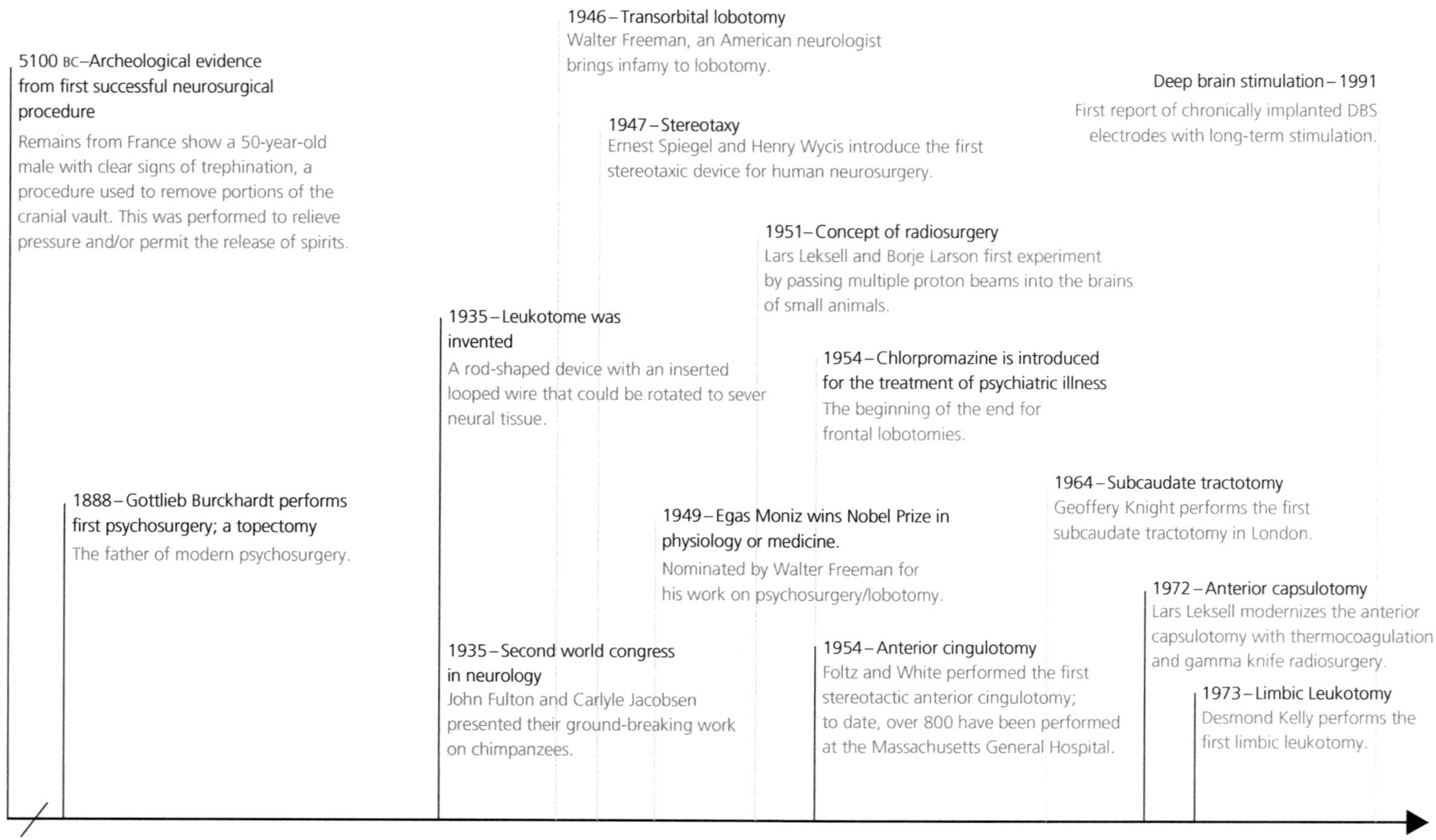

Figure 22.1 Timeline of major advancements in psychiatric neurosurgery. Source: From Patel *et al.* [4]. Reproduced with permission of Elsevier.

depression as the leading cause of disability worldwide [5]. In the United States, lifetime prevalence rates of depression among adults exceed 16%, with women being affected nearly twice as often as men [6]. *The Diagnostic and Statistical Manual of Mental Disorders* (DSM-IV-TR) characterizes the disorder as a depressed mood or loss of interest or pleasure, with other symptoms including changes in sleep or appetite, feelings of worthlessness or guilt, loss of energy, impaired concentration and recurrent thoughts of death or suicide. Although tremendous advances have been made in pharmacotherapy for depression, many patients fail to adequately respond to initial treatment. Quantifying the fraction of patients affected by 'treatment-resistant' or the more severe 'treatment-refractory' depression is difficult, largely because the terms have been inconsistently defined [7]. Despite this, it is estimated that between 30 and 45% of patients diagnosed with depression do not exhibit an adequate response to initial antidepressant treatment [8].

Cognitive models

Introduced in 1967, Aaron Beck's cognitive model of depression has served as a framework for studying the disorder and informing treatment [9, 10]. Beck's model posits the existence of latent schemas – negative self-referential beliefs or representations of stimuli, ideas or experiences formed by adverse experiences – which are activated by later life events [9]. These activated schemas alter the processing of incoming stimuli via creation of maladaptive beliefs and attitudes regarding the self, the external world/environment and the future, termed Beck's cognitive triad, thereby increasing an individual's vulnerability to depression. Since Beck's model was introduced, discoveries regarding the brain's structural and functional architecture have permitted a greater understanding of the model's neurobiological underpinnings. Patients with depression exhibit maladaptive changes in multiple domains, including attention, emotional processing and memory, which researchers have been able to correlate with specific regions of neural dysfunction [10].

Depression circuitry

Converging research suggests that depression emerges from dysfunction in 'bottom-up' emotional processing centres such as the thalamus, ventral striatum and amygdala, combined with loss of 'top-down' modulatory control from cortex [10–12]. Balance between these networks is disrupted in depressed patients, causing negative aspects of incoming stimuli to be overrepresented. Functional neuroimaging of depressed and healthy subjects demonstrates activity differences following emotional stimuli within many of the brain structures listed above [12–14]. These differences are thought to underlie a biasing of multiple domains, including emotional processing, memory and attentional engagement [10]. A diagram of the main circuitry affected in depression may be seen in Figure 22.2.

Amygdala

The amygdala is a crucial structure in the detection and interpretation of emotional quality in the incoming stimuli [15–18]. In a meta-analysis of functional magnetic resonance imaging (fMRI) and positron emission tomography (PET) studies examining amygdala activation during emotional processing, Costafreda *et al.* demonstrated an increased probability of amygdala activation following exposure to emotional versus neutral stimuli in normal subjects [15]. Fear and disgust were most likely to elicit amygdala activation and were significantly more likely to do so than happiness. Disruption of amygdala activity has been demonstrated in depressed patients, in whom negative stimuli assume an increased salience. Patients with MDD shown pictures of fearful human faces exhibit haemodynamic responses of increased magnitude and duration within the amygdala compared with healthy controls [12, 19].

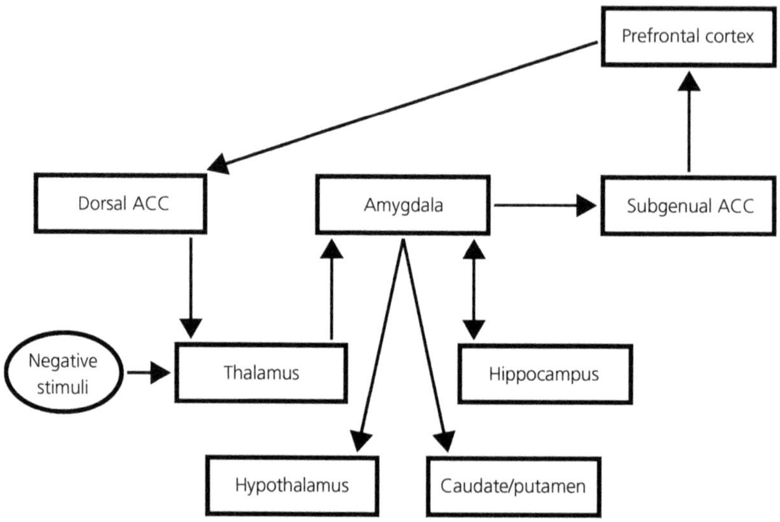

Figure 22.2 Diagram of primary neural structures implicated in depression. Emotional stimuli travel via the thalamus to the amygdala. They are processed there, and information is sent to prefrontal cortex by way of the subgenual anterior cingulate cortex. In turn, prefrontal cortex indirectly modulates activity within the amygdala via top-down projections, which exert cognitive control over subcortical emotional processing. Abnormal activity within subcortical emotional processing regions, coupled with disruption of cortical signalling, provides the basis for the deficits seen in depression. Amygdala projections to other areas such as the hippocampus, caudate, putamen and hypothalamus mediate other deficits including biased memory processing, ruminative thought and neuroendocrine abnormalities. ACC, anterior cingulate cortex.

The amygdala serves as a major hub of emotional processing, maintaining connections with a variety of structures and sending emotional information to prefrontal cortex (PFC) by route of the subgenual anterior cingulate cortex (sgACC) [20]. This pathway constitutes a bottom-up signal that is posited to maladaptively bias emotional processing within higher cortical areas in depressed patients [10]. Normally, this signal is balanced by indirect modulation arising from areas of PFC, particularly left dorsolateral PFC (DLPFC) [12, 21]. In depressed individuals, this modulating neural tone is attenuated, leading to an abnormally increased signal from the amygdala [14, 19]. The increase in amygdala activity has been positively correlated with depression severity, as measured by well-validated metrics such as the Hamilton Depression Scale [22, 23]. Pharmacological treatment with selective serotonin reuptake inhibitors has been shown to attenuate amygdala hyperactivity in depressed subjects, perhaps lending insight into the effect of these medications at the circuit level [24–26].

Studies analysing amygdala size in depressed patients have yielded mixed results, with different studies reporting increased and reduced amygdala volumes in depressed patients [27–29]. Accumulating evidence suggests that these differences are dependent on the acute or chronic nature of the illness, with acute depression being variably defined as the first major depressive episode, or as short illness duration and a small number of previous episodes [30]. Eijndhoven *et al.* reported results of magnetic resonance imaging (MRI) studies comparing patients in their first depressive episode, patients recovered from their first depressive episode and healthy controls [16].

They found amygdala size to be increased in patients experiencing their first episode compared with the other two groups. Other imaging studies have found that patients suffering from chronic depression or with several previous depressive episodes demonstrate reductions in amygdala size compared with healthy controls [31, 32]. These findings suggest that size variances within the amygdala of depressed patients are related to disease chronicity and reconcile increased amygdala sizes during acute depression with the observed correlation between long-term depression and grey matter reductions within this structure.

Prefrontal cortex

Although the amygdala serves as a central component of the 'bottom-up' pathway in emotional processing, converging research also indicates that dysfunction in PFC plays a major role in depression [10, 11]. PFC generally plays a top-down regulatory role in emotional processing and has been divided into several functionally defined regions, many of which are implicated in the neural circuits disrupted during depression. As stated above, the DLPFC is thought to play a role in modulating activity within the amygdala. Functional imaging of healthy subjects reveals DLPFC activity that varies inversely with that of amygdala [14, 19, 33, 34]. Depressed patients show decreased DLPFC activity when cued with emotional stimuli, coinciding with increased amygdala activation [12, 35, 36]. Reduced DLPFC grey matter volume in depressed versus healthy subjects has also been documented in structural studies [37, 38]. In contrast to left DLPFC hypoactivity, right DLPFC often demonstrates increased activity following emotional stimuli in depressed patients [39]. This hyperactivity has been associated with anticipation of negative stimuli, potentially biasing attentional resources towards negative aspects of the environment [10, 40]. Disengagement from negative stimuli is also impaired in depression and is thought to be linked to dysfunction within the DLPFC and the rostral ACC (rACC) [41–43].

Like the DLPFC, ventrolateral PFC (vLPFC) is involved in cognitive control of emotional processing and cognitive reappraisal [44]. Decreased vLPFC activity in depressed patients is associated with poor control of stimulus selection as well as depressive rumination [10, 33, 44, 45]. DLPFC and vLPFC modulate activity within the hippocampus and amygdala, areas implicated in emotional recall, and lowered activity in these cortical areas permits sustained hippocampal and amygdala activation seen in rumination [10]. Another cortical area, medial PFC (mPFC), is thought to be active during self-referent and autobiographical thought, and impaired mPFC function is thought to contribute to the tendency of depressed patients to interpret incoming stimuli as self-referential [46–48]. Within the mPFC, MRI and PET studies have demonstrated increased sgACC activity during ruminative thought in depressed patients compared with healthy controls, despite an apparent decrease in subgenual PFC volume [46, 49–51]. This elevated activity has also been observed during transient sadness in healthy patients [52]. On a cellular level, brains of depressed patients have been shown to possess decreased glial cell density within the supracallosal and subgenual ACC [50, 53, 54].

One of the least understood areas of the brain the orbitofrontal cortex (OFC) has been implicated in a range of functions including sensory integration, encoding reward value, goal-directed behaviour and decision-making [55]. OFC maintains connections with many regions implicated in emotional processing, including DLPFC, ACC, ventral striatum, hippocampus and the amygdala, and it is perhaps unsurprising that this area has been implicated in depressive disease [55–60]. Comparison of unmedicated, primary MDD patients with healthy controls at rest has demonstrated increased OFC blood flow and metabolism in the depressed group [61]. PET and fMRI comparisons of depressed and remitted patients reveal relatively increased OFC blood flow and metabolism during active depression [22, 62]. Similar to the role of DLPFC, it has been hypothesized that the OFC acts in depression to attenuate increased activity within the limbic circuit [13]. Unlike DLPFC, however, OFC activity is increased in depression, which is suggested to represent increased 'effort' on the part of OFC to mitigate limbic hyperactivity. Antidepressant therapy, which inhibits overactive limbic structures, decreases OFC activation [13]. This has been posited to represent a 'relaxation' of the area following limbic normalization.

Anterior cingulate cortex

The ACC is associated with cognitive tasks such as motivation, problem-solving and attention, and growing evidence has implicated this region in depression. rACC dysfunction is implicated along with DLPFC in faulty attentional disengagement from negative stimuli [41–43]. As mentioned previously, functional imaging studies of the sgACC, which acts as an intermediary between the amygdala and higher cortical areas, have demonstrated increased metabolic levels in depressed patients despite an apparent reduction in size. While sgACC carries information from the amygdala to cortex in a bottom-up fashion, modulatory signals from DLPFC reach the limbic system by way of the dorsal ACC. The dorsal ACC projects to the thalamus, which maintains connections with the amygdala crucial to emotional processing [10, 63]. Compared to healthy controls, depressed patients show reduced dorsal ACC-thalamic connectivity, manifesting as limbic hyperactivity and impaired control of emotional processing [64].

Additional brain regions

In addition to the above-mentioned areas, dysfunction in other brain regions has also been implicated in depression. Depressed patients demonstrate biased memory encoding and recall for negative stimuli. This effect has been linked to abnormal function within the amygdala, which is thought to be involved in encoding emotional aspects of memory [65, 66]. The amygdala also projects to the hippocampal and caudoputamen regions, where evidence suggests that it modulates memory encoding as well [67]. The hippocampus plays a significant role in episodic and spatial memory, while the caudate and putamen are involved in skill learning. Using fMRI, Hamilton and Gotlib [68] found that the right amygdala exhibits elevated activity and greater functional connectivity to the hippocampus and caudoputamen during encoding of subsequently remembered negative stimuli, compared with healthy controls. Increased amygdala activity is further associated with elevated hippocampal and caudoputamen activation during the recall of negative information. Collectively, elevated activity in these regions is thought to underlie the biasing of memory encoding and retrieval of negative stimuli in depressed patients.

The nucleus accumbens (NAc) shares connections with PFC, both of which are activated in healthy subjects following positive stimuli and during positive reappraisal [69]. PFC-regulated dopamine release within the NAc is thought to contribute to affective responses to pleasure and reward [70]. These effects are blunted in depression, both in response to positive stimuli and when patients are asked to maintain a positive mood [71, 72]. Dysfunction in the PFC and NAc is associated with decreased activity in the caudate, an area implicated in reinforcement of behaviours potentially leading to reward [73]. As a result, patients with depression manifest a failure to pursue rewarding behaviours, due to an inability to trigger proper reinforcement following positive stimuli [10, 73, 74].

The amygdala also connects to the hypothalamus via the stria terminalis, and abnormal activity within this pathway is thought to mediate the neuroendocrine abnormalities seen in depression [38]. Patients with depression demonstrate elevated cortisol levels, secondary to increased anterior hypothalamic release of corticotropin-releasing hormone.

Bipolar disorder

Bipolar disorder (BPD) is a disabling mood disorder characterized by affective swings between major depressive and manic (Type I) or hypomanic (Type 2) episodes. The DSM IV-TR describes mania as a distinct period of abnormally and persistently elevated, expansive or irritable mood, lasting at least 1 week. Specific symptoms include increases in distractibility and goal-directed activity, decreased need for sleep, elevated self-esteem or grandiosity and excessive pursuit of pleasurable behaviours with high risk of adverse consequences. Hypomanic episodes are similar, but last only 4 days, do not cause severe social or occupational impairment or necessitate hospitalization and lack psychotic features. Lifetime prevalence of BPD has been estimated at 1.0 and 1.1% for Types 1 and 2, respectively [75]. Among individuals with BPD who reported a manic or hypomanic episode in the past 12 months, 70% reported severe impairment in psychosocial functioning. During the depressive episodes, these patients reported severely impaired functioning in approximately 90% of cases [76]. As in the case of MDD, quantifying treatment resistance is difficult due to lack of standard criteria. It is estimated that approximately half of patients treated with monotherapy fail to respond; this figure drops to 30% when combination pharmacotherapy is employed [77].

Studies examining areas of dysfunction in BPD have largely implicated the same areas as discussed above in MDD. As in MDD, patients with BPD demonstrate similar increased activity in limbic areas, combined with loss of 'top-down' regulation from cortex. [78] There are, however, a few key differences highlighted in imaging studies of bipolar patients. Diffusion tensor imaging has revealed abnormalities in large white matter tracts, including the left superior longitudinal fasciculus and right uncinate fasciculus in BPD, but not MDD, patients [79]. These white matter tracts interconnect key emotional regulatory centres, and their degradation in BPD may suggest a more widespread effect on white matter connectivity [80]. MRI studies comparing BPD and MDD patients also demonstrate decreased habenula volume in BPD patients [81]. The habenula exerts an inhibitory influence over dopaminergic transmission from the ventral tegmental area (VTA), and loss of this activity may lead to heightened reward sensitivity, possibly underlying the manic/hypomanic episodes that separate the two conditions [80, 82].

During investigating the neural basis of manic/hypomanic episodes, one key finding that has emerged in BPD patients is hyperactivation of the striatum [78, 83], as well as the globus pallidus and thalamus [84, 85]. Activity in these areas is elevated in BPD patients compared to that in both MDD patients and healthy controls and is broadly correlated with an increased intensity of affective experience. Loss of differential striatal activation in response to receipt versus omission of reward has been implicated in faulty reward processing, hypothesized to predispose towards impaired judgement and increased pleasure-seeking behaviours in mania [78, 86].

Obsessive-compulsive disorder

Obsessive-compulsive disorder (OCD) is a chronic psychiatric disorder defined by recurrent obsessions and/or compulsions that cause significant impairments in daily functioning. The global prevalence of OCD is 1–2% [87, 88], with a slight female gender predominance among adults, but 2:1 male to female ratio among paediatric patients [88]. The DSM IV-TR defines obsessions as recurrent and persistent thoughts or impulses that cause marked distress, with the person driven to perform repetitive, excessive compulsions to reduce or neutralize the distress or dreaded consequence. Importantly, these obsessions and compulsions interfere with the person's normal functioning and social relationships. The severity of symptoms varies considerably between patients and during the course of the disease. While most patients experience continuous symptoms, many suffer a relapsing/remitting course with periods of only subclinical symptoms. In a prospective study of 293 patients with a diagnosis of OCD seeking treatment, enrollment interviews revealed that 27% of patients were unable to work due to psychopathology and more than 70% were categorized as moderate to severe severity using the well-described Yale-Brown Obsessive Compulsive Scale (Y-BOCS) [89].

Cortico-striato-thalamo-cortical (CSTC) circuits

CSTC circuits have been demonstrated via non-invasive imaging to be fundamental to cognitive and motor functions [90]. CSTC circuits are organized in a loop, in which circuits project from specific territories in frontal cortex to targets within the striatum, and via direct and indirect pathways, through specific areas in the basal ganglia to the thalamus, and finally back to the original frontal territory [91]. A diagram of a typical CSTC circuit may be seen in Figure 22.3. Functional neuroimaging allows comparison of CSTC circuit function in OCD and normal patients. Delineation of the involved fibre tracts, nuclei and cortical regions is critical to understanding the pathophysiology of OCD, as no single neurotransmitter, genetic abnormality or brain region is likely to provide a complete explanation of the disease pathology resulting from CSTC dysfunction [93, 94].

CSTC circuits convey information flow from cortical and limbic regions to modulate a number of processes that include motivation, attention and motor function [92, 95, 96]. The key nodes within these circuits include DLPFC, OFC, ACC and striatum (specifically the caudate). Corrupting information flow between these structures can result in disordered behavioural and emotional processing, core pathophysiological features of OCD [97].

Striatum

At the cellular level, the striatum is composed of two main neural components, smaller patchy compartments called striosomes, which are surrounded by a larger compartment called the matrix [98]. The ventral and anterior regions of the striatum are highly concentrated with striosomes and receive cortical afferents from the OFC and ACC [56]. Studies that have evaluated the neuroanatomy of this frontal–subcortical circuit suggest that the striosomes are neurochemically specialized to exert a strong inhibitory influence on dopaminergic input, thus influencing negative feedback inhibition on the main frontal–subcortical circuits [99]. Frontal projections that pass through the striatum are believed to contribute to the execution of complex and emotional response behaviours that are typically executed quickly in response to stimuli [100]. Therefore, dysfunction involving striosomes, commonly manifested as hyperactivity in the caudate nucleus, might result in overactive inhibition of the negative feedback processes that affect frontal cortices. This may lead to elevated cortical excitability, producing brain activation patterns in the frontal–subcortical circuits that may underlie mechanisms for cognitive (e.g. learning) and emotional deficits observed in OCD patients [101].

Prefrontal cortices

The OFC plays an important role in emotion and social behaviour. This brain region is involved in the mediation of emotional responses as well as allows for integration of emotional information [102, 103]. Hyperactivity

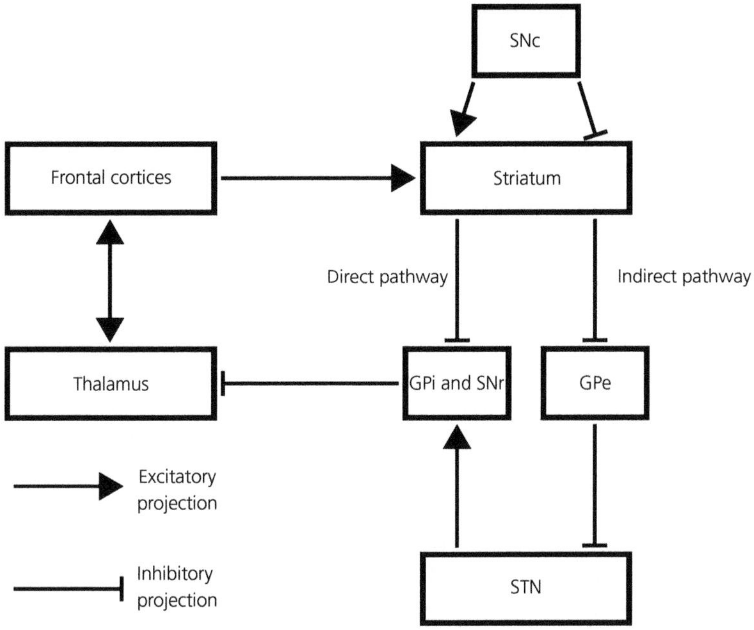

Figure 22.3 Conceptual cortico-striato-thalamo-cortical circuit. The block diagram shows direct and indirect loop pathways between cortical and subcortical structures. The direct pathway has projections from frontal cortex to the striatum, which then project to the internal segment of the globus pallidus and substantia nigra pars reticulata, which in turn projects back to the cortex via the thalamus. The indirect pathway differs by having projections from the striatum to the external segment of the globus pallidus, which then projects to the subthalamic nucleus before connecting with the globus pallidus interna and substantia nigra pars reticulata. Prefrontal cortex and thalamus have mutual excitatory projections. Under this framework, the direct pathway disinhibits the thalamus to generate a positive feedback loop, whereas the indirect pathway inhibits the thalamus to generate a negative feedback. GPe, Globus pallidus externa; GPi, Globus pallidus interna; SNc, Substantia nigra pars compacta; SNr, Substantia nigra pars reticulata; STN, Subthalamic nucleus. Source: From Aronson *et al.* [92]. Reproduced with permission of Elsevier.

in the OFC can corrupt the weighing of emotional information, thereby skewing the consequences of immediate action to generate uncontrolled thoughts and behaviour [104]. Different subregions of the OFC have also been evaluated with respect to OCD. Lateral orbitalfrontal cortex (lOFC) and medial orbitalfrontal cortex (mOFC) play distinct roles in processing behavioural control. Specifically, activation in the lOFC appears to correlate with ritualized behavioural responses [105, 106], while the mOFC appears more involved in emotion regulation and reward processing [107]. This regional distinction in the OFC provides a new level of detail that can help elucidate the complexities of the disorder.

The DLPFC is a high-order brain region that is implicated in executive processes needed for voluntary, goal-directed behaviour. The region is also associated with different aspects of cognitive control including the ability to focus thoughts and actions, enabling shifting of focus according to environmental input [108]. Hyperactive brain patterns observed in the DLPFC of OCD patients may corrupt these cognitive resources and impair executive function to cause compulsive behaviour and obsessive thoughts.

The ACC is associated with cognitive processes such as attention, motivation, problem-solving, detecting the presence of cognitive conflict and error monitoring and detection [104]. Cognitive conflict behaviour studies, where congruent conditions require an expected, reflexive response while incongruent conditions require the inhibition of reflexive behaviour, cause a large degree of activation in the ACC. Patients with OCD who are tested on such tasks show hyperactivation of the ACC in response to the incongruent relative to the congruent conditions [109, 110]. Similar studies in OCD patients support a role for abnormal cortico-cortical interactions affecting error processing in patients with OCD, and ultimately adversely affecting decision-making. In summary, hyperactivation of the ACC may facilitate faulty error detection that contributes to cognitive difficulties and obsessions.

Addiction

Addiction is a chronic disease characterized by cravings, impaired behavioural control and inability to abstain from certain behaviours despite adverse consequences, often leading to inability to fulfill social, work and home obligations. This disorder is highly prevalent – epidemiological studies of substance use report that 2% of US adults had a drug use disorder in the previous year, with 10.4% reporting a drug use disorder during their lifetime [111]. The neurobiology of addiction involves dysfunction within the brain's reward pathways and disruption of executive function, particularly in the realms of motivation and self-control.

Early investigations into addiction circuitry focused upon the mesolimbic pathway [112]. Dopaminergic neurons project from the VTA to the NAc within the ventral striatum. Addition of VTA neurons projecting to PFC forms the expanded mesocorticolimbic pathway. Common to addictive drugs is their general ability to induce dopamine release within the NAc [113]. Initial theories held that increases in NAc dopamine during drug administration were indicative of an elevated sensitization to the dopamine-enhancing effects of drugs, increasing the perceived reward and thus creating motivation to procure more of the drug [112]. However, more recent fMRI studies have shown that acute administration of cocaine to drug abusers correlates with *de*activation of the ventral striatum – an apparent contradiction [114]. Similarly, stimulant administration to detoxified drug addicts leads to marked attenuation of striatal dopamine release compared with non-drug using controls, and a more recent study administering stimulants to active cocaine addicts found striatal dopamine release to be indistinguishable from placebo [112, 115].

The change appears to be due to a conditioning response within the brain after repeated administration of the drug, such as is the case in chronic dependency. While non-chronic drug users experience dopamine increases in the NAc secondary to the drug's pharmacological effect, following repeated administration, dopamine release shifts to occur as a result of reward anticipation [112]. Drug abusers who were shown craving-eliciting videos demonstrated significant striatal dopamine increases, whose magnitude correlated with the subjective experience of craving [116, 117]. On the other hand, striatal dopamine changes following administration of the drug itself were significantly blunted [118]. Cue-elicited cravings in addicts have been shown to activate not only mesolimbic structures but also cortical areas involved in motivation and executive control, including the ACC and OFC [119–121].

In addition to the mesolimbic pathway, other circuits have been implicated in addiction. Dopaminergic neurons connecting the substantia nigra and dorsal striatum form the nigrostriatal pathway, which displays

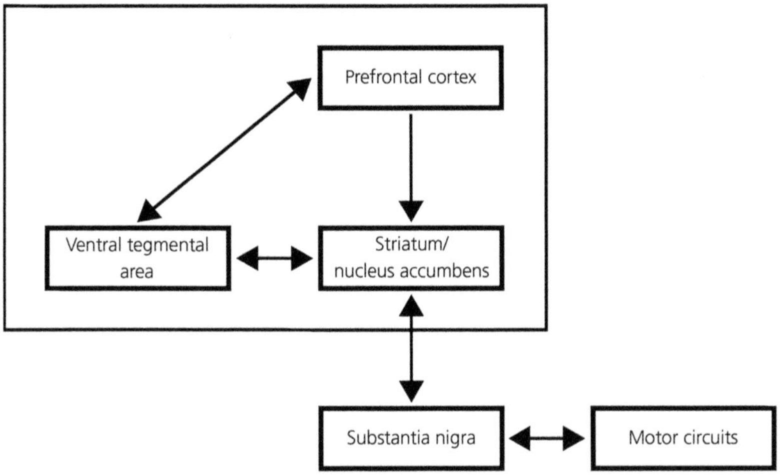

Figure 22.4 Schematic drawing of neural structures implicated in addiction. Limbic regions (boxed) include the prefrontal cortex, ventral tegmental area and striatum (specifically the nucleus accumbens). These areas are responsible for determining the adaptive value of behavioural change in response to novel stimuli (e.g. acquiring a drug to experience its effects). If repetition of this behaviour continues to produce the desired effect, neural activity during the behaviour migrates from limbic areas to motor regions organized around task performance. Nigrostriatal projections to and from the substantia nigra have been proposed to mediate this shift in activity. Addiction has been characterized by the disrupted ability of limbic structures to modulate the motor circuit.

enhanced reactivity during conditioned responses [112, 122]. Yin and Knowlton propose a role for these neurons in facilitating the propagation of activity between cortico-basal ganglia circuits during habit formation [123]. Functional imaging studies in drug addicts have shown local increases in dopamine within the dorsal striatum in response to cue-elicited cravings, with the magnitude of increase correlated with addiction severity [117]. The dorsal striatum is implicated in the selection and initiation of action, as well as habit learning, and its increased reactivity has been proposed to reflect the automatized nature of craving in worsening addiction, as well as the habitual aspects of compulsive drug seeking.

With control over functions such as motivation, decision-making, goal-directed behaviour and inhibitory control, cortical areas play a vital role in addiction [124]. Areas of PFC project to striatal structures including the NAc, which is proposed to serve as a gateway between limbic circuits responsible for processing motivational value and motor circuits that guide ongoing behaviour [125]. Initial exposure to a novel stimulus (e.g. a drug) engages limbic structures such as the PFC, VTA and NAc, which determine the adaptive value of implementing behavioural strategies (e.g. acquiring the drug). Repetition of this behaviour to obtain the desired outcome leads to migration of activity away from limbic regions, with elevated activation of motor circuits organized around behavioural performance reflecting the behaviour's increasing automaticity [125, 126]. This migration is thought to be mediated by nigrostriatal projections interconnecting the limbic and motor circuits [123]. If the action ceases to produce a reward, the limbic areas again show high activity, thought to reflect reassessment of the behaviour's value. Figure 22.4 illustrates this interplay between limbic and motor regions. Addiction and relapse have been characterized by loss of the limbic circuit's ability to process and utilize negative environmental contingencies to regulate drug-seeking behaviour mediated by the motor circuit [123, 125]. Reduction of striatal D2 receptors has been observed n drug addicts, with low levels of these receptors persisting for months following detoxification [127]. Loss of these receptors is further associated with a decrease in activity within OFC, ACC and DLPFC [128–130]. OFC plays a role in salience attribution and goal-directed behaviour. Reduced activity in this area is associated with disrupted temporal discounting (subjects are more likely to prefer smaller, immediate rewards over larger delayed ones) [131, 132]. These subjects also show difficulty inhibiting behaviours formerly associated with reward, thought to explain why addicts may continue to repeat destructive behaviours even after reward for such behaviours has been abolished [133]. ACC is associated with inhibitory control, and loss of activity in this area is thought to be associated with impulsive behaviour. DLPFC is associated with higher cognition, as well as decision-making.

Recent studies have also implicated dysfunction within other areas in addiction. The supramammillary nucleus (SUM), located in the posterior hypothalamic area, is thought to act as a 'trigger zone' for the mesolimbic reward circuit [134]. Structural studies have identified reciprocal connections between the VTA-NAc circuit and the SUM, and stimulation of the SUM has been shown to activate the VTA-NAc dopamine system [135]. Other notable structures include the midbrain raphe nuclei and the rostromedial tegmental nucleus. Both of these structures have been described as having possible inhibitory control over the reward circuitry. Studies in rats have shown that inhibition of the midbrain raphe nuclei is perceived as rewarding [136]. The rostromedial tegmental nucleus contains inhibitory GABAergic neurons, whose major projections target the dopaminergic neurons of the VTA [134].

Currently, there are no approved psychosurgical procedures used for the treatment of addiction. However, past reports have indicated that certain techniques may be effective in ameliorating addiction symptoms. In 1978, Kanaka and Balasubramaniam described 73 patients undergoing anterior cingulotomy for drug addiction [137]. During 6 years of follow-up, the relapse rate was 22%, with no significant psychological deficits or procedural complications. Reported results of 335 bilateral anterior cingulotomies in 2003 for heroin addiction indicated total immediate remission in 30% of patients, with an additional 30% entering remission after 2 months [138].

Several studies from China have recently emerged that have examined the use of bilateral NAc ablation to treat addiction. Gao *et al.* [139] in 2003 described 28 heroin addicts undergoing this operation. Although limited by lack of blinding, and poor assessment instruments and controls, the study reported complete remission in seven patients, while six others relapsed but reported reduced withdrawal symptoms. Side effects included personality changes (two patients) and temporary memory loss (four patients). In 2010, Wu *et al.* [140] reported results of NAc ablation in 12 patients with alcohol dependence with an average follow-up of 16.6 months. In the first year, 25% of the patients relapsed, with the only side effect being temporary anosmia in one patient. Severity of dependence and cravings was reported to be decreased from preoperative baseline.

Surgical approaches to therapy

Currently, application of ablative psychosurgery is limited to patients suffering from severe, disabling, chronic and treatment-refractory

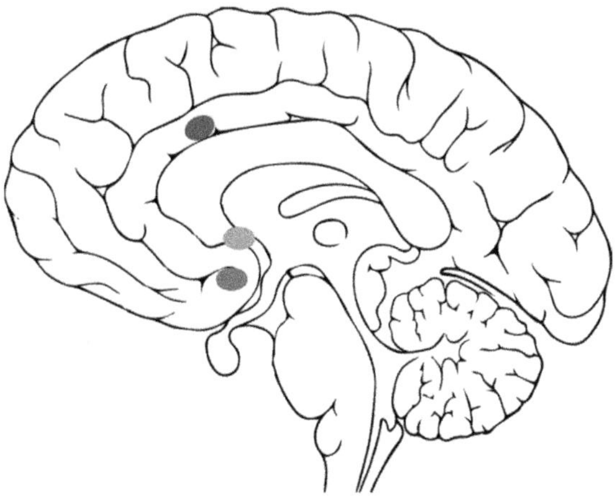

Figure 22.5 Targets in psychosurgery. For anterior capsulotomy, fibres of the internal capsule (middle dot) are interrupted via thermocoagulation or ionizing radiation. Cingulotomy targets the anterior cingulate (upper dot) using thermocoagulation. For subcaudate tractotomy, lesions are placed within the substantia innominata (lower dot), inferior to the head of the caudate. Limbic leucotomy combines the targets of both anterior cingulotomy and subcaudate tractotomy (upper and lower dots). Though dots representing capuslotomy and leukotomy are portrayed in this midline section, we note tat the actual targets are lateral to include the structures described in the text. Source: From Patel *et al.* [4]. Reproduced with permission of Elsevier.

psychiatric illness. Surgical intervention is considered an option after pharmacological, psychological and (when applicable) electroconvulsive therapies have failed to produce an adequate response, and as with all surgical procedures, the potential risks and benefits to the patient must be weighed before the decision to proceed is made. Following the introduction of stereotaxis, four neurosurgical procedures have emerged as the safest and the most effective for the treatment of psychiatric disease. These are the anterior capsulotomy, anterior cingulotomy, subcaudate tractotomy and limbic leucotomy (Figure 22.5, Table 22.1). All are performed bilaterally and under stereotactic conditions. Although they target different structures, these procedures share the underlying goal of modulating activity within the limbic system, as well as interconnected structures including areas of the basal ganglia, and PFC and ACC. A summary of information regarding the efficacy of these procedures organized by psychiatric disorder may be found in Tables 22.2, 22.3, and 22.4.

Anterior capsulotomy

Lars Leksell and Jean Talairach developed the anterior capsulotomy in the 1940s, targeting the anterior limb of the internal capsule just superior to the ventral striatum [161–163]. This operation is indicated today in the treatment of OCD. The goal is to interrupt fibres traversing the internal capsule, connecting the orbitalfrontal and sgACC with the thalamic nuclei and the caudate, by ablating the area between the anterior and middle of third of the anterior limb of the internal capsule at approximately the level of the foramen of Monro (Figure 22.6). Bilateral lesions were originally placed through burr holes in the skull using thermocoagulation, resulting in roughly 15–18 mm long and 4 mm wide lesions. Subsequent imaging studies have suggested that limiting the lateral extent of capsulotomy lesions may increase the efficacy, while limiting the posterior and medial extent of the lesions may lessen the side effects [152]. More recently, capsulotomy has been performed using the Leksell Gamma Knife, stereotactically focusing ionizing radiation onto the target site. Although it is a relatively new procedure, the efficacy is similar to thermocoagulation and the need for open surgery is eliminated. A controlled study of gamma knife capsulotomy for OCD is currently in progress at the University of Sao Paulo, Brazil.

In the 1950s, Leksell reported the results of anterior capsulotomy in 116 patients, with 50% improvement in patients with OCD. More recent outcome studies of capsulotomy for intractable OCD report an approximate

Table 22.1 Ablative procedures for psychiatric disorders.

Procedure	Indications	Method	Target	Side effects
Anterior capsulotomy	OCD	Thermocoagulation, Gamma Knife	Anterior limb of internal capsule	Short term: headache, confusion, incontinence Long term: weight gain, fatigue, memory loss, incontinence, seizure
Anterior cingulotomy	OCD, MDD, BPD	Electrocoagulation	Anterior cingulate	Short-term: Headache, confusion, disinhibition, urinary incontinence, fatigue, memory loss, seizure
Subcaudate tractotomy	OCD, MDD, BPD, anxiety	Yttrium-90 rods, electrocoagulation, ` Knife	Substantia innominate	Short term: oedema, disorientation Long term: seizure
Limbic leucotomy	OCD, MDD, BPD	Mechanical disruption, heat, radioactive material, radiofrequency thermocoagulation	Anterior cingulate, substantia innominate	Short term: headache, confusion, lethargy, perseveration, incontinence, somnolence, apathy, seizure

Source: From Patel *et al.* [4]. Reproduced with permission of Elsevier.
BPD, bipolar disorder; MDD, major depressive disorder; OCD, obsessive-compulsive disorder.

Table 22.2 Case studies of lesioning procedures for major depressive disorder.

Study	Procedure	*n*	Responders (%)
Spangler *et al.* [141]	Cingulotomy	10	60*
Steele *et al.* [142]	Cingulotomy	8	63†
Shields *et al.* [143]	Cingulotomy	17	41‡
Göktepe *et al.* [144]	Subcaudate tractotomy	78	68§
Sachdev and Sachdev [145]¶	Subcaudate tractotomy	22	73§
Mitchell-Heggs *et al.* [146]	Limbic leucotomy	9	56§
Montoya *et al.* [147]	Limbic leucotomy	6	50*

Responder defined as:
*Score of 1 or 2 on Clinical Global Improvement Scale (CGI) and 3, 4 or 5 on the Current Global Psychiatric Social Status Scale (CGPSS).
†Patients were either a responder (≥50% reduction in baseline Hamilton Rating Scale for Depression (HRSD-17) and Montgomery-Asberg Depression Rating Scale (MADRS)) or in remission (HRSD-17 ≤7 and MADRS ≤10).
‡50% improvement in Beck Depression Inventory (BDI) score and CGI score of 1–2 and improvement attributed to surgical intervention.
§Investigators' determination of completely recovered or only mild residual symptoms.
¶Seventy-six patients were examined in the study, but follow-up data were available only for 22. Of these, an unknown number met the criteria for BPD, although the indication for surgery in all patients was MDD.

Table 22.3 Case studies of lesioning procedures for bipolar disorder.

Study	Procedure	*n*	Responders (%)
Ballantine *et al.* [148]	Cingulotomy	26	77*
Spangler *et al.* [141]	Cingulotomy	5	40†
Poynton *et al.* [149]	Subcaudate tractotomy	9	44‡
Cho *et al.* [150]	Limbic leucotomy	18	69§

Responder defined as:
*Investigators' determination of significantly improved.
†Score of 1 or 2 on Clinical Global Improvement Scale (CGI) and 3, 4 or 5 on the Current Global Psychiatric Social Status Scale (CGPSS).
‡Investigators' determination of completely recovered or only mild residual symptoms.
§CPGSS ≥ 3.

Table 22.4 Case studies of lesioning procedures for OCD.

Study	Procedure	*n*	Responders (%)
Liu *et al.* [151]	Anterior capsulotomy	35	86*
Rück *et al.* [152]	Anterior capsulotomy	25	48†
Ballantine *et al.* [153]	Cingulotomy	32	25‡
Jenike *et al.* [154]	Cingulotomy	33	27§
Dougherty *et al.* [155]	Cingulotomy	44	32¶
Sheth *et al.* [156]	Cingulotomy	34	38¶
Bourne *et al.* [157]‡‡	Cingulotomy	8	76**
Yang *et al.* [158]	Cingulotomy	11	18¶
Hodgkiss *et al.* [159]	Subcaudate tractotomy	15	33††
Bourne *et al.* [157]‡‡	Subcaudate tractotomy	11	73**
Kelly *et al.* [160]	Limbic leucotomy	17	41††
Mitchell-Heggs *et al.* [146]	Limbic leucotomy	27	67††
Yang *et al.* [158]	Limbic leucotomy	8	50¶

Responder defined as decrease in Y-BOCS of:
*Greater than or equal to 50%
†Greater than or equal to 33%
‡Investigators' determination of normal with or without pharmacological or behavioural treatment.
§Greater than or equal to 25% or investigators' determination of at least moderate improvement based on clinical record review.
¶Greater than or equal to 35%.
**Greater than or equal to 25%.
††Investigators' determination of completely recovered or only mild residual symptoms.
‡‡These surgeries represent reoperations following failure to respond to initial cingulotomy for refractory OCD, with failure to respond being defined as Y-BOCS reduction less than 25%.

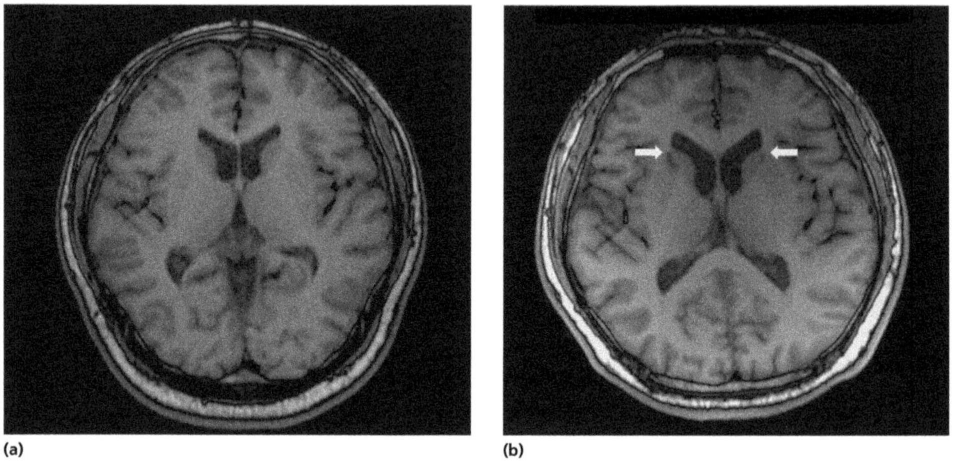

Figure 22.6 T1-weighted coronal MR images before (**a**) and after (**b**) undergoing anterior capsulotomy. Arrows in (**b**) indicate bilateral lesions in the mid-third of the anterior limb of the internal capsule. Source: From Zhan *et al.* [164]. Reproduced with permission of Elsevier.

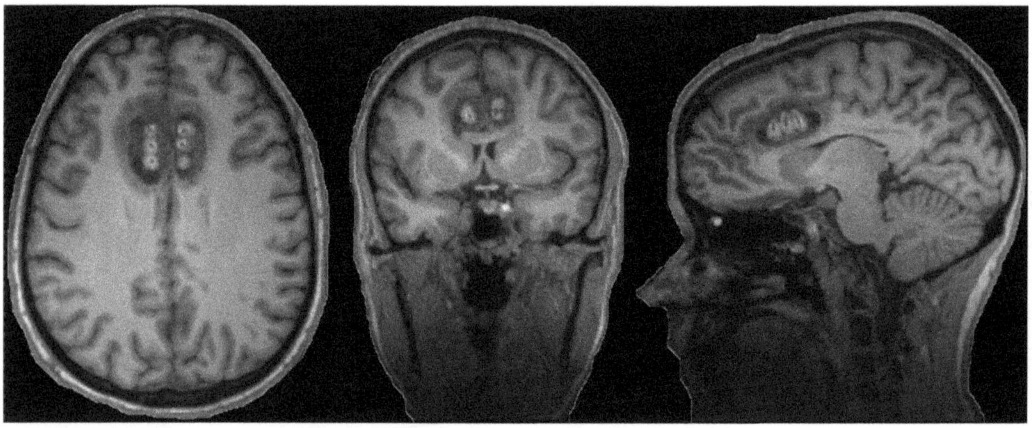

Figure 22.7 Representative cingulotomy images. Axial, coronal and sagittal T1-weighted MR images (left to right).

70% improvement [4, 165, 166]. Short-term side effects included headache, confusion, disinhibition and urinary incontinence. Weight gain, fatigue, memory loss, incontinence and seizure have been reported as rare but long-lasting side effects [167]. Therapeutic responses for gamma knife capsulotomy, defined as greater than 35% improvement in the Yale-Brown Obsessive Compulsive Scale (YBOCS) at follow-up, have been reported in 60% of OCD patients [168], and no significant difference between thermocoagulation and radiosurgery has been reported [152].

Anterior cingulotomy

Walter Freeman and James Watts detailed the earliest reports of cingulotomies in the 1940s [169]. In 1948, Hugh Cairns began targeting the anterior cingulum for anxiety, pain and mood disorders. Foltz and White reported on their use of anterior cingulotomy for the treatment of intractable pain in 1962, where they noted that the best outcomes were obtained in patients with comorbid anxiety conditions [170]. Currently, anterior cingulotomy is the most common neurosurgical procedure for refractory psychiatric illness in the United States and Canada and is indicated for the treatment of depression and BPD, as well as OCD [1, 4].

In this procedure, two or three stereotactic lesions of approximately 1.0 cm^3 are made bilaterally in the anterior cingulate (Brodmann area 24) via thermocoagulation. Lesions are typically made 2–2.5 cm from the tip of the frontal horns, 7 mm lateral from the midline and 1 mm above the room of the ventricles (Figure 22.7). The goal of this procedure is interrupt fibre tracts in the anterior cingulate that carry information from the cingulate cortex to the OFC and the limbic system.

In 1967, H. Thomas Ballantine published the results of 69 patients undergoing bilateral cingulotomy [148]. Ballantine utilized monopolar radiofrequency electrocoagulation, with needles placed 3–4 cm from the tip of frontal horns to within 5 mm of the midline, to destroy the medial portion of the cingulum. Of these subjects, 26 suffered from manic-depressive symptoms consistent with a modern BPD diagnosis. Post-operatively, 20 patients (77%) showed significant improvement and were followed up between 3 months up to 4 years. There were no deaths or major complications attributed to surgery, although three patients (4%) experienced post-operative seizures [148].

Ballantine's work played a major role in establishing the safety and effectiveness of anterior cingulotomy. In 1987, he published another study characterizing the safety and efficacy of anterior cingulotomy in 198 patients suffering from a range of psychiatric disorders [153]. A 56% improvement in OCD patients was reported using a subjective functional/symptomatic rating scale. In 2000, these data were reanalysed using more rigid criteria, and a 33% improvement from cingulotomy was reported [171].

Stereotaxic cingulotomy results from Massachusetts General Hospital performed between 1991 and 1995 were reported by Spangler *et al.* in 1996 [141]. A total of 34 patients, 10 with MDD and 5 with BPD, were followed up for 6–38 months (mean 17 months), and the outcome was assessed via the Clinical Global Improvement (CGI) scale and the Current Global Psychiatric Social Status Scale (CGPSS). Patients were considered responders if they improved on the CGI scale and were no longer institutionalized and usually working to some extent (CGPSS score 3 or greater). Partial responders were minimally improved or better on the CGI scale, or showed at least some improvement while still requiring intensive care or institutionalization on the CGPSS scale (score 2 or better). Of the MDD patients, 60% were characterized as responders, 10% possible responders and 30% non-responders. For the BPD patients, 40% were responders, 40% were partial responders and 20% failed to respond. The authors stated that cingulotomy is associated with mild, transient side effects and reported no major long-term complications. More recently, long-term prospective studies have found a 32–48% reduction in baseline Y-BOCS scores following cingulotomy [155, 172]. A report on the safety of the more than 800 cingulotomies performed at the Massachusetts General Hospital over a 40-year period resulted in no deaths and only two infections [173]. Recent evidence also suggests that in cases of depression, placement of smaller lesions more anteriorly within the ACC is associated with superior outcomes [142].

Patients who do not respond to initial surgical intervention may sometimes elect to undergo reoperation to enlarge the original lesion or to create a new, distinct lesion. A 2013 study reported on 31 patients at Massachusetts General Hospital with refractory OCD who failed to respond to initial cingulotomy [157], with failure to respond defined as a reduction of less than 25% in Y-BOCS score post-operatively. In total, 19 patients underwent reoperation, 8 undergoing repeat cingulotomy and 11 receiving a subcaudate tractotomy. The remaining 12 patients were observed. Of those receiving a second operation, 10 were considered full responders (Y-BOCS decrease ≥35%), and 4 were considered partial responders (Y-BOCS decease between 25 and 34%). In contrast, of the 12 patients who were observed after initial surgery, 2 were eventually classified as full responders and 3 as partial responders. Between the two reoperative groups, the proportion of patients meeting the criteria for full or partial responder status and the mean reduction in Y-BOCS scores did not differ significantly. However, there was a higher proportion of full responders versus partial responders in the subcaudate tractotomy group compared with the cingulotomy group. In both the reoperative groups, complications included one intraoperative seizure, as well as transient abulia and memory deficits, which resolved after a short time.

Subcaudate tractotomy

Used in the treatment of MDD, BPD, OCD and other anxiety disorders, the subcaudate tractotomy seeks to interrupt white matter tracts connecting the orbitofrontal and subcortical limbic structures by targeting the substantia innominata located just inferior to the head of the caudate nucleus. Subcaudate tractotomies were first performed in 1961 by Geoffrey Knight, who focused on the last 2 cm of the lesion created by orbital undercutting, where the lesion entered the subcaudate region. This selective cortical undercutting led to improved results over orbital undercutting [174], although freehand procedures often led to suboptimal lesion localization. The introduction of stereotaxis permitted standardized lesion localization, and the result was termed stereotactic subcaudate tractotomy. Knight inserted seeds of radioactive yttrium-90 into the bilateral white matter just below and anterior to the caudate. Beta-radiation from the seeds destroyed white matter up to 2 mm from the seed surface. In 1995, the unavailability of yttrium led to its replacement with thermo-controlled high-frequency electrocoagulation [175]. Currently, lesions are stereotactically created via Leksell frame localization in a manner mimicking the size and location of lesions originally created using yttrium.

Göktepe *et al.* reported on 208 patients undergoing subcaudate tractotomy in 1975, with a mean follow-up of 2.5 years [144]. They found a 50% improvement in OCD patients following subcaudate tractotomy using a categorical outcome scale. Response rates for intractable depression ranged from 55 to 66%. Since 1970, the Brook General Hospital in London has performed more than 1300 subcaudate tractotomies for affective disorders, OCD and chronic anxiety [176]. They reported 40–60% of patients leading 'normal or near-normal lives' following 1-year post-surgical assessments. Similar to cingulotomy, subcaudate tractotomy is relatively free of major complications. Oedema-induced disorientation is observed in approximately 10% of patients post-operatively, usually dissipating within a month. Seizures are the most common long-term complication, seen in about 1.6% of patients. Knight *et al.* reported only one death from the more than 1300 cases examined, attributed to yttrium bead migration resulting in destruction of the hypothalamus [177]. Recently, there has been a case report of one OCD patient improving following a frameless stereotactic subcaudate tractotomy [178].

Hodgkiss *et al.* reported subcaudate tractotomy results for 286 patients treated from 1979 to 1991 at the Geoffrey Knight National Unit for Affective Disorders in London [159]. Of the 249 patients for whom diagnostic and follow-up data were available, 183 carried a diagnosis of depression. Outcome was assessed 12 months after surgery and categorized as recovered (no symptoms, no additional treatment), well (mild residual symptoms, little to no interference with everyday life, may require medication), improved (significant residual symptoms), unchanged and worse. Of the depressed patients, 64 (34%) were recovered or well, 58 (32%) improved and 57 (31%) were unchanged or worse. Detailed complications were not disclosed, although five patients in the depression group (3%) died within the 12-month follow-up period.

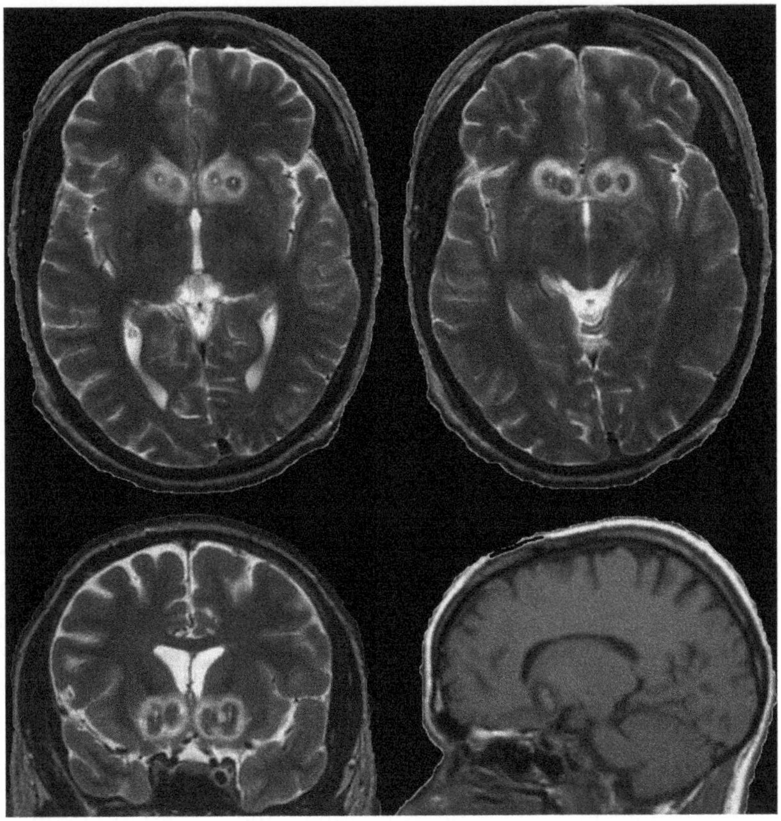

Figure 22.8 Representative limbic leucotomy images. Upper images, T2 axial views of lesions; lower left, T2 coronal view; lower right, T1 sagittal view.

Limbic leucotomy

Unlike the above-mentioned surgical techniques, which focus upon a single discrete area for lesioning, limbic leucotomy is designed to disrupt two fibre tracts. Kelly *et al.* reported in 1973 a new surgical approach focusing on discrete lesions within the lower medial quadrant of the frontal lobe to interrupt frontolimbic connections and the cingulum bundle running above the corpus callosum to interrupt the Papez circuit (Figure 22.8) [160]. Wire loops, blunt instruments, heat or radioactive materials were used to create lesions approximately 8 mm large. Confusion and drowsiness were reported for the initial 24–48 post-operative hours, with slow recovery and return to psychiatric care. This operation effectively produces a combination of the anterior cingulotomy and the subcaudate tractotomy and is used in the treatment of MDD, BPD and OCD.

Kelly *et al.* assessed 66 limbic leucotomy patients with a mean follow-up of 16 months, reporting an 89% improvement in OCD patients [179, 180]. In 1993, Hay *et al.* reported on 26 OCD patients following limbic leucotomy, with an improvement in 38% [181]. In 2002, Kim *et al.* reported a decrease in the mean Y-BOCS scores from 34 to 3 in 12 patients treated with limbic leucotomy for OCD; at 45 months post-surgery, 10 of the 12 patients had returned to their previous normal state of function.

Mitchell-Heggs *et al.* reported their results of 66 patients followed up post-operatively for 16 months. Of the nine patients with depression, all were improved at 6 weeks [146]. However at 16 months, three (33%) were symptom free, two (22%) had minimal residual symptoms, two (22%) were improved with significant residual symptoms and two (22%) were unchanged. The authors commented on 100 patients who underwent the procedure as of publication date that the only serious complication was post-operative memory deficit in one patient. Transient confusion, headache, incontinence and lethargy were reported, which resolved within a few weeks of surgery.

Montoya *et al.* reported on the results of 21 patients who underwent MRI-guided limbic leucotomy at Massachusetts General Hospital from 1993 to 1999 [147]. Six patients (29%) were diagnosed with refractory depression. Four patients had previously undergone bilateral anterior cingulotomy as well as a second surgery to expand these lesions. The mean follow-up time was 26 months. By physician-rated assessments of global functioning, three (50%) of the six depressed patients were considered responders to surgery. One committed suicide post-operatively. Complications in all 21 patients included one wound infection, one patient with persistent complex partial seizures, two patients with short-term memory disorder and one with persistent headaches. Other post-operative symptoms included somnolence in six patients (29%), apathy in five patients (24%) and seizures in three patients (14%). These symptoms were minor and resolved shortly after surgery.

A report of 16 patients treated between 1997 and 1998 evaluated the use of limbic leucotomy for BPD. Radiofrequency thermocoagulation was utilized to create the lesions, and the patients were followed up for 7 years [150]. Outcome was assessed using the CGPSS, as well as a variety of other psychiatric metrics. Tests were administered annually throughout the follow-up period. Results showed that 68.8% of the patients experienced a marked response (CGPSS >3, improved and usually working, or better), 18.8% a possible response (CGPSS 2) and 12.6% did not improve or declined. Evaluating the entire battery of outcome scales revealed significant improvement in depressive, anxiety and negative symptoms, with no significant change in mania and active symptoms. Three patients experienced minor complications including local infection, transient hallucinations and extra-pyramidal symptoms.

Conclusions

Psychiatric neurosurgery has withstood a turbulent history, at different times being embraced and rejected within the medical community. Once broadly utilized as a treatment for psychiatric illness, ablative psychosurgery is now employed in patients with specific disorders and only when these conditions have proven refractory to medical treatment and psychotherapy. As the field continus to progress, several lessons become apparent. First, it is imperative to adhere to carefully considered guidelines on the ethical selection of patients for these procedures. A multidisciplinary team of psychiatrists, neurologists and neurosurgeons is necessary to assess candidacy before the surgery is offered. There are currently no established criteria governing the determination of candidacy for ablative psychosurgery. Institutions that offer these procedures typically have established their own criteria, which usually include refractoriness to conventional therapies, as well as lack of psychotic or Axis II features. In the authors' opinion, the consensus reached in the late 1970s by the Congressional Commission provides an excellent framework to determine the eligibility for psychiatric surgery [4, 182].

Second, the success of ablative neurosurgery in the treatment of psychiatric disease highlights the role of advancing technology in increasing our understanding of how these conditions disrupt normal brain function. This understanding stands in contrast to how these disorders are currently diagnosed, which relies upon symptom-based, rather than physiologically based criteria. Many disorders, including MDD and BPD, are diagnosed based upon patients exhibiting a minimum number of symptoms from a given list for a certain amount of time. This raises the question of whether different permutations of symptoms, although currently falling under the same disease umbrella, may in fact represent different disruptions of function at the neurobiological level. Investigating this question may in turn shed light on why patients with the 'same' condition exhibit varying responses to intervention, psychosurgical or otherwise. Nonetheless, recent lesioning studies continue to demonstrate the efficacy and durability of outcomes in patients severely disabled by psychiatric illness. As such, the judicious application of lesion techniques should continue to be considered for appropriately selected patients with severe, refractory psychiatric disorders.

References

1 Lapidus K, Kopell B, Ben-Haim S, Rezai A, Goodman W. History of psychosurgery: a psychiatrist's perspective. World Neurosurgery 2013; 80:16.

2 Braslow JT. History and evidence-based medicine: lessons from the history of somatic treatments from the 1900s to the 1950s. Mental Health Services Research 1999;1:231–40.

3 The Nobel Prize in Physiology or Medicine 1949. Nobel Media. At http://www.nobelprize.org/nobel_prizes/medicine/laureates/1949/. (accessed 27 April 2015).

4 Patel S, Aronson J, Sheth S, Eskandar E. Lesion procedures in psychiatric neurosurgery. World Neurosurgery 2013;80:16.

5 Depression Fact Sheet 2012 World Health Organization. At http://www.who.int/mediacentre/factsheets/fs369/en/. (accessed 27 April 2015).

6 Kessler RC, Berglund P, Demler O, *et al.* The epidemiology of major depressive disorder: results from the National Comorbidity Survey Replication (NCS-R). JAMA 2003;289:3095–105.

7 Keller MB. Issues in treatment-resistant depression. The Journal of Clinical Psychiatry 2005;66 Suppl 8:5–12.

8 Fava M, Davidson KG. Definition and epidemiology of treatment-resistant depression. The Psychiatric Clinics of North America 1996;19: 179–200.

9 Beck A. Depression: Clinical, Experimental, and Theoretical Aspects. New York: Harper & Row; 1967.

10 Disner S, Beevers C, Haigh E, Beck A. Neural mechanisms of the cognitive model of depression. Nature Reviews Neuroscience 2011;12: 467–77.

11 Diener C, Kuehner C, Brusniak W, Ubl B, Wessa M, Flor H. A meta-analysis of neurofunctional imaging studies of emotion and cognition in major depression. NeuroImage 2012;61: 677–85.

12 Drevets W. Neuroimaging and neuropathological studies of depression: implications for the cognitive-emotional features of mood disorders. Current Opinion in Neurobiology 2001;11:240–9.

13 Drevets W. Neuroimaging studies of mood disorders. Biological Psychiatry 2000;48:813–29.

14 Siegle GJ, Steinhauer SR, Thase ME, Stenger VA, Carter CS. Can't shake that feeling: event-related fMRI assessment of sustained amygdala activity in response to emotional information in depressed individuals. Biological Psychiatry 2002;51:693–707.

15 Costafreda S, Brammer M, David A, Fu C. Predictors of amygdala activation during the processing of emotional stimuli: a meta-analysis of 385 PET and fMRI studies. Brain Research Reviews 2008;58:57–70.

16 van Eijndhoven P, van Wingen G, van Oijen K, *et al.* Amygdala volume marks the acute state in the early course of depression. Biological Psychiatry 2009;65:812–8.

17 LeDoux JE. Emotion circuits in the brain. Annual Review of Neuroscience 2000;23:155–84.

18 Phelps EA, LeDoux JE. Contributions of the amygdala to emotion processing: from animal models to human behavior. Neuron 2005;48:175–87.

19 Fales C, Barch D, Rundle M, *et al.* Altered emotional interference processing in affective and cognitive-control brain circuitry in major depression. Biological Psychiatry 2008;63:377–84.

20 Greicius M, Flores B, Menon V, *et al.* Resting-state functional connectivity in major depression: abnormally increased contributions from subgenual cingulate cortex and thalamus. Biological Psychiatry 2007;62:429–37.
21 Davidson R. Affective style, psychopathology, and resilience: brain mechanisms and plasticity. The American Psychologist 2000;55: 1196–214.
22 Drevets WC, Videen TO, Price JL, Preskorn SH, Carmichael ST, Raichle ME. A functional anatomical study of unipolar depression. The Journal of Neuroscience 1992;12:3628–41.
23 Abercrombie HC, Schaefer SM, Larson CL, *et al.* Metabolic rate in the right amygdala predicts negative affect in depressed patients. Neuroreport 1998;9:3301–7.
24 Anand A, Li Y, Wang Y, Gardner K, Lowe M. Reciprocal effects of antidepressant treatment on activity and connectivity of the mood regulating circuit: an FMRI study. The Journal of Neuropsychiatry and Clinical Neurosciences 2007;19:274–82.
25 Delaveau P, Jabourian M, Lemogne C, Guionnet S, Bergouignan L, Fossati P. Brain effects of antidepressants in major depression: a meta-analysis of emotional processing studies. Journal of Affective Disorders 2011;130:66–74.
26 Fu CH, Williams SC, Cleare AJ, *et al.* Attenuation of the neural response to sad faces in major depression by antidepressant treatment: a prospective, event-related functional magnetic resonance imaging study. Archives of General Psychiatry 2004;61:877–89.
27 Frodl T, Meisenzahl E, Zetzsche T, *et al.* Enlargement of the amygdala in patients with a first episode of major depression. Biological Psychiatry 2002;51:708–14.
28 Frodl T, Meisenzahl EM, Zetzsche T, *et al.* Larger amygdala volumes in first depressive episode as compared to recurrent major depression and healthy control subjects. Biological Psychiatry 2003;53:338–44.
29 Hastings RS, Parsey RV, Oquendo MA, Arango V, Mann JJ. Volumetric analysis of the prefrontal cortex, amygdala, and hippocampus in major depression. Neuropsychopharmacology 2004;29:952–9.
30 Sacher J, Neumann J, Fünfstück T, Soliman A, Villringer A, Schroeter M. Mapping the depressed brain: a meta-analysis of structural and functional alterations in major depressive disorder. Journal of Affective Disorders 2012;140:142–8.
31 Sheline YI, Gado MH, Price JL. Amygdala core nuclei volumes are decreased in recurrent major depression. Neuroreport 1998;9:2023–8.
32 Hamilton JP, Siemer M, Gotlib IH. Amygdala volume in major depressive disorder: a meta-analysis of magnetic resonance imaging studies. Molecular Psychiatry 2008;13:993–1000.
33 Ochsner KN, Ray RD, Cooper JC, *et al.* For better or for worse: neural systems supporting the cognitive down- and up-regulation of negative emotion. NeuroImage 2004;23:483–99.
34 Drevets WC. Prefrontal cortical-amygdalar metabolism in major depression. Annals of the New York Academy of Sciences 1999;877:614–37.
35 Baxter LR, Jr., Schwartz JM, Phelps ME, *et al.* Reduction of prefrontal cortex glucose metabolism common to three types of depression. Archives of General Psychiatry 1989;46:243–50.
36 Bench CJ, Friston KJ, Brown RG, Frackowiak RS, Dolan RJ. Regional cerebral blood flow in depression measured by positron emission tomography: the relationship with clinical dimensions. Psychological Medicine 1993;23:579–90.
37 Li CT, Lin CP, Chou KH, *et al.* Structural and cognitive deficits in remitting and non-remitting recurrent depression: a voxel-based morphometric study. NeuroImage 2010;50:347–56.
38 Drevets W, Price J, Furey M. Brain structural and functional abnormalities in mood disorders: implications for neurocircuitry models of depression. Brain Structure & Function 2008;213:93–118.
39 Liotti M, Mayberg HS, McGinnis S, Brannan SL, Jerabek P. Unmasking disease-specific cerebral blood flow abnormalities: mood challenge in patients with remitted unipolar depression. The American Journal of Psychiatry 2002;159: 1830–40.
40 Ueda K, Okamoto Y, Okada G, Yamashita H, Hori T, Yamawaki S. Brain activity during expectancy of emotional stimuli: an fMRI study. Neuroreport 2003;14:51–5.
41 Mitterschiffthaler MT, Williams SC, Walsh ND, *et al.* Neural basis of the emotional Stroop interference effect in major depression. Psychological Medicine 2008;38:247–56.

42 Eugene F, Joormann J, Cooney RE, Atlas LY, Gotlib IH. Neural correlates of inhibitory deficits in depression. Psychiatry Research 2010;181: 30–5.

43 Shafritz KM, Collins SH, Blumberg HP. The interaction of emotional and cognitive neural systems in emotionally guided response inhibition. NeuroImage 2006;31:468–75.

44 Ray RD, Ochsner KN, Cooper JC, Robertson ER, Gabrieli JD, Gross JJ. Individual differences in trait rumination and the neural systems supporting cognitive reappraisal. Cognitive, Affective, & Behavioral Neuroscience 2005;5: 156–68.

45 Beevers CG, Clasen P, Stice E, Schnyer D. Depression symptoms and cognitive control of emotion cues: a functional magnetic resonance imaging study. Neuroscience 2010;167: 97–103.

46 Cooney RE, Joormann J, Eugene F, Dennis EL, Gotlib IH. Neural correlates of rumination in depression. Cognitive, Affective, & Behavioral Neuroscience 2010;10:470–8.

47 McDonald AJ, Mascagni F, Guo L. Projections of the medial and lateral prefrontal cortices to the amygdala: a Phaseolus vulgaris leucoagglutinin study in the rat. Neuroscience 1996;71:55–75.

48 Gusnard DA, Akbudak E, Shulman GL, Raichle ME. Medial prefrontal cortex and self-referential mental activity: relation to a default mode of brain function. Proceedings of the National Academy of Sciences of the United States of America 2001;98:4259–64.

49 Drevets WC, Ongur D, Price JL. Neuroimaging abnormalities in the subgenual prefrontal cortex: implications for the pathophysiology of familial mood disorders. Molecular Psychiatry 1998;3:220–6, 190–1.

50 Hamani C, Mayberg H, Stone S, Laxton A, Haber S, Lozano AM. The subcallosal cingulate gyrus in the context of major depression. Biological Psychiatry 2011;69:301–8.

51 Coryell W, Nopoulos P, Drevets W, Wilson T, Andreasen NC. Subgenual prefrontal cortex volumes in major depressive disorder and schizophrenia: diagnostic specificity and prognostic implications. The American Journal of Psychiatry 2005;162:1706–12.

52 Mayberg HS, Liotti M, Brannan SK, *et al.* Reciprocal limbic-cortical function and negative mood: converging PET findings in depression and normal sadness. The American Journal of Psychiatry 1999;156:675–82.

53 Ongur D, Drevets WC, Price JL. Glial reduction in the subgenual prefrontal cortex in mood disorders. Proceedings of the National Academy of Sciences of the United States of America 1998;95:13290–5.

54 Cotter D, Mackay D, Landau S, Kerwin R, Everall I. Reduced glial cell density and neuronal size in the anterior cingulate cortex in major depressive disorder. Archives of General Psychiatry 2001;58:545–53.

55 Kringelbach M. The human orbitofrontal cortex: linking reward to hedonic experience. Nature Reviews Neuroscience 2005;6:691–702.

56 Eblen F, Graybiel AM. Highly restricted origin of prefrontal cortical inputs to striosomes in the macaque monkey. The Journal of Neuroscience 1995;15:5999–6013.

57 Ongur D, Price JL. The organization of networks within the orbital and medial prefrontal cortex of rats, monkeys and humans. Cerebral Cortex 2000;10:206–19.

58 Cavada C, Company T, Tejedor J, Cruz-Rizzolo RJ, Reinoso-Suarez F. The anatomical connections of the macaque monkey orbitofrontal cortex. A review. Cerebral Cortex 2000;10:220–42.

59 Carmichael ST, Price JL. Limbic connections of the orbital and medial prefrontal cortex in macaque monkeys. The Journal of Comparative Neurology 1995;363:615–41.

60 Carmichael ST, Price JL. Sensory and premotor connections of the orbital and medial prefrontal cortex of macaque monkeys. The Journal of Comparative Neurology 1995;363:642–64.

61 Biver F, Goldman S, Delvenne V, *et al.* Frontal and parietal metabolic disturbances in unipolar depression. Biological Psychiatry 1994;36: 381–8.

62 Drevets W. Orbitofrontal cortex function and structure in depression. Annals of the New York Academy of Sciences 2007;1121:499–527.

63 Ochsner KN, Gross JJ. The cognitive control of emotion. Trends in Cognitive Sciences 2005;9:242–9.

64 Anand A, Li Y, Wang Y, *et al.* Activity and connectivity of brain mood regulating circuit in depression: a functional magnetic resonance study. Biological Psychiatry 2005;57:1079–88.

65 Adolphs R, Cahill L, Schul R, Babinsky R. Impaired declarative memory for emotional material following bilateral amygdala damage in humans. Learning & Memory 1997;4: 291–300.

66 Cahill L, Babinsky R, Markowitsch HJ, McGaugh JL. The amygdala and emotional memory. Nature 1995;377:295–6.

67 Packard MG, Cahill L, McGaugh JL. Amygdala modulation of hippocampal-dependent and caudate nucleus-dependent memory processes. Proceedings of the National Academy of Sciences of the United States of America 1994;91:8477–81.

68 Hamilton JP, Gotlib IH. Neural substrates of increased memory sensitivity for negative stimuli in major depression. Biological Psychiatry 2008;63:1155–62.

69 Wager TD, Davidson ML, Hughes BL, Lindquist MA, Ochsner KN. Prefrontal-subcortical pathways mediating successful emotion regulation. Neuron 2008;59:1037–50.

70 Del Arco A, Mora F. Prefrontal cortex-nucleus accumbens interaction: in vivo modulation by dopamine and glutamate in the prefrontal cortex. Pharmacology, Biochemistry and Behavior 2008; 90:226–35.

71 Heller AS, Johnstone T, Shackman AJ, *et al.* Reduced capacity to sustain positive emotion in major depression reflects diminished maintenance of fronto-striatal brain activation. Proceedings of the National Academy of Sciences of the United States of America 2009;106: 22445–50.

72 Epstein J, Pan H, Kocsis JH, *et al.* Lack of ventral striatal response to positive stimuli in depressed versus normal subjects. The American Journal of Psychiatry 2006;163:1784–90.

73 Tricomi EM, Delgado MR, Fiez JA. Modulation of caudate activity by action contingency. Neuron 2004;41:281–92.

74 Pizzagalli DA, Holmes AJ, Dillon DG, *et al.* Reduced caudate and nucleus accumbens response to rewards in unmedicated individuals with major depressive disorder. The American Journal of Psychiatry 2009;166:702–10.

75 Merikangas KR, Jin R, He JP, *et al.* Prevalence and correlates of bipolar spectrum disorder in the world mental health survey initiative. Archives of General Psychiatry 2011;68:241–51.

76 Merikangas KR, Akiskal HS, Angst J, *et al.* Lifetime and 12-month prevalence of bipolar spectrum disorder in the National Comorbidity Survey replication. Archives of General Psychiatry 2007;64:543–52.

77 Gajwani P. Treatment-refractory bipolar disorder: classification to aid in clinical management. Expert Opinion on Pharmacotherapy 2009;10: 1907–15.

78 Kuiper S, McLean L, Malhi G. To BD or not to BD: functional neuroimaging and the boundaries of bipolarity. Expert Review of Neurotherapeutics 2013;13:75.

79 Versace A, Almeida JR, Quevedo K, *et al.* Right orbitofrontal corticolimbic and left corticocortical white matter connectivity differentiate bipolar and unipolar depression. Biological Psychiatry 2010;68:560–7.

80 Cardoso de Almeida J, Phillips M. Distinguishing between unipolar depression and bipolar depression: current and future clinical and neuroimaging perspectives. Biological Psychiatry 2013;73:111–8.

81 Savitz JB, Nugent AC, Bogers W, *et al.* Habenula volume in bipolar disorder and major depressive disorder: a high-resolution magnetic resonance imaging study. Biological Psychiatry 2011;69:336–43.

82 Ranft K, Dobrowolny H, Krell D, Bielau H, Bogerts B, Bernstein HG. Evidence for structural abnormalities of the human habenular complex in affective disorders but not in schizophrenia. Psychological Medicine 2010;40: 557–67.

83 Marchand WR, Yurgelun-Todd D. Striatal structure and function in mood disorders: a comprehensive review. Bipolar Disorders 2010;12: 764–85.

84 Malhi GS, Lagopoulos J, Sachdev P, Mitchell PB, Ivanovski B, Parker GB. Cognitive generation of affect in hypomania: an fMRI study. Bipolar Disorders 2004;6:271–85.

85 Caligiuri MP, Brown GG, Meloy MJ, Eberson S, Niculescu AB, Lohr JB. Striatopallidal regulation of affect in bipolar disorder. Journal of Affective Disorders 2006;91:235–42.

86 Abler B, Greenhouse I, Ongur D, Walter H, Heckers S. Abnormal reward system activation in mania. Neuropsychopharmacology 2008;33: 2217–27.

87 Sasson Y, Zohar J, Chopra M, Lustig M, Iancu I, Hendler T. Epidemiology of obsessive-compulsive disorder: a world view. The Journal of Clinical Psychiatry 1997;58 Suppl 12:7–10.
88 Franklin ME, Foa EB. Treatment of obsessive compulsive disorder. Annual Review of Clinical Psychology 2011;7:229–43.
89 Pinto A, Mancebo MC, Eisen JL, Pagano ME, Rasmussen SA. The Brown Longitudinal Obsessive Compulsive Study: clinical features and symptoms of the sample at intake. The Journal of Clinical Psychiatry 2006;67: 703–11.
90 Di Filippo M, Picconi B, Tantucci M, *et al.* Short-term and long-term plasticity at corticostriatal synapses: implications for learning and memory. Behavioural Brain Research 2009;199: 108–18.
91 Alexander GE, DeLong MR, Strick PL. Parallel organization of functionally segregated circuits linking basal ganglia and cortex. Annual Review of Neuroscience 1986;9:357–81.
92 Aronson J, Katnani H, Eskandar E. Neuromodulation for obsessive-compulsive disorder. Neurosurgery Clinics of North America 2014;25: 85–101.
93 Nestler EJ, Barrot M, DiLeone RJ, Eisch AJ, Gold SJ, Monteggia LM. Neurobiology of depression. Neuron 2002;34:13–25.
94 Ressler KJ, Mayberg HS. Targeting abnormal neural circuits in mood and anxiety disorders: from the laboratory to the clinic. Nature Neuroscience 2007;10:1116–24.
95 Goto Y, Grace AA. Limbic and cortical information processing in the nucleus accumbens. Trends in Neurosciences 2008;31:552–8.
96 Redgrave P, Gurney K, Reynolds J. What is reinforced by phasic dopamine signals? Brain Research Reviews 2008;58:322–39.
97 Saxena S, Rauch SL. Functional neuroimaging and the neuroanatomy of obsessive-compulsive disorder. The Psychiatric Clinics of North America 2000;23:563–86.
98 Graybiel AM. Neurotransmitters and neuromodulators in the basal ganglia. Trends in Neurosciences 1990;13:244–54.
99 Besson MJ, Graybiel AM, Nastuk MA. [3H]SCH 23390 binding to D1 dopamine receptors in the basal ganglia of the cat and primate: delineation of striosomal compartments and pallidal and nigral subdivisions. Neuroscience 1988;26: 101–19.
100 Baxter LR, Jr., Saxena S, Brody AL, *et al.* Brain mediation of obsessive-compulsive disorder symptoms: evidence From functional brain imaging studies in the human and nonhuman primate. Seminars in Clinical Neuropsychiatry 1996;1:32–47.
101 Rossi S, Bartalini S, Ulivelli M, *et al.* Hypofunctioning of sensory gating mechanisms in patients with obsessive-compulsive disorder. Biological Psychiatry 2005;57:16–20.
102 Zald DH, Kim SW. Anatomy and function of the orbital frontal cortex, I: anatomy, neurocircuitry; and obsessive-compulsive disorder. Journal of Neuropsychiatry and Clinical Neurosciences 1996;8:125–38.
103 Krawczyk DC. Contributions of the prefrontal cortex to the neural basis of human decision making. Neuroscience and Biobehavioral Reviews 2002;26:631–64.
104 Aouizerate B, Guehl D, Cuny E, *et al.* Pathophysiology of obsessive-compulsive disorder: a necessary link between phenomenology, neuropsychology, imagery and physiology. Progress in Neurobiology 2004;72:195–221.
105 Elliott R, Agnew Z, Deakin JF. Hedonic and informational functions of the human orbitofrontal cortex. Cerebral Cortex 2010;20 :198–204.
106 O'Doherty J, Critchley H, Deichmann R, Dolan RJ. Dissociating valence of outcome from behavioral control in human orbital and ventral prefrontal cortices. The Journal of Neuroscience 2003;23:7931–9.
107 Graham BM, Milad MR. The study of fear extinction: implications for anxiety disorders. The American Journal of Psychiatry 2011;168: 1255–65.
108 Kunde W, Reuss H, Kiesel A. Consciousness and cognitive control. Advances in Cognitive Psychology/University of Finance and Management in Warsaw 2012;8:9–18.
109 Fitzgerald KD, Stern ER, Angstadt M, *et al.* Altered function and connectivity of the medial frontal cortex in pediatric obsessive-compulsive disorder. Biological Psychiatry 2010;68:1039–47.
110 Fitzgerald KD, Welsh RC, Gehring WJ, *et al.* Error-related hyperactivity of the anterior

cingulate cortex in obsessive-compulsive disorder. Biological Psychiatry 2005;57: 287–94.
111 Schulden JD, Thomas YF, Compton WM. Substance abuse in the United States: findings from recent epidemiologic studies. Current Psychiatry Reports 2009;11:353–9.
112 Volkow N, Wang G-J, Fowler J, Tomasi D. Addiction circuitry in the human brain. Annual Review of Pharmacology and Toxicology 2012;52:321–36.
113 Di Chiara G, Imperato A. Drugs abused by humans preferentially increase synaptic dopamine concentrations in the mesolimbic system of freely moving rats. Proceedings of the National Academy of Sciences of the United States of America 1988;85:5274–8.
114 Kufahl PR, Li Z, Risinger RC, *et al.* Neural responses to acute cocaine administration in the human brain detected by fMRI. NeuroImage 2005;28:904–14.
115 Martinez D, Narendran R, Foltin RW, *et al.* Amphetamine-induced dopamine release: markedly blunted in cocaine dependence and predictive of the choice to self-administer cocaine. The American Journal of Psychiatry 2007;164:622–9.
116 Wong DF, Kuwabara H, Schretlen DJ, *et al.* Increased occupancy of dopamine receptors in human striatum during cue-elicited cocaine craving. Neuropsychopharmacology 2006;31: 2716–27.
117 Volkow ND. Cocaine cues and dopamine in dorsal striatum: mechanism of craving in cocaine addiction. Journal of Neuroscience 2006;26:6583–8.
118 Risinger RC, Salmeron BJ, Ross TJ, *et al.* Neural correlates of high and craving during cocaine self-administration using BOLD fMRI. NeuroImage 2005;26:1097–108.
119 Wang GJ, Volkow ND, Fowler JS, *et al.* Regional brain metabolic activation during craving elicited by recall of previous drug experiences. Life Sciences 1999;64:775–84.
120 Garavan H, Pankiewicz J, Bloom A, *et al.* Cue-induced cocaine craving: neuroanatomical specificity for drug users and drug stimuli. The American Journal of Psychiatry 2000;157: 1789–98.
121 Hommer DW. Functional imaging of craving. Alcohol Research & Health 1999;23: 187–96.
122 Wise R. Roles for nigrostriatal – not just mesocorticolimbic – dopamine in reward and addiction. Trends in Neurosciences 2009;32: 517–24.
123 Yin HH, Knowlton BJ. The role of the basal ganglia in habit formation. Nature Reviews Neuroscience 2006;7:464–76.
124 Volkow ND, Fowler JS. Addiction, a disease of compulsion and drive: involvement of the orbitofrontal cortex. Cerebral Cortex 2000;10: 318–25.
125 Kalivas PW. The glutamate homeostasis hypothesis of addiction. Nature Reviews Neuroscience 2009;10:561–72.
126 Poldrack RA, Sabb FW, Foerde K, *et al.* The neural correlates of motor skill automaticity. The Journal of Neuroscience 2005;25:5356–64.
127 Volkow ND, Fowler JS, Wang GJ, Baler R, Telang F. Imaging dopamine's role in drug abuse and addiction. Neuropharmacology 2009;56 Suppl 1:3–8.
128 Volkow ND, Chang L, Wang GJ, *et al.* Low level of brain dopamine D2 receptors in methamphetamine abusers: association with metabolism in the orbitofrontal cortex. The American Journal of Psychiatry 2001;158: 2015–21.
129 Volkow ND, Fowler JS, Wang GJ, *et al.* Decreased dopamine D2 receptor availability is associated with reduced frontal metabolism in cocaine abusers. Synapse 1993;14:169–77.
130 Volkow ND, Wang GJ, Telang F, *et al.* Profound decreases in dopamine release in striatum in detoxified alcoholics: possible orbitofrontal involvement. The Journal of Neuroscience 2007;27:12700–6.
131 Reynolds B. A review of delay-discounting research with humans: relations to drug use and gambling. Behavioural Pharmacology 2006;17:651–67.
132 Berlin HA, Rolls ET, Kischka U. Impulsivity, time perception, emotion and reinforcement sensitivity in patients with orbitofrontal cortex lesions. Brain 2004;127:1108–26.
133 Schoenbaum G, Saddoris MP, Stalnaker TA. Reconciling the roles of orbitofrontal cortex in

reversal learning and the encoding of outcome expectancies. Annals of the New York Academy of Sciences 2007;1121:320–35.

134 Ikemoto S. Brain reward circuitry beyond the mesolimbic dopamine system: a neurobiological theory. Neuroscience and Biobehavioral Reviews 2010;35:129–50.

135 Ikemoto S, Witkin BM, Zangen A, Wise RA. Rewarding effects of AMPA administration into the supramammillary or posterior hypothalamic nuclei but not the ventral tegmental area. The Journal of Neuroscience 2004;24: 5758–65.

136 Liu ZH, Ikemoto S. The midbrain raphe nuclei mediate primary reinforcement via GABA(A) receptors. The European Journal of Neuroscience 2007;25:735–43.

137 Kanaka TS, Balasubramaniam V. Stereotactic cingulumotomy for drug addiction. Applied Neurophysiology 1978;41:86–92.

138 Medvedev SV, Anichkov AD, Poliakov IuI. Physiological mechanisms of the effectiveness of bilateral stereotactic cingulotomy in treatment of strong psychological dependence in drug addiction. Fiziologiia Cheloveka 2003;29: 117–23.

139 Gao G, Wang X, He S, *et al.* Clinical study for alleviating opiate drug psychological dependence by a method of ablating the nucleus accumbens with stereotactic surgery. Stereotactic and Functional Neurosurgery 2003;81:96–104.

140 Wu HM, Wang XL, Chang CW, *et al.* Preliminary findings in ablating the nucleus accumbens using stereotactic surgery for alleviating psychological dependence on alcohol. Neuroscience Letters 2010;473:77–81.

141 Spangler WJ, Cosgrove GR, Ballantine HT, Jr., *et al.* Magnetic resonance image-guided stereotactic cingulotomy for intractable psychiatric disease. Neurosurgery 1996;38:1071–6; discussion 6–8.

142 Steele JD, Christmas D, Eljamel MS, Matthews K. Anterior cingulotomy for major depression: clinical outcome and relationship to lesion characteristics. Biological Psychiatry 2008;63: 670–7.

143 Shields D, Asaad W, Eskandar E, *et al.* Prospective assessment of stereotactic ablative surgery for intractable major depression. Biological Psychiatry 2008;64:449–54.

144 Göktepe EO, Young LB, Bridges PK. A further review of the results of stereotactic subcaudate tractotomy. The British Journal of Psychiatry 1975;126: 270–280.

145 Sachdev PS, Sachdev J. Long-term outcome of neurosurgery for the treatment of resistant depression. Journal of Neuropsychiatry and Clinical Neurosciences 2005;17:478–85.

146 Mitchell-Heggs N, Kelly D, Richardson A. Stereotactic limbic leucotomy – a follow-up at 16 months. The British Journal of Psychiatry 1976;128:226–40.

147 Montoya A, Weiss A, Price B, *et al.* Magnetic resonance imaging-guided stereotactic limbic leukotomy for treatment of intractable psychiatric disease. Neurosurgery 2002;50: 1043.

148 Ballantine H, Cassidy W, Flanagan N, Marino R. Stereotaxic anterior cingulotomy for neuropsychiatric illness and intractable pain. Journal of Neurosurgery 1967;26:488–95.

149 Poynton A, Bridges PK, Bartlett JR. Resistant bipolar affective disorder treated by stereotactic subcaudate tractotomy. The British Journal of Psychiatry 1988;152:354–8.

150 Cho D-Y, Lee W-Y, Chen C-C. Limbic leukotomy for intractable major affective disorders: a 7-year follow-up study using nine comprehensive psychiatric test evaluations. Journal of Clinical Neuroscience 2008;15: 138–42.

151 Liu K, Zhang H, Liu C, *et al.* Stereotactic treatment of refractory obsessive compulsive disorder by bilateral capsulotomy with 3 years follow-up. Journal of Clinical Neurosciences 2008;15:622–9.

152 Rück C, Karlsson A, Steele JD, *et al.* Capsulotomy for obsessive-compulsive disorder: long-term follow-up of 25 patients. Archives of General Psychiatry 2008;65:914–21.

153 Ballantine HT, Jr., Bouckoms AJ, Thomas EK, Giriunas IE. Treatment of psychiatric illness by stereotactic cingulotomy. Biological Psychiatry 1987;22:807–19.

154 Jenike MA, Baer L, Ballantine T, *et al.* Cingulotomy for refractory obsessive-compulsive disorder. A long-term follow-up of 33 patients.

Archives of General Psychiatry 1991;48: 548–55.
155 Dougherty DD, Baer L, Cosgrove GR, *et al.* Prospective long-term follow-up of 44 patients who received cingulotomy for treatment-refractory obsessive-compulsive disorder. The American Journal of Psychiatry 2002;159: 269–75.
156 Sheth S, Neal J, Tangherlini F, *et al.* Limbic system surgery for treatment-refractory obsessive-compulsive disorder: a prospective long-term follow-up of 64 patients. Journal of Neurosurgery 2013;118:491–7.
157 Bourne SK, Sheth SA, Neal J, *et al.* Beneficial effect of subsequent lesion procedures after nonresponse to initial cingulotomy for severe, treatment-refractory obsessive-compulsive disorder. Neurosurgery 2013;72:196–202; discussion.
158 Yang J, Ginat D, Dougherty D, Makris N, Eskandar E. Lesion analysis for cingulotomy and limbic leucotomy: comparison and correlation with clinical outcomes. Journal of Neurosurgery 2014;120:152–63.
159 Hodgkiss AD, Malizia AL, Bartlett JR, Bridges PK. Outcome after the psychosurgical operation of stereotactic subcaudate tractotomy, 1979–1991. Journal of Neuropsychiatry and Clinical Neurosciences 1995;7: 230–4.
160 Kelly D, Richardson A, Mitchell-Heggs N. Stereotactic limbic leucotomy: neurophysiological aspects and operative technique. British Journal of Psychiatry 1973;123: 133–40.
161 Greenberg BD, Price LH, Rauch SL, *et al.* Neurosurgery for intractable obsessive-compulsive disorder and depression: critical issues. Neurosurgery Clinics of North America 2003;14 :199–212.
162 Talairach J, Hecaen H, David M. Lobotomie prefrontale limitee par electrocoagulation des fibres thalamo-frontalis leur emergence du bras anterior de la capsule interne. In: Proceedings of the Fourth Congress Neurologique Internationale 1949; p. 141.
163 Leksell L. The stereotaxic method and radiosurgery of the brain. Acta chirurgica Scandinavica 1951;102:316–9.
164 Zhan S, Liu W, Li D, *et al.* Long-term follow-up of bilateral anterior capsulotomy in patients with refractory obsessive-compulsive disorder. Clinical Neurology and Neurosurgery 2014;119: 91–5.
165 Leiphart J, Valone F. Stereotactic lesions for the treatment of psychiatric disorders. Journal of Neurosurgery 2010;113:1204–11.
166 Mindus P. Present-day indications for capsulotomy. Acta Neurochirurgica Supplementum 1993;58:29–33.
167 Feldman RP, Goodrich JT. Psychosurgery: a historical overview. Neurosurgery 2001; 48:647–57; discussion 57–9.
168 Greenberg BD, Rauch SL, Haber SN. Invasive circuitry-based neurotherapeutics: stereotactic ablation and deep brain stimulation for OCD. Neuropsychopharmacology 2010;35: 317–36.
169 Watts JW, Freeman W. Psychosurgery for the relief of unbearable pain. The Journal of the International College of Surgeons 1946;9: 679–83.
170 Foltz EL, White LE. Pain "relief" by frontal cingulumotomy. Journal of Neurosurgery 1962; 19:89–94.
171 Cosgrove GR. Surgery for psychiatric disorders. CNS Spectrums 2000;5:43–52.
172 Jung HH, Kim CH, Chang JH, Park YG, Chung SS, Chang JW. Bilateral anterior cingulotomy for refractory obsessive-compulsive disorder: long-term follow-up results. Stereotactic and Functional Neurosurgery 2006;84: 184–9.
173 Cosgrove GR, Rauch SL. Stereotactic cingulotomy. Neurosurgery Clinics of North America 2003;14:225–35.
174 Knight G. Stereotactic tractotomy in the surgical treatment of mental illness. Journal of Neurology, Neurosurgery and Psychiatry 1965;28:304–10.
175 Malhi GS, Bartlett JR. Depression: a role for neurosurgery? British Journal of Neurosurgery 2000;14:415–22; discussion 23.
176 Bridges PK, Bartlett JR, Hale AS, Poynton AM, Malizia AL, Hodgkiss AD. Psychosurgery: stereotactic subcaudate tractomy. An indispensable treatment. British Journal of Psychiatry 1994;165:599–611; discussion 2–3.

177 Knight G. Further observations from an experience of 660 cases of stereotactic tractotomy. Postgraduate Medical Journal 1973;49:845–54.

178 Woerdeman PA, Willems PW, Noordmans HJ, Berkelbach van der Sprenkel JW, van Rijen PC. Frameless stereotactic subcaudate tractotomy for intractable obsessive-compulsive disorder. Acta Neurochirurgica 2006;148:633–7; discussion 7.

179 Kelly D, Mitchell-Heggs N. Stereotactic limbic leucotomy – a follow-up study of thirty patients. Postgraduate Medical Journal 1973;49:865–82.

180 Kelly D, Richardson A, Mitchell-Heggs N, Greenup J, Chen C, Hafner RJ. Stereotactic limbic leucotomy: a preliminary report on forty patients. British Journal of Psychiatry 1973;123:141–8.

181 Hay P, Sachdev P, Cumming S, *et al.* Treatment of obsessive-compulsive disorder by psychosurgery. Acta Psychiatrica Scandinavica 1993;87:197–207.

182 The National Commission for the Protection of Human Subjects of Biomedical and Behavioral Research. Psychosurgery: Report and Recommendations. U.S. Department of Health, Education, and Welfare. Washington, DC; 1977.

CHAPTER 23

Electroconvulsive therapy: Introduction and technical aspects

Sandarsh Surya, Peter B. Rosenquist and W. Vaughn McCall
Medical College of Georgia, Georgia Regents University, Augusta, USA

Introduction

The origin of electrical stimuli as a treatment for neuropsychiatric conditions can be traced to the use of the torpedo fish by ancient Greeks and Romans to treat intractable headaches [1, 2]. In the 16th century, a Jesuit missionary in Ethiopia used electric catfish to expel devils from humans [1]. Chemically induced convulsions in the history of psychiatry dates back to the 16th century when the Swiss physician Paracelsus induced seizures by administration of camphor by mouth to treat mental illness [3, 4]. Several somatic therapies were investigated for the treatment of mental illness in the first half of the 19th century [3]. An Austrian physician Julius Wagner-Jauregg inoculated patients with malaria to induce fever as a therapy for neurosyphilis; these fevers were occasionally associated with convulsions. He was awarded the Nobel Prize in Medicine in 1927 for his work on the treatment of patients with general paresis with the goal of reducing psychotic and physical symptoms by injecting patients with blood from patients who suffered from active malaria [1, 3].

Manfred Sakel, an Austrian psychiatrist, is credited with developing insulin shock treatment in 1927 [3]. Insulin-induced hypoglycaemic coma and occasional hypoglycaemia-induced convulsions were noted to have favourable outcomes in patients with schizophrenia [3]. Ladislas Meduna, a Hungarian psychiatrist, proposed the existence of biological antagonism between convulsions and schizophrenia after the observation that patients with catatonia and schizophrenia improved after having an epileptic attack [3, 4]. Meduna then used intramuscular injections of camphor-in-oil in a patient with schizophrenia [1]. Meduna later introduced pentylenetetrazol or metrazol as a substitute for camphor because of the difficulty in inducing seizures with camphor [1, 3]. Metrazol therapy was painful and induced intense anxiety and frightening experiences in the time between the injection of metrazol and the onset of the convulsions [3]. An inadequate dose of metrazol left the patient with severe fright without the benefits of the convulsion. Ugo Cerletti and Lucio Bini are credited for the use of electric currents to induce seizures in a 39-year-old male with psychosis in 1938 and demonstrated the efficacy of this new method [1, 3, 5]. Use of electric current to induce seizure gained popularity and replaced chemical injection for seizure induction, because of the reliability of the electrical stimulus in inducing seizures, and the immediate unconsciousness that followed

Neuromodulation in Psychiatry, First Edition. Edited by Clement Hamani, Paul Holtzheimer, Andres M. Lozano and Helen Mayberg.

the electrical stimulus, thus eliminating the frightening interval seen with metrazol between injection and the onset of the convulsion.

Abram Bennett, an American psychiatrist, reports in regard to convulsive therapy 'this revolutionary psychiatric treatment has been seriously condemned by many workers and totally abandoned by some' due to musculoskeletal injuries and fractures associated with convulsive therapy [6, 7]. In 1939, Bennett used the paralytic drug curare to modify metrazol-induced convulsive therapy that greatly reduced the incidence of musculoskeletal injuries [6]. Soon seizure modification by muscle paralysis and anaesthesia became a common practice. Curare was then replaced in the 1950s by the synthetic drug succinylcholine as the preferred choice of skeletal muscle relaxant [4] and succinylcholine remains the drug of choice today for this purpose[8]. This technique of modifying electroconvulsive therapy (ECT) using a muscle relaxant and a sedative is now known as modified ECT. Unmodified ECT, which is the administration of ECT without use of anaesthesia and muscle relaxant, is no longer recommended for use [9], but it is still practised in some developing countries that do not have access to anaesthesia services [10]. An American psychiatrist Max Fink was the first to apply rigorous scientific methods to ECT and gave the treatment scientific legitimacy [11].

Indications of ECT

ECT was first introduced and used to treat a person who suffered from a psychotic disorder by Cerletti and Bini in 1938 [1, 5]. As the treatment gained popularity, the benefits of ECT in other psychiatric conditions became evident. In the United States, ECT is usually used as a second-line treatment option for depression and is considered when there is resistance to first-line treatments, such as psychotherapy and pharmacotherapy. However, the presence of certain conditions such as suicidal thoughts, catatonia, neuroleptic malignant syndrome (NMS), psychosis associated with mania or depression make psychiatrists rely on ECT during earlier phases of illness for rapid recovery. The American Psychiatric Association (APA) task force [9] recommends that ECT be used earlier in the course of the illness to curtail the suffering of the patients and to reduce treatment resistance.

Major depression

Unipolar and bipolar depression is the most common indication for administration of ECT in the Western Hemisphere. ECT has a high success rate in both conditions with reported response rates of 91.4% in patients receiving ECT as a first-line treatment and 63.1% in patients with medication resistance [12]. Even though antidepressant-resistant major depression tends to have poorer response to ECT, the remission rates are still very high when compared to antidepressant remission rates of patients who were previously treated with antidepressants as a first-line treatment [13]. Depressive illness with symptoms such as psychomotor retardation, catatonia and psychosis tends to have a favourable response [9] while the presence of a personality disorder is an indicator of poorer response [14]. Suicidality is a common symptom in patients with major depression, and ECT has acute benefits in reducing suicidal ideations in patients with depression [15–17]. ECT also normalizes abnormal sleep architecture in depressed patients and the changes persist even after completion of the treatment [3, 18].

Mania

Mood stabilizers and atypical antipsychotics are the recommended first-line agents for the treatment of acute mania [19]. Poor response to pharmacological treatment is an indication for ECT in mania. The superiority of ECT over lithium and neuroleptics was reported in an extensive review that included 50 years of research on ECT in the treatment of mania [20]. ECT had a more rapid response when compared to lithium in one study [21], and in another study, the group that received chlorpromazine and ECT had more rapid improvement in symptoms when compared to the group that received chlorpromazine alone [22]. ECT is the treatment of choice in delirious mania, which is a severe form of mania with delirium, mania, psychosis and catatonia [23]. Daily ECT can be considered for patients with a severe form of mania [3, 15]. Patients with rapid cycling bipolar disorder generally tend to have poor response to psychotropic drugs and maintenance ECT has been shown to have a long-term prophylactic effect [24, 25].

Schizophrenia

The first use of ECT was in a person with psychosis, but subsequent ECT practice showed that its benefits were more consistent in mood disorders versus psychotic disorders [1]. Western countries use ECT predominantly to treat depression, whereas in Asian countries ECT is still predominantly used for the treatment of schizophrenia [10, 26]. Patients with schizophrenia who have prominent depression, positive symptoms and catatonic symptoms of recent onset are suggested to be the best candidates for ECT [9]. There are also studies reporting an improvement in classic schizophrenic symptoms, but only intermediate or even no improvement in depressive symptoms in patients with schizophrenia [27, 28]. Zervas *et al.* suggest that patients with refractory schizophrenia should be considered for a trial of ECT, especially if positive symptoms are present, and should not be excluded only on the basis of lack of affective symptoms [28]. A common indication for use of ECT in schizophrenia is to augment pharmacotherapy and the combined use of ECT with risperidone or clozapine was found to be most effective [29]. The available literature suggests that the combination of ECT with antipsychotic medications is superior to either treatment in monotherapy. While each treatment contributes uniquely and has the potential for independent adverse effects, the combination appears to be safe, without generating unusual, additive effects in adults or adolescents with schizophrenia [30].

Catatonia and NMS

Catatonia can manifest in many medical conditions, neurological disorders, mood disorders and psychotic disorders [31]. Catatonia requires a special mention when discussing the uses of ECT because it is highly responsive to ECT with 80–100% resolution and the response to treatment is irrespective of the aetiology [32, 33]. NMS and catatonia are considered syndromes with common pathophysiological mechanisms [28]. NMS is not consistently responsive to pharmacotherapy and ECT is the treatment of choice [34].

Parkinson's disease

It is not a conventional practice to use ECT for the treatment of the motor symptoms of Parkinson's disease (PD). Psychiatric comorbidities are common in PD and approximately 40% of patients suffer from depression [35]. ECT is beneficial for depression [36] and psychotic symptoms [37], and there is also evidence of improvement in motor symptoms of PD [38, 39]. ECT particularly showed benefits with 'on' phase of 'on–off phenomenon' in PD [40, 41]. The beneficial effects of ECT in PD persist for a variable period [39]. Further research is needed to explore the beneficial effects of ECT on the motor symptoms of PD.

Status epilepticus

ECT has anticonvulsive properties and raises the seizure threshold (see mechanism of action for more details) [42]. These properties of ECT can benefit patients with refractory status epilepticus [43]. Several case reports have been published regarding the use of ECT in refractory status epilepticus and the outcomes varied from reduction and cessation of seizures to total recovery [43–45]. ECT should be considered as an option for patients with medication refractory status epilepticus [46].

Technical aspects

Apparatus

Stimulus

The efficacy and side effects of ECT are dependent on all individual characteristics of the stimulus and the choice of electrode placement [9, 47]. The benefits of ECT may not be solely from seizure induction and there are various other biological changes that are triggered by the electrical stimulus (see 'Therapeutic mechanisms of ECT'). Research has shown that different strengths of individual parameters may influence the biological changes in different ways, making treatment more or less effective and decreasing or increasing the adverse events of the treatment [9, 47–49]. In this section, we will discuss the relationship of the parameters of a stimulus and the influence of all the individual parameters on the therapeutic efficacy and the adverse-effect profile of ECT.

Stimulus waveforms used in ECT are sine-wave and rectangular pulses (Figure 23.1) with biphasic alternating current. Sine-wave pulse was first used by Cerletti and Bini [1, 50] and it is characterized by slow rise and fall of the wave. Most ECT devices in the early years were 'constant voltage'. These are no longer recommended. Instead, safer 'constant current' devices are preferred [9] (more details can be found in a Section "ECT device"). As compared with brief-pulse constant current ECT, sine-wave ECT requires a higher energy stimulus for seizure induction with poor efficiency. This is because much of the stimulus of the sine-wave during the rise and fall of the wave is at levels below those required for seizure induction. During the slow rise and fall of the wave, there is a continuous flow of current that results in delivery of far more electric charge than is necessary [51]. Weiner and colleagues [49] has shown that to induce an adequate seizure (generally believed to be greater than 25 s duration), the sine-wave

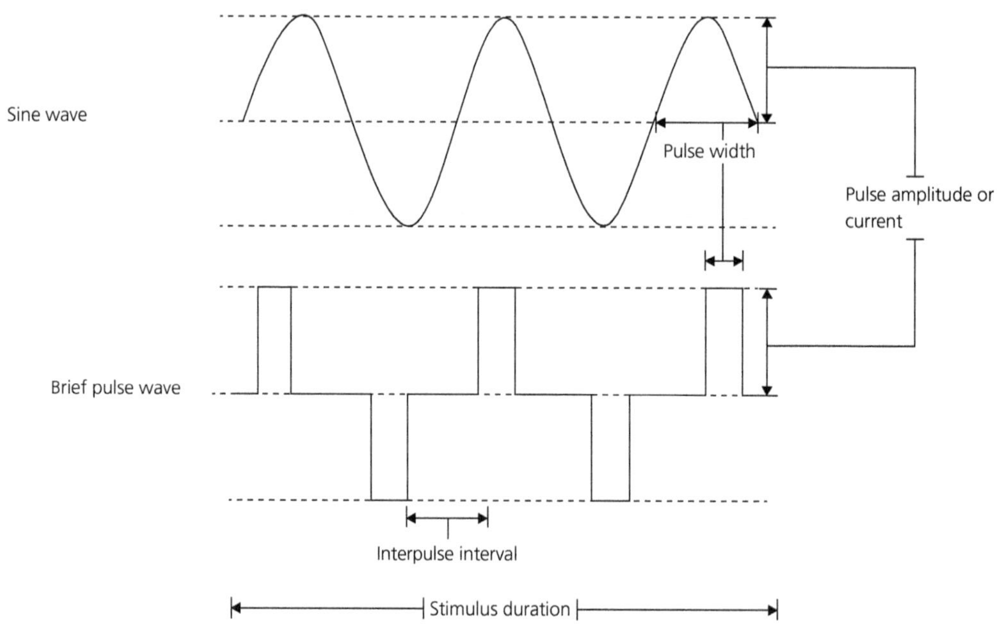

Figure 23.1 Stimulus waveforms.

stimulus is associated with 2.6 times higher stimulus energy, 3.1 times higher applied charge and 6.9 times higher mean current, as compared to brief-pulse stimulus. The extra charge delivered increases the cognitive adverse effects [51]. Hence, the sub-threshold levels of stimulation with sine-wave are believed to contribute to cognitive side effects without contributing to efficacy [51]. Brief-pulse constant current stimulus is used in modern ECT devices and is characterized by trains of monophasic rectangular pulses with alternating polarity. Brief pulses have instantaneous rise and fall time, unlike a sine-wave, which contributes to its better adverse-effect profile and more efficient neuronal excitation [47, 52]. Bidirectional pulses, which include alternating positive and a negative phase, are commonly used in practice. However, there is interest in the use of unidirectional pulse trains for improving the specificity of stimulation [47].

Charge, pulse amplitude, pulse width, pulse frequency and stimulus duration are the different parameters of an alternating brief-pulse, constant current stimulus. Charge is the total dose of electrons administered during the treatment as measured in millicoulombs. Total charge delivered is the most frequently used and recommended summary metric for expressing stimulus dose. Pulse amplitude is the current reported in amperes or milliamperes in a constant current device. Pulse width is the duration of each pulse and is reported in milliseconds. Pulse frequency is the number of pulse cycles in 1 s of the stimulus, which determines the recovery time allowed to the neurons between pulses and is reported in hertz or cycles per second. Stimulus duration is the total duration of the stimulus train, including all the time required to deliver the pulses plus all the 'silent' time in between pulses and is measured in seconds. The total charge of the stimulus is the product of pulse amplitude, pulse width, pulse frequency and stimulus duration:

$$\text{Charge} = \text{pulse amplitude} \times \text{pulse width} \times \text{pulse frequency} \times \text{stimulus duration}$$

Selecting the stimulus dose is an important step as it impacts the efficacy and side effects of ECT. Seizure threshold is unknown for patients who are undergoing treatment for the first time and varies between individuals depending on age, sex, electrode placement, head size and so on [53]. The chosen dose of the stimulus should be appropriately above the seizure threshold to induce an adequate seizure (believed to be at least 25 s of electroencephalogram (EEG) seizure [54, 55]). At the same time, the dose of the stimulus should not be so high to increase the likelihood of cognitive side effects. There are three approaches used in practice to calculate the stimulus dose [47]. In the first approach, the dose is calculated based on various factors that influence the seizure threshold, such as electrode placement, sex, age, anaesthetic dose and concomitant medication, and this is called the 'formula-based approach'. Of course, the formula for predicting the seizure threshold can be erroneous, resulting in a delivered stimulus dose that is sub-threshold or markedly supra-therapeutic. Sub-threshold stimuli are well known to increase the parasympathetic outflow and hence predispose to bradycardia or even asystole [56, 57] and with supra-therapeutic dosing, the patient is exposed to dose-related excess cognitive side effects [58]. The second approach depends on empiric estimation of the seizure threshold via the *dose titration method* [59]. The dose titration method involves selecting an initial dose based on patient's age [9, 60]. If there is no seizure activity noted with the first stimulus, the dose should be increased by 50–100% and restimulated after an interval of 20 s with a maximum of five trials [9]. Once the seizure threshold is determined at the first session, the future treatments are dosed as multiples of the seizure threshold. Recommended doses are 1.5–2.5 times the threshold for bitemporal

ECT and five to eight times the threshold for right unilateral (RUL) ECT [9, 55, 61]. The dose titration method to calculate seizure threshold is somewhat cumbersome and requires multiple stimulations, potentially increasing the cardiovascular risk associated with sub-threshold stimulus administration [62]. The third approach is administration of fixed high charge to all subjects. The problems with this approach are similar to the first approach where there is the possibility that the dose can be sub-threshold or markedly supra-therapeutic (and therefore associated with more cognitive side effects without additional efficacy). This approach is used mostly with unilateral electrode placement [63]. The current recommendation is that the dosage be individualized for each subject by adjusting it relative to either age/sex or seizure threshold [9].

Charge is a key metric when calculating the dose of a stimulus and the same value of charge can be obtained by varying the values of other individual parameters. Hence, it is very important to understand the influence of other individual stimulus parameters on seizure threshold and clinical outcomes of the treatment. Modern ECT devices being constant current devices with an amplitude of 800–900 mA, very few studies have looked at the influence of pulse amplitude variation. Pulse amplitude has greater influence on depolarization and hyperpolarization of the neural membranes compared with other parameters of a stimulus [47], but the clinical relevance of this effect has not been studied. Hence, the role of varying pulse amplitude on the therapeutic effects of ECT and side-effect profile needs further investigation.

Pulses are separated by an interval when there is no passage of any current to the patient, which is termed the inter-pulse interval (Figure 23.1) and is embodied in the frequency. Actual duration of current passage during ECT is the product of pulse width and total number of pulses in the stimulus train. A pulse width range of 8.33–10 ms was used with sine-wave cycle [47]. Sine-wave was largely withdrawn from ECT practice in the Western Hemisphere for reasons discussed earlier in the chapter. For ECT devices being manufactured today, only rectangular pulses are used, and the pulse width ranging from 0.5 to 2 ms is termed brief-pulse stimulus and pulse width below 0.5 ms is termed ultra-brief-pulse stimulus. The recommended pulse width duration for ultra-brief pulse is between 0.2 and 0.5 ms [47]. Brief-pulse stimulus replaced sine-wave because of its more efficient seizure induction and lesser cognitive side-effect profile [64–66]. There is now interest in ultra-brief-pulse stimulus, which has shown fewer short- and long-term cognitive side effects compared to brief-pulse stimulus [64]. Some studies have shown that ultra-brief-pulse RUL treatments have comparable remission rates to brief-pulse RUL treatments [64, 67, 68] and ultra-brief-pulse bi-frontal treatments have comparable remission rates to brief-pulse bi-frontal treatments [65, 66]. But, the remission rate with ultra-brief bitemporal ECT was not significant [64]. Another recent study concluded that both brief-pulse and ultra-brief-pulse stimuli are effective treatments for depression; however, the brief-pulse unilateral stimulus showed better efficacy and faster response compared to ultra-brief-pulse stimulus with no difference in the cognitive side-effect profile [69].

In modern ECT devices, stimulus duration and frequency may be adjusted to vary the total dose of the stimulus. Lower pulse frequencies are noted to be more efficient in seizure induction and frequencies above 50 Hz are shown to suppress ongoing ictal activity. The optimal pulse frequency dosage suggested for use during stimulus dosing in ECT range from 20 to 40 Hz [47]. In a study with frequencies ranging from 20 to 91 Hz using RUL ECT, 32 Hz was noted to be optimal because the convulsive activity was initiated at this interval [70]. In a study using bitemporal ECT, lower frequencies (50 Hz) were also noted to be associated with lower seizure thresholds, requiring fewer subconvulsive stimulations during dose titration when compared to higher frequencies (200 Hz) [71]. Similarly in other studies with RUL ECT, lower frequency stimuli compared to high-frequency stimuli produced seizures at a lower stimulus dose and also showed significantly better improvement in depression scores [72, 73].

Stimulus train duration is another key parameter adjusted during stimulus dosing in modern ECT devices, as stimulation with longer stimulus train duration is associated with lower seizure threshold compared to stimuli with shorter stimulus train duration of equal charge [74, 75]. This suggests that the seizure can be induced at lower total charge if longer stimulus train duration is used in the stimulus. Longer stimulus train duration prolongs the seizure duration and is also reported to have better therapeutic efficacy [74–76]. In other words, having longer stimulus train duration allows for the pulse amplitude and pulse width to be lowered to reduce the cognitive side effects, while preserving the total charge delivered. Recognizing the importance of longer stimulus train duration, modern ECT devices are designed to allow stimulus duration of up to 8 s [47].

ECT device

Three types of ECT devices exist, designed based on the principles of having constant energy, constant voltage or constant current. Constant energy devices deliver the stimulus dose as total energy measured in joules rather than the currently recommended metric total charge. In constant energy devices, as the name suggests, the stimulus is delivered keeping a fixed dose of energy. The impedance between the electrodes is of two types static impedance and dynamic impedance. Static impedance is largely determined by the skin electrode interface, which can be placed in a desired range by mildly excoriating the skin and applying conducting solutions between the skin and the stimulating electrode. The dynamic impedance is determined by the skin, hair, skull, blood vessels, meninges, brain and cerebrospinal fluid (CSF) whose electrical properties vary between individuals [50]. Hence, as (i) the dynamic impedance cannot be controlled during the treatment and (ii) energy is inversely proportional to the impedance during the treatment, then (iii) a fixed dose of energy delivered means that the ECT provider cannot predict the voltage or charge required during the stimulus that will be necessary to deliver a fixed dose of energy. Consider a scenario where the impedance is low and to deliver a fixed amount of charge the stimulus duration may be lowered to an extent that the treatment may not be effective as discussed in the above section about the importance of duration of the stimulus. The total energy as a metric is also questioned in terms of its reliability and sensitivity for stimulus dosing [55].

Constant voltage devices are designed to deliver a fixed dose of voltage. As per Ohm's law (voltage = current × resistance), the strengths of the current and the impedance between the electrodes vary inversely to attain a fixed dose of voltage. We discussed earlier that the impedance cannot be controlled during the ECT and will vary among individuals. Hence, the constant voltage devices have a similar limitation as that of the constant energy device where the possibility of total current delivered may be minimized at times of high impedance. Inadequate strength of current may not induce therapeutically effective seizure. Another possibility is the risk of overdosing with high current under circumstances of low impedance. Thus, the constant energy devices and constant voltage devices are no longer recommended for use [9]. However, these are still used in some countries in eastern hemisphere.

The ECT device that is recommended for use is the constant current, brief-pulse device that delivers the predetermined dose of current while varying the dose of voltage depending on the impedance between the electrodes. When current is constant, the output voltage increases proportional to the increase in the impedance. Modern devices are equipped with the ability to limit the voltage surge in times of abnormally high-impedance conditions. This is very important to prevent burns to the skin, which can result from high-voltage stimulus delivery. Some of the ECT devices are now equipped with a feature that disables the device before delivery of the stimulus in the case when the impedance reading is above a certain level. With constant current devices, the desired total stimulus dose (i.e. charge) can be assured by varying total duration of stimulation by adjusting pulse width, pulse frequency and stimulus duration. Some devices also have an option of delivering pulses in unidirectional or bidirectional mode and ability to deliver the pulses that are uniformly distributed or intermittently distributed [9]. Modern devices are equipped with either a single dial to adjust the dose of the stimulus that proportionately increases different variables of the stimulus as set by the manufacturer, or multiple dials for each parameter so that all individual parameters can be independently adjusted (Figure 23.2). Single-dial equipped devices are easy to use without the ability to adjust each individual parameter. The maximum output of the ECT device in the United States is set at 504–576 ms or 100 J at 220-Ω impedance [9] whereas, in Europe, Canada and other countries, twice this maximum output is allowed [9, 77]. The maximum output allowed in the United States was reported to be therapeutically insufficient in 5% of the patients studied when using a standard brief pulse, which arguably might justify the use of higher maximum output allowed in countries other than the United States [78].

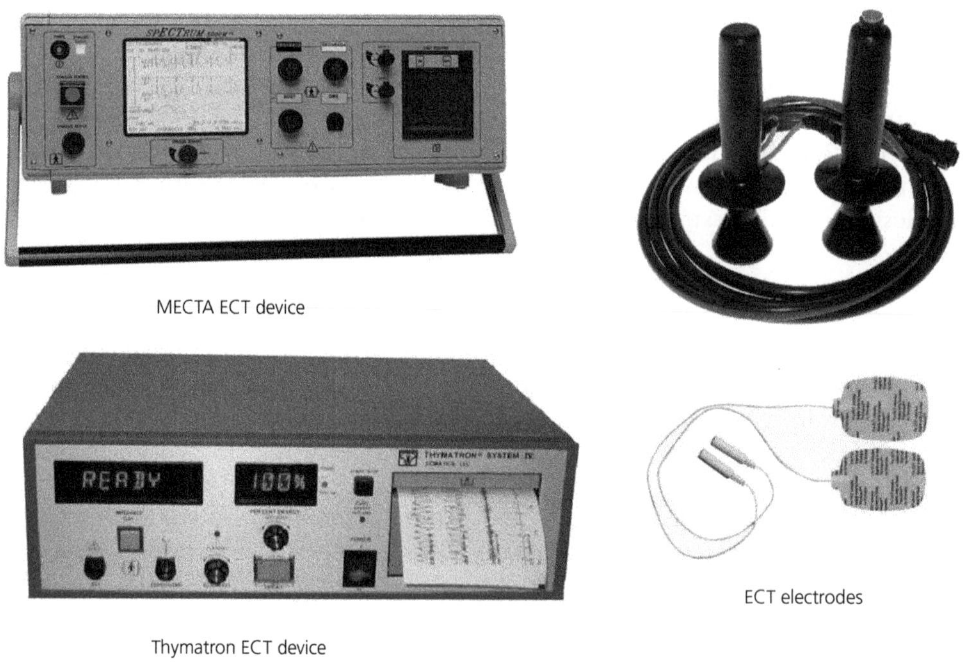

Figure 23.2 ECT device and electrodes. Source: Top left image used with permission of MECTA Corporation; bottom left and right images used with permission of Somatics, LLC. (*See insert for colour representation of the figure.*)

Electrodes

Two electrodes are placed on the scalp during ECT to pass the electrical stimulus, and the location of these electrodes on the scalp plays a critical role in determining the efficacy and side effects of ECT. There are predominantly three different electrode placements in the practice of the ECT. Bitemporal and RUL (d'Elia) electrode placements have been used extensively, and there has been significant research done on these two types of placements. *Bifrontal* electrode placement has gained popularity over the last two decades. There are many other electrode placements that are recognized in recent years (but are not commonly used), including *left anterior right temporal* (LART), *frontovertex*, *right frontoparietal* and *right fronto (small electrode)-parietal (large electrode)* [47]. The clinical evidence on these later new electrode placements is meager.

In bitemporal ECT, electrodes are placed in both temples of the skull, which correspond to the point just above the midpoint on an imaginary line connecting outer canthus of an eye and the external auditory meatus (Figure 23.3a). Bitemporal electrode placement is the oldest and most widely used electrode placement for ECT. It is also still the gold standard when comparing the treatment efficacy of other types of electrode placement. Bitemporal ECT is criticized for higher risk of acute and long-term cognitive impairment [48, 58, 64, 79] and increased risk of delirium during immediate post-treatment [64] compared to other electrode placements. Despite the fact that bitemporal ECT has higher cognitive side effects, it retains an important place for the treatment of certain severe psychiatric conditions where the speed of recovery is crucial such as catatonia, acute mania and suicidality [15, 33, 63, 80–82]. Fink [15, 33] has recommended more frequent (i.e. daily) bitemporal ECT for the treatment of catatonia and delirious mania. Because of the lack of research data for ECT in suicidal patients, Fink *et al.* [15] recommends that the best approach

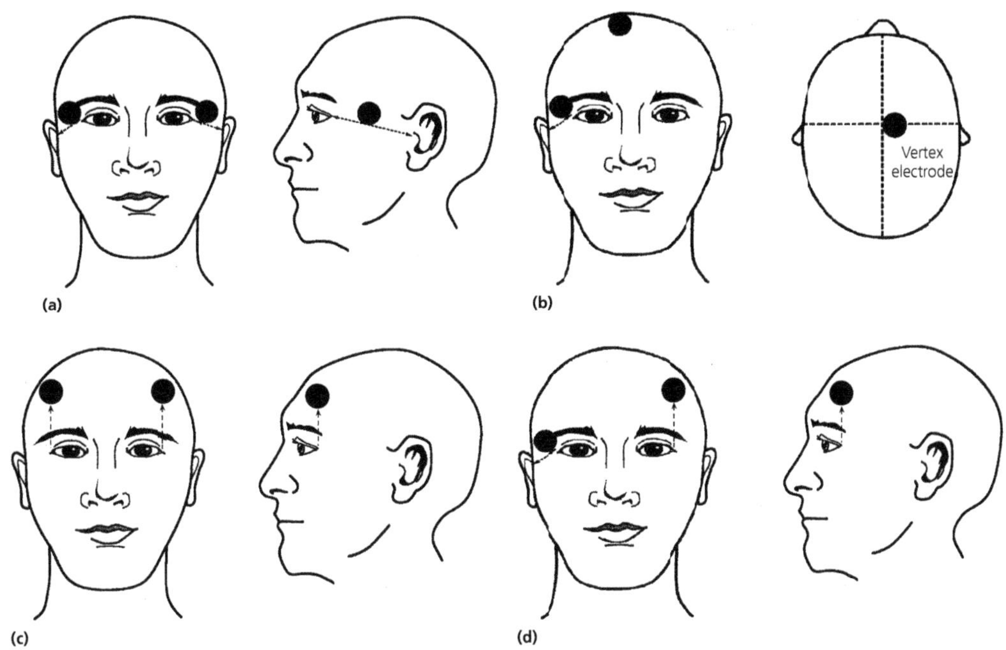

Figure 23.3 ECT stimulus electrode placement: **(a)** Bilateral, **(b)** right unilateral, **(c)** bifrontal and **(d)** left anterior right temporal. Source: From Kellner *et al.* [119]. Reproduced with permission of Charles Kellner.

is to maximize the antidepressant efficacy by using bitemporal ECT treatments. Bitemporal ECT has been reported to have greater efficacy compared to RUL ECT in the treatment of major depression in some studies [48, 80]. However, other studies have noted that bitemporal ECT may have a comparable efficiency when compared with 'high-dose' (e.g. greater than five times seizure threshold) RUL ECT [61, 63, 79, 82]. One study reported that high-dose RUL ECT is not inferior but superior in efficacy in the treatment of depression and also reported lesser cognitive side effects, when compared to moderate-dose bitemporal ECT [83]. Recent studies have also shown comparable efficacy between bitemporal and bifrontal electrode placements in the treatment of major depression [82, 84]. Bitemporal ECT has comparable effects to RUL ECT in the treatment of patients with schizophrenia [85].

The concept of RUL ECT came into existence in late 1940s and gained popularity after d'Elia [86] introduced a wide inter-electrode distance electrode placement for RUL ECT, which is known as the 'd'Elia placement'. In this technique, one electrode is placed on the right temple, which is a point just above the midpoint of an imaginary line drawn from outer cantus of the eye to the external auditory meatus (which is similar to bitemporal electrode placement) and another electrode is placed on a point just to the right of the point of intersection between a perpendicular line connecting two external auditory canals and a line running between nasion and inion (Figure 23.3b). RUL ECT has a superior cognitive side-effect profile compared with bitemporal ECT. Some earlier studies questioned the use of RUL ECT because of its lower efficacy compared to bitemporal ECT [59, 80]. However, it is now known that the antidepressant efficacy of RUL ECT depends on the degree to which the dose exceeds above the seizure threshold [5, 61]. The studies, which used high-dose RUL compared to moderately supra-threshold RUL ECT, showed comparable efficacy when compared against bitemporal ECT [61, 63, 79, 82, 83]. However, with the use of markedly supra-threshold stimuli, the cognitive advantages may be lost [61]. The standard for the treatment of acute mania is bitemporal electrode placement but there is evidence that RUL placement is effective in some studies [20]. Comparative efficacy of bitemporal placement versus RUL placement needs further research. Unilateral ECT is administered on the right side in view of having less influence on the language centre, which has adverse consequences on memory. Left unilateral ECT can be used in an individual with language centre localized to right side [87]. In left-handed individuals, the laterality of the language centre can be either right or left. One method proposed to identify the side of language centre is to compare the cognitive measures for the individual after the individual received right and left unilateral ECT [87]. The efficacy of left unilateral ECT was reported to be similar to RUL ECT [88]. Given the dearth of evidence regarding the cognitive effects of left unilateral ECT, this is not generally recommended, although it may be used judiciously where there is right-sided structural defect such as a skull defect, or cerebral encephalomalacia [89].

Inglis [90] recognized that the amnestic side effects associated with bitemporal and unilateral ECT were possibly caused by direct stimulation of the temporal lobes and suggested a trial of placement of electrodes in the frontal regions. Following this suggestion, Abrams and Taylor introduced bifrontal ECT in 1972 and one earlier study showed therapeutic efficacy intermediate to bitemporal and RUL ECT with memory effects similar to unilateral ECT [91]. Bifrontal ECT was later studied by Lawson *et al.* [92] and Letemendia *et al.* [93] who suggested placement of electrodes 5 cm above the lateral angle of the orbits bilaterally and this has now become a standard practice (Figure 23.3c). There are many studies published comparing the efficacy in major depression and memory effects of bifrontal ECT with bitemporal and RUL ECT. The results of the studies are variable, with one study showing better therapeutic effects of bifrontal ECT over bitemporal and RUL ECT in major depression [93]. However, the findings in other studies, including the most recent largest head-to-head comparison between bifrontal, bitemporal and RUL placements, the therapeutic efficacy of bifrontal ECT was comparable to bitemporal and RUL ECT [65, 82, 84, 94, 95]. In a double-blinded randomized controlled study, Hiremani *et al.* [96] noted that bifrontal ECT is associated with a faster response compared to bitemporal ECT in the treatment of acute mania with comparable cognitive side effects. Bifrontal ECT and bitemporal ECT were compared in a randomized double-blinded controlled study on clinical effects and cognitive profile in patients with schizophrenia, and this study showed superior clinical effects and cognitive outcomes with bifrontal ECT [97]. Data from Phutane *et al.* [97] study were used to analyse any differences in haemodynamic changes and found no difference between bifrontal and bitemporal ECT [98]. Most studies on major depression have reported better cognitive profile of bifrontal ECT over bitemporal ECT [92, 94, 95], which was not replicated in the recent large randomized controlled trial [82], whereas bifrontal and RUL ECT are shown to have comparable cognitive profile [66, 82].

Swartz [99] introduced LART electrode placement in 1996 with the intention to reduce cognitive side effects. In LART, the electrode on the right side is placed at the bitemporal electrode placement site and the electrode on the left side is placed 5 cm anterior to the left bitemporal electrode placement site (Figure 23.3d) [100]. Swartz and colleagues have noted comparable efficacy and better cognitive profile using LART placement compared with bitemporal placement in studies with small sample sizes [99, 101, 102]. Spellman and colleagues introduced FEAST (focal electrically administered seizure therapy), a novel form of ECT in 2009 [103]. Two different sizes of electrodes are used and the placement of electrodes is unique. An anode (small electrode, 0.75″ diameter) is placed above the centre of the right eyebrow and a cathode (large electrode, 1 × 2.5″) is placed tangential to the midline and extended across the right supplementary motor cortex [104]. The stimulus used is an unidirectional stimulus, which creates a current flow in one direction (anode → cathode) [104]. This technique facilitates the stimulation to be localized to the subcallosal cingulate (SCC) gyrus and frontal pole [104]. SCC gyrus is one of the neuroanatomical targets in the treatment of depression [105]. The temporal lobe stimulation is also reduced with this technique compared to the bilateral (BL) stimulation and this could possibly reduce the cognitive side effects [104]. In a feasibility study, safety and tolerability of the FEAST were demonstrated and its efficacy in the treatment of depression was noted [104]. Further research is needed before LART and FEAST would be recommended in general clinical practice.

Adjunctive apparatus

Monitoring of certain physiological parameters such as the EEG, cardiovascular status and measure of adequacy of oxygenation is important during the ECT procedure, and to accomplish this, modern ECT devices are equipped to monitor some of these important physiological parameters. The medical equipment used in modern ECT practice is listed in Table 23.1. Monitoring of seizure activity is essential during ECT, which aids in (i) confirming that a seizure adequate for therapeutic purposes occurred and (ii) confirming that the EEG seizure terminated within a sufficient period of time. Seizure activity and duration can be monitored either by EEG monitoring or merely visualizing the motor seizure. General consensus is that the EEG seizure duration of

Table 23.1 Therapeutic mechanisms of ECT – highlights.

• Diencephalic and neuroendocrine hypothesis
• Anticonvulsant hypothesis
• Regional cerebral blood flow changes
• Effect on a wide range of neurotransmitters
• Neurogenesis and synaptogenesis
• Immunomodulation

at least 25 s should be achieved for the treatment to be effective [54]. The motor seizure duration tends to be shorter than the EEG seizure. EEG recording of the seizure activity is more reliable than the motor seizure activity because the motor seizure is influenced by the muscle relaxant used during the treatment, and the relaxant can completely suppress the motor seizure. This can happen in spite of use of the cuff technique where a BP cuff is inflated around the ankle before the injection of muscle relaxant to isolate the limb from the effect of muscle relaxant for monitoring the motor seizure. Some ECT devices are equipped with electromyography to detect motor seizure activity. However, the reliability of this approach is not clearly superior to visual observation. For these reasons, EEG monitoring of the seizure is considered a standard practice for modern ECT. A nerve stimulator is also an optional but useful device to check for adequacy of skeletal muscle relaxation. Checking for deep tendon reflexes or plantar response is an alternative when there is no nerve stimulator.

Cardiovascular complications account for a large proportion of the more serious side effects associated with the treatment, especially in a population with comorbid cardiovascular conditions [106, 107]. The initial cardiovascular response after ECT is bradycardia or even asystole due to initial parasympathetic outflow associated with autonomic nervous system stimulation related to the stimulus, followed by a sympathetic release resulting in tachycardia, hypertension and dysrhythmia related to seizure induction [108]. Modern ECT devices are equipped to record the electrocardiogram (ECG). Automated blood pressure monitoring is a helpful adjunctive apparatus.

Monitoring of oxygenation is essential for any procedure that requires general anaesthesia and hence pulse oximetry is routinely used and is essential to monitor adequacy of oxygenation during ECT. Desaturation can occur during the ECT or in the recovery phase [109] and arterial carbon dioxide (CO_2) levels may rise as a result of hypoventilation. Resulting hypercapnia can decrease the seizure duration [110] and can also disturb the haemodynamics contributing to cardiovascular morbidity. End tidal CO_2 monitoring is a non-invasive method of monitoring ventilation efficacy and use of this method was shown to improve the haemodynamics (heart rate, mean blood pressure and flow velocityin middle cerebral artery) during ECT when compared to ECT without end tidal CO_2 monitoring [111].

Treatment

Pre-treatment

The psychiatrist trained in the administration of ECT should evaluate prospective patients for comorbid medical conditions and current medications. Common practice includes basic investigations such as complete blood count, basic metabolic panel and ECG. A more parsimonious approach to laboratories is justifiable in young and healthy individual scheduled for ECT. Patients should undergo pre-ECT anaesthesia evaluation, and if necessary, referral should be made to other medical specialties for guidance on optimizing the safety of ECT. After educating the patient about the risks and benefits of the treatment, an informed consent should be obtained. Certain severe psychiatric conditions such as catatonia, acute suicidality, mania or psychosis can affect the patient's capacity to consent for the treatment. During such times, local legal policies should be followed regarding consent for the treatment.

Consultation is required regarding whether the patient will receive ECT as an inpatient or as an outpatient, during the acute phase, continuation phase and maintenance phase. In acute-phase treatment, patients are severely ill and may require admission to an inpatient psychiatry unit; this also gives an opportunity to closely monitor patient for any side effects of the treatment. In the United States, acute-phase ECT sessions are typically performed on alternate days with three treatments per week and the numbers of treatments often approach 12 treatments. Continuation treatment is administered to prevent relapse of the condition after the conclusion of the acute phase of the treatment. Continuation treatments are usually administered on an outpatient basis and the frequency of the treatments is decided on a case-to-case basis. Patients who are in remission for 6 months or more are considered recovered from that episode of the illness. Maintenance phase of ECT is offered to a patient who has recovered from an episode of the psychiatric condition to prevent a recurrence of another episode. Patients should be instructed to withhold food or drink for at least 8 h before ECT. Medications pre-approved by the ECT psychiatrist and anaesthesiologist should be instructed to be taken with a sip of water before the treatment. In the ECT suite preparation area, the patient should be interviewed by the treating psychiatrist to obtain a brief interval history and a mental status examination should be performed. Vital signs should be monitored and intravenous access line should be obtained.

Procedure

ECT team members typically consist of an ECT psychiatrist, anaesthetist, one or two recovery nurses and an ECT treatment nurse [9]. On arrival of the patient in the ECT suite, preparations are made to monitor heart rate, blood pressure, pulse oximetry and ECG. Pre-anaesthetic oxygenation is standard [112]. ECT electrodes should be affixed to the predetermined electrode placement positions after gentle cleansing of the area of the electrode placement on the scalp using electrode gel. The impedance between ECT electrodes and scalp should be confirmed to be within the acceptable range. A baseline EEG tracing should be obtained through the ECT device.

Patients are occasionally pre-medicated with anticholinergic medication to decrease salivation and to prevent bradycardia and asystole that may result from immediate postictal parasympathetic discharge [113]. Intravenous glycopyrrolate (0.2–0.4 mg) and atropine (0.4–0.8 mg) are commonly used anticholinergic drugs [9]. Glycopyrrolate does not cross the blood–brain barrier and does not cause post-ECT tachycardia but atropine is a more effective vagolytic and has a shorter half-life [8, 113]. Short general anaesthesia is recommended for ECT, often with barbiturates [108]. Higher doses of barbiturates can increase the seizure threshold and they have the potential to make treatment less effective [8, 108]. Hence, the dose used should have minimal effect on increasing the seizure threshold and at the same time should attain adequate anaesthesia. An anaesthetic with minimal seizure antagonistic properties should be used. Methohexital is the drug of choice for ECT anaesthesia due to its long safety record and low cost [8, 9]. Methohexital is epileptogenic at low dose (0.5–1 mg/kg), which makes it an ideal anaesthetic [8]. Methohexital shortage of supply has been a problem at times forcing ECT practitioners rely on other anaesthetic agents [114]. Thiopental is a second choice barbiturate when methohexital is not available. One limitation of thiopental is its potential to suppress seizure [113]. Similarly, propofol can also suppress the seizure activity [8, 113]. Etomidate is sometimes used when the ECT-induced seizure is inadequate and the seizure threshold is high, and it is a preferred drug in patients with congestive heart failure [9, 113]. Etomidate is associated with increased postictal confusion and delayed recovery [8].

Similar to etomidate, ketamine is also used in patients who have inadequate seizure and have high seizure threshold [9, 113]. It also has analgesic properties [112]. Another unique property of ketamine is its independent and rapid antidepressant properties [115]. Ketamine can cause postictal confusion, psychosis and dissociative symptoms [9, 113]. Sevoflurane is the only inhalational anaesthetic in use for ECT [113]. Remifentanil is a short acting opioid analgesic that can be used either as a sole anaesthetic or as an adjunct to other anaesthetics, and it is indicated in patients with inadequate seizure and high seizure threshold [116].

Bag mask ventilation with 100% oxygen is maintained after the intravenous anaesthetic is administered [112]. The patient should be completely unconscious before administration of the skeletal muscle relaxant because the patient's experience of being unable to breathe while still conscious can be a terrifying experience. A blood pressure cuff is inflated around the ankle with pressure slightly above the systolic blood pressure to isolate the limb from the muscle relaxant. The depolarizing muscle relaxant succinylcholine is preferred for skeletal muscle relaxation because it has a rapid onset of action and is very short acting, with rapid spontaneous recovery [9]. Non-depolarizing muscle relaxants are used when succinylcholine is contraindicated in patients with pseudocholinesterase deficiency, organophosphate poisoning, hypercalcaemia, severe neuromuscular disease, severe osteoporosis, personal or family history of malignant hyperthermia, prolonged bed rest from any cause (such as catatonia) and severe burns [8, 9]. Mivacurium, atracurium and rocuronium are the commonly used non-depolarizing muscle relaxants for ECT [9, 112]. Mivacurium cause histamine release and can induce bronchospasm [8, 112]. Rocuronium has a good safety profile [117, 118]. When rocuronium is used with selective relaxant binding agent sugammadex, rocuronium-induced neuromuscular blockade is rapidly reversed. Hence, the duration of action of the combination of rocuronium and sugammadex is comparable to succinylcholine [117, 118].

A bite block is placed to prevent injury to patient's teeth and tongue since muscle relaxants do not protect against clamping action of the jaw [9]. A predetermined dose of electrical stimulus is delivered. Motor and EEG seizure should be monitored and the duration of the seizure is recorded. Patients who did not have a seizure should be restimulated (as discussed previously). Some patients may have prolonged seizures and it should be terminated using a barbiturate or midazolam or lorazepam if the seizure duration exceeds 2–3 min [119]. Ventilation through bag mask should be resumed after the seizure is terminated. Patients should be making respiratory efforts soon after the end of the seizure and spontaneous respiration will resume within a few minutes. Patients should be monitored for ictal and postictal haemodynamic changes, which are due to sympathetic discharge typically manifesting as tachycardia and hypertension. This may lead to arrhythmias or myocardial ischaemia in susceptible patients, and this may be treated with intravenous administration of labetalol or esmolol, or other anti-hypertensive drugs such as nitrates, hydralazine, calcium channel blockers and ganglionic blockers [8, 9, 108]. Haemodynamic parameters and oxygen saturation should be monitored for 15–30 min after ECT. Patient should be shifted to the recovery room for further monitoring after regaining consciousness. Most common side effects during the recovery period are confusion, agitation, amnesia and headaches [108]. Ketorolac prophylaxis may be beneficial in patients with post-ECT headaches [9].

Therapeutic mechanisms of ECT

ECT has been used in the treatment of people with mental illness for over eight decades. Psychiatrists are well aware of the benefits and risks of ECT but the precise mechanism of how ECT works remains unknown. ECT has a number of demonstrable effects on the brain that may provide support for theories of mechanism of action, when combined with what is known about pathophysiology of various neuropsychiatric conditions. During the earlier years of ECT, several theories were put forth to explain the therapeutic effects of ECT. However, there is a lack of evidence in support of these theories. The Hungarian neuropsychiatrist Ladislas Meduna was the first to attempt to chemically induce convulsions in humans with therapeutic purposes [1, 3]. This was based on neuropathologic observation that the brains of the patients with schizophrenia appeared to have a lower concentration of glia, compared with those of patient with epilepsy, and the clinical observation that patients with psychosis who had seizures seemed to improve [3]. This notion led to the hypothesis that seizure therapy might increase glial cells, which could be therapeutic in schizophrenia. The 'gliosis theory' was discarded after the coexistence of schizophrenia and epilepsy was demonstrated [3]. Another hypothesis was based on the concept that an increased accumulation of toxic substances in the brain could cause psychosis and that by increasing permeability of the blood–brain barrier, ECT could enhance the removal of these toxic substances. Along this line, research has shown a transient increase in permeability of the blood–brain barrier after ECT lasting less than 15 min, which is secondary to transient systemic hypertension and cerebral vasodilation [120]. Twenty-four hours after the last seizure, there seems to be no change in blood–brain barrier permeability and no evidence of damage to glial cells, neurons or subcellular structures on electron microscopy [121].

Over the years, several psychogenic and psychological theories have been proposed to elucidate the mechanism of ECT. In 1948, Gordon published 'Fifty shock therapy theories' in which he categorizes the effects of ECT into somatogenic and psychogenic theories [122]. Under somatogenic theories, Gordon hypothesized the effects of ECT on the diencephalon, hippocampus and glial tissue, and there is now evidence that ECT does affect these structures. Some of the psychological theories described are the theory of punishment, the denial theory and the amnesia theory, which lack scientific evidence in their support [3].

Cerletti hypothesized that the mode of induction of the seizure was not the essential part of the treatment, but rather the resultant changes in the endocrine systems [123]. Abrams and Taylor [124] similarly argued that the benefits of bilateral ECT over unilateral ECT are due to the stimulation of the diencephalon directly by the electrical current and indirectly through frontal lobe efferents. RUL ECT also stimulates the diencephalon but to a lesser extent compared to bilateral ECT, as evidenced in a study on changes of prolactin levels pre- and post-ECT with unilateral versus bilateral treatments [125]. Theories of mechanism of action focusing on ECT's stimulation of the deep brain structures that regulate the hypothalamic pituitary axis activity leading to the release of pituitary hormones such as adrenocorticotropic hormone, thyrotropin, prolactin, oxytocin and vasopressin include the *diencephalic hypothesis* and the *neuroendocrine hypothesis* [126]. Patients with severe depression experience abnormalities in mood, sleep, appetite and libido and all of these can be related to neuroendocrine dysfunction, which is reversed after treatment with ECT. CSF analysis in patients with depression has revealed abnormal levels of various neuroendocrine hormone levels, which normalize after treatment with ECT [126].

Sleep disturbance is very common in psychiatric illnesses. Neural sleep control centres are located in the brainstem, and an improvement in sleep following ECT provides additional evidence for the diencephalic hypothesis. Sleep studies show abnormal patterns of rapid eye movement (REM) activity during severe depression and reversal with ECT [127]. After ECT, patients with major depressive disorder and schizophrenia showed increased duration of sleep, increased REM latency, reduced sleep latency, decreased night-time awakenings, decreased REM sleep and increased time of slow wave sleep, which portrays shift of sleep pattern towards normality [127–129]. These changes persists even after stopping the ECT [3] unlike with antidepressants where there is rebound of abnormal sleep architecture [130].

Sackeim introduced the *anticonvulsant hypothesis* to show the link between anticonvulsant property of ECT and its antidepressant effects [42]. The seizure threshold increases and the seizure duration decreases during the course of ECT due to the anticonvulsant effect, and the changes in seizure threshold and seizure duration are independent of each other [42, 127, 131–133]. In animal models, the increase in seizure threshold during ECT is shown to be consistent with alterations in gamma-Aminobutyric acid (GABA), opioid and peptide neurotransmission [42]. Transfer of the intraventricular CSF from a cat treated with electroconvulsive shock (ECS) to a naive cat raised the seizure threshold to ECS in naive cats. This effect of raising seizure threshold was blocked by pre-treatment of the naive animals with naloxone [134]. Proconvulsant drugs such as strychnine and quizapine did not alter the seizure threshold after ECS in rats, which raise the question that the ECS may have a very specific action via a particular substrate by which it increases the seizure threshold [135]. Therapeutic effects of ECT are shown to have characteristic expressions in seizure, which include earlier onset of slow wave activity with higher amplitude, and lower frequency of the slow wave activity, and are followed by postictal suppression [42]. Hence, RUL ECT dosage close to seizure threshold lacks therapeutic benefits that may be due to delayed onset of slow wave activity, reduced slow wave amplitude and reduced likelihood of postictal suppression [42]. Sackeim reported an increase in seizure threshold during the course of ECT correlates with the therapeutic outcome in patients, and the seizure threshold reverts to pre-treatment baseline once ECT is terminated, which is independent of current mood state [42]. However, there is no correlation between the change in seizure duration and the therapeutic outcome of the ECT [42, 132]. Despite the intuitive appeal of the anticonvulsant hypothesis, an association between ECT-related change in seizure threshold and corresponding change in depression scores has not been found [127, 131, 133].

Cerebral blood flow (CBF) and cerebral metabolic rate (CMR) for glucose increase markedly during the ictus and decrease below baseline values in postictal and interictal states, which is similar to patients with epilepsy [136]. Patients treated with RUL ECT showed significant postictal CBF reductions largely restricted to right-sided frontal regions whereas bilateral ECT had symmetric reduction in BL anterior prefrontal regions. Responders to ECT showed more marked global reductions in CBF after the treatments, as well as greater reductions in a specific topography involving anterior frontal regions. Post-ECT PET imaging showed CBF decreases in the anterior cingulate and medial frontal cortex, areas involved in the pathophysiology of depression [136, 137]. CBF levels in the thalamus after ECT are reported to be elevated, and some symptoms of depression may be associated with diencephalic disturbances [124, 136]. ECT results in regional increases in CBF 5–8 days after the treatment, and this was mostly marked in ECT responders [136]. The seizure threshold change was significantly associated with a global change in CBF [136].

ECT and antidepressants share some commonalities in their effects on neurotransmitters. Both are known to affect a wide range of neurotransmitters systems, including serotonin, norepinephrine and dopamine [138].

However, ECT goes further in its effects on neurotransmitters by directly impacting GABA, glutamate and cholinergic systems [138]. These additional effects of the ECT surpass the effects of antidepressants and may explain its broader therapeutic efficacy in mania, catatonia, NMS, schizophrenia and Parkinsonism [139, 140].

Neurogenesis is implicated in antidepressant effect and also thought to strengthen hippocampal inhibitory control over the hypothalamic–pituitary–adrenal axis [141]. Major depression is associated with suppression of neurogenesis in the hippocampus, hippocampal volume loss and dysfunction [141]. Neurogenesis is a process that consists of proliferation of stem cells and progenitor cells, determination of the fate of neurons and how the new neurons develop and integrate into neural circuitry [142]. Repeated administration of antidepressants and ECS has been shown to promote cell proliferation and neurogenesis in adult hippocampus of rats and monkeys [141, 143]. ECS induced proliferation of the normally quiescent type-1 cells in the hippocampus that ultimately determines the increase in newborn neurons [142]. Also, ECS for 5 consecutive days was associated with a massive increase in neurogenesis that was detectable even 3 months later, whereas ECS every 2 weeks elicited a slower but identical increase in net hippocampal neurogenesis after 3 months [142]. The combination of both daily ECS for 5 days and continuation ECS every 2 weeks had a synergistic effect and approximately doubled the number of newborn neurons [142]. Unlike ECT, antidepressant medication transiently amplified progenitor cells and did not acutely stimulate progenitor proliferation in the dentate gyrus [144, 145]. MRI scans in patients with treatment-resistant depression after ECT have shown a significant volume increase in the hippocampus and amygdala [146]. Interestingly, increased neurogenesis is shown to be a general response to seizure activity and is not specific to seizures induced by electrical stimulus [147].

Increased dendritic arbourization and synaptogenesis in the amygdala is suggested to represent fear – learning and explain the anxiety, fear and related dysfunctional moods experienced by depressed patient [148]. A high-dose ECS stimulus in animal models is shown to correct the aberrant amygdalar neuro-plasticity that characterizes depression and stress [147]. Transmission electron microscopy study examining the sections of basolateral amygdala of rats treated with ECS showed a reduced number of excitatory synapses [148]. Synaptic dysfunction and a decreased number of synapses have been implicated in certain brain regions in depressed patients [149]. ECS has been reported to increase the total number of synapses in the adult rat hippocampus [149]. Glial reduction has been found in several brain regions in patients with depression and pharmacological ablation of astrocytes induces depressive-like behaviours [150]. Thrombospondin-1 (TSP-1) has been shown to be secreted by astrocytes and to regulate synaptogenesis, which is specifically shown to be increased by repeated ECS in the hippocampus. This finding has not been seen after chronic treatment with antidepressants [151].

Tissue plasminogen activator (tPA) and plasmin are proteins whose main role are in coagulation. These proteins, however, have also been shown to play a role in synaptic plasticity, long-term potentiation and neurogenesis [152]. Decreased levels of tPA has been described in patients with major depression and schizophrenia [152]. Hoirisch-Clapauch and colleagues hypothesize that the mechanism of ECT may increase the synthesis and release of tPA by various converging pathways [152]. These include the activation of both brain-derived neurotrophic factor and vascular endothelial growth factor, improved NMDA receptor-mediated signalling, increased bioavailability of zinc, purinergic release and increased mobility of dendritic spines [152]. ECT also increases the expression of glutamate decarboxylase isoforms in GABAergic neurons and p11, a protein that increases the amount of serotonin receptor 1B [152].

There is evidence suggesting elevated cytokine levels in mood disorders. Some of the critical mediators are interleukin (IL)-6, IL-1β and tumour necrosis factor (TNF)-α [153]. Similarly, in schizophrenia, elevation of cytokines such as IL-1β, IL-6, IL-12, TNF-α, transforming growth factor-β and interferon-γ is implicated [154]. ECT seems to change the expression of several inflammatory markers and this may be another mechanism for the therapeutic effects of ECT [155].

A principal concern of ECT is the associated cognitive side effects [156]. Several preclinical and clinical studies implicate effects on multiple biochemical and neurotransmitter systems in the pathophysiology of cognitive side effects [157, 158]. Research has shown that ECT results in the release of endogenous opioids, glutamate, excitatory amino acids, cortisol and prostaglandins, and each chemical have been independently linked with cognitive side effects [157, 158]. The glutamate excitotoxicity may impair long-term potentiation and synaptic plasticity, which may explain the amnestic effects of ECT [157]. ECT-induced hypercortisolemia over-stimulates glucocorticoid receptors and may result in the loss of dendritic spines and synapses in the hippocampus, and these structural changes are reversible, and it is a plausible explanation why cognitive difficulties associated with ECT are transient [157]. Calcium channel blockers verapamil and felodipine attenuated ECS-induced retrograde amnesia in an animal model. It remains uncertain whether these benefits are due to their effects on calcium-mediated neural functioning or due to prevention of ECS-induced hypertensive surge [157]. ECS induced muscarinic–cholinergic receptor down-regulation in an animal model and a possible causal relationship with ECS-induced anterograde amnesia was suggested as another possible mechanism of cognitive side effects [159]. There is limited electrophysiology and neuroimaging research regarding the mechanism of cognitive side effects of ECT. To date, evidence has suggested that a greater reduction of CBF in the prefrontal cortex after ECT was associated with greater inconsistent recall of historical information, while reduction in post-ECT CBF and CMR in certain temporal lobe regions was associated with anterograde amnesia [158]. In one study, correlation of electrophysiological activity collected with 19-lead EEG and cognitive outcome showed (i) accentuated delta power in anterior frontal and temporal regions during the period of disorientation immediately following RUL ECT, and increased theta activity in frontotemporal regions was associated with longer time taken to recover orientation, (ii) increased delta power relative to theta across the cortex correlated with post-ECT poor global cognitive function and (iii) increased theta activity in frontotemporal regions correlated with the magnitude of inconsistent recall of autobiographical events [160]. The mechanisms of ECT-related induced cognitive side effects must be considered still preliminary and uncertain. A recent review [161] suggested that the mechanisms underlying the association

Table 23.2 Medical equipment used in modern ECT practice.

Necessary equipment
- Constant current brief-pulse ECT device
- ECT stimulus electrodes
- Electroencephalogram
- Electrocardiogram
- Automated blood pressure and heart rate monitor
- Pulse oximetry

Optional equipment
- Electromyogram
- Nerve stimulator
- End tidal CO_2 monitor

between ECT and cognitive outcome are complex and involve a combination of both moderating and mediating factors. Further research is warranted to elucidate the mechanisms of ECT-associated cognitive side effects.

In conclusion, ECT induces a myriad of changes in neuroendocrine system, neural tissues, neurotransmitter systems, neurophysiology and immune system (Table 23.2). However, the exact mechanism by which ECT exerts its therapeutic and adverse effects remains unknown. Considering the benefits of ECT benefits in various neuropsychiatric conditions with different pathophysiologies, it is possible that the therapeutic mechanisms may vary in different neuropsychiatric conditions.

Acknowledgement

The authors thank Charles H. Kellner and American Psychiatric Press, Inc. for giving permission to use the drawing. The authors also thank Shawn M. McClintock for reviewing the section on mechanism of ECT-induced cognitive side effects and Adarsh S. Reddy for proofreading the manuscript.

References

1 Endler NS. The origins of electroconvulsive therapy (ECT). Convuls Ther. 1988; 4: 5–23.

2 Higgins ES, George MS. The Neuroscience of Clinical Psychiatry: The Pathophysiology of Behavior and Mental Illness. Philadelphia, PA: Wolters Kluwer Health/Lippincott Williams & Wilkins, 2007.

3 Fink M. Convulsive Therapy: Theory and Practice. New York: Raven, 1979.

4 Prudic J. Electroconvulsive therapy. In: Sadock BJ, Sadock VA eds. Kaplan & Sadock's Comprehensive Textbook of Psychiatry, 8th ed. Philadelphia, PA: Lippincott Williams &Wilkins, 2005: 2968–2983.

5 Cerletti U. Old and new information about electroshock. Am J Psychiatry. 1950; 107: 87–94.

6 Bennett AE. Curare: a preventive of traumatic complications in convulsive shock therapy (including a preliminary report on a synthetic curare-like drug). 1940. Convuls Ther. 1997; 13: 93–107.

7 Kelly JP. Fractures complicating electro-convulsive therapy and chronic epilepsy. J Bone Joint Surg (Br). 1954; 36-B: 70–79.

8 Wagner KJ, Möllenberg O, Rentrop M *et al.* Guide to anaesthetic selection for electroconvulsive therapy. CNS Drugs. 2005; 19: 745–758.

9 American Psychiatric Association. Treatment procedures. In: The Practice of Electroconvulsive Therapy: Recommendations for Treatment, Training, and Privileging: A Task Force Report of the American Psychiatric Association. Washington, DC: American Psychiatric Association, 2001: 125–196.

10 Chanpattana W, Kramer BA, Kunigiri G *et al.* A survey of the practice of electroconvulsive therapy in Asia. J ECT. 2010; 26: 5–10.

11 Taylor S. Electroconvulsive therapy: a review of history, patient selection, technique, and medication management. South Med J. 2007; 100: 494–498.

12 Prudic J, Haskett RF, Mulsant B *et al.* Resistance to antidepressant medications and short-term clinical response to ECT. Am J Psychiatry. 1996; 153: 985–992.

13 Rush AJ, Trivedi MH, Wisniewski SR *et al.* Acute and longer-term outcomes in depressed outpatients requiring one or several treatment steps: a STAR*D report. Am J Psychiatry. 2006; 163: 1905–1917.

14 Thase ME. The role of axis II comorbidity in the management of patients with treatment-resistant depression. Psychiatr Clin North Am. 1996; 19: 287–309.

15 Fink M, Kellner CH, McCall WV. The role of ECT in suicide prevention. J ECT. 2014; 30: 5–9.

16 Kellner CH, Fink M, Knapp R *et al.* Relief of expressed suicidal intent by ECT: a consortium for research in ECT study. Am J Psychiatry. 2005; 162: 977–982.

17 Sharma V. The effect of electroconvulsive therapy on suicide risk in patients with mood disorders. Can J Psychiatry. 2001; 46: 704–799.

18 Coffey CE, McCall WV, Hoelscher TJ *et al.* Effects of ECT on polysomnographic sleep: a prospective investigation. Convuls Ther. 1988; 4: 269–279.

19 Nivoli AM, Murru A, Goikolea JM *et al.* New treatment guidelines for acute bipolar mania: a critical review. J Affect Disord. 2012; 140: 125–141.

20 Mukherjee S, Sackeim HA, Schnur DB. Electroconvulsive therapy of acute manic episodes: a review of 50 years' experience. Am J Psychiatry. 1994; 151: 169–176.

21 Small JG, Klapper MH, Kellams JJ *et al.* Electroconvulsive treatment compared with lithium in the management of manic states. Arch Gen Psychiatry. 1988; 45: 727–732.

22 Sikdar S, Kulhara P, Avasthi A *et al.* Combined chlorpromazine and electroconvulsive therapy in mania. Br J Psychiatry. 1994; 164: 806–810.

23 Jacobowski NL, Heckers S, Bobo WV. Delirious mania: detection, diagnosis, and clinical management in the acute setting. J Psychiatr Pract. 2013; 19: 15–28.

24 Minnai GP, Salis PG, Oppo R. Effectiveness of maintenance electroconvulsive therapy in rapid-cycling bipolar disorder. J ECT. 2011; 27: 123–126.

25 Vanelle JM, Loo H, Galinowski A *et al.* Maintenance ECT in intractable manic-depressive disorders. Convuls Ther. 1994; 10: 195–205.

26 Leiknes KA, Jarosh-von Schweder L, Høie B. Contemporary use and practice of electroconvulsive therapy worldwide. Brain Behav. 2012; 2: 283–344.

27 Chanpattana W, Sackeim HA. Electroconvulsive therapy in treatment-resistant schizophrenia: prediction of response and the nature of symptomatic improvement. J ECT. 2010; 26: 289–298.

28 Zervas IM, Theleritis C, Soldatos CR. Using ECT in schizophrenia: a review from a clinical perspective. World J Biol Psychiatry. 2012; 13: 96–105.

29 Pompili M, Lester D, Dominici G *et al.* Indications for electroconvulsive treatment in schizophrenia: a systematic review. Schizophr Res. 2013; 146: 1–9.

30 Braga RJ, Petrides G. The combined use of electroconvulsive therapy and antipsychotics in patients with schizophrenia. J ECT. 2005; 21: 75–83.

31 American Psychiatric Association. Diagnostic and Statistical Manual of Mental Disorders, 5th ed. Arlington, VA: American Psychiatric Publishing, 2013.

32 Bush G, Fink M, Petrides G *et al.* Catatonia. II. Treatment with lorazepam and electroconvulsive therapy. Acta Psychiatr Scand. 1996; 93: 137–143.

33 Fink M. The intimate relationship between catatonia and convulsive therapy. J ECT. 2010; 26: 243–245.

34 Strawn JR, Keck PE Jr, Caroff SN. Neuroleptic malignant syndrome. Am J Psychiatry. 2007; 164: 870–876.

35 Cummings JL. Depression and Parkinson's disease: a review. Am J Psychiatry. 1992; 149: 443–454.

36 Kramer BA. A naturalistic review of maintenance ECT at a university setting. J ECT. 1999; 15: 262–269.

37 Usui C, Hatta K, Doi N *et al.* Improvements in both psychosis and motor signs in Parkinson's disease, and changes in regional cerebral blood flow after electroconvulsive therapy. Prog Neuropsychopharmacol Biol Psychiatry. 2011; 35: 1704–1708.

38 Pridmore S, Pollard C. Electroconvulsive therapy in Parkinson's disease: 30 month follow up. J Neurol Neurosurg Psychiatry. 1996; 60: 693.

39 Popeo D, Kellner CH. ECT for Parkinson's disease. Med Hypotheses. 2009; 73: 468–469.

40 Andersen K, Balldin J, Gottfries CG *et al.* A double-blind evaluation of electroconvulsive therapy in Parkinson's disease with 'on-off' phenomena. Acta Neurol Scand. 1987; 76: 191–199.

41 Pintor LP, Valldeoriola F, Fernández-Egea E *et al.* Use of electroconvulsive therapy in Parkinson disease with residual axial symptoms partially unresponsive to l-dopa: a pilot study. J ECT. 2012; 28: 87–91.

42 Sackeim HA. The anticonvulsant hypothesis of the mechanisms of action of ECT: current status. J ECT. 1999; 15: 5–26.

43 Lambrecq V, Villéga F, Marchal C *et al.* Refractory status epilepticus: electroconvulsive therapy as a possible therapeutic strategy. Seizure. 2012; 21: 661–664.

44 Kamel H, Cornes SB, Hegde M *et al.* Electroconvulsive therapy for refractory status epilepticus: a case series. Neurocrit Care. 2010; 12: 204–210.

45 Lisanby SH, Bazil CW, Resor SR *et al.* ECT in the treatment of status epilepticus. J ECT. 2001; 17: 210–215
46 Rossetti AO, Lowenstein DH. Management of refractory status epilepticus in adults: still more questions than answers. Lancet Neurol. 2011; 10: 922–930.
47 Peterchev AV, Rosa MA, Deng ZD *et al.* Electroconvulsive therapy stimulus parameters: rethinking dosage. J ECT. 2010; 26: 159–174.
48 Sackeim HA, Prudic J, Devanand DP *et al.* Effects of stimulus intensity and electrode placement on the efficacy and cognitive effects of electroconvulsive therapy. N Engl J Med. 1993; 328: 839–846.
49 Weiner RD, Rogers HJ, Davidson JR *et al.* Effects of stimulus parameters on cognitive side effects. Ann N Y Acad Sci. 1986; 462: 315–325.
50 Robertson C, Fergusson G. Electroconvulsive therapy machines. Adv Psychiatr Treat. 1996; 2: 24–31.
51 Andrade C. Dose calculation with brief-pulse ECT demystified. Indian J Psychiatry. 2010; 52: 276–278.
52 Squire LR, Zouzounis JA. ECT and memory: brief pulse versus sine wave. Am J Psychiatry. 1986; 143: 596–601.
53 McCall WV, Shelp FE, Weiner RD *et al.* Convulsive threshold differences in right unilateral and bilateral ECT. Biol Psychiatry. 1993; 34: 606–611.
54 Abrams R. Stimulus titration and ECT dosing. J ECT. 2002; 18: 3–9.
55 Sackeim H, Decina P, Prohovnik I *et al.* Seizure threshold in electroconvulsive therapy. Effects of sex, age, electrode placement, and number of treatments. Arch Gen Psychiatry. 1987; 44: 355–360.
56 Andrade C. ECT and cardiovascular disorders. Arch Indian Psychiatry. 1995; 2: 105–109.
57 McCall WV, Reid S, Ford M. Electrocardiographic and cardiovascular effects of subconvulsive stimulation during titrated right unilateral ECT. Convuls Ther. 1994; 10: 25–33.
58 Semkovska M, Keane D, Babalola O *et al.* Unilateral brief-pulse electroconvulsive therapy and cognition: effects of electrode placement, stimulus dosage and time. J Psychiatr Res. 2011; 45: 770–780.
59 Sackeim HA, Decina P, Kanzler M *et al.* Effects of electrode placement on the efficacy of titrated, low-dose ECT. Am J Psychiatry. 1987; 144: 1449–1455.
60 Petrides G, Braga RJ, Fink M *et al.* Seizure threshold in a large sample: implications for stimulus dosing strategies in bilateral electroconvulsive therapy: a report from CORE. J ECT. 2009; 25: 232–237.
61 McCall WV, Reboussin DM, Weiner RD *et al.* Titrated moderately suprathreshold vs fixed high-dose right unilateral electroconvulsive therapy: acute antidepressant and cognitive effects. Arch Gen Psychiatry. 2000; 57: 438–444.
62 Petrides G, Fink M. The 'half-age' stimulation strategy for ECT dosing. Convuls Ther. 1996; 12: 138–146.
63 Abrams R, Swartz CM, Vedak C. Antidepressant effects of high-dose right unilateral electroconvulsive therapy. Arch Gen Psychiatry. 1991; 48: 746–748.
64 Sackeim HA, Prudic J, Nobler MS *et al.* Effects of pulse width and electrode placement on the efficacy and cognitive effects of electroconvulsive therapy. Brain Stimul. 2008; 1: 71–83.
65 Sienaert P, Vansteelandt K, Demyttenaere K *et al.* Randomized comparison of ultra-brief bifrontal and unilateral electroconvulsive therapy for major depression: clinical efficacy. J Affect Disord. 2009; 116: 106–112.
66 Sienaert P, Vansteelandt K, Demyttenaere K *et al.* Randomized comparison of ultra-brief bifrontal and unilateral electroconvulsive therapy for major depression: cognitive side-effects. J Affect Disord. 2010; 122: 60–67.
67 Loo C, Sheehan P, Pigot M *et al.* A report on mood and cognitive outcomes with right unilateral ultrabrief pulsewidth (0.3 ms) ECT and retrospective comparison with standard pulsewidth right unilateral ECT. J Affect Disord. 2007; 103: 277–281.
68 Loo CK, Sainsbury K, Sheehan P *et al.* A comparison of RUL ultrabrief pulse (0.3 ms) ECT and standard RUL ECT. Int J Neuropsychopharmacol. 2008; 11: 883–890.
69 Spaans HP, Verwijk E, Comijs HC *et al.* Efficacy and cognitive side effects after brief pulse and ultrabrief pulse right unilateral electroconvulsive

therapy for major depression: a randomized, double-blind, controlled study. J Clin Psychiatry. 2013; 74: e1029–e1036.
70 Weaver LA Jr, Ives J, Williams R. Studies in brief-pulse electroconvulsive therapy: the voltage threshold, interpulse interval, and pulse polarity parameters. Biol Psychiatry. 1982; 17: 1131–1143.
71 Girish K, Gangadhar BN, Janakiramaiah N *et al.* Seizure threshold in ECT: effect of stimulus pulse frequency. J ECT. 2003; 19: 133–135.
72 Kotresh S, Girish K, Janakiramaiah N *et al.* Effect of ECT stimulus parameters on seizure physiology and outcome. J ECT. 2004; 20: 10–12.
73 Roepke S, Luborzewski A, Schindler F *et al.* Stimulus pulse-frequency-dependent efficacy and cognitive adverse effects of ultrabrief-pulse electroconvulsive therapy in patients with major depression. J ECT. 2011; 27: 109–113.
74 Andrade C, Kurinji S, Sudha S *et al.* Effects of pulse amplitude, pulse frequency, and stimulus duration on seizure threshold: a laboratory investigation. J ECT. 2002; 18: 144–148.
75 Andrade C, Sudha S, Jyothsna K, *et al.* Effects of stimulus parameters on seizure duration and ECS-induced retrograde amnesia. J ECT. 2002; 18: 31–37.
76 Swartz CM, Larson G. ECT stimulus duration and its efficacy. Ann Clin Psychiatry. 1989; 1: 147–152.
77 Scott AIF. Practical administration of ECT. In: The ECT Handbook: The Third Report of the Royal College of Psychiatrists' Special Committee of ECT, 2nd ed. London: Royal College of Psychiatrists, 2005: 144–158.
78 Krystal AD, Dean MD, Weiner RD *et al.* ECT stimulus intensity: are present ECT devices too limited? Am J Psychiatry. 2000; 157: 963–967.
79 Sackeim HA, Prudic J, Devanand DP, *et al.* A prospective, randomized, double-blind comparison of bilateral and right unilateral electroconvulsive therapy at different stimulus intensities. Arch Gen Psychiatry. 2000; 57: 425–434.
80 Gregory S, Shawcross CR, Gill D. The Nottingham ECT Study. A double-blind comparison of bilateral, unilateral and simulated ECT in depressive illness. Br J Psychiatry. 1985; 146: 520–524.
81 Kellner CH, Tobias KG, Wiegand J. Electrode placement in electroconvulsive therapy (ECT): a review of the literature. J ECT. 2010; 26: 175–180.
82 Kellner CH, Knapp R, Husain MM *et al.* Bifrontal, bitemporal and right unilateral electrode placement in ECT: randomised trial. Br J Psychiatry. 2010; 196: 226–234.
83 Sackeim HA, Dillingham EM, Prudic J *et al.* Effect of concomitant pharmacotherapy on electroconvulsive therapy outcomes: short-term efficacy and adverse effects. Arch Gen Psychiatry. 2009; 66: 729–737.
84 Dunne RA, McLoughlin DM. Systematic review and meta-analysis of bifrontal electroconvulsive therapy versus bilateral and unilateral electroconvulsive therapy in depression. World J Biol Psychiatry. 2012; 13: 248–258.
85 Tharyan P, Adams CE. Electroconvulsive therapy for schizophrenia. Cochrane Database Syst Rev. 2005; 2: 1–74.
86 d'Elia G. Unilateral electroconvulsive therapy. Acta Psychiatr Scand Suppl. 1970; 215: 1–98.
87 Kellner CH. Left unilateral ECT: still a viable option? Convuls Ther. 1997; 13: 65–67.
88 Abrams R, Swartz CM, Vedak C. Antidepressant effects of right versus left unilateral ECT and the lateralization theory of ECT action. Am J Psychiatry. 1989; 146: 1190–1192.
89 Popeo DM, Aloysi AS, Kellner CH. Left unilateral electroconvulsive therapy (ECT) after oligodendroglioma resection. J ECT. 2011; 27: 273–274.
90 Inglis J. Shock, surgery and cerebral asymmetry. Br J Psychiatry. 1970; 117: 143–148.
91 Abrams R, Taylor MA. Anterior bifrontal ECT: a clinical trial. Br J Psychiatry. 1973; 122: 587–590.
92 Lawson JS, Inglis J, Delva NJ *et al.* Electrode placement in ECT: cognitive effects. Psychol Med. 1990; 20: 335–344.
93 Letemendia FJ, Delva NJ, Rodenburg M *et al.* Therapeutic advantage of bifrontal electrode placement in ECT. Psychol Med. 1993; 23: 349–360.
94 Bailine SH, Rifkin A, Kayne E *et al.* Comparison of bifrontal and bitemporal ECT for major depression. Am J Psychiatry. 2000; 157: 121–123.

95 Ranjkesh F, Barekatain M, Akuchakian S. Bifrontal versus right unilateral and bitemporal electroconvulsive therapy in major depressive disorder. J ECT. 2005; 21: 207–210.
96 Hiremani RM, Thirthalli J, Tharayil BS *et al.* Double-blind randomized controlled study comparing short-term efficacy of bifrontal and bitemporal electroconvulsive therapy in acute mania. Bipolar Disord. 2008; 10: 701–707.
97 Phutane VH, Thirthalli J, Muralidharan K *et al.* Double-blind randomized controlled study showing symptomatic and cognitive superiority of bifrontal over bitemporal electrode placement during electroconvulsive therapy for schizophrenia. Brain Stimul. 2013; 6: 210–217.
98 Abhishekh HA, Anusha M, Thirthalli J *et al.* Cardiovascular responses are similar in bifrontal and bitemporal ECT. J ECT. 2012; 28: 194.
99 Swartz CM, Evans CM. Beyond bitemporal and right unilateral electrode placements. Psychiatr Ann. 1996; 26: 705–708.
100 Swartz CM, Nelson AI. Rational electroconvulsive therapy electrode placement. Psychiatry (Edgmont). 2005; 2: 37–43.
101 Swartz CM. Asymmetric bilateral right frontotemporal left frontal stimulus electrode placement for electroconvulsive therapy. Neuropsychobiology. 1994; 29: 174–178.
102 Manly DT, Swartz CM. Asymmetric bilateral right frontotemporal left frontal stimulus electrode placement: comparisons with bifrontotemporal and unilateral placements. Convuls Ther. 1994; 10: 267–270.
103 Spellman T, Peterchev AV, Lisanby SH. Focal electrically administered seizure therapy: a novel form of ECT illustrates the roles of current directionality, polarity, and electrode configuration in seizure induction. Neuropsychopharmacology. 2009; 34: 2002–2010.
104 Nahas Z, Short B, Burns C. A feasibility study of a new method for electrically producing seizures in man: focal electrically administered seizure therapy [FEAST]. Brain Stimul. 2013; 6: 403–438.
105 Williams NR, Okun MS. Deep brain stimulation (DBS) at the interface of neurology and psychiatry. J Clin Invest. 2013; 123: 4546–4556.
106 Rice EH, Sombrotto LB, Markowitz JC *et al.* Cardiovascular morbidity in high-risk patients during ECT. Am J Psychiatry. 1994; 151: 1637–1641.
107 Zielinski RJ, Roose SP, Devanand DP *et al.* Cardiovascular complications of ECT in depressed patients with cardiac disease. Am J Psychiatry. 1993; 150: 904–909.
108 Gaines GY 3rd, Rees DI. Anesthetic considerations for electroconvulsive therapy. South Med J. 1992; 85: 469–482.
109 McCormick AS, Saunders DA. Oxygen saturation of patients recovering from electroconvulsive therapy. Anaesthesia. 1996; 51: 702–704.
110 Crawford CD, Butler P, Froese A. Arterial PaO_2 and $PaCO_2$ influence seizure duration in dogs receiving electroconvulsive therapy. Can J Anaesth. 1987; 34: 437–441.
111 Saito S, Kadoi Y, Nihishara F *et al.* End-tidal carbon dioxide monitoring stabilized hemodynamic changes during ECT. J ECT. 2003; 19: 26–30.
112 Ding Z, White PF. Anesthesia for electroconvulsive therapy. Anesth Analg. 2002; 94: 1351–1364.
113 Deiner S, Frost EA. Electroconvulsive therapy and anesthesia. Int Anesthesiol Clin. 2009; 47: 81–92.
114 Kellner C. Lessons from the methohexital shortage. J ECT. 2003; 19: 127–128.
115 Ghasemi M, Kazemi MH, Yoosefi A *et al.* Rapid antidepressant effects of repeated doses of ketamine compared with electroconvulsive therapy in hospitalized patients with major depressive disorder. Psychiatry Res. 2014; 215: 355–361.
116 Chen ST. Remifentanil: a review of its use in electroconvulsive therapy. J ECT. 2011; 27: 323–327.
117 Kadoi Y, Hoshi H, Nishida A *et al.* Comparison of recovery times from rocuronium-induced muscle relaxation after reversal with three different doses of sugammadex and succinylcholine during electroconvulsive therapy. J Anesth. 2011; 25: 855–859.
118 Turkkal DC, Gokmen N, Yildiz A *et al.* A cross-over, post-electroconvulsive therapy comparison of clinical recovery from rocuronium versus succinylcholine. J Clin Anesth. 2008; 20: 589–593.
119 Kellner CH, Pritchett JT, Beale MD *et al.* Handbook of ECT. Washington, DC: American Psychiatric, 1997.

120 Bolwig TG, Hertz MM, Paulson OB *et al.* The permeability of the blood-brain barrier during electrically induced seizures in man. Eur J Clin Invest. 1977; 7: 87–93.
121 Devanand DP, Dwork AJ, Hutchinson ER *et al.* Does ECT alter brain structure? Am J Psychiatry. 1994; 151: 957–970.
122 Gordon HL. Fifty shock therapy theories. Mil Surg. 1948; 103: 397–401.
123 Fink M. Meduna and the origins of convulsive therapy. Am J Psychiatry. 1984; 141: 1034–1041.
124 Abrams R, Taylor MA. Diencephalic stimulation and the effects of ECT in endogenous depression. Br J Psychiatry. 1976; 129: 482–485.
125 McCall WV, Weiner RD, Carroll BJ *et al.* Serum prolactin, electrode placement, and the convulsive threshold during ECT. Convuls Ther. 1996; 12: 81–85.
126 Fink M, Nemeroff CB. A neuroendocrine view of ECT. Convuls Ther. 1989; 5: 296–304.
127 Coffey CE, Lucke J, Weiner RD *et al.* Seizure threshold in electroconvulsive therapy (ECT) II. The anticonvulsant effect of ECT. Biol Psychiatry. 1995; 37: 777–788.
128 Ren YP, Jiang W, Cotes RO *et al.* Electroconvulsive therapy in China (II): research on the technical parameters and mechanism of action. J ECT. 2012; 28: 213–218.
129 Zhang ZJ, Chen YC, Wang HN *et al.* Electroconvulsive therapy improves antipsychotic and somnographic responses in adolescents with first-episode psychosis–a case-control study. Schizophr Res. 2012; 137: 97–103.
130 Feige B, Voderholzer U, Riemann D *et al.* Fluoxetine and sleep EEG: effects of a single dose, subchronic treatment, and discontinuation in healthy subjects. Neuropsychopharmacology. 2002; 26: 246–258.
131 Fink M, Petrides G, Kellner C *et al.* Change in seizure threshold during electroconvulsive therapy. J ECT. 2008; 24: 114–116.
132 Kales H, Raz J, Tandon R *et al.* Relationship of seizure duration to antidepressant efficacy in electroconvulsive therapy. Psychol Med. 1997; 27: 1373–1380.
133 Shapira B, Lidsky D, Gorfine M *et al.* Electroconvulsive therapy and resistant depression: clinical implications of seizure threshold. J Clin Psychiatry. 1996; 57: 32–38.
134 Tortella FC, Long JB. Characterization of opioid peptide-like anticonvulsant activity in rat cerebrospinal fluid. Brain Res. 1988; 456: 139–146.
135 Nutt DJ, Cowen PJ, Green AR. Studies on the post-ictal rise in seizure threshold. Eur J Pharmacol. 1981; 71: 287–295.
136 Takano H, Motohashi N, Uema T *et al.* Changes in regional cerebral blood flow during acute electroconvulsive therapy in patients with depression: positron emission tomographic study. Br J Psychiatry. 2007; 190: 63–68.
137 Drevets WC. Functional anatomical abnormalities in limbic and prefrontal cortical structures in major depression. Prog Brain Res. 2000; 126: 413–431.
138 Wahlund B, von Rosen D. ECT of major depressed patients in relation to biological and clinical variables: a brief overview. Neuropsychopharmacology. 2003; 28 Suppl 1: S21–S26.
139 Fink M. Convulsive therapy: a review of the first 55 years. J Affect Disord. 2001; 63: 1–15.
140 Lichtenberg P, Lerer B. Implications of clinical spectrum for mechanisms of action: ECT and antidepressants reconsidered. Convuls Ther. 1989; 5: 216–226.
141 Perera TD, Coplan JD, Lisanby SH *et al.* Antidepressant-induced neurogenesis in the hippocampus of adult nonhuman primates. J Neurosci. 2007; 27: 4894–4901.
142 Weber T, Baier V, Lentz K *et al.* Genetic fate mapping of type-1 stem cell-dependent increase in newborn hippocampal neurons after electroconvulsive seizures. Hippocampus. 2013; 23: 1321–1330.
143 Nakamura K, Ito M, Liu Y *et al.* Effects of single and repeated electroconvulsive stimulation on hippocampal cell proliferation and spontaneous behaviors in the rat. Brain Res. 2013; 1491: 88–97.
144 Encinas JM, Vaahtokari A, Enikolopov G. Fluoxetine targets early progenitor cells in the adult brain. Proc Natl Acad Sci U S A. 2006; 103: 8233–8238.
145 Segi-Nishida E, Warner-Schmidt JL, Duman RS. Electroconvulsive seizure and VEGF increase the proliferation of neural stem-like cells in rat hippocampus. Proc Natl Acad Sci U S A. 2008; 105: 11352–11357.

146 Tendolkar I, van Beek M, van Oostrom I *et al.* Electroconvulsive therapy increases hippocampal and amygdala volume in therapy refractory depression: a longitudinal pilot study. Psychiatry Res. 2013; 214: 197–203.
147 Khaleel N, Roopa R, Smitha JS *et al.* Electroconvulsive therapy attenuates dendritic arborization in the basolateral amygdala. J ECT. 2013; 29: 156–157.
148 Khaleel N, Ravindranath R, Sagar BK *et al.* Images in electroconvulsive therapy: pilot impressions suggesting that ECT reduces excitatory synapses in the basolateral amygdala. Indian J Psychiatry. 2013; 55: 204–205.
149 Chen F, Madsen TM, Wegener G *et al.* Repeated electroconvulsive seizures increase the total number of synapses in adult male rat hippocampus. Eur Neuropsychopharmacol. 2009; 19: 329–338.
150 Banasr M, Duman RS. Glial loss in the prefrontal cortex is sufficient to induce depressive-like behaviors. Biol Psychiatry. 2008; 64: 863–870.
151 Okada-Tsuchioka M, Segawa M, Kajitani N *et al.* Electroconvulsive seizure induces thrombospondin-1 in the adult rat hippocampus. Prog Neuropsychopharmacol Biol Psychiatry. 2014; 48: 236–244.
152 Hoirisch-Clapauch S, Mezzasalma MA, Nardi AE. Pivotal role of tissue plasminogen activator in the mechanism of action of electroconvulsive therapy. J Psychopharmacol. 2014; 28: 99-105.
153 Rosenblat JD, Cha DS, Mansur RB *et al.* Inflamed moods: a review of the interactions between inflammation and mood disorders. Prog Neuropsychopharmacol Biol Psychiatry. 2014; 53: 23–34.
154 Kirkpatrick B, Miller BJ. Inflammation and schizophrenia. Schizophr Bull. 2013; 39: 1174–1179.
155 Rotter A, Biermann T, Stark C *et al.* Changes of cytokine profiles during electroconvulsive therapy in patients with major depression. J ECT. 2013; 29: 162–169.
156 Semkovska M, McLoughlin DM. Objective cognitive performance associated with electroconvulsive therapy for depression: a systematic review and meta-analysis. Biol Psychiatry. 2010; 68: 568–577.
157 Andrade C, Singh NM, Thyagarajan S *et al.* Possible glutamatergic and lipid signalling mechanisms in ECT-induced retrograde amnesia: experimental evidence for involvement of COX-2, and review of literature. J Psychiatr Res. 2008; 42: 837–850.
158 Nobler MS, Sackeim HA. Neurobiological correlates of the cognitive side effects of electroconvulsive therapy. J ECT. 2008; 24: 40–45.
159 Lerer B, Stanley M, McIntyre I *et al.* Electroconvulsive shock and brain muscarinic receptors: relationship to anterograde amnesia. Life Sci. 1984; 35: 2659–2664.
160 Sackeim HA, Luber B, Moeller JR *et al.* Electrophysiological correlates of the adverse cognitive effects of electroconvulsive therapy. J ECT. 2000; 16: 110–120.
161 McClintock SM, Choi J, Deng ZD *et al.* Multifactoral determinants of the neurocognitive effects of electroconvulsive therapy. J ECT. 2014; 30: 165–176.

CHAPTER 24
Electroconvulsive therapy: Clinical results

Malek Bajbouj

Charité and Freie Universitaet Berlin, Berlin, Germany

Indication

The indication spectrum of electroconvulsive therapy (ECT) varies enormously throughout the world. In some regions, ECT is only considered under specific circumstances while in others, it is either a first-line treatment or largely disclaimed (e.g. the Kanton Geneva and Jura, Swiss Society for Psychiatry, Switzerland [1]). Based on existing evidence, national guidelines have been developed for the usage of ECT in different disease entities. For the sake of clarity, we will focus on four representative guidelines, namely the recommendations of the American Psychiatric Association (APA), the British guidelines of the National Institute of Clinical Excellence (NICE), the guidelines of the German Chamber of Physicians and the guidelines of the Canadian Psychiatric Association. A summary of key aspects is depicted in Table 24.1. In the following paragraphs, we will mainly focus on the disease entities mentioned in these guidelines and will ignore other less frequent and less evidence-based indications.

According to the APA, ECT should be generally used in severely depressed patients when other forms of therapy, such as medications and psychotherapy, are not effective or practical. In addition, ECT may also be recommended as a first-line treatment in patients with psychotic symptoms, catatonic features, suicide risk and patients in need for a rapid treatment response (e.g. those who refuse to ingest food). With respect to schizophrenia, the APA recommends ECT only as an add-on treatment to antipsychotics when a quick response is needed, and in patients with affective and/or catatonic symptoms. According to the guidelines of the Canadian Psychiatric Association, the main diagnostic indications are limited to unipolar major depression, bipolar disorder (depressed, manic or mixed), non-chronic schizophrenia, especially with affective or catatonic symptoms, schizoaffective disorder and schizophreniform disorder. Individual factors such as the patient's prior treatment response, disease severity, need for rapid therapeutic response and the individual risk-benefit ratio should be taken into account. The British NICE recommends ECT only to achieve rapid and short-term improvement after an ineffective trial with other treatment modalities and/or when the disorder (severe depression, catatonia and prolonged or severe manic episodes) is considered to be potentially life-threatening. The German Medical Association ('Bundesärztekammer') states that ECT should be used if a quick response to a severe condition

Neuromodulation in Psychiatry, First Edition. Edited by Clement Hamani, Paul Holtzheimer, Andres M. Lozano and Helen Mayberg.

Table 24.1 The five main fields of indication and contraindication of electroconvulsive therapy.

Indication	Contraindication
Depression with psychotic features	High intracerebral pressure
Depression with therapy resistance	Recent myocardial infarction
Depression with suicidality	Recent cerebral infarction
Acute catatonic syndrome	Increased anaesthetic risk
Life-threatening condition	Increased risk for intracerebral haemorrhage

The selection of the five conditions is based on recommendations of the guidelines of the American Psychiatric Association, the Canadian Psychiatric Association, the British National Institute for Clinical Excellence and the German Medical Association. Please note that only the German guidelines classify the contraindication as being absolute.

is needed, if risks are lower than those with other treatments, if the patient had both a medication resistance and a good response to ECT in the past and if the individual patient has a past history of severe adverse events with medications. Under these circumstances, the guidelines recommend ECT as a first-line treatment in psychotic depression, depressive stupor, schizoaffective disorder with severe depressive symptoms, major depression with suicidality or refusal to eat and in acute life-threatening catatonia. In addition, the German guidelines list three conditions in which ECT is recommended as a second-line treatment: (i) Therapy-resistant depression (characterized by failure to respond to two antidepressant treatment trials and sleep deprivation), (ii) therapy-resistant, non-life-threatening catatonia and other forms of schizophrenia with an acute course and (iii) therapy-resistant mania after treatment failure with antipsychotics, lithium or carbamazepine. For a summary of the indications, please see Table 24.1.

Contraindications

A summary of the contraindications to ECT may be found in Table 24.1. According to the APA, there are no absolute contraindications for ECT. Relative contraindications comprise medical conditions that may substantially increase the risk of ECT, such as unstable or severe cardiovascular conditions, cerebral aneurysm or vascular malformation, increased intracranial pressure, cerebral infarction, pulmonary insufficiency and a patient medical status rated as ASA (American Society of Anesthesiologists) level 4 or 5. These guidelines describe three specific patient populations with relative contraindications: (i) Those with coexisting medical illness who, despite being prone to complications related to anaesthesia, electrical stimulation and seizure activity, will likely have a bad outcome if not treated; (ii) patients in which the risk of medical complications with pharmacotherapy surpasses that of ECT and (iii) pregnant women during all trimesters of pregnancy and puerperium and nursing mothers in whom the risks of receiving medical therapy or not being treated may surpass that of ECT. According to the Canadian Psychiatric Association, there is no absolute contraindication to ECT. Relative contraindications comprise a variety of specific conditions, such as space-occupying intracranial lesions, elevated intracranial pressure, recent myocardial infarction with cardiac decompensation, severe underlying hypertension (e.g. due to pheochromocytoma), evolving strokes and other risk factors for intracerebral haemorrhage, retinal detachment and any condition with an anaesthetic risk rated as ASA 4 or 5. The NICE guidelines do not specify contraindications to the procedure. However, they state that the decision for or against ECT should be based on the documented assessment of potential benefits and risks to the individual, including those associated with anaesthesia, comorbid disorders, anticipated adverse events, cognitive impairment and the risks of not having treatment. In contrast to the three guidelines described above, the one by the German Medical Association does provide a list of absolute contraindications, including recent myocardial or cerebral infarction (<3 months old), severe cardiopulmonary disease, severe hypertonia, increased intracerebral pressure, intracerebral tumours with oedema and acute glaucoma. Relative contraindications comprise cerebral aneurysms and angiomas.

Efficacy

Acute clinical efficacy

A meta-analysis by the United Kingdom ECT Group [2] revealed an effect size of 0.91 based on six randomized controlled trials involving 256 patients comparing ECT with sham treatment. In another 18 randomized controlled trials including 1144 patients that compared ECT with pharmacotherapy, the effect size was 0.80. Bilateral electrode placement was more effective than right unilateral (RUL) ECT, and high-dose ECT (minimum 2.5 × seizure threshold and higher) was more effective than ECT at low doses (see Figures 24.1 and 24.2). The Consortium for Research on ECT (CORE) demonstrated a 75% remission rate in 217 patients suffering from an acute episode of depression who completed 10 ECT treatments, 65% of whom remitted by the fourth week of therapy [4]. Another recent systematic meta-analysis that reviewed trials with different stimulus parameters reported positive results with the use of RUL ECT in depression. Patients were randomized to receive RUL (six times suprathreshold (ST) or bifrontotemporal ECT (2.5 times ST)) at pulse widths of 0.3 or 1.5 ms [5, 6]. For RUL ECT, efficacy was maintained while cognitive side effects were markedly reduced with the use of 0.3 ms pulse width. After bifrontotemporal ECT, both cognitive side effects and efficacy were reduced with short pulse widths. Recent research has confirmed the application procedure of ST dosing for RUL ECT, with studies [6] demonstrating increasing efficacy with increasing dose (up to 12 times ST). The use of high doses, however, is limited by a commensurate increase in cognitive side effects. In addition, efficacy has also been demonstrated for bifrontotemporal ECT, with results suggesting that dosing should be between 1.5 and 2.5 times ST for optimal results in terms of efficacy and cognitive side effects. In a recent double-blinded randomized controlled trial, 92 patients diagnosed with pharmaco-resistant major depression received either six RUL ECT (2.5 stimulus intensity of titrated threshold) or six bifrontal ECT (1.5 of threshold) treatments over a 3-week period [7] with comparable efficacy and tolerability effects.

Depending on the combination of stimulus intensity and electrode position, antidepressant response rates with ECT vary from 20% to more than 70% [8, 9]. In the United States, and in most European countries, ECT treatments are usually administered three times per week for approximately 4–6 weeks (12–18 treatments), depending on the severity of the patient's symptoms and the rapidity of the response [10]. Predictors of non-remission for an acute ECT trial in a multi-centre study conducted for 7 years were chronicity of depression (i.e. time since illness onset), long current episode duration and medication resistance [11].

A study on patients with major depressive disorder and comorbid personality disorders showed that patients with borderline personality had less symptomatic improvement 8 days after ECT than patients with other or no personality disorders [12]. In other words, patients with personality disorders other than borderline seem to respond well to ECT.

Efficacy of ECT highly depends on various stimulation parameters (see Figure 24.2) Double-blinded, randomized, controlled trials have shown the importance of electrode placement (RUL, bifrontal, bitemporal) and dosage (relative to seizure threshold) for the efficacy and side effects. In a double-masked study with 90 depressed patients [13], subjects

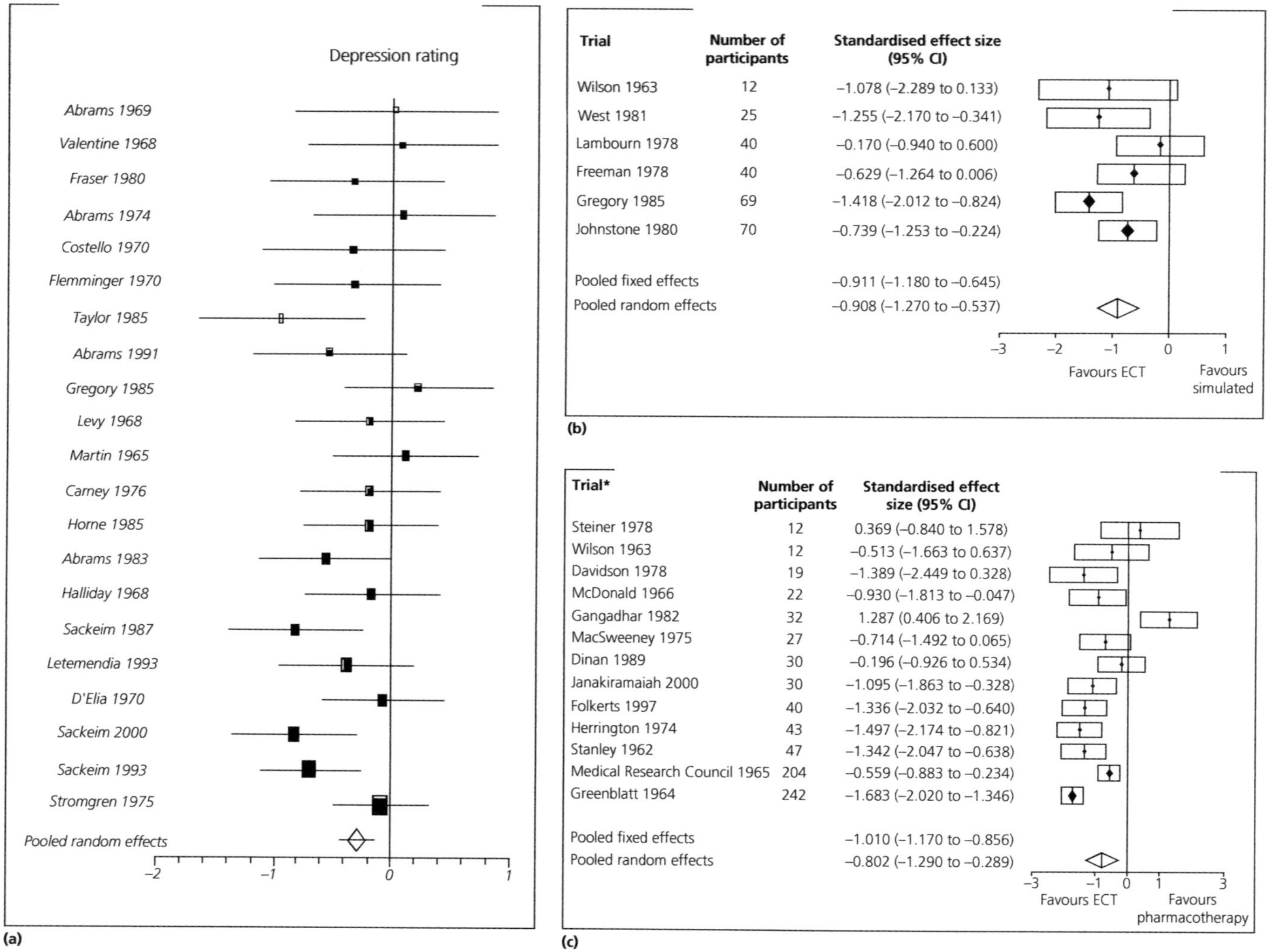

Figure 24.1 Clinical effects of electroconvulsive therapy: (**a**) ECT efficacy as a function of electrode placement: standardized effect size between the two types of electrode placement was −0.289 (−0.428 to −0.151), which significant favours bilateral ECT; 3.4 point (95% CI: 2.0–4.8) change in HAMD depression score in favour of bilateral ECT. (**b**) ECT versus sham: standardized difference between real and simulated ECT was −0.91 (95% CI=−1.27 to −0.54) indicating a statistically significant effect of real ECT; mean HAMD difference of 9.67 (95% CI=5.72–13.53) in favour of real ECT. (**c**) ECT versus drug treatment: treatment with ECT led to a significantly greater decrease in depressive symptoms than drug treatment (standardized effect size −0.80; 95% CI=−1.29 to −0.29); mean HAMD difference of 5.20 (95% CI=1.37–8.87) in favour of ECT. Source: The UK ECT Review Group [3]. Reproduced with permission of Elsevier.

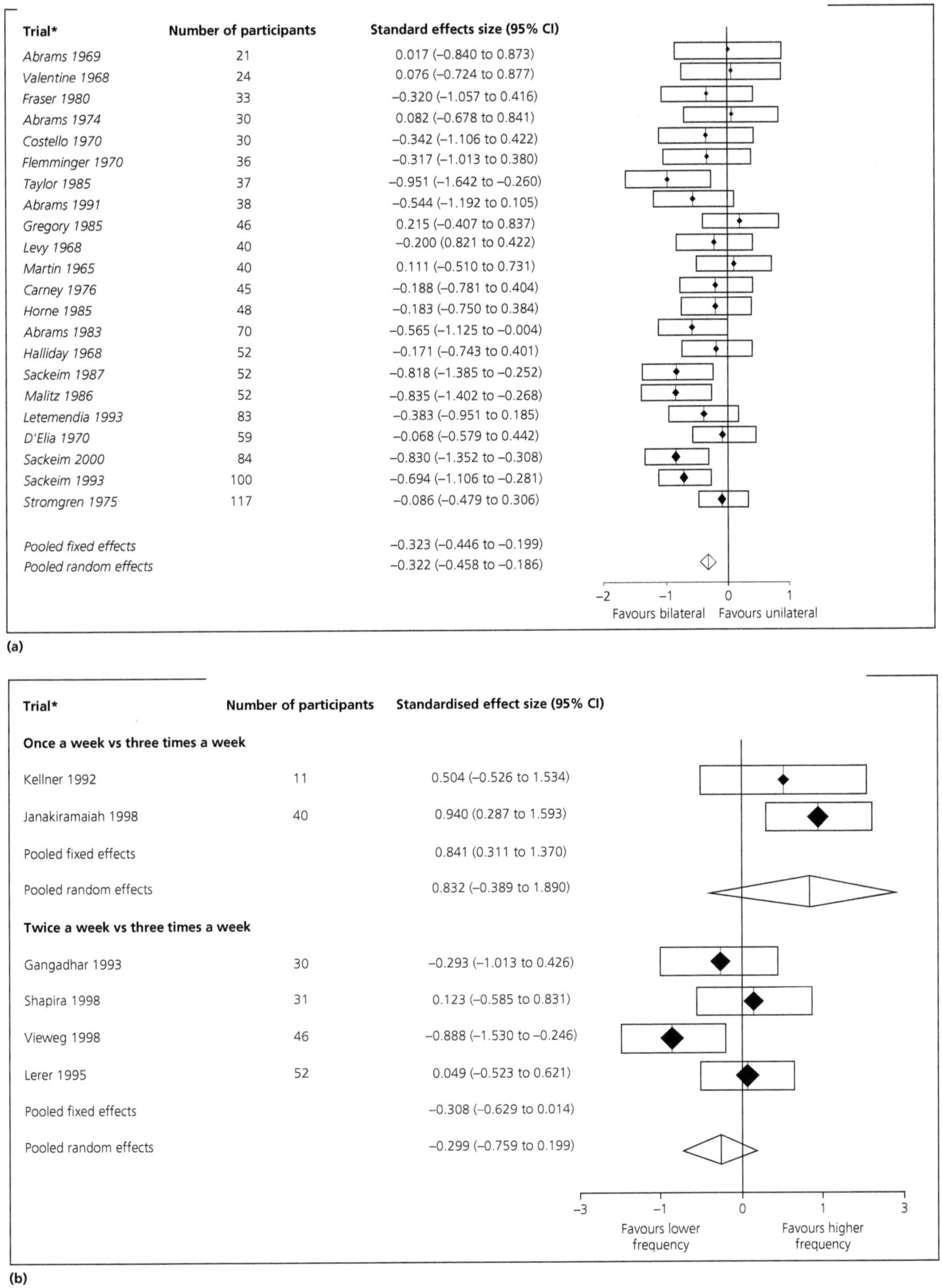

Figure 24.2 ECT efficacy with different (**a**) electrode placements (standardized effect size: 0.387 (95% CI=−0.09 to 0.87); HAMD difference: 3.87 points (95% CI=−0.90 to 8.70)), (**b**) stimulation frequency (standardized effect size −0.30 (95% CI −0.76 to 0.20); HAMD difference 0.40 (95% CI=−5.26 to 6.30),

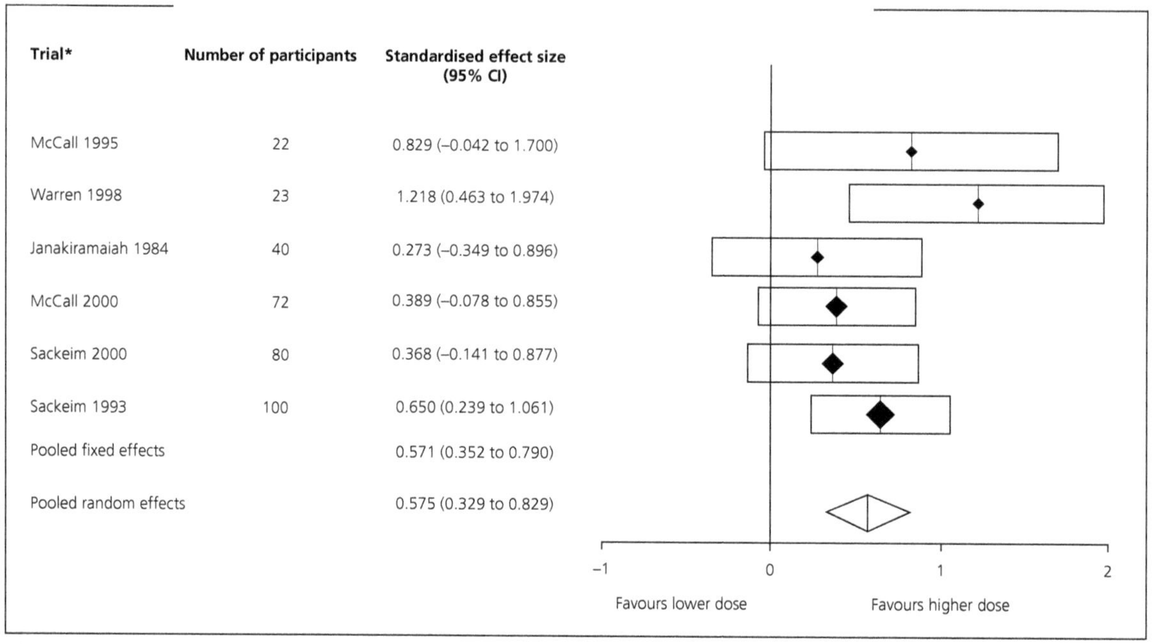

(c)

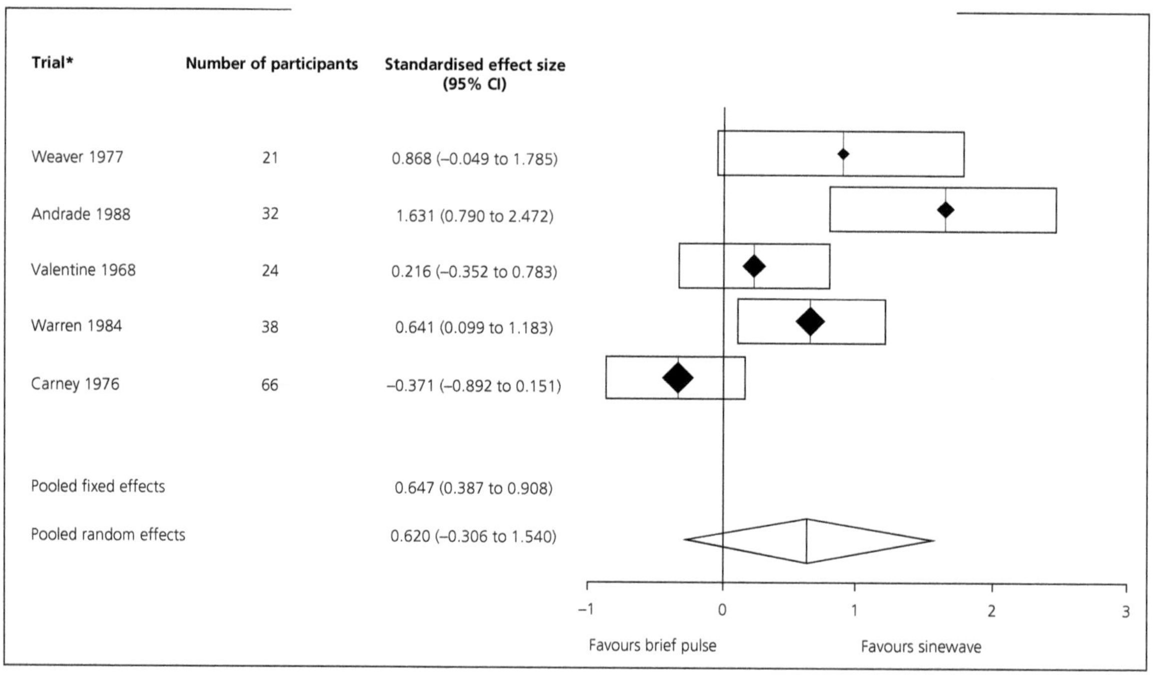

(d)

Figure 24.2 (continued) (**c**) stimulation intensity (standardized treatment effect 0.73 (95% CI=0.41–1.08); HAMD difference 5.24 (95% CI=2.94–7.75), and (**d**) pulse width (standardized effect size: 0.62 (95% CI=–0.31 to 1.54); HAMD difference 4.21 (95% CI=–2.08 to 10.5)). Source: The UK ECT Review Group [3]. Reproduced with permission of Elsevier.

were randomly assigned to RUL ECT (6x ST) or bilateral ECT (2x ST) after either traditional brief pulses (1.5 ms) or ultrabrief pulses (0.3 ms). Antidepressant efficacy was assessed immediately after treatment and 2 and 6 months later. The final remission rate for ultrabrief RUL ECT was higher (73%) than that observed after ultrabrief bilateral (BL) (35%), standard pulse BL (65%) and standard pulse RUL ECT (59%). It is noteworthy that cognitive side effects were markedly reduced after ultrabrief pulse ECT. Overall, these interesting results give rise to the concept that seizure duration may be less important than the amount of ST stimulation and electrode placement for efficacy of ECT.

Management of ECT patients

Patients referred to ECT initially undergo the following three steps:

1. **Individual risk-benefit evaluation:** the first step in most ECT centres is the evaluation of the individual indication, predictors of response and tolerability. (see Table 24.1). The decision to offer ECT should be based on a shared decision-making process that also includes thorough physical and neuropsychological evaluations. Factors such as history of the illness, past treatment responses and the preferences of the patient are all taken into account. A frequent reason for not offering ECT is pseudo-therapy resistance, that is, patients referred to the ECT unit without having had sufficient antidepressant trials in the current episode due to underdosing and/or short treatment duration.
2. **General risk assessment:** after the psychiatric evaluation, cardiac and anaesthesia risks are assessed. Medications and clinical treatments to be offered prior to and during ECT are appraised (e.g. antihypertensives). This assessment is particularly important in patients with cardiovascular and cerebrovascular disorders.
3. **Risk reduction:** although little is known about the complex interactions of pharmacological treatment and ECT, changes in the medication regimen are usually required if patients receive drugs such as lithium or compounds with anticholinergic properties, since they may increase the likelihood for delirium and/or prolonged seizures. In some centres, additional electroencephalographic recordings as well as brain imaging are performed to detect structural abnormalities and to evaluate the individual seizure risk prior to ECT.

Both efficacy (e.g. with weekly Hamilton Depression Rating Scale assessments) and tolerability of ECT (e.g. with a brief neuropsychological test battery at baseline and at fixed time points) should be regularly monitored. In general, patients who show no antidepressant effects after 12 treatment sessions should be classified as ECT non-responders [14]. Patients with a partial response (25–49% Hamilton Depression Rating Scale (HAMD) reduction) should receive unilateral ECT at higher intensities or bilateral ECT. Finally, patients with remission should receive a maintenance therapy with medication, continuation ECT and/or psychotherapy (see next paragraph).

Continuation therapy

Although ECT is the most effective acute antidepressant intervention, sustained response rates are relatively low. A variety of different forms of maintenance therapies, including cognitive-behavioural therapy, continuation ECT or pharmacotherapy, have been investigated in the last decades. Sackeim *et al.* [15] have studied the effects of different continuation pharmacotherapies after ECT in a placebo-controlled randomized trial. The relapse rate for placebo-treated patients was 84% after discontinuation of ECT, with 55% initially classified as remitters. Continuation therapy in that study was carried out with either nortriptyline alone or combined with lithium. The authors found that the abrupt discontinuation of effective ECT was associated with a high risk of relapse. In this context, they note that tapering ECT over a few weeks, as is commonly done with pharmacological treatments, could provide symptom suppression during the most vulnerable post-treatment period. Finally, they suggest that antidepressant medications used in continuation therapies may be started during the course of ECT, followed, for example, by the addition of lithium. In another study including 201 unipolar depression patients who remitted after bilateral ECT, Kellner *et al.* [16] randomly assigned patients to receive maintenance ECT or nortriptyline plus lithium for 6 months. Both treatments were associated with a relapse rate of almost 50%. In contrast to previous reports, data from this study suggest that melancholia, as defined by Structured Clinical Interview for DSM Disorders (SCID-1) criteria, was not a predictor of successful ECT [17]. In a retrospective trial, Gagne *et al.* [18] studied 29 patients who had a positive response to acute ECT treatment followed by continuation treatment with either antidepressant alone or ECT plus antidepressants. They showed that outcome was significantly better in the continuation ECT group, with a cumulative probability of surviving without relapse or recurrence at 2 years of 93% (vs. 52% in antidepressant-alone-treated patients). At 5 years, the survival rate in these two groups declined to 73 and 18%, respectively. In a recently published study, Brakemeier and colleagues investigated 90 depressive patients and distributed them into three different arms: medication, ECT and psychotherapy. After 6 and 12 months, sustained response rates in the cognitive-behavioural therapy, ECT or medication treatment arms were 77, 40 and 44%, respectively. The authors conclude that cognitive-behavioural group therapy combined with antidepressants might be an effective continuation treatment to sustain response after successful ECT in depressive patients [19]. As a consequence, some centres such as the Berlin Charité use cognitive-behavioural therapy as a standard continuation therapy in depressive patients after successful ECT.

Tolerability

Beside high relapse rates, cognitive adverse effects are a second major limitation of ECT, particularly retrograde and anterograde amnesia. Overall, retrograde amnesia often improves within the first few months of treatment [3]. While most studies comparing ECT-treated patients with controls have shown that anterograde amnesia does not last longer than 4 weeks [3, 20], significant loss of recall, that is retrograde amnesia, may persist for up to 1 year [9, 21]. In general, autobiographic memory is less affected than memory for impersonal events [21]. Pre-treatment cognitive impairment has been thought to be a predictor of amnesia after ECT. In addition, amnesia may be more likely in the elderly [22, 23].

A single case report found no evidence of neuronal cell death in a post-mortem specimen of a depressive patient who had 91 ECT administrations. [24] This finding, although not representative, is in agreement with previous studies that examined the neuronal effects of ECT in autopsies in patients who received ECT [25]. In addition, studies in non-human primates have also shown a lack of neuropathological damage after chronic exposure to electroconvulsive shock and magnetic seizure therapy (MST) [26]. A proton magnetic resonance spectroscopic (MRS) imaging study [27] demonstrated that ECT is not likely to induce hippocampal atrophy or cell death in patients with depression, which would be reflected by a decrease in the *N*-acetylaspartate signal in MRS. Nevertheless, neurons in the pyramidal cell layer of the hippocampus seem to be exposed to high degrees of potentially cytotoxic calcium influx during seizure activity, which per se may lead to neuronal atrophy [28]. Although studies in some experimental models do sometimes reveal neuronal death, seizure severity under these artificial conditions is far greater than that associated with modern ECT. Furthermore, the different electrode applications of the ECT itself can substantially reduce the incidence and severity of retrograde amnesia, particularly RUL and ultrabrief pulse width (0.3 μs) [6]. In fact, RUL ECT at high dosage (>400 mC) was shown to be as effective as bilateral ECT at a lower fixed dosage and was reported to produce less severe and persistent cognitive effects [9]. In a more recent study [13] that compared ultrabrief with a wide pulse width ECT (1.5 ms), a lower rate of cognitive side effects and amnesia compared with the former was observed.

Another relevant issue is the interaction between medications and stimulation treatment. The reason for combining both is not only to provide optimal therapeutic responses but also to carefully plan discharge and maintenance therapy. So far, no prospective randomized double-blind controlled trial has been reported on the neurobiological augmentation of ECT by psychopharmacological treatments. In general, the same guidelines for combination therapy with ECT and drugs during the acute and maintenance ECT treatment are applied. The combination of antipsychotics and ECT is well tolerated and may be beneficial. Neuroleptics are allowed during the course of ECT due to their synergistic effects on lowering seizure threshold [29]. In a study combining ECT and clozapine, 67% of patients were improved but 17% developed side effects (e.g. cardiac arrhythmias) [30]. Antipsychotics with strong antihistaminic effects should be carefully applied due to an increased risk of delirious states and disorientation when co-administered with anaesthetics [31]. With regard to the antidepressants, tricyclic antidepressants and ECT can be combined safely and beneficially. More care is required when ECT is administered in the setting of a monoamine oxidase inhibitor (MAOI), especially the older irreversible classes and in patients recently treated with MAOI therapy [31]. When lithium is given concomitant to ECT, patients have a significant risk of developing delirious syndromes. Otherwise, ECT can be safely and effectively administered to patients receiving other mood stabilizers such as valproic acid and carbamazepine, however, without evidence that there are additive effects [32]. One also has to be careful with anticonvulsants because they may inhibit seizure activity. In addition, carbamazepine may prolong the action of suxamethonium (succinylcholine) [33]. As far as anxiolytics are concerned, benzodiazepines have anticonvulsant properties that might interfere with the therapeutic efficacy of ECT. Calcium channel blockers should be used with a great degree of caution to avoid significant cardiovascular depression. In a retrospective study on the possible therapeutic advantages of combination therapies versus ECT alone, seizure duration was unaffected by most of the antidepressants [34]. However, with respect to interaction between ECT and antidepressants, there are a couple of observations and reports, which might be of relevance in the evaluation of individual seizure characteristics: selective serotonin reuptake inhibitors (SSRIs) may increase seizure duration. Post-ictal suppression seems to be lower with mirtazapine than with SSRI and selective noradrenaline reuptake inhibitors (SNRI). Buproprion might produce prolonged seizures when combined with ECT, especially when given at high doses. A study has found that patients taking high doses of venlafaxine (i.e. more than 300 mg/day) are at an increased risk of developing asystole [35]. As for the combination lithium/ECT, a few studies have reported on patients who developed side effects (e.g. seizures and a serotonin syndrome) while serum lithium levels were still within a sub-therapeutic range [36]. In summary, in most cases, one does not need to taper antidepressants while patients receive ECT. At the Berlin Charité, we only discontinue Lithium and Buproprion during ECT and reduce Venlafaxin to 225 mg/day. Venlafaxine has shown to be safe in a non-controlled trial with a very small sample size [37]. However, the doses of venlafaxine used seem to be important for possible side effects, as one study [35] found four cases of asystole, all of them in patients treated with more than 300 mg/day.

Perspective

ECT is highly effective for the treatment of depression. However, improving the adverse effect profile and finding treatment algorithms to maintain response are the two main research questions for the future. There will be at least two approaches to improve tolerability: (i) the better understanding of the clinical effects of different electrode configuration and stimulation parameters, such as ultrabrief pulse ECT, non-dominant hemispheric stimulation and pulsed square wave stimulation. This already led to new stimulation techniques such as MST [38]) and focal electrically administered seizure therapy (FEAST) [5] and (ii) the investigation of the complex interactions of ECT with concomitant pharmacological and even psychotherapeutic treatments. The second challenge will be to find therapeutic interventions capable of maintaining the outstanding clinical effects of acute ECT. From my perspective, the combination of psychotherapeutic and neuromodulatory interventions does have the biggest potential to change ECT towards a treatment that not only have acute but also good longer term effects.

References

1 Swiss Society for Psychiatry. 2012. Electroconvulsive therapy: Psychiatric associations in four countries recommend its timely and appropriate use. http://www.psychiatrie.ch/sgpp/ueber-uns/stellungnahmen-und-positionspapiere/therapie-und-diagnostik/. (accessed 24 April 2015).

2 Group, U. E. 2003. Efficacy and safety of electroconvulsive therapy in depressive disorders: a systematic review and meta-analysis. Lancet 361: 799–808.

3 UK ECT Review Group. 2003. Efficacy and safety of electroconvulsive therapy in depressive disorders: a systematic review and meta-analysis. Lancet 361: 799–808.

4 Husain, M. M., Rush, A. J., Fink, M., Knapp, R., Petrides, G., Rummans, T., Biggs, M. M., O'Connor, K., Rasmussen, K., Litle, M., Zhao, W., Bernstein, H. J., Smith, G., Mueller, M., McClintock, S. M., Bailine, S. H. and Kellner, C. H. 2004. Speed of response and remission in major depressive disorder with acute electroconvulsive therapy (ECT): a Consortium for Research in ECT (CORE) report. J Clin Psychiatry 65: 485–491.

5 Loo, C. K., Schweitzer, I. and Pratt, C. 2006. Recent advances in optimizing electroconvulsive therapy. Aust N Z J Psychiatry 40: 632–638.

6 Sackeim, H. A., Prudic, J., Devanand, D. P., Kiersky, J. E., Fitzsimons, L., Moody, B. J., McElhiney, M. C., Coleman, E. A. and Settembrino, J. M. 1993. Effects of stimulus intensity and electrode placement on the efficacy and cognitive effects of electroconvulsive therapy. N Engl J Med 328: 839–846.

7 Eschweiler, G. W., Vonthein, R., Bode, R., Huell, M., Conca, A., Peters, O., Mende-Lechler, S., Peters, J., Klecha, D., Prapotnik, M., DiPauli, J., Wild, B., Plewnia, C., Bartels, M. and Schlotter, W. 2007. Clinical efficacy and cognitive side effects of bifrontal versus right unilateral electroconvulsive therapy (ECT): a short-term randomised controlled trial in pharmaco-resistant major depression. J Affect Disord 101: 149–157.

8 McCall, W. V., Reboussin, D. M., Weiner, R. D. and Sackeim, H. A. 2000. Titrated moderately suprathreshold vs fixed high-dose right unilateral electroconvulsive therapy: acute antidepressant and cognitive effects. Arch Gen Psychiatry 57: 438–444.

9 Sackeim, H. A., Prudic, J., Devanand, D. P., Nobler, M. S., Lisanby, S. H., Peyser, S., Fitzsimons, L., Moody, B. J. and Clark, J. 2000. A prospective, randomized, double-blind comparison of bilateral and right unilateral electroconvulsive therapy at different stimulus intensities. Arch Gen Psychiatry 57: 425–434.

10 Lisanby, S. H. 2007. Electroconvulsive therapy for depression. N Engl J Med 357: 1939–1945.

11 Dombrovski, A. Y., Mulsant, B. H., Haskett, R. F., Prudic, J., Begley, A. E. and Sackeim, H. A. 2005. Predictors of remission after electroconvulsive

therapy in unipolar major depression. J Clin Psychiatry 66: 1043–1049.
12 Feske, U., Mulsant, B. H., Pilkonis, P. A., Soloff, P., Dolata, D., Sackeim, H. A. and Haskett, R. F. 2004. Clinical outcome of ECT in patients with major depression and comorbid borderline personality disorder. Am J Psychiatry 161: 2073–2080.
13 Sackeim, H. A., Prudic, J., Nobler, M. S., Fitzsimons, L., Lisanby, S. H., Payne, N., Berman, R. M., Brakemeier, E.-L., Perera, T. and Devanand, D. P. 2008. Effects of pulse width and electrode placement on the efficacy and cognitive effects of electroconvulsive therapy. Brain Stimul 1: 71–83.
14 Merkl, A., Heuser, I. and Bajbouj, M. 2009. Antidepressant electroconvulsive therapy: mechanism of action, recent advances and limitations. Exp Neurol 219(1): 20–26.
15 Sackeim, H. A., Haskett, R. F., Mulsant, B. H., Thase, M. E., Mann, J. J., Pettinati, H. M., Greenberg, R. M., Crowe, R. R., Cooper, T. B. and Prudic, J. 2001. Continuation pharmacotherapy in the prevention of relapse following electroconvulsive therapy: a randomized controlled trial. JAMA 285: 1299–1307.
16 Kellner, C. H., Knapp, R. G., Petrides, G., Rummans, T. A., Husain, M. M., Rasmussen, K., Mueller, M., Bernstein, H. J., O'Connor, K., Smith, G., Biggs, M., Bailine, S. H., Malur, C., Yim, E., McClintock, S., Sampson, S. and Fink, M. 2006. Continuation electroconvulsive therapy vs pharmacotherapy for relapse prevention in major depression: a multisite study from the Consortium for Research in Electroconvulsive Therapy (CORE). Arch Gen Psychiatry 63: 1337–1344.
17 Fink, M., Rush, A. J., Knapp, R., Rasmussen, K., Mueller, M., Rummans, T. A., O'Connor, K., Husain, M., Biggs, M., Bailine, S. and Kellner, C. H. 2007. DSM melancholic features are unreliable predictors of ECT response: a CORE publication. J ECT 23: 139–146.
18 Gagne, G. G., Jr., Furman, M. J., Carpenter, L. L. and Price, L. H. 2000. Efficacy of continuation ECT and antidepressant drugs compared to long-term antidepressants alone in depressed patients. Am J Psychiatry 157: 1960–1965.
19 Brakemeier, E. L., Merkl, A., Wilbertz, G., Quante, A., Regen, F., Bührsch, N., van Hall, F., Kischkel, E., Anghelescu, I., Danker-Hopfe, H., Heuser, I., Kathmann, N. and Bajbouj, M. 2014. Cognitive behavioral therapy as continuation treatment after electroconvulsive therapy in patients with unipolar depression. Biol Psychiatry 76(3): 194–202. in press.
20 Nobler, M. S. and Sackeim, H. A. 2008. Neurobiological correlates of the cognitive side effects of electroconvulsive therapy. J ECT 24: 40–45.
21 Lisanby, S. H., Maddox, J. H., Prudic, J., Devanand, D. P. and Sackeim, H. A. 2000. The effects of electroconvulsive therapy on memory of autobiographical and public events. Arch Gen Psychiatry 57: 581–590.
22 Donahue, A. B. 2000. Electroconvulsive therapy and memory loss: a personal journey. J ECT 16: 133–143.
23 Mulsant, B. H., Rosen, J., Thornton, J. E. and Zubenko, G. S. 1991. A prospective naturalistic study of electroconvulsive therapy in late-life depression. J Geriatr Psychiatry Neurol 4: 3–13.
24 Scalia, J., Lisanby, S. H., Dwork, A. J., Johnson, J. E., Bernhardt, E. R., Arango, V., McCall, W. V. 2007. Neuropathologic examination after 91 ECT treatments in a 92-year-old woman with late-onset depression. J ECT 23(2): 96–98.
25 Devanand, D. P. 1995. Does electroconvulsive therapy damage brain cells? Semin Neurol 15: 351–357.
26 Dwork, A. J., Arango, V., Underwood, M., Ilievski, B., Rosoklija, G., Sackeim, H. A. and Lisanby, S. H. 2004. Absence of histological lesions in primate models of ECT and magnetic seizure therapy. Am J Psychiatry 161: 576–578.
27 Ende, G., Braus, D. F., Walter, S., Weber-Fahr, W. and Henn, F. A. 2000. The hippocampus in patients treated with electroconvulsive therapy: a proton magnetic resonance spectroscopic imaging study. Arch Gen Psychiatry 57: 937–943.
28 DeLorenzo, R. J. and Sun, D. A. 2006. Basic mechanisms in status epilepticus: role of calcium in neuronal injury and the induction of epileptogenesis. Adv Neurol 97: 187–197.
29 Sackeim, H. A. 1994. Continuation therapy following ECT: directions for future research. Psychopharmacol Bull 30: 501–521.
30 Kupchik, M., Spivak, B., Mester, R., Reznik, I., Gonen, N., Weizman, A. and Kotler, M. 2000.

Combined electroconvulsive-clozapine therapy. Clin Neuropharmacol 23: 14–16.
31 Baghai, T. C., Frey, R., Kasper, S. and Möller, H-J. 2004. Elektrokonvulsionstherapie: Klinische und wissenschaftliche Aspekte. Springer, Wien, New York.
32 Sienaert, P. and Peuskens, J. 2007. Anticonvulsants during electroconvulsive therapy: review and recommendations. J ECT 23(2): 120–123.
33 Naguib, M. and Koorn, R. 2002. Interactions between psychotropics, anaesthetics and electroconvulsive therapy: implications for drug choice and patient management. CNS Drugs 16: 229–247.
34 Baghai, T. C., Marcuse, A., Brosch, M., Schule, C., Eser, D., Nothdurfter, C., Steng, Y., Noack, I., Pietschmann, K., Moller, H. J. and Rupprecht, R. 2006. The influence of concomitant antidepressant medication on safety, tolerability and clinical effectiveness of electroconvulsive therapy. World J Biol Psychiatry 7: 82–90.
35 Gonzalez-Pinto, A., Gutierrez, M., Gonzalez, N., Elizagarate, E., Perez de Heredia, J. L. and Mico, J. A. 2002. Efficacy and safety of venlafaxine-ECT combination in treatment-resistant depression. J Neuropsychiatry Clin Neurosci 14: 206–209.
36 Sartorius, A., Wolf, J. and Henn, F. A. 2005. Lithium and ECT – concurrent use still demands attention: three case reports. World J Biol Psychiatry 6: 121–124.
37 Bernardo, M., Navarro, V., Salva, J., Arrufat, F. J. and Baeza, I. 2000. Seizure activity and safety in combined treatment with venlafaxine and ECT: a pilot study. J ECT 16: 38–42.
38 Rosa, M. A. and Lisanby, S. H. 2012. Somatic treatments for mood disorders. Neuropsychopharmacology 37(1):102–116.

CHAPTER 25

Neuromodulation in psychiatry: Conclusions

Paul Holtzheimer[1], Helen Mayberg[2], Andres M. Lozano[3] and Clement Hamani[3]
[1] *Geisel School of Medicine at Dartmouth, Hanover, USA*
[2] *Emory University School of Medicine, Atlanta, USA*
[3] *Toronto Western Hospital, University of Toronto, Toronto, Canada*

Psychiatric disorders are among the most prevalent, disabling and lethal medical conditions worldwide. Approximately 30% of Americans will meet criteria for an anxiety disorder during their lifetime, more than 20% will develop a clinically significant depressive disorder and approximately 50% will meet diagnostic criteria for any psychiatric disorder [1]. Major depressive disorder is currently the leading cause of years lost due to disability worldwide, followed by alcohol use disorders [2]. Major depression is the third largest contributor to global burden of disease and is projected to be the greatest contributor within 10–15 years [2]. Suicide, which is nearly always associated with a psychiatric disorder, is the 10th leading cause of death in the United States (http://www.cdc.gov/violenceprevention/suicide). Beyond suicide, individuals with mental illness die sooner compared to those without, despite using more healthcare resources over their lifetime [3].

Effective treatments for psychiatric disorders are available. For most of the major mental illnesses, medications and psychotherapy result in clinically significant improvement in more than half of patients. However, for many disorders, response is not complete and relapse rates are high. Strikingly, for most of the major psychiatric disorders (e.g. depression and schizophrenia), pharmacologic options today are no more efficacious than in the 1950s [4]. For depression, ECT (available since the early part of the 20th century) remains the most effective treatment available. Clearly, new treatment approaches for psychiatric disorders are needed.

The concept of treating psychiatric illness within the context of a neural circuit model is by no means new. Beginning in the late 19th century and continuing into the early 20th century, neurosurgical interventions were attempted with limited success [5]. These techniques were based on a crude understanding of the neural networks involved in the regulation of mood and behaviour (e.g. [6]). This work culminated in the advent of the prefrontal leucotomy – a procedure to sever the white matter connections connecting the prefrontal cortex to deeper cortical and subcortical structures [7]. Due to notable side effects and the development of the first psychotropic medications, use of the prefrontal leucotomy essentially disappeared in the latter part of the 20th century. However, more focused ablative procedures for severe, intractable psychiatric conditions have remained in use to this day.

Over the last few decades, there has been renewed interest in focal neuromodulation as

Neuromodulation in Psychiatry, First Edition. Edited by Clement Hamani, Paul Holtzheimer, Andres M. Lozano and Helen Mayberg.

a treatment approach for neuropsychiatric conditions. This has been supported by the relative success of certain techniques in the treatment of patients with neurological disorders (e.g. deep brain stimulation (DBS) for patients with Parkinson's disease or essential tremor; vagus nerve stimulation (VNS) for patients with epilepsy). In addition, with the emergence of high-resolution structural and functional neuroimaging methods, much more sophisticated models of the neural networks underlying psychiatric illness have been developed (e.g. [8]).

As described in this book, the field of neuromodulation in psychiatry is at a very exciting stage. There have been multiple successes and certain techniques have already made their way into clinical use: transcranial magnetic stimulation for depression, VNS for depression and DBS for obsessive–compulsive disorder (OCD). Beyond this, efforts are underway to optimize the ways we can focally stimulate the brain and methods for identifying the best patients (e.g. through the development of biomarkers). Interest in the use of neuromodulation in psychiatry continues to grow and offers a completely different paradigm for treatment (versus medications and psychotherapy).

However, there are some reasons for caution within the field as well. For example, although TMS and VNS were approved by the US FDA for the treatment of depression, many feel that the clinical trial data are not particularly strong, and neither treatment has, as of yet, received a national coverage determination from the Centers for Medicare and Medicaid Services (though some patients have been successful in getting coverage for these treatments on a case-by-case basis). Concerning DBS for depression, and despite very encouraging preliminary data reviewed within this book, two industry-sponsored, Phase III trials have been halted presumably due to lack of demonstrated efficacy. There are many potential explanations for the available data not showing a more clear treatment advantage for active neuromodulation (e.g. patient selection, targeting errors, time of endpoints and efficacy measures). However, there is significant concern that these studies will be simply interpreted as failures of neuromodulation and thereby stunt growth within the field.

We feel strongly that this would be a mistake. Instead, an even stronger and better funded effort should be made to develop and test these interventions. This would involve more carefully and creatively designed clinical trials, the integration of various approaches (e.g. imaging and electrophysiology) within clinical trials to better test for evidence of target engagement as well as to identify biomarkers for response, and potentially a review of what constitutes a successful trial. For example, and especially for interventions that require an implanted device, the classic 12-week clinical trial design may be inappropriate. Also, the most accepted rating scales used as efficacy measures within psychiatry may not be most appropriate when evaluating the effects of focal neuromodulation – it is possible that the initial behavioural effects of stimulation may be more subtle and/or behaviourally specific than what can be captured with, say, the Hamilton Depression Rating Scale, first introduced in 1960 [9]. These challenges should be addressed directly by the field.

Going forward, there are many directions for ongoing research. Current techniques should continue to be tested, and a broader range of indications should be considered. Most of the data presented in this book are for neuromodulation for treating depression. Where available, data for other indications (e.g. OCD and addictions) are presented. As we better understand the neural circuitry of various psychiatric conditions, it is appropriate to hypothesize and test and contrast/compare the effects of focal stimulation of 'key nodes' as a potential therapy for these disorders. This has the important caveat that this work should be balanced by a consideration of the prevalence and severity of the condition, the clarity of knowledge about the neural circuitry underlying its pathophysiology and treatment and the invasiveness of the neuromodulation technique under consideration. In addition, it should be considered that neuromodulation may only be effective in altering one aspect of what is otherwise a complex, neurobehavioural syndrome. For example, DBS of the nucleus accumbens may be able to attenuate cue-reactive craving for an addictive disorder, but multimodal treatment involving psychotherapy, medications and group support will likely be required for full remission. Finally, while the vast majority of treatment studies within psychiatry have focused on acute resolution of symptoms, very few have addressed symptom recurrence over time in what are known to be chronic, highly recurrent illnesses. Ideally, future trials will develop mechanisms for assessing benefit over months to years, perhaps incorporating metrics to better capture longitudinal efficacy (e.g. the Illness Density Index [10]).

References

1 Kessler RC, Berglund P, Demler O, Jin R, Merikangas KR, Walters EE. Lifetime prevalence and age-of-onset distributions of DSM-IV disorders in the National Comorbidity Survey Replication. Arch Gen Psychiatry. 2005;62(6):593–602.
2 WHO. The Global Burden of Disease: 2004 Update. Geneva: World Health Organization; 2008.
3 Miller BJ, Paschall CB, 3rd, Svendsen DP. Mortality and medical comorbidity among patients with serious mental illness. Psychiatr Serv. 2006;57(10):1482–1487.
4 Holtzheimer PE, Mayberg HS. Stuck in a rut: rethinking depression and its treatment. Trends Neurosci. 2011;34(1):1–9.
5 Hamani C, Snyder B, Laxton A, Holtzheimer P, Mayberg H, Lozano A. Surgical Treatment of Major Depression. In: Winn HR, ed. Youmans Neurological Surgery. Elsevier: Saunders; 2011: 1018–1025.
6 Papez JW. A proposed mechanism of emotion. Arch Neurol Psychiatry. 1937;38:725–743.
7 Jasper HH. A historical perspective. The rise and fall of prefrontal lobotomy. Adv Neurol. 1995;66: 97–114.
8 Mayberg HS. Modulating dysfunctional limbic-cortical circuits in depression: towards development of brain-based algorithms for diagnosis and optimised treatment. Br Med Bull. 2003;65:193–207.
9 Hamilton M. A rating scale for depression. J Neurol Neurosurg Psychiatry. 1960;23:56–62.
10 Kelley ME, Franco AR, Mayberg HS, Holtzheimer PE. The Illness Density Index (IDI) : a longitudinal measure of treatment efficacy. Clin Trials. 2012;9:596–604.

Index

Page numbers in *italics* refer to illustrations; those in **bold** refer to tables

Neuromodulation in Psychiatry, First Edition. Edited by Clement Hamani, Paul Holtzheimer,
Andres M. Lozano and Helen Mayberg.

www.ingramcontent.com/pod-product-compliance
Ingram Content Group UK Ltd.
Pitfield, Milton Keynes, MK11 3LW, UK
UKHW050842101026
15624UKWH00018B/445

9 781118 801048